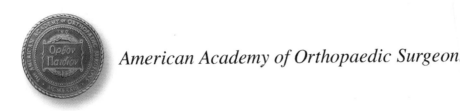

American Academy of Orthopaedic Surgeon

OKU
Orthopaedic Knowledge Update:

Shoulder and Elbow

2

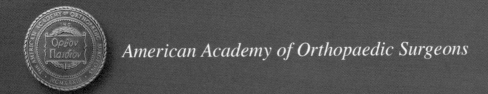

American Academy of Orthopaedic Surgeons

OKU

Orthopaedic Knowledge Update:

Shoulder and Elbow
2

Edited by
Tom R. Norris, MD

Developed by the
American Shoulder and Elbow Surgeons

Published 2002
by the American Academy of Orthopaedic Surgeons
6300 North River Road
Rosemont, Illinois   60018
1-800-626-6726

The material presented in *Orthopaedic Knowledge Update: Shoulder and Elbow 2* has been made available by the American Academy of Orthopaedic Surgeons for educational purposes only. This material is not intended to present the only, or necessarily best, methods or procedures for the medical situations discussed, but rather is intended to represent an approach, view, statement, or opinion of the author(s) or producer(s), which may be helpful to others who face similar situations.

Some drugs or medical devices demonstrated in Academy courses or described in Academy print or electronic publications have not been cleared by the Food and Drug Administration (FDA) or have been cleared for specific uses only. The FDA has stated that it is the responsibility of the physician to determine the FDA clearance status of each drug or device he or she wishes to use in clinical practice.

The U.S. FDA has expressed concern about potential serious patient care issues involved with the use of polymethylmethacrylate (PMMA) bone cement in spine. A physician might insert the PMMA bone cement into vertebrae by various procedures, including vertebroplasty and kyphoplasty.

PMMA bone cement is considered a device for FDA purposes. In October 1999, the FDA reclassified PMMA bone cement as a Class II device for its intended use "in arthroplastic procedures of the hip, knee, and other joints for the fixation of polymer or metallic prosthetic implants to living bone." The use of a device for other than its FDA-cleared indication is an off-label use. Physicians may use a device off-label if they believe, in their best medical judgment, that its use is appropriate for a particular patient (eg, tumors).

The use of PMMA bone cement in the spine is described in Academy educational courses, videotapes, and publications for educational purposes only. As is the Academy's policy regarding all of its educational offerings, the fact that the use of PMMA bone cement in the spine is discussed does not constitute an Academy endorsement of this use.

Furthermore, any statements about commercial products are solely the opinion(s) of the author(s) and do not represent an Academy endorsement or evaluation of these products. These statements may not be used in advertising or for any commercial purpose.

Second Edition
Copyright © 2002 by the
American Academy of Orthopaedic Surgeons

ISBN 0-89203-255-3

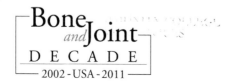

Bone *and* Joint
DECADE
— 2002 - USA - 2011 —

Acknowledgments

Contributors

Jeffrey S. Abrams, MD
Attending Orthopaedic Surgeon
Department of Surgery
Princeton Medical Center
Associate Medical Director
Princeton Orthopaedic and Rehabilitative
　Associates
Princeton, New Jersey

Answorth A. Allen, MD
Assistant Attending Orthopaedic Surgeon
Department of Sports Medicine
Hospital for Special Surgery
New York, New York

David W. Altchek, MD
Head Team Physician, New York Mets
Associate Attending Orthopaedic Surgeon
Hospital for Special Surgery
Sports Medicine and Shoulder Service
New York, New York

Maria Apreleva, PhD
Research Director
Shoulder Biomechanics Group
Orthopedic Biomechanics Laboratory
Beth Israel Deaconess Medical Center
Boston, Massachusetts

Carl J. Basamania, MD, FACS
Assistant Professor of Surgery
Chief, Orthopaedic Surgery Service
Durham Veterans Administration Medical
　Center
Division of Orthopaedic Surgery
Duke University Medical Center
Durham, North Carolina

Louis U. Bigliani, MD
Frank E. Stinchfield Professor and Chairman
Department of Orthopaedic Surgery
Columbia University
New York Presbyterian Hospital
　Columbia Campus
New York, New York

Theodore A. Blaine, MD
Assistant Professor of Orthopaedic Surgery
Associate Director, The Shoulder Service
Department of Orthopaedic Surgery
Columbia-Presbyterian Medical Center
New York, New York

John J. Brems, MD
Section Head, Upper Extremity Surgery
Department of Orthopaedic Surgery
Cleveland Clinic Foundation
Cleveland, Ohio

Stephen S. Burkhart, MD
Clinical Associate Professor
Department of Orthopaedic Surgery
University of Texas Health Science Center
San Antonio, Texas

Alan Buschman, MD
Attending Anesthesiologist
Department of Anesthesia
California Pacific Medical Center
San Francisco, California

Brian D. Cameron, MD
Stevens Orthopedic Group
Stevens Memorial Hospital
Edmonds, Washington

Robert H. Cofield, MD
Professor of Orthopedics
Mayo Medical School
Chair, Department of Orthopedic Surgery
Mayo Clinic
Rochester, Minnesota

Brian S. Cohen, MD
Center for Advanced Orthopaedics and
　Sports Medicine
Chillicothe, Ohio

Brian J. Cole, MD, MBA
Assistant Professor
Section of Shoulder Surgery
Department of Orthopedic Surgery
Rush-Presbyterian-St. Luke's
　Medical Center
Rush University
Chicago, Illinois

David N. Collins, MD
Clinical Assistant Professor
Department of Orthopaedic Surgery
University of Arkansas for Medical Sciences
Little Rock, Arkansas

William C. Doukas, MD, LTC
Chief, Orthopaedic Surgery Service
Department of Orthopaedics and
　Rehabilitation
Walter Reed Army Medical Center
Washington, District of Columbia

Mark C. Drakos, BA
Research Assistant
Hospital for Special Surgery
Sports Medicine and Shoulder Service
New York, New York

Roger C. Dunteman, MD
Sports Medicine Fellow
Southern California Orthopedic Institute
Van Nuys, California

Stephen Fealy, MD
Assistant Attending Orthopaedic Surgeon
Department of Sports Medicine and
　Shoulder Service
Hospital for Special Surgery
New York, New York

Evan L. Flatow, MD
Chief of Shoulder Surgery
Department of Orthopaedics
The Mount Sinai Hospital
New York, New York

Richard J. Friedman, MD, FRCSC
Clinical Professor of Orthopaedic Surgery
Medical University of South Carolina
Charleston, South Carolina

Hiroaki Fukuda, MD
Professor and Chairman
Department of Orthopaedic Surgery
Tokai University School of Medicine
Isehara, Kanagawa, Japan
Leesa M. Galatz, MD

Shoulder and Elbow Service
Department of Orthopaedic Surgery
Washington University School of Medicine
Barnes-Jewish Hospital
St. Louis, Missouri

Gary M. Gartsman, MD
Clinical Associate Professor
Department of Orthopaedics
University of Texas
Houston Health Science Center
Houston, Texas

Ariane Gerber, MD
Clinical Fellow
Harvard Shoulder Service
Partners Orthopaedics
Massachusetts General Hospital
Boston, Massachusetts

Christian Gerber, MD
Professor and Chairman
Department of Orthopaedics
University of Zurich
Zurich, Switzerland

David L. Glaser, MD
The Cali Family Assistant Professor of
　Orthopaedic Surgery
Shoulder and Elbow Service
University of Pennsylvania
Philadelphia, Pennsylvania

Andrew Green, MD
Assistant Professor Orthopaedic Surgery
Department of Orthopaedic Surgery
Brown Medical School
Providence, Rhode Island

Sean Griggs, MD
Clinical Assistant Professor
Department of Orthopedic Surgery
Brown University
Providence, Rhode Island

R. Michael Gross, MS, MD
Clinical Instructor
Department of Orthopaedics and
　Rehabilitation
Creighton/University of Nebraska
　Medical Centers
Omaha, Nebraska

Stephen B. Gunther, MD
Chief, University of California,
　San Francisco Shoulder and
　Elbow Service
Co-Director, Sports Medicine
Department of Orthopedic Surgery
University of California
San Francisco, California

Armodios M. Hatzidakis, MD
Western Orthopaedics P.C.
Denver, Colorado

Patrick Hayes, MD
Orthopedic Surgeon
Shoulder and Elbow Service
Miller Orthopedic Clinic
Shelby, North Carolina

Yassamin Hazrati, MD
Department of Orthopaedic Surgery
Kaiser Permanente Medical Center
Vallejo, California

Robert E. Hunter, MD
Clinical Professor
Department of Orthopaedics
University of Colorado
Aspen, Colorado

Joseph P. Iannotti, MD, PhD
Chairman, Department of Orthopaedic
    Surgery
The Cleveland Clinic Foundation
Cleveland, Ohio

Kirk L. Jensen, MD
Assistant Clinical Professor
University of California, San Francisco
Peralta Orthopaedic Associates
Oakland, California

Christopher M. Jobe, MD
Professor, Orthopaedic Surgery
Chairman, Department of Orthopaedic
    Surgery
Department of Orthopaedic Surgery
Loma Linda University School of Medicine
Loma Linda, California

Lloyd Johnson III, MD
Orthopaedic Surgery Chief Resident
Washington University School of Medicine
Department of Orthopaedic Surgery
St. Louis, Missouri

Thomas A. Joseph, MD
Director, Sports Medicine and Shoulder
    Surgery
St. Elizabeth's Hospital
Youngstown, Ohio

Jesse B. Jupiter, MD
Chief, Hand and Upper Extremity Service
Department of Orthopaedic Surgery
Massachusetts General Hospital
Boston, Massachusetts

Ronald P. Karzel, MD
Orthopaedic Surgeon
Southern California Orthopedic Institute
Van Nuys, California

W. Ben Kibler, MD
Medical Director
Sports Medicine Center
Lexington Clinic
Lexington, Kentucky

Graham J.W. King, MD, MSc, FRCSC
Associate Professor
Hand and Upper Limb Centre
University of Western Ontario
London, Ontario, Canada

Cyrus J. Lashgari, MD
Shoulder and Elbow Fellow
Washington University
Department of Orthopaedics
St. Louis, Missouri

Mark D. Lazarus, MD
Associate Professor Orthopaedic Surgery
Chief, Shoulder and Elbow Service
Department of Orthopaedic Surgery
MCP Hahnemann University
Philadelphia, Pennsylvania

Robert D. Leffert, MD
Professor of Orthopaedic Surgery
Harvard Medical School
Boston, Massachusetts

Brian T. McDermott, MD
Department of Orthopaedic Surgery
The Cleveland Clinic Foundation
Cleveland, Ohio

J. B. McMullen, MS, ATC
Manager, Lexington Clinic Sports Medicine
    Center
Lexington Clinic
Lexington, Kentucky

Suzanne L. Miller, MD
Chief Resident
Department of Orthopaedics
The Mount Sinai Hospital
New York, New York

Tom R. Norris, MD
Past President, American Shoulder and
    Elbow Surgeons
Department of Orthopaedic Surgery
California Pacific Medical Center
San Francisco, California

Wesley M. Nottage, MD
Associate Clinical Professor, Orthopaedic
    Surgery
University of California, Irvine
The Sports Clinic Orthopaedic Medical
    Associates, Inc.
Laguna Hills, California

Shawn W. O'Driscoll, PhD, MD
Professor of Orthopedic Surgery
Department of Orthopedic Surgery
Mayo Clinic
Mayo Foundation
Rochester, Minnesota

Michael L. Pearl, MD
Orthopaedic Surgeon
Department of Orthopaedic Surgery
Kaiser Permanente
Los Angeles, California

Mark Pinto, MD
Chelsea Orthopedic Specialists
Chelsea Community Hospital
Chelsea, Michigan

Roger C. Pollock, MD
Assistant Professor
Department of Orthopaedic Surgery
Columbia University
New York, New York

Matthew L. Ramsey, MD
Assistant Professor of Orthopaedic Surgery
Penn Orthopaedic Institute
University of Pennsylvania School of
    Medicine
Philadelphia, Pennsylvania

Paul R. Reynolds, MD
Orthopaedic Surgery Resident
McKay Orthopaedic Research Laboratory
University of Pennsylvania
Philadelphia, Pennsylvania

Robin R. Richards, MD, FRCSC
Professor of Surgery
Department of Surgery
Division of Orthopaedic Surgery
University of Toronto and St. Michael's
    Hospitals
Toronto, Ontario, Canada

David Ring, MD
Hand and Upper Extremity Service
Department of Orthopaedic Surgery
Massachusetts General Hospital
Boston, Massachusetts

Paul S. Robinson, MS
Research Engineer
McKay Orthopaedic Research Laboratory
University of Pennsylvania
Philadelphia, Pennsylvania

Charles A. Rockwood, Jr, MD
Professor and Chairman Emeritus
Department of Orthopaedics
University of Texas Health Science Center
San Antonio, Texas

Joel T. Rohrbough, MD
Fellow, Sports Medicine Service
Hospital for Special Surgery
New York, New York

Anthony A. Romeo, MD
Associate Professor
Department of Orthopaedic Surgery
Rush Presbyterian-St. Luke's Medical
    Center
Chicago, Illinois

Richard K.N. Ryu, MD
Chairman
Department of Orthopaedic Surgery
Cottage Hospital
Santa Barbara, California

Edward Baldwin Self, Jr, MD
Chairman, Department of Orthopaedic
    Surgery
The Valley Hospital
Ridgewood, New Jersey

Stephen J. Snyder, MD
Attending Surgeon
Orthopedic Shoulder Service
Southern California Orthopedic Institute
Van Nuys, California

Louis J. Soslowsky, PhD
Associate Professor of Orthopaedic Surgery
  and Bioengineering
Director of Orthopaedic Research
McKay Orthopaedic Research Laboratory
University of Pennsylvania
Philadelphia, Pennsylvania

Scott P. Steinmann, MD
Assistant Professor of Orthopedic Surgery
Department of Orthopedic Surgery
Mayo Clinic
Rochester, Minnesota

Jeffrey L. Swisher, MD
Staff Anesthesiologist
Department of Anesthesia
California Pacific Medical Center
San Francisco, California

James P. Tasto, MD
Clinical Professor
Orthopaedic Department
University of California, San Diego
San Diego, California

C. Thomas Vangsness, Jr, MD
Professor, Orthopaedic Surgery
Chief of Sports Medicine
Keck School of Medicine
University of Southern California
Los Angeles, California

Gilles Walch, MD
Orthopaedic Surgery Department
Clinique St. Anne-Lumiere
Lyon, France

Jon J.P. Warner, MD
Associate Professor
Head, Harvard Shoulder Service
Partners Orthopaedics
Massachusetts General Hospital
Boston, Massachusetts

Stephen C. Weber, MD
Sacramento Knee and Sports Medicine
Sacramento, California

Gerald R. Williams, Jr, MD
Associate Professor
Chief, Shoulder and Elbow Service
Chairman, Department of Orthopaedic
  Surgery
Presbyterian Hospital
University of Pennsylvania
Philadelphia, Pennsylvania

Karyn A. Wong, PT, OCS
Physical Therapy Clinical Specialist
Department of Physical Medicine
Kaiser Permanente
Los Angeles, California

Kirk L. Wong, MD
Fellow
The Hand Center of San Antonio
San Antonio, Texas

Ken Yamaguchi, MD
Assistant Professor
Chief, Shoulder and Elbow Service
Department of Orthopaedic Surgery
Washington University School of Medicine
St. Louis, Missouri

Preface

The second edition of *Orthopaedic Knowledge Update: Shoulder and Elbow*, like the first edition, was developed in response to the explosion of knowledge and interest in the field of shoulder and elbow disorders. The book is written for the general orthopaedist as well as residents and fellows in training. It provides a concise review and update on recent developments in the field of shoulder and elbow disorders. Along with sections on basic science, instability and athletic injuries, rotator cuff impingement, trauma/fracture, and arthroplasty, there are new sections on miscellaneous shoulder topics and arthroscopy. As always, it has been difficult to know whether to assign arthroscopy treatments to the general fields or to cover each of these fields separately with an arthroscopic approach. Fortunately, and without unnecessary redundancy, both have been accomplished.

I would like to thank all of the section editors and authors for volunteering their time and expertise in developing this book. It has been a pleasure to include section editors from the international community of experts. This volume has been truly enriched with the expertise of Gilles Walch and Christian Gerber. Their contributions are invaluable. I also wish to thank Shawn O'Driscoll who came in late and undertook the work of several contributors to head up the elbow section in superb style. In addition, many thanks to the publications staff at the American Academy of Orthopaedic Surgeons for their coordinated efforts in the editing, production, and overall management of this project. I would especially like to acknowledge the tireless efforts of Susan Baim, Lisa Moore, Lynne Shindoll, Marilyn Fox, PhD, and Alan Levine, MD. Without their encouragement and diligence, this new edition would not have much of the timely information now available. I know that this book will be a useful resource in the study of the shoulder and elbow.

Tom R. Norris, MD
Editor

Table of Contents

Preface .... *ix*

Section 1: Basic Science
Section Editor: Louis J. Soslowsky, PhD

1 Tissues of the Shoulder and Their Structure. . 3
Roger G. Pollock, MD

2 Basic Science of Glenohumeral Instability . . . 13
Ariane Gerber, MD
Maria Apreleva, PhD
Jon J.P. Warner, MD

3 Basic Science of the Rotator Cuff. 23
Paul S. Robinson, MS
Paul R. Reynolds, MD
Louis J. Soslowsky, PhD

4 Shoulder Kinematics and Kinesiology 37
Michael L. Pearl, MD
Karyn A. Wong, PT

*5 Basic Science Considerations in
Glenohumeral Arthroplasty and Proximal
Humeral Fractures. 49*
Brian D. Cameron, MD
Matthew L. Ramsey, MD
Gerald R. Williams, Jr, MD

Section 2: Instability and Athletic Injuries
Section Editor: Michael A. Wirth, MD

*6 Glenohumeral Instability: Classification,
Clinical Assessment, and Imaging 65*
Kirk L. Jensen, MD
Charles A. Rockwood, Jr, MD

*7 Acute and Chronic Dislocations of the
Shoulder 71*
Mark D. Lazarus, MD

8 Recurrent Anterior Shoulder Instability 83
Stephen S. Burkhart, MD

*9 Multidirectional and Posterior Shoulder
Instability 91*
Thomas A. Joseph, MD
John J. Brems, MD

*10 Arthroscopic Anterior Glenohumeral
Ligament Reconstruction 103*
Brian J. Cole, MD, MBA
Jon J.P. Warner, MD

*11 Athletic Injuries and the Throwing Athlete:
Shoulder 117*
Stephen Fealy, MD
David W. Altchek, MD

*12 Complications and Failures in Instability
Repair 129*
Patrick Hayes, MD
Yassamin Hazrati, MD
Evan L. Flatow, MD

Section 3: Rotator Cuff Impingement

Section Editors: Christian Gerber, MD, and Gilles Walch, MD

13 *Rotator Cuff Disorders: Anatomy, Function, Pathogenesis, and Natural History* 143

Christopher M. Jobe, MD

14 *Natural History and Nonsurgical Treatment of Rotator Cuff Disorders* 155

Cyrus J. Lashgari, MD
Ken Yamaguchi, MD

15 *Surgical Treatment of Partial-Thickness Tears* 163

Roger C. Dunteman, MD
Hiroaki Fukuda, MD
Stephen J. Snyder, MD

16 *Surgical Treatment of Full-Thickness Tears* 171

Robert H. Cofield, MD
Gary M. Gartsman, MD

17 *Complications of Rotator Cuff Surgery* 181

Brian S. Cohen, MD
Armodios M. Hatzidakis, MD
Anthony A. Romeo, MD

18 *Massive Rotator Cuff Tears* 191

Christian Gerber, MD
Gilles Walch, MD

19 *Cuff Tear Arthropathy* 197

Evan L. Flatow, MD
David L. Glaser, MD
Armodios M. Hatzidakis, MD
Suzanne L. Miller, MD
Tom R. Norris, MD
Matthew L. Ramsey, MD
Gerald R. Williams, Jr, MD

Section 4: Trauma/Fracture

Section Editor: Andrew Green, MD

20 *Proximal Humeral Fractures* 209

Andrew Green, MD

21 *Clavicular Fractures and Sternoclavicular Dislocations* 219

Andrew Green, MD
Sean Griggs, MD
William C. Doukas, MD, LTC
Carl J. Basamania, MD, FACS

22 *Scapular Fractures* 227

Kirk L. Wong, MD
Matthew L. Ramsey, MD
Gerald R. Williams, Jr, MD

23 *Diaphyseal Fractures of the Humerus* 237

David Ring, MD
Jesse B. Jupiter, MD

American Academy of Orthopaedic Surgeons

Section 5: Arthritis/Arthroplasty

Section Editor: Joseph P. Iannotti, MD, PhD

24 *Inflammatory Arthritis of the Shoulder* 251
David N. Collins, MD

25 *Management of Osteoarthritis of the Shoulder* 257
John J. Brems, MD

26 *Osteonecrosis and Other Noninflammatory Degenerative Diseases of the Glenohumeral Joint* 267
Lloyd Johnson III, MD
Leesa M. Galatz, MD

27 *Proximal Humeral Malunions, Posttraumatic Arthritis, and Postcapsulorrhaphy Arthritis* 275
Joseph P. Iannotti, MD, PhD
Brian T. McDermott, MD

28 *Shoulder Arthroplasty: Complications and Revision* 285
Stephen B. Gunther, MD
Tom R. Norris, MD

Section 6: Elbow Trauma, Fracture, and Reconstruction

Section Editor: Shawn W. O'Driscoll, PhD, MD

29 *Athletic Injuries and the Throwing Athlete: Elbow* 297
Stephen Fealy, MD
Joel T. Rohrbough, MD
Answorth A. Allen, MD
David W. Altchek, MD
Mark C. Drakos, BA

30 *Acute, Recurrent, and Chronic Elbow Instabilities* 313
Shawn W. O'Driscoll, PhD, MD

31 *Elbow Stiffness* 325
Scott P. Steinmann, MD

32 *Elbow Arthritis* 333
Scott P. Steinmann, MD

33 *Radial Head Fractures* 343
Graham J.W. King, MD, MSc, FRCSC

34 *Fractures of the Distal Humerus* 357
David Ring, MD
Jesse B. Jupiter, MD

35 *Proximal Ulnar Fractures and Fracture-Dislocations* 369
David Ring, MD
Jesse B. Jupiter, MD

36 *Coronoid Fractures* 379
Shawn W. O'Driscoll, PhD, MD

Section 7: Miscellaneous Shoulder Topics
Section Editor: Robert D. Leffert, MD

37 *Brachial Plexus Injuries in the Adult* 387
Robert D. Leffert, MD

38 *Thoracic Outlet Syndrome* 397
Robert D. Leffert, MD

39 *Accelerated Postoperative Shoulder Rehabilitation* 403
W. Ben Kibler, MD
J.B. McMullen, MS, ATC

40 *CPT® and ICD-9-CM Coding for the Shoulder Surgeon* 411
Richard J. Friedman, MD, FRCSC

41 *Outcomes Analysis in the Shoulder and Elbow* 421
Robin R. Richards, MD, FRCSC

42 *Regional Anesthesia for Shoulder Surgery* ..433
Alan Buschman, MD
Jeffrey L. Swisher, MD

43 *Clinical Guidelines for Shoulder Pain* 443
Edward Baldwin Self, Jr, MD

Section 8: Arthroscopy
Section Editors: James C. Esch, MD, and Armodios M. Hatzidakis, MD

44 *Arthroscopic Rotator Cuff Repair* 471
Jeffrey S. Abrams, MD

45 *Recurrent Anterior Dislocations* 479
Richard K. N. Ryu, MD

46 *The Role of Arthroscopy for Acute Shoulder Dislocations* 487
Robert E. Hunter, MD

47 *Arthroscopic Pancapsular Plication for Multidirectional Instability* 495
Stephen J. Snyder, MD
Roger C. Dunteman, MD

48 *Thermocapsulorrhaphy* 501
C. Thomas Vangsness, Jr, MD

49 *Arthroscopic Subacromial Decompression* ..507
Armodios M. Hatzidakis, MD
R. Michael Gross, MD

50 *Arthroscopic Acromioclavicular Joint Resection* 519
James P. Tasto, MD

51 *Arthroscopy for the Arthritic Shoulder* 525
Theodore A. Blaine, MD
Louis U. Bigliani, MD

52 *Arthroscopic Treatment of Calcific Tendinitis* 533
Stephen C. Weber, MD

53 *Shoulder Ganglion Cysts* 539
Mark Pinto, MD
Ronald P. Karzel, MD

54 *Superior Labrum Anterior and Posterior Lesions* 543
Stephen S. Burkhart, MD

55 *Complications of Arthroscopic Shoulder Surgery* 551
Wesley M. Nottage, MD

Index 559

American Academy of Orthopaedic Surgeons

Section 1

Basic Science

Section Editor:
Louis J. Soslowsky, PhD

Chapter 1

Tissues of the Shoulder and Their Structure

Roger G. Pollock, MD

Introduction

The shoulder is a complex joint, consisting of the gleno-humeral, acromioclavicular, and sternoclavicular joints and the subacromial and scapulothoracic spaces. Each of these components consists of osseous structures surrounded and stabilized by nonosseous elements, including muscles, tendons, ligaments, cartilage, and fibrocartilage. These structures interact to produce a complex joint that possesses the greatest degree of mobility of all the major joints in the human body. Basic research has led to a continually evolving understanding of the gross and microanatomy of these tissues and of their physiology and biochemical composition. This chapter reviews current understanding of these tissues and their structure, with emphasis on recent studies in this field.

The Glenohumeral Joint

Osseous Structures

Interest in the development of third-generation anatomic shoulder prosthetic designs has resulted in a number of recent studies on the bony geometry of the gleno-humeral joint. The authors of these studies contend that prosthetic arthroplasty that most nearly restores the original geometry of the glenohumeral articular surfaces should allow the most physiologic motion. Various methodologies involving plain radiography, calipers, MRI, stereophotogrammetry, CT, and three-dimensional computer modeling have been used to accurately measure the morphologic features of the proximal humerus and glenoid.

One recent study used CT data and three-dimensional computer modeling to analyze both extramedullary and intramedullary humeral morphology. In this study, the humeral head radius averaged 23 mm (range, 17 to 28 mm), and the humeral head thickness averaged 19 mm (range, 15 to 24 mm). These values are in close agreement with those reported previously. Moreover, the humeral head thickness and the length of the humerus were found

to be proportionately linked, as were the head radius and the head thickness. On average, the humeral head center was offset 7 mm medially and 2 mm posteriorly from the humeral axis. Humeral head inclination averaged 41° (range, 34° to 47°), and the neck-shaft angle averaged 131°. The superior aspect of the humeral head was 6 mm (range, 3 to 8 mm) higher than the superior aspect of the greater tuberosity. Proximal humeral retroversion was found to be quite variable, averaging 19° (range, 9° to 31°). Prior studies had reported even greater ranges for retroversion, up to 50° and 60°, respectively. This variability in geometric parameters of the proximal humerus has led recent investigators to emphasize the need for surgeons to carefully consider prosthetic component size and version during an arthroplasty to recreate the native anatomy.

Another earlier study provided valuable information about the size and shape of the glenoid. The superoinferior dimension of the glenoid averaged 39 mm (range, 30 to 48 mm), and the anteroposterior dimension of the lower half of the glenoid averaged 29 mm (range, 21 to 35 mm). The anteroposterior measurement of the upper half of the glenoid was consistently less than that of the lower half, with a ratio of the lower half to the upper half of 1:0.8, giving the glenoid a pear-shaped appearance. The radius of curvature of the glenoid, as measured in the coronal plane, averaged 2.3 mm greater than that of the humeral head.

The articular surface of the glenoid is concave and is covered with hyaline cartilage, which is thinner in the center and thicker toward the periphery. The articular surface of the glenoid is only one third to one fourth the area of the humeral articular surface. The glenoid has a normal superior tilt of 5° and is retroverted between 2° and 10° in relation to the long axis of the scapula. The version also changes slightly from the upper third to the lower third of the glenoid.

Clinical concerns about glenoid component loosening after total shoulder arthroplasty have stimulated further studies on glenoid bone architecture. In one study, glenoid subchondral plate thickness averaged 1.9 mm (range, 1.2 to 2.9 mm). The volume fraction of trabecular bone varied from 11% to 45%, with peak values at the posterior glenoid vault. The middle portion of the glenoid appeared as transverse, isotropic, platelike trabeculae, which were radially oriented perpendicular to the subchondral plate. The peripheral zones tended to be more anisotropic, demonstrating regional variations in the trabecular bone architecture. Another recent study found that values of the mechanical properties were significantly higher at the center and at the posterior edge of the glenoid.

The clinical problem of osteonecrosis has inspired renewed interest in the vascularization of the humeral head. The major source of blood for the humeral head has been shown to be the anterolateral branch of the anterior circumflex artery, which crosses under the tendon of the long head of the biceps, runs proximally just adjacent to the lateral aspect of the intertubercular groove, and enters the humeral head at the proximal end of the transition from the greater tuberosity to the intertubercular groove. This vessel vascularizes nearly the entire humeral head as the arcuate artery. The posterior circumflex artery vascularizes only the posterior portion of the greater tuberosity and a small posteroinferior part of the head. There are also abundant anastomoses between the thoracoacromial, suprascapular, subscapular, and circumflex scapular arteries and the anterior and posterior circumflex arteries.

Labrum

The labrum is the peripheral rim of tissue surrounding the glenoid. It consists largely of fibrous tissue, with a fibrocartilaginous transition zone at its attachment to the articular cartilage. Structurally, the superior portion of the labrum differs from the inferior portion. The superior and anterosuperior portions of the labrum are loosely attached to the glenoid, and these regions resemble the meniscus of the knee with its triangular shape. The superior part of the labrum inserts directly into the biceps tendon distal to the insertion of the tendon at the supraglenoid tubercle. At the 12 o'clock position, there is a synovial recess between the superior part of the labrum and the glenoid rim. The past decade has seen significant interest in so-called SLAP (superior labrum, anterior-to-posterior) lesions, especially in throwing athletes.

In contrast, the inferior portion of the labrum is firmly attached to the glenoid rim and appears as a rounded fibrous elevation. A consistent fibrocartilaginous transition zone lies between the hyaline articular cartilage and the fibrous tissue of the labrum. The inferior glenohumeral ligament (IGHL) is intimately attached to both the glenoid rim and the labrum. Measurements have shown that the labrum increases the depth of the glenoid fossa by approximately 216% at the anterior portion, 227% at the posterior portion, 180% at the superior portion, and 175% at the inferior portion. A biomechanical study of the mechanism by which compression of the humeral head into the glenoid concavity provides stability against translation forces found that resection of the glenoid labrum reduced the effectiveness of compression stabilization by approximately 20%.

The glenoid labrum receives its vascular supply from branches of the suprascapular artery, the circumflex scapular branch of the subscapular artery, and the posterior circumflex humeral artery. Branches from these capsular and periosteal vessels supply the glenoid throughout its peripheral attachment but not from the underlying glenoid bone. In general, the superior and anterosuperior regions of the labrum are less vascular than the posterior and inferior portions.

Glenohumeral Ligaments

The glenohumeral ligaments are collagenous thickenings of the joint capsule. They are thought to play an important role in stabilizing the glenohumeral joint, particularly at the end range of motion. Besides acting as a structural barrier against instability, these ligaments are believed to have proprioceptive function, interacting through nerve receptors in their substance with the overlying shoulder muscles to facilitate dynamic stabilization through concerted muscle action. Studies of these ligaments have focused on their anatomy; their biomechanical role as glenohumeral stabilizers; and, recently, their ability to be altered (shrunk) by a variety of energy sources, including laser, thermal, and radiofrequency devices.

The superior glenohumeral ligament (SGHL) is fairly consistently present, though its size is quite variable. The SGHL usually originates from the glenoid labrum near the biceps tendon and inserts just superior to the lesser tuberosity. A recent anatomic study found the SGHL to be present in 94% of cadavers, although its diameter was greater than 2 mm in only two thirds of these; it was only a rudimentary structure in the remaining one third. In 73% of the shoulders, the ligament had contact with the long head of the biceps tendon, while in 17% the SGHL originated together with the middle glenohumeral ligament (MGHL). Ligament-sectioning studies have suggested that the SGHL contributes to stability against inferior translations in the adducted shoulder.

The MGHL is present less frequently than the SGHL and IGHL and is the most variable in size. In a recent anatomic study, the MGHL was found in 85% of the specimens, but it was only rudimentary in 11% of these shoulders. The diameter of the MGHL averaged 3.6 mm (range, 2 to 5 mm) and its width averaged 18 mm (range, 6 to 25 mm). The MGHL usually arises from the labrum just below the SGHL, and it inserts onto the humerus just medial to the lesser tuberosity. This ligament appears to contribute to stability against anterior translations in abduction to 45° and also helps to limit external rotation.

The IGHL comprises the portion of the capsule that originates between the 3 o'clock and 9 o'clock positions on the glenoid labrum. It inserts in an approximately 90° arc just below the articular margin of the humeral head in either a V-shaped or a collarlike attachment. Some researchers have used the terms superior band, anterior axillary pouch, and posterior axillary pouch to describe the three regions of this ligament, while others have described its anatomy as resembling a hammock, with a thick anterior band and a thin posterior band surrounding the axillary pouch. In a recent anatomic study, the IGHL was a clearly defined structure in 72% of cadaver specimens; in another 21% it was present but only as a thickening of the inferior joint capsule rather than a structure with definite anterior and posterior bands. Based on quantitative measurements, the superior band is the thickest region of the IGHL (average, 2.8 mm), while the posterior portion of the axillary pouch is the thinnest region (average, 1.7 mm). The IGHL is also thicker near its glenoid origin (average, 2.3 mm) than near its humeral insertion (average 1.6 mm). In a histologic study, the collagen fibers of the IGHL were found to have a complex structure, with predominantly radial fibers linked to each other by circular elements.

A number of biomechanical ligament-sectioning studies have shown that the IGHL is a primary stabilizer against anterior and posterior translations of the humeral head at greater degrees of abduction. One study demonstrated that this anterior band of the ligament is the primary stabilizer in abduction to 90° and 30° of horizontal extension or zero degrees of flexion/extension (neutral flexion/extension), while the posterior band is the primary stabilizer in abduction to 90° and 30° of horizontal flexion. Other studies have shown that the IGHL is an effective contributor to posterior stability when the shoulder is internally rotated. The IGHL also has been found to serve as a secondary restraint against inferior translations of the humeral head when the shoulder is in abduction.

Other studies have focused on the mechanical response of the IGHL to various types of loading. Earlier studies of this type examined the ligament response to failure testing protocols. A more recent study examined the effects of repetitive subfailure strains on the mechanical behavior of the IGHL. In this study, repetitive loading of the IGHL was found to induce laxity in the ligament, as manifested in the peak load response

and measured elongations. The mechanical response of the ligament was affected by both the magnitude of the cyclic strain and the frequency of loading at the higher levels. An increase in length was seen in all of the specimens and appeared to be largely unrecoverable. This was thought to result from accumulated microdamage caused by repetitively applied subfailure strains. This mechanism may contribute to the acquired type of glenohumeral instability, which is seen predominantly in the shoulders of young athletes who participate in sports activities requiring repetitive overhead motion.

Further studies have addressed the strain fields in the anterior capsule in a two-dimensional manner rather than simply measuring one-dimensional strains from bone-ligament-bone tests. These studies demonstrated that strains on the glenoid side of the capsule were significantly greater than those on the humeral side and that the principal strain directions were not aligned along the superior band of the IGHL.

Another area of recent research is thermal capsular shrinkage. The collagen of the shoulder capsule is predominantly type I, which is organized in a triple-helical configuration with intramolecular hydrogen bonding stabilizing the triple helix. Heating the collagen to temperatures of greater than 60°C with a laser or radiofrequency device causes the heat-labile intramolecular hydrogen bonds to break, resulting in denaturation and shrinkage of the tissue. Early work in this field has shown that the capsule is significantly weakened and made more compliant immediately after treatment but that mechanical properties of the tissue can approach normal by 12 weeks after the thermal shrinkage procedures. This technique may be an effective means of correcting excessive capsular redundancy in patients with glenohumeral instability, though published long-term outcome studies judging its efficacy are presently lacking.

Rotator Interval

The triangular-shaped region between the supraspinatus and subscapularis tendons is referred to as the rotator interval. Lesions involving the rotator interval have been described in association with rotator cuff tears, and this has stimulated recent interest in the anatomy of this region. One recent histoanatomic study found that the SGHL forms an anterior suspension sling for the long head of the biceps tendon. The roof of this sling is composed of three different layers: the SGHL, the coracohumeral ligament (CHL) and the fasciculus obliquus. The histologic appearance of this sling suggests that these structures function to protect the long head of the biceps against anterior shearing stress.

Another recent anatomic study found the rotator interval to be composed of parts of the supraspinatus,

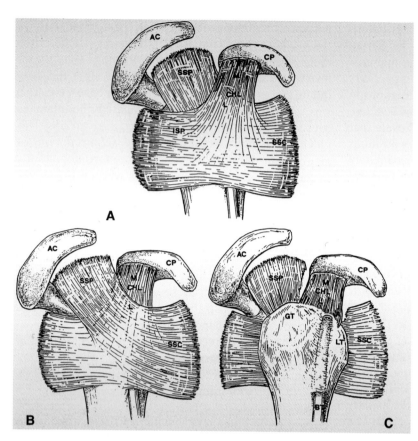

Figure 1 The rotator interval. **A,** Superficial layer of the lateral rotator interval (L), consisting of superficial fibers of the coraco-humeral ligament (CHL), which extend to the insertions of the supraspinatus (SSP) and subscapularis (SSC). **B,** Second layer of the lateral rotator interval (L), consisting of fibers of the SSP and SSC, which criss-cross through the lateral interval and blend with each other and the CHL. **C,** Third layer of the lateral rotator interval (L), consisting of deep fibers of the CHL, which insert mainly at the greater tuberosity (GT) but also at the lesser tuberosity (LT). AC = acromion, CP = coracoid process, M = medial rotator interval, ISP = infraspinatus, LT = lesser tuberosity. *(Reproduced with permission from Jost B, Koch PP, Gerber C: Anatomy and functional aspects of the rotator interval.* J Shoulder Elbow Surg *2000;9:336-341.)*

subscapularis, CHL, SGHL, and glenohumeral joint capsule. These investigators divided the rotator interval into a lateral part (ie, lateral to the cartilage-bone transition of the humeral head) and a medial part (ie, the portion covering the cartilaginous humeral head). The lateral part consists of four layers, and the medial part consists of two layers. Layers 1 through 3 are pictured in Figure 1. Layer 4 consists of the SGHL and joint capsule. The superficial layer of the medial part of the rotator interval consists of the CHL, and the deep layer consists of the SGHL and joint capsule. Sectioning studies of the components of the rotator interval showed that the medial part, especially the CHL, limits inferior translation and, to a much lesser extent, external rotation. The lateral part mainly limits external rotation of the adducted arm.

Long Head of the Biceps Tendon

The origin of the long head of the biceps tendon is variable. In a recent anatomic study, the tendon originated from the supraglenoid tubercle in 30% of shoulders; in 45%, it originated directly from the glenoid labrum; in the remaining 25%, it originated from both the supraglenoid tubercle and the labrum. The tendon travels obliquely within the shoulder joint and turns sharply inferiorly to exit the joint beneath the transverse

humeral ligament along the intertubercular sulcus or bicipital groove. The tendon is covered by a reflection of the synovial sheath, which ends as a blind pouch at the distal part of the bicipital groove, thus making the tendon an intra-articular but extrasynovial structure. On average, the total length of this tendon is 102 mm (range; 89 to 146 mm). The size and shape of the tendon change from proximal to distal. Near its origin on the glenoid, the tendon has an average cross-sectional area of 8.4 mm × 3.4 mm. As it exits the bicipital groove, the cross-sectional area decreases to 4.5 mm × 2.1 mm. When degenerative lesions are present in this tendon, they are most commonly found in the distal bicipital groove and near the origin of the tendon at the glenoid labrum.

The function of the long head of the biceps tendon at the shoulder remains a topic of debate. It has long been assumed to act as a humeral head depressor, especially in the presence of a rotator cuff tear. In one biomechanical cadaver model using simulated muscle forces, it was shown that biceps tendon force restrains superior humeral translation, most significantly when a large rotator cuff defect is present. Another study using a cadaver model demonstrated that the biceps contributes to anterior stability of the glenohumeral joint by increasing the resistance to torsional forces. Several electromyographic studies, however, have suggested that the biceps shows little action during shoulder motion and acts mainly to control the elbow. Thus, controversy remains over the functional role of the long head of the biceps tendon for the shoulder, and further studies are necessary to determine whether it plays a role at this joint.

The Subacromial Space
Osseous Structures

The major osseous structure of this region is the acromion, which extends from the spine of the scapula anteriorly and laterally and articulates with the distal clavicle. The acromion forms from two and occasionally three ossification centers that appear during puberty and normally fuse approximately at the age of 22 years. In an anatomic study of 420 scapulae, differences in the size of the acromion were found between men and women. In men, the average length was 48.5 mm, the average anterior width was 19.5 mm, and the average anterior thickness was 7.7 mm. In women, acromial length averaged 40.6 mm, anterior width averaged 18.4 mm, and anterior thickness averaged 6.7 mm. The acromial facet of the acromioclavicular joint was noted to be medially inclined (superolateral to inferomedial) in 49% of shoulders, vertical in 48%, and laterally inclined in 3%. An unfused acromial epiphysis was found in 8%.

Lateral radiographs with a 10° caudal tilt (outlet views) have been used to classify the acromion into three morphologic patterns: flat (type I), curved (type II), and hooked (type III). In cadavers and in a clinical population, a higher incidence of rotator cuff tears has been found in shoulders with a hooked acromion, which compromises the subacromial space. A recent study of 420 scapulae from cadavers of various ages found that basic acromial morphology (flat, curved, or hooked) is a primary anatomic characteristic that is independent of age. However, spur formation on the anterior acromion appears to be age related as these spurs appeared in only 7% of specimens from patients younger than 50 years of age and in 30% of specimens from patients older than 50 years of age. This study suggests that variations in acromial shape contribute to impingement both independently of age-related degenerative processes (eg, by a native hooked morphology) and through age-related degenerative spurring.

The coracoid process projects anteriorly and laterally from the neck of the scapula and forms the anterior boundary of the subacromial space. Its size, shape, and angle of inclination can vary widely. It serves as the site of origin of the short head of the biceps and the coracobrachialis tendons and as the insertion site for the pectoralis minor tendon and the coracohumeral, coracoclavicular, and coracoacromial ligaments. The coracoid provides an easily palpable landmark for determining the rotator interval between the supraspinatus and subscapularis tendons during rotator cuff surgery.

Coracoacromial Ligament

The coracoacromial ligament (CAL) forms the anterosuperior boundary of the coracoacromial arch. A recent anatomic report identified several morphologic types: quadrangular (48%), Y-shaped with a broader lateral band and a thinner medial band (42%), broad-banded (8%), and multiple bands (2%). The length of the coracoid attachment averaged 32 mm, and the length of the acromial attachment of this ligament averaged 19 mm. The thickness of the ligament at the midpoint between its attachment sites was 1.3 mm. Other investigators have found that the length of the lateral ban was significantly shorter and its cross-sectional area was significantly larger in specimens with a rotator cuff tear, perhaps resulting in a smaller subacromial space in these shoulders. Significant differences in the material properties of the lateral band were also found in the specimens with a rotator cuff tear, as the elastic modulus was much lower in these ligaments. Other recent biomechanical studies of the CAL have shown that there is an appreciable resting load of 20 N, demonstrating that this ligament is under tension in situ. There were no differences in this parameter between normal shoulders and those with a rotator cuff tear. However, cyclic loading of the CAL in shoulders with cuff tears showed a larger drop in peak stress than in normal shoulders but no significant differences in stress relaxation. Finally, a histologic study of the coracoacromial arch found age-related degenerative changes in the CAL, degeneration of the acromial bone-ligament junction, and acromial spur formation, and these changes were not dependent on the presence of a rotator cuff tear.

Subacromial Bursa

Between the structures of the coracoacromial arch and the tendons of the rotator cuff lies the subacromial bursa, a synovium-lined thin structure that can become quite thickened in disease. This structure has been shown to contain numerous free nerve endings, indicating that it may be involved with pain perception in pathologic conditions. A recent study of the anatomic boundaries of the subacromial bursa found that the bursal margins were always 2 cm or more from the anterolateral corner of the bursal acromial surface and the bursa lined the anterior half of the acromial undersurface. The mean minimum distance from the subdeltoid bursal reflection to the axillary nerve was 0.8 cm, with a range of 0 to 1.4 cm. Thus, these investigators urged caution when approaching the inferior boundary of the subdeltoid bursal reflection, because of the proximity of the axillary nerve.

Deltoid Muscle

Although the deltoid is not a subacromial structure, it interfaces with the coracoacromial arch and has its origin on the acromion. Recent histologic studies of the deltoid origin may have implications for surgical procedures aimed at decompressing the subacromial space. One study showed that a combination of tendon and muscle fibers of the deltoid attached it to part of the superior surface and to the entire anterior surface of the anterior acromion. The fibrous insertion of the CAL covered the inferior surface of the acromion. When an acromioplasty was performed with a burr, 70% of the origin of the deltoid from the anterior acromion was detached, but the superior and anterosuperior attachments were preserved, and there was little retraction of the muscle fibers. Another histologic study of the deltoid origin found that the deltoid attaches to the anterior and lateral acromion primarily by direct tendinous attachment. The deltoid tendon attaches indirectly by periosteal fiber attachment only on the superior surface of the acromion. According to a computer simulation of an acromioplasty, removal of 4 mm of bone would release more than 40% of the direct fiber attachment; removal of 6 mm of bone would release nearly 70% of the direct tendinous fibers. The authors point out that although arthroscopic acromioplasty results in the release of a portion of the direct tendon fibers at the deltoid origin, the functional effect of this is not known and requires further study.

Rotator Cuff

The rotator cuff consists of the tendons of the supraspinatus, infraspinatus, teres minor, and subscapularis muscles. These muscles play an important role in providing dynamic stability for the glenohumeral joint by compressing the humeral head against the glenoid and by depressing the humeral head, thereby opposing the upward pull of the deltoid. The infraspinatus and teres minor also provide active external rotation for the shoulder, and the subscapularis acts as an internal rotator. The supraspinatus assists the deltoid in elevating the arm. Rotator cuff disorders represent a wide spectrum of disease, including tendon inflammation, tendon and bursal fibrosis, and both partial- and full-thickness tendon tears. These disorders constitute a large percentage of the shoulder pathologies that require surgical treatment by orthopaedic surgeons. Basic research on the anatomy, biomechanical properties, and function of the rotator cuff, as well as on models for the pathogenesis of rotator cuff disease, has been extensive.

A recent anatomic study examined the relationship of the supraspinatus and infraspinatus tendons to the three facets of the greater tuberosity. In all of the specimens, the authors found that the supraspinatus tendon attached to the superior facet of the greater tuberosity as well as to the superior half of the middle facet. The infraspinatus tendon attached to the entire length of the middle facet, covering a portion of the supraspinatus tendon. The superior margin of the anatomic neck without articular cartilage or sulcus was found to be located not at the interval between the supraspinatus and the infraspinatus tendons but 4 mm posterior to the posterior margin of the supraspinatus tendon.

The architecture of the supraspinatus muscle and tendon was recently studied. The supraspinatus was found to consist of an anterior muscle belly with a thick, tubular anterior tendon and a posterior muscle belly with a flatter, wider tendon. The anterior muscle belly is fusiform, originating entirely from the supraspinous fossa. An internal tendon runs within the muscle like an intramuscular core, and the larger anterior muscle mass inserts onto this core. The internal tendon then thickens and runs as a tubular, extramuscular tendon, which comprises 40% of the total width of the supraspinatus tendon (Fig. 2). The posterior muscle belly is a smaller strap muscle, which originates from the scapular spine and glenoid neck. It has no tendinous core and inserts onto a flatter, wider posterior tendon, which comprises 60% of the total width of the supraspinatus. The physiologic cross-sectional areas of the anterior and posterior muscle bellies were calculated to be 140 mm^2 and 62 mm^2, respectively, and their tendon cross-sectional areas were 26.4 mm^2 and 31.2 mm^2, respectively. Thus, while the anterior muscle mass is greater, it pulls through a smaller cross-sectional area of tendon, subjecting the anterior tendon to nearly three times greater stress than the posterior tendon. This architecture suggests that the anterior supraspinatus is responsible for the bulk of the contractile force of the supraspinatus.

Other studies have focused on the histologic and intrinsic biomechanical properties of the rotator cuff tendons. One study reported on histologic evidence of degeneration in the supraspinatus, infraspinatus, and subscapularis tendons. Degenerative changes were seen in all three tendons to an equal extent. The degeneration was more pronounced in the articular half than in the bursal half in all three tendons. These data suggest that intrinsic tendon degeneration is an important factor in the pathogenesis of rotator cuff tears. Another study found histologic differences between the bursal-side and joint-side layers of the supraspinatus tendon, as well as differences in their biomechanical properties. The bursal-side layer was composed of tendon bundles with a decreasing muscular component near the insertion, while the joint-side layer was a complex of tendon, ligament, and joint capsule. The strain to yield point for the bursal-side layer was 0.15 versus 0.07 for the joint-side layer, and the ultimate fail-

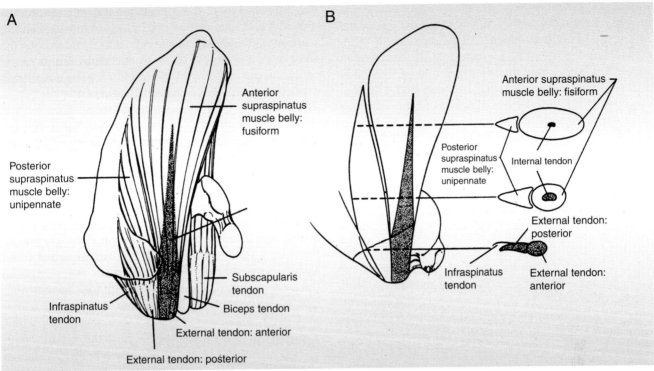

Figure 2 A, Schematic representation of the anterior and posterior musculotendinous anatomy of the supraspinatus. **B,** Cross-sectional views. *(Reproduced with permission from Roh MS, Wang VM, April EW, Pollock RG, Bigliani LU, Flatow EL: Anterior and posterior musculotendinous anatomy of the supraspinatus. J Shoulder Elbow Surg 2000; 9:436-440.)*

ure stress for the bursal-side layer was 6.3 N/mm^2 versus 2.8 N/mm^2 for the joint-side layer. Because it is composed primarily of longitudinal tendon fibers, the bursal-side layer generates greater resistance when loaded in tension than does the joint-side layer. The thinner, heterogenously composed joint-side layer appears more vulnerable to tensile loads.

An important biomechanical study used the technique of stereophotogrammetry to investigate the relationship of the rotator cuff to the acromion during scapular elevation. Subacromial contact started at the anterolateral edge of the acromion at 0° of elevation and shifted medially on the acromion with elevation. On the humeral side, contact shifted from proximal to distal on the supraspinatus tendon with elevation. The acromial undersurface and rotator cuff were in closest proximity between 60° and 120° of elevation. Specimens with a type III (hooked) acromion had consistently more pronounced contact, and contact was consistently centered on the supraspinatus insertion. The results of this study suggest that some degree of contact between the rotator cuff and coracoacromial arch is normal (ie, a normal buffering or stabilizing role for the arch is implicated), but markedly increased or focused contact may be harmful to the tendon.

Other recent studies using animal models have investigated mechanisms of injury to the rotator cuff tendons. Overuse activity was found to produce significant changes in the supraspinatus tendons in the rat shoulder model. An increase in cellularity and a loss of the normal collagen fiber organization was seen, similar to what has been seen in human tendinopathy. The tendons in the overuse group were thicker but had inferior mechanical properties compared with normal controls, as the modulus of elasticity and maximum stress at failure decreased by nearly half. Other work in the field has shown that damage to the supraspinatus tendon can be caused by intrinsic injury and extrinsic compression, as well as by overuse alone.

The Acromioclavicular Joint

The acromioclavicular joint is a diarthrodial joint and is the only articulation between the clavicle and the scapula. It has a variable inclination, ranging from near vertical to angled downward medially up to 50°. The shallow concave facet on the acromion averages 17 mm in length and 9 mm in height. A fibrocartilaginous disk, which undergoes degeneration with advancing age and the function of which is not well understood, is contained in the joint. Motion at the normal acromioclavicular joint appears to be small, involving small translations and mainly rotation between the clavicle and acromion.

Recent ligament-sectioning studies have provided additional information about the two major sets of ligaments that stabilize the acromioclavicular joint: the capsular acromioclavicular ligaments and the coracoclavicular ligaments (consisting of the conoid and trapezoid ligaments). In one study of 10 shoulders, the average length of the conoid ligament was 15.1 mm and that of the trapezoid ligament was 11.5 mm; the average widths of the conoid and trapezoid ligaments were 10.7 mm and 11.0 mm, respectively. The inferior acromioclavicular capsular ligament appeared to be the major restraint against anterior joint translations. The trapezoid ligament provided a significantly greater contribution to stability against posterior translations than did the other ligaments, providing 56% of the resisting force. The trapezoid and conoid ligaments were the major stabilizers against superior displacement of the joint. Another biomechanical study considered the importance to anteroposterior stability of the different portions of the acromioclavicular joint capsule. Sectioning the anterior and inferior ligaments had no significant effect on posterior translation of the joint. On the other hand, the superior and posterior ligaments provided significant stability against posterior translations, contributing 56% and 25% of the stabilizing forces, respectively. These authors recommended sparing the posterior and superior capsular ligaments when performing distal clavicle excision to prevent excessive posterior clavicular translations after resection.

The Sternoclavicular Joint

The sternoclavicular joint is the only true joint that connects the upper extremity to the axial skeleton. Half of the medial end of the clavicle articulates with the sternum, and the other half forms a portion of the sternal notch. The sternoclavicular joint has very little inherent bony stability and relies almost completely on a number of surrounding ligaments for its stability. These include the anterior and posterior sternoclavicular or capsular ligaments, the interclavicular ligament, and the anterior and posterior costoclavicular ligaments. The posterior capsular ligament is the most important stabilizer, preventing upward displacement of the medial clavicle caused by downward forces on the lateral end of the clavicle. These ligaments allow the clavicle to move approximately 30° upward and 30° in the anteroposterior direction and to rotate 45° about its long axis.

The Scapulothoracic Articulation

The scapulothoracic articulation is not a true joint but rather is a space between the concave surface of the anterior scapula and the convex surface of the posterior chest wall. The stability of this articulation is maintained by the muscular and ligamentous attachments to the scapula. The scapula protracts, retracts, and rotates as it glides along the chest wall in a smooth scapulohumeral rhythm. A recent report on the anatomy of the scapulothoracic articulation divided the structures of this articulation into three layers. The superficial layer includes the trapezius and latissimus dorsi muscles and an inconsistent bursa between the inferior angle of the scapula and the latissimus dorsi. The intermediate layer consists of the rhomboid major and minor muscles, the levator scapulae muscle, the spinal accessory nerve, and a consistent bursa between the superomedial scapula and the trapezius. The spinal accessory nerve traveled intimately along the wall of this bursa, an average of 2.7 cm lateral to the superomedial scapular angle. Finally, the deep layer is composed of the serratus anterior and subscapularis muscles, the scapulothoracic bursa (between the serratus anterior and the thorax), and the subscapularis bursa (between the serratus and subscapularis).

Annotated Bibliography

The Glenohumeral Joint

Boileau P, Walch G: The three-dimensional geometry of the proximal humerus: Implications for surgical technique and prosthetic design. *J Bone Joint Surg Br* 1997; 79:857-865.
This landmark study is the basis for the third generation of prosthetic design with more accurate appreciation of humeral version and head offset. A mathematical relationship exists between the articular segment diameter removed in surgery and the head height (neck length).

Frich LH, Odgaard A, Dalstra M: Glenoid bone architecture. *J Shoulder Elbow Surg* 1998;7:356-361.
This study of six glenoid specimens found regional variations in the trabecular bone architecture of the glenoid. Subchondral plate thickness averaged 1.9 mm (range, 1.2 to 2.9 mm), and the volume fraction of trabecular bone varied from 11% to 45%. Bone density was greatest in the posterior glenoid.

Jost B, Koch PP, Gerber C: Anatomy and functional aspects of the rotator interval. *J Shoulder Elbow Surg* 2000;9:336-341.
The anatomy of the rotator interval was studied in 22 cadaveric shoulders. A medial part, consisting of two layers, and a lateral part, consisting of four layers, were identified. The medial part was found to limit inferior translation primarily, and the lateral part mainly limited external rotation.

Pollock RG, Wang VM, Bucchieri JS, et al: Effects of repetitive subfailure strains on the mechanical behavior of the inferior glenohumeral ligament. *J Shoulder Elbow Surg* 2000;9:427-435.

The mechanical response of the IGHL to varying subfailure cyclic strains was studied in 33 cadaveric shoulders. Repetitive loading was found to induce laxity in the IGHL. The residual length increase appeared to be largely unrecoverable and was thought to result from accumulated microdamage within the ligament substance.

Malicky DM, Soslowsky LJ, Mouro CM, et al: Total strain fields of the glenohumeral joint capsule under shoulder subluxation. *J Biomech Eng*, in press.

Using a stereoradiogrammetry method, two-dimensional strain fields were obtained for the anteroinferior glenohumeral capsule. These studies demonstrated higher strains near the glenoid. Interestingly, principal strain directions were not aligned along the superior band of the IGHL.

Robertson DD, Yuan J, Bigliani LU, Flatow EL, Yamaguchi K: Three-dimensional analysis of the proximal part of the humerus: Relevance to arthroplasty. *J Bone Joint Surg Am* 2000; 82:1594-1602.

The extramedullary and intramedullary humeral morphology was studied in 60 cadaveric humeri, using CT data and three-dimensional computer modeling. The humeral head center was offset 7 mm medially and 2 mm posteriorly from the humeral axis. Humeral head thickness averaged 19 mm, and head thickness and head radius were proportionately linked. Marked variability was seen in proximal humeral morphology.

Steinbeck J, Liljenqvist U, Jerosch J: The anatomy of the glenohumeral ligamentous complex and its contribution to anterior shoulder stability. *J Shoulder Elbow Surg* 1998;7:122-126.

The anatomy of the glenohumeral ligaments was studied in 104 cadaveric shoulders. The SGHL was seen in 94%, the MGHL in 85%, and the IGHL in 93%. Synovial recesses in the capsule were also studied, using the classification system described previously by DePalma.

Wallace AL, Hollinshead RM, Frank CB: The scientific basis of thermal capsular shrinkage. *J Shoulder Elbow Surg* 2000;9:354-360.

This article reviews much of the scientific literature on thermal capsular shrinkage. Biomechanical data show that significant alterations in the length of ligaments may be achieved by thermal treatment, though there may be adverse effects of the strength and stiffness of the tissues, at least during the acute period after treatment.

Werner A, Mueller T, Boehm D, Gohlke F: The stabilizing sling for the long head of the biceps tendon in the rotator cuff interval: A histoanatomic study. *Am J Sports Med* 2000;28:28-31.

A histoanatomic study of the rotator interval was performed in 13 cadaveric shoulders. A stabilizing fibrous sling for the long head of the biceps was found to consist mainly of fibers from the SGHL with lesser contributions from the coracohumeral ligament and fasciculus obliquus.

The Subacromial Space

Nicholson GP, Goodman DA, Flatow EL, Bigliani LU: The acromion: Morphologic condition and age-related changes: A study of 420 scapulas. *J Shoulder Elbow Surg* 1996;5:1-11.

This study of acromial morphology evaluated 420 scapulae from an osteologic collection. Acromial morphology was found to be independent of age and appeared to be a primary anatomic characteristic. Spur formation on the undersurface of the anteroinferior acromion, however, was found to be an age-dependent process.

Roh MS, Wang VM, April EW, Pollock RG, Bigliani LU, Flatow EL: Anterior and posterior musculotendinous anatomy of the supraspinatus. *J Shoulder Elbow Surg* 2000;9:436-440.

The architecture of the supraspinatus was studied in 25 cadaveric shoulders. Structural differences were seen between the anterior and posterior musculotendinous parts of the supraspinatus: the anterior supraspinatus has a larger muscle size, a fusiform structure, and a thicker, tubular tendon; the posterior part is a smaller strap muscle with a flatter, wider tendon, which is subjected to much less stress.

Sano H, Ishii H, Trudel G, Uhthoff HK: Histologic evidence of degeneration at the insertion of 3 rotator cuff tendons: A comparative study with human cadaveric shoulders. *J Shoulder Elbow Surg* 1999;8:574-579.

During a histologic examination of 76 cadaveric shoulders, the authors determined the degree of degeneration at the insertion of three rotator cuff tendons. Degeneration was more prominent on the articular side than on the bursal side. In addition, degeneration of partially torn tendons was greater than that of intact tendons.

Soslowsky LJ, An CH, DeBano CM, Carpenter JE: Coracoacromial ligament: In situ load and viscoelastic properties in rotator cuff disease. *Clin Orthop* 1996;330:40-44.

The biomechanical properties of CALs from 16 cadaveric shoulders were evaluated. An in situ tensile load of nearly 20 N was found. Cyclic loading of the ligaments demonstrated a greater drop in peak stress in shoulders with rotator cuff tears than in normal shoulders; however, the stress relaxation response was not different.

Soslowsky LJ, Thomopoulos S, Tun S, et al: Overuse activity injures the supraspinatus tendon in an animal model: A histologic and biomechanical study. *J Shoulder Elbow Surg* 2000;9:79-84.

The authors discussed implications of overuse injuries as an etiologic factor in rotator cuff injuries, particularly injury to the supraspinatus tendon. They compared the effects of overuse running in 36 rats with those in rats that were allowed normal cage activity. The supraspinatus tendons in the rats in the exercised group demonstrated significant histologic and biomechanical changes when compared with the rats in the control group. This study provides a reliable animal model for understanding the etiology and pathogenesis of overuse injuries in humans.

Torpey BM, Ikeda K, Weng M, et al: The deltoid muscle origin: Histologic characteristics and effects of subacromial decompression. *Am J Sports Med* 1998;26:379-383.

The histologic appearance of the deltoid attachment to the acromion was studied in nine cadaveric shoulders. The deltoid muscle attaches to the anterior and lateral acromion primarily by direct tendinous attachment, whereas it attaches to the dorsal surface of the acromion by periosteal fiber attachment.

The Acromioclavicular Joint

Klimkiewicz JJ, Williams GR, Sher JS, Karduna A, Des Jardins J, Iannotti JP: The acromioclavicular capsule as a restraint to posterior translation of the clavicle: A biomechanical analysis. *J Shoulder Elbow Surg* 1999;8:119-124.

A biomechanical analysis of the acromioclavicular capsule in six cadaveric shoulders was performed. Sectioning of the anterior and inferior capsular ligaments had no significant effect on posterior translation of the clavicle, whereas sectioning of the superior and posterior ligaments allowed significantly greater posterior translations.

Lee K-W, Debski RE, Chen C-H, Woo SL, Fu FH: Functional evaluation of the ligaments at the acromioclavicular joint during anteroposterior and superoinferior translation. *Am J Sports Med* 1997;25:858-862.

The anatomy and biomechanical function of the ligaments at the acromioclavicular joint were studied in 10 cadaveric shoulders. The inferior acromioclavicular capsular ligament was the primary restraint against anterior displacement, while the trapezoid was the primary restraint against posterior displacement.

The Scapulothoracic Articulation

Williams GR, Shakil M, Klimkiewicz J, Iannotti JP: Anatomy of the scapulothoracic articulation. *Clin Orthop* 1999;359:237-246.

The structures of the scapulothoracic articulation were divided into three anatomic layers: a superficial layer consisting of the trapezius and latissimus dorsi; an intermediate layer consisting of the levator scapulae, rhomboids, spinal accessory nerve, and scapulotrapezial bursa; and a deep layer consisting of the serratus anterior, subscapularis, the scapulothoracic bursa, and the subscapularis bursa.

Classic Bibliography

Clark JM, Harryman DT II: Tendons, ligaments, and capsule of the rotator cuff: Gross and microscopic anatomy. *J Bone Joint Surg Am* 1992;74:713-725.

Cooper DE, Arnoczky SP, O'Brien SJ, Warren RF, DiCarlo E, Allen AA: Anatomy, histology, and vascularity of the glenoid labrum: An anatomical study. *J Bone Joint Surg Am* 1992;74:46-52.

Flatow EL, Soslowsky LJ, Ticker JB, et al: Excursion of the rotator cuff under the acromion: Patterns of subacromial contact. *Am J Sports Med* 1994;22:779-788.

Gerber C, Schneeberger AG, Vinh TS: The arterial vascularization of the humeral head: An anatomical study. *J Bone Joint Surg Am* 1990;72:1486-1494.

Gohlke F, Essigkrug B, Schmitz F: The pattern of the collagen fiber bundles of the capsule of the glenohumeral joint. *J Shoulder Elbow Surg* 1994;3:111-128.

Iannotti JP, Gabriel JP, Schneck SL, Evans BG, Misra S: The normal glenohumeral relationships: An anatomical study of 140 shoulders. *J Bone Joint Surg Am* 1992;74:491-500.

Nakajima T, Rokuuma N, Hamada K, Tomatsu T, Fukuda H: Histologic and biomechanical characteristics of the supraspinatus tendon: Reference to rotator cuff tearing. *J Shoulder Elbow Surg* 1994;3:79-87.

O'Brien SJ, Neves MC, Arnoczky SP, et al: The anatomy and histology of the inferior glenohumeral ligament complex of the shoulder. *Am J Sports Med* 1990;18:449-456.

Refior HJ, Sowa D: Long tendon of the biceps brachii: Sites of predilection for degenerative lesions. *J Shoulder Elbow Surg* 1995;4:436-440.

Chapter 2

Basic Science of Glenohumeral Instability

Ariane Gerber, MD

Maria Apreleva, PhD

Jon J.P. Warner, MD

Introduction

The glenohumeral joint is a synovial joint formed by the articulation of the large, nearly spherical humeral head with the smaller, shallow glenoid surface of the scapula. The joint has minimal bony constraints as well as a unique anatomic architecture and functional arrangements that allow for a large range of motion during everyday and sports activities. Despite its minimally constrained nature, the glenohumeral joint can carry both small and large loads at various speeds of arm motion while maintaining stability because of soft-tissue support. Instability is defined as abnormal or painful excessive movement of the humeral head out of the glenoid during active shoulder motion. Instability should be distinguished from laxity, which is a passive characteristic inherent in both normal and unstable joints.

The control of glenohumeral stability is achieved by the complex interaction between the static restraints (ligaments and tendons) and dynamic restraints (muscular contraction) acting across the joint. In the middle range of rotation, joint stability is provided by the dynamic action of the rotator cuff and the biceps muscles through compression of the humeral head in the glenoid socket. The ligamentous structures function passively at the extreme positions of rotation, preventing excessive translation of the humeral head on the glenoid. Contraction of the muscles around the shoulder may also have the secondary effect of protecting the smaller ligamentous structures from injury at end-range positions. Articular surface conformity, articular version, negative intra-articular pressure, and adhesion-cohesion, either singly or in combination, also affect the stabilization of the glenohumeral joint. Additional factors that determine susceptibility to glenohumeral instability are patient age and gender, congenital capsular insufficiency, and strength and conditioning of the rotator cuff and axioscapular muscles of the shoulder complex.

The goal of the contemporary therapeutic approach to glenohumeral instability is the restoration of anatomy. This approach requires a thorough and clear understanding of the anatomy and biomechanics of this articulation.

Static Stability Factors

Articular Anatomy

Orientation of the Articular Surfaces

The anatomy of the proximal humerus is variable. The humeral head articular inclination, or the angle formed by the neck and shaft axes, varies from 114° to 147°. It is also retroverted from –6.5° to 47.5° (average, 18°) relative to the axis passing through the humeral condyles.

The orientation of the glenoid in the space depends on the position of the scapula and the orientation of the articular surface in relation to the scapular body. The horizontal (glenoid version) and vertical (glenoid inclination) orientation of the glenoid is not defined by a simple geometric relationship, as is demonstrated by CT morphometric analysis, which has shown that the superior part of the articular surface is retroverted, while the inferior portion may be anteverted. Therefore, the perception of glenoid version depends on the level of the cross-sectional image. In a midglenoid transverse CT scan, the image to be used is the first inferior image, on which the tip of the coracoid process is no longer visible. At that level, glenoid retroversion between –2° and –8° is considered to be normal, although the literature reports a wide range of values. One anthropometric study of more than 1,000 scapulae found that in the superoinferior plane, 50% of the glenoids were inclined inferiorly, 20% were vertical, and 30% were inclined superiorly. Articular geometry plays an important role in the motion and stability of the shoulder.

Articular Conformity

An understanding of the humerus and the glenoid as separate but interdependent congruent structures is required to appreciate how the joint surfaces can maintain stability while at the same time permitting a large range of motion.

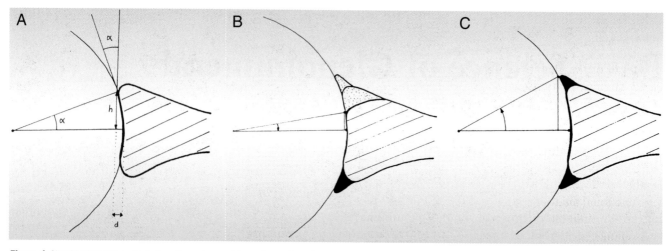

Figure 1 Glenoid constraint angle. **A,** In a given plane and for a given radius of curvature, the angle α enclosed between the deepest point of the articular surface and the edge of the glenoid rim defines the maximal slope, the depth (d), and the length (h) of the articular surface. If α increases, the glenoid constraint increases and the joint becomes more stable. **B,** Effect of a defect of the articular surface on glenoid constraint. **C,** Effect of the labrum on glenoid constraint.

The glenohumeral joint can be compared to a golf ball sitting on a tee because of the smaller area and larger radius of curvature of the glenoid compared with that of the humeral head. This is true as far as the skeletal (radiologic) anatomy of the joint is considered without the cartilage. However, because the cartilage of the glenoid is thicker at the periphery than in the center and because the humeral head has a converse anatomic relationship, the articular surfaces are almost perfectly conforming. Recent anatomic, CT, and MRI studies found that in most shoulders, the glenoid and humeral head have similar radii of curvature. In one study, stereophotogrammetry was used to define the surface topography of the glenohumeral joint. The authors found not only that the articulation showed less than 1% deviation from sphericity but also that the radii of curvature of the glenoid and humeral head matched in 88% of cases. This finding is consistent with kinematic analysis that has shown the glenohumeral joint to function analogously to a ball-and-socket articulation during glenohumeral rotation.

The articular surface area of the humeral head is three times that of the glenoid. In any position of joint rotation, only 25% to 30% of the humeral head is in contact with the glenoid. This relationship has been referred to as the glenohumeral index and is defined as the maximum glenoid diameter divided by the maximum head diameter. Another way to define the amount of humeral articular surface in contact with the glenoid is to consider the glenoid constraint angle α. Assuming that the glenohumeral articulation is congruent, the radius of curvature of the glenoid and that of the humeral head in a defined plane will be identical. For a given radius of curvature, the angle α is enclosed between the deepest point of the articular surface and the edge of the glenoid rim. This angle defines the maximal slope, the depth, and the length of the articular surface (Fig. 1). If α increases, the maximal slope at the edge, the depth, and the length of the articular surface increase. Consequently, the surface area increases and the joint becomes more constrained. In the case of a glenoid rim fracture, this mechanism of stability is disrupted. Experimental modeling of an anterior glenoid rim fracture involving 20% of the length of the anterior glenoid resulted in significant reduction of stability. If only a soft-tissue Bankart repair was performed following the creation of a 1.5-cm defect of the anterior-inferior rim, the joint remained up to 50% less stable than the normal joint. In such cases, reconstruction of the anteroinferior glenoid articular surface with bone graft is indicated.

Glenoid Labrum

The glenoid labrum is a wedge-shaped fibrous structure that consists of densely packed collagen bundles. Located between the articular cartilage and the labrum, this narrow fibrocartilaginous transition zone is composed of dense collagen fibers in a woven pattern within the hyaline cartilage. Below the glenoid equator, the inferior labrum is firmly continuous with the articular cartilage, whereas above the glenoid equator, the superior labrum is quite variable and is often loosely attached and more mobile.

The labrum is vascularized throughout its peripheral attachment to the joint capsule and acts as an anchor for the glenohumeral ligaments and the biceps tendon. Lesions in the centrifugal vascular portion of the labrum are thus more likely to heal after injury than are those close to the articular surface.

The contribution of the labrum to glenohumeral stability has been clearly established: it acts as the anchor point for the capsuloligamentous structures, increases the depth of the glenoid socket, and facilitates the concavity-compression mechanism as the humeral head is compressed in the glenoid during rotator cuff contraction. Loss of the labrum (Bankart lesion) has been reported to result in a 50% decrease in the glenoid depth. A 1993 study demonstrated that the translational force required to dislocate the humeral head was 20% smaller after removal of the glenoid labrum. Although the functional anatomy of the glenoid labrum is becoming better understood, its role in the glenohumeral restraining mechanism, particularly at the extremes of motion, remains unclear.

Capsuloligamentous Structures

Similar to other joints in the body, the shoulder capsule is composed primarily of type I collagen, with lesser amounts of types II and III. The secondary structure of collagen is that of an α-helix in which the individual collagen molecules are held in an extended conformation by both intramolecular and intermolecular forces (hydrogen bonds, salt links, and covalent crosslinks). This highly ordered (crystalline) arrangement of collagen in the extended conformation is the structural basis for the viscoelastic properties of collagenous tissues.

Localized thickenings of the joint capsule have traditionally been described as the glenohumeral ligaments (Fig. 2). Whereas the anatomy of the inferior glenohumeral complex is relatively constant, the configuration of the superior and middle glenohumeral ligaments is variable. Numerous intraoperative observations and cadaveric studies have improved understanding of the anatomy and biomechanics of these structures (Table 1). Because of the orientation of these ligaments, portions of the capsule reciprocally tighten and loosen as the glenohumeral joint rotates, thus limiting translation and rotation by load sharing. In the middle range of rotation, these structures are relatively lax, and stability is maintained primarily by the action of the rotator cuff muscles compressing the humeral head into the conforming glenoid socket. However, recent investigations have shown that the static restraints may lead to small amounts of obligate translation in positions of extreme rotation. In normal subjects, the humeral head translated posteriorly up to several millimeters when the shoulder was extended and externally rotated; this coupled posterior translation does not occur in patients with anterior instability. An experimental cadaveric study has shown that anterior translation of several millimeters normally occurs with flexion beyond 55°, while posterior translation occurs with extension beyond 35°. With experimental

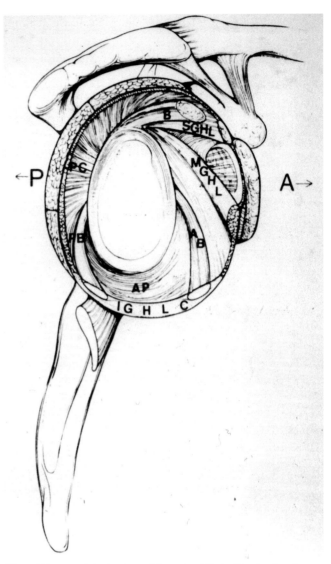

Figure 2 Anatomy of the glenohumeral ligaments: right shoulder, view from the side. B = biceps tendon, SGHL = superior glenohumeral ligament, MGHL = middle glenohumeral ligament, AB = anterior band, AP = axillary pouch, PB = posterior band, PC = posterior capsule, IGHLC = inferior glenohumeral complex. *(Reproduced with permission from O'Brien SJ, Neves MC, Arnoczky SP, et al: The anatomy and histology of the inferior glenohumeral ligament complex of the shoulder. Am J Sports Med 1990;18:449.)*

tightening of the posterior capsule or of the rotator interval capsular region, obligate anterior translation during flexion both increased and occurred earlier than in the normal shoulder. That is, tightening of a portion of the capsule can cause excessive translation of the humeral head during glenohumeral rotation. This translation usually occurs in the opposite direction of the capsular tightening and can lead to instability, articular damage, and even symptoms of impingement. Such impingement symptoms may occur through nonoutlet mechanisms because a tight posterior capsule or rotator interval capsule causes the humeral head to move superiorly during flexion. This has been termed the capsular constraint mechanism.

TABLE 1 | Anatomy and Function of the Glenohumeral Ligaments and Capsule

	Structure	Origin	Insertion	Anatomic Relationships	Function
Coracohumeral ligament (CHL)	Dense, fibrous, 1- to- 2-cm wide; thin structure	Lateral surface of the coracoid process	Greater and lesser tuberosities adjacent to the bicipital groove	Extra-articular, intermingled with the edges of the supraspinatus and subscapularis tendons; reinforcement of the rotator interval	Limits inferior translation and external rotation when the arm is adducted and posterior translation when the shoulder is in a position of forward flexion, adduction, and internal rotation
Superior glenohumeral ligament (SGHL)	Variable in size; present in 90% of individuals	Superior glenoid tubercle just inferior to the biceps tendon	Superior aspect of the lesser tuberosity just medial to the bicipital groove	Intra-articular, lies deep to the CHL; reinforcement of the rotator interval	Same as the CHL
Middle glenohumeral ligament (MGHL)	Great variation in size and presence; absent or poorly defined in 40% of individuals	Superior glenoid tubercle and anterosuperior labrum, often along with the SGHL	Anterior to the lesser tuberosity	Intra-articular, blending with the posterior aspect of the subscapularis tendon	Passive restraint to both anterior and posterior translation when the arm is abducted in the range of 60° to 90° in external rotation and limits inferior translation when the arm is adducted at the side
Inferior glenohumeral complex (IGHLC)	Consists of three components: anterior band, posterior band, axillary pouch; decreases in thickness from anterior to posterior	Anteroinferior labrum neck of the glenoid adjacent to the labrum	Inferior to the MGHL at the humeral neck	Can be sheetlike and confluent with the SGHL or cordlike with a foraminal separation between it and the anterior band of the IGHL complex	Functions as a hammock of the humeral head: in adduction, it acts as a secondary restraint, limiting large inferior translations; in abduction, it becomes taut under the humeral head, limiting inferior translation; in internal rotation, it moves posteriorly, and in external rotation, it moves anteriorly, forming a barrier to posterior and anterior dislocation, respectively
Posterior capsule	Thinnest region of the joint capsule without discrete ligamentous reinforcements	Posterior band of the IGHLC postero-superior labrum to the insertion of the biceps	Posterior humeral neck	Blends with the posterior aspect of the infraspinatus and teres minor	Limits posterior translation when the arm is forward flexed, adducted, and internally rotated

Negative Intra-articular Pressure

The stabilizing effect of intra-articular pressure is the result of the vacuum effect, which exists within a sealed joint compartment. Any force that tends to displace the articular surfaces is resisted by the negative pressure created within that compartment. When a 25-N inferior force was applied to the cadaveric shoulder, the intra-articular pressure doubled compared with the pressure in the relaxed adducted shoulder (arm hanging at the side). In a 1985 study, it was reported that if this pressure is equalized by venting the joint with a small puncture, inferior subluxation of the glenohumeral joint readily occurs. However, this effect has been shown to be minimal compared with the stabilizing effect of joint compression from dynamic muscle action.

Adhesion-Cohesion

The glenohumeral joint contains a small amount of synovial fluid that provides cartilage nourishment. Viscous and intermolecular forces between the fluid and the joint surfaces create an adhesion-cohesion effect analogous to that seen when two glass plates are separated by a thin film of water: the plates slide easily over one another but are difficult to separate.

Rotator Cuff

Experimentally, the rotator cuff has been shown to have a passive effect on stability. The subscapularis statically limits anterior translation in the lower ranges of abduction similar to the way the infraspinatus and teres minor limit posterior translation. This mechanism is probably less important in vivo than the contribution of the rotator cuff during active motion.

Dynamic Stability Factors

Several dynamic factors play important roles in enhancing glenohumeral stability. Active contraction of the rotator cuff contributes to stabilization by the joint compression mechanism from coordinated muscular activity and by secondary tightening of ligamentous constraints through direct attachments to the rotator cuff muscles. This effect works in combination with the concavity-compression mechanism, the compression of nearly congruent articular surfaces into one another by muscle contraction. The contraction of the long head of the biceps, coordinated scapulothoracic rhythm, and the proprioceptive modulation of all dynamic factors also contribute to dynamic stabilization of the glenohumeral joint.

The Rotator Cuff and the Deltoid Muscle

The deltoid is a very large muscle with a large moment arm, which allows it to produce torque at the gleno-humeral joint. Many authors describe this muscle as one of the primary contributors to glenohumeral abduction, and loss of deltoid function is considered a disaster. The rotator cuff consists of the subscapularis, supraspinatus, infraspinatus, and teres minor muscles, the tendons of which blend in with the adjacent capsule and insert onto the greater and lesser tuberosities of the humerus. The supraspinatus muscle is important because it is active with any motion involving elevation. The line of action of the supraspinatus is oriented directly toward the glenoid, therefore providing joint compression and contributing to the stability of the glenohumeral joint. The infraspinatus and teres minor muscles function together to externally rotate and extend the humerus. The infraspinatus also functions as a depressor of the humeral head and has been reported to be an important contributor to the anterior and posterior stability of the glenohumeral joint. The subscapularis functions as an internal rotator of the humerus and a passive stabilizer to anterior subluxation and external rotation. Its lower fibers serve as a humeral head depressor. Together with the infraspinatus muscle, the subscapularis provides a downward force on the humeral head, resisting the shear forces and superior pull of the deltoid. The rotator cuff muscles attach very close to the axis of rotation and provide joint compression. Thus, coordinated function of the rotator cuff muscles is required to counteract the shearing force of the deltoid while still allowing the spinning motion of the humerus on the glenoid and maintaining stability. Furthermore, experimental studies of various capsulolabral injuries demonstrated that muscle action maintained joint stability even after a large Bankart lesion was created or the entire capsule and glenohumeral ligaments were sectioned. Therefore, it seems that instability requires a sudden failure not only of static ligamentous components but also of the dynamic stabilizing effect of the rotator cuff muscles.

Long Head of the Biceps

The biceps maintains stability of the glenohumeral joint through the intra-articular orientation of its long head. Electromyographic analysis has demonstrated that the biceps muscle is active only with elbow flexion, so it is likely that it functions as an important stabilizing mechanism only during elbow motion, as in the throwing motion, and not during simple actions such as abduction. This is an important concept as it has been suggested that the biceps may prevent superior displacement of the humeral head in the case of a massive rotator cuff tear. This is not supported by experimental observations. During shoulder motion when the elbow is also moving, the biceps contributes to stability by the following mechanisms: in internal rotation, the biceps stabilizes the humeral head

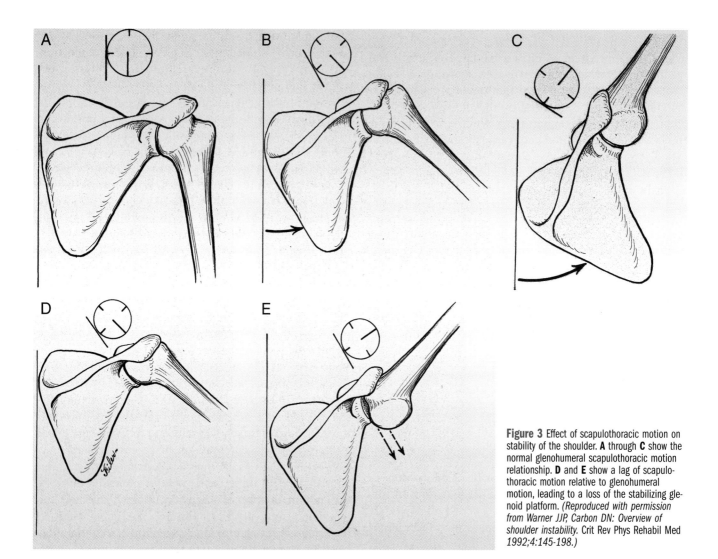

Figure 3 Effect of scapulothoracic motion on stability of the shoulder. **A** through **C** show the normal glenohumeral scapulothoracic motion relationship. **D** and **E** show a lag of scapulothoracic motion relative to glenohumeral motion, leading to a loss of the stabilizing glenoid platform. *(Reproduced with permission from Warner JJP, Carbon DN: Overview of shoulder instability. Crit Rev Phys Rehabil Med 1992;4:145-198.)*

anteriorly; in external rotation, the biceps acts to restrain posterior translation. Superoinferior translation is also reduced with simulated contraction of the biceps. One study suggested that contraction of the biceps enhances stability during the throwing motion by increasing the torsional rigidity of the joint. In so doing, it reduces strain in the inferior glenohumeral ligament when the shoulder is in the cock-up position. Additionally, it has been suggested that because the biceps inserts onto the relatively mobile superior labrum, tension could be transmitted by the labrum to the superior and middle glenohumeral ligaments.

Scapular Rotators

The axioscapular muscles or scapular rotators include the trapezius, rhomboids, serratus anterior, and levator scapulae. Of these, the serratus anterior and trapezius are primarily responsible for scapulothoracic rotation, which maintains the normal overall rhythm of shoulder motion. The ratio of normal glenohumeral to scapulothoracic motion is 2:1 (glenohumeral rotation to scapulothoracic rotation) (Fig. 3). This normal relationship is important because it maintains the glenoid as a stable platform underneath the humeral head as the shoulder rotates into positions required for overhead motions such as throwing. Because the axioscapular muscles tend to fatigue first during repetitive overhead motions such as throwing and swimming, a lag in normal scapulothoracic rotation has been implicated as a contributing factor for instability and pain during shoulder motion in these sports activities. This is the rationale for supplementing rotator cuff strengthening with an axioscapular strengthening program when treating shoulder instability.

Proprioception

Proprioception, defined as the perception of joint motion and position, is mediated by mechanoreceptors that transduce mechanical deformation into electric neural signals. Highly specialized nerve endings have been identified in the joint capsule, in ligaments of the glenohumeral joint, and in tendons surrounding the joint. The transmitted signal is thought to be the afferent component of a reflex arc, the efferent component being the motoneurons supplying the dynamic stabilizer. In other words, capsular stretch produces an afferent signal, which results in an efferent signal, causing a protective muscle contraction that enhances the stability of the joint when the shoulder suddenly rotates into extreme positions or translates. This stabilizing mechanism has been shown to be disrupted in patients with shoulder instability but is restored after capsulolabral repair. Proprioception seems to play a role in low-energy situations, when the dynamic stabilizers have time to react to changes in the capsular tension. Furthermore, it has been postulated that proprioception may help protect the capsuloligamentous structures from failure caused by repetitive trauma.

Voluntary asynchronous contraction of the rotator cuff muscles can lead to dislocation of the glenohumeral joint and is an extreme example of the effect of cortical modulation of this reflex arc. Therefore, biofeedback training may be a useful therapeutic option in rehabilitation after surgical stabilization in these complex situations.

The Effect of Structural Lesions on Instability

Skeletal Lesions

The osteometry of the proximal humerus and the glenoid have been studied extensively and have implications for shoulder arthroplasty design as well as glenohumeral stability. The relationship between pathologic articular version and clinical instability remains unclear.

Decreased humeral retroversion might play a role in predisposing the shoulder to a recurrent anterior instability. Also, excessive glenoid retroversion may be a contributing factor in posterior instability. For example, some individuals with atraumatic posterior instability have been found on CT analysis to have posterior glenoid dysplasia. In practice, however, excessive retroversion is not frequently associated with posterior instability but is seen in osteoarthritis with eccentric wear of the posterior articular surface as a result of posterior subluxation of the humeral head. For these rare cases, derotational osteotomy of the humerus or glenoid opening wedge osteotomy has been proposed. Unfortunately, these procedures have been associated with an increased incidence of arthritis.

The Hill-Sachs lesion, an impression fracture of the humeral articular surface caused by translation of the humeral head over the glenoid rim, is present in 80% of

anterior dislocations, 25% of anterior subluxations, and in almost 100% of cases of recurrent anterior instability. With posterior instability, a reverse Hill-Sachs lesion results from impaction of the anterior articular surface when the humeral head dislocates over the posterior glenoid rim. These humeral articular lesions rarely contribute to instability, as they are usually small; however, when a lesion that includes more than 30% of the articular surface is associated with instability, it may be an important indication for surgery. Such large lesions occur only after recurrent dislocations or in the case of a chronic locked dislocation. Recent clinical experience has demonstrated that one option in treating these kinds of injuries is restoration of normal articular conformity by allograft reconstruction of the articular defect.

Bony lesions of the anterior or posterior glenoid rim decrease glenoid constraint. These lesions may result from an osseous (anterior or posterior) Bankart lesion, a displaced glenoid fracture, or wear of the glenoid rim related to recurrent instability.

Clinical experience has suggested that a defect that involves more than 25% of the glenoid surface should be repaired intra-articularly with a bone graft. The goal of such surgery is to increase glenoid constraint and provide support for the joint capsule.

Bankart Lesions

Bankart lesions were originally described as lesions of the labrum corresponding to the detachment of the anchoring point of the inferior glenohumeral and middle glenohumeral ligaments from the glenoid rim. They have been considered the primary and most common pathology leading to recurrent anterior dislocations. Although an arthroscopic assessment of initial traumatic dislocations showed that 97% were associated with isolated detachment of the capsuloligamentous complex, recurrent dislocation is believed to require an additional lesion within the capsule. This lesion may represent a stretch injury or plastic deformation from a microscopic ultrastructural failure.

A Bankart lesion usually presents as a partial or complete detachment of the capsuloligamentous complex from the anterior glenoid. In recurrent dislocations, the detached capsulolabral origin may heal medially along the scapular neck, requiring anatomic reattachment at the articular margin.

Lesions of the Superior Labrum

Isolated lesions of the superior labrum occur as a result of a sudden eccentric force from biceps contraction. Cadaveric studies of complete lesions of the superior portion of the labrum have shown destabilization of the biceps insertion and significant increases in anteroposterior and superoinferior glenohumeral translations in the lower and middle ranges of elevation. These lesions should be identified and repaired at the time of instability repair, as the biceps is an important stabilizing mechanism for the shoulder during overhead motion.

Capsular Lesions

The range of capsular laxity considered normal overlaps the pathologic laxity associated with instability. An individual's capsular laxity may be congenital. Arthroscopic or open surgical evaluation of the capsule in an atraumatic unstable shoulder may demonstrate dysplastic glenohumeral ligaments and an insufficient rotator interval. This may explain why instability develops in some individuals without a traumatic episode.

As previously described, traumatic intrasubstance injury of the joint capsule is commonly associated with anterior dislocation. Depending on the magnitude of the anterior shear force, either a plastic deformation or a complete tear of the joint capsule can occur. The recognition of a concomitant posttraumatic capsular laxity or rupture and a Bankart lesion is essential to select the correct surgical procedure. A traumatic capsular rupture or an open rotator interval leads to venting of the joint, which increases glenohumeral translation. A positive sulcus sign in external rotation is the clinical sign for an open rotator interval.

Repetitive stresses in the capsule occurring with subluxation may lead to microtrauma, causing acquired laxity in overhead throwing athletes and gymnasts. Those patients present with symptoms of impingement, which are secondary to instability. Nevertheless, the primary pathology is the capsular laxity, and this should be addressed first if surgical treatment becomes an option.

Disruption of the capsule from the humerus is rare but has been reported in association with anterior dislocation. Rarely, humeral avulsion of the glenohumeral ligaments may occur in conjunction with a Bankart lesion. Thus, appreciation of the humeral capsular insertion is important at the time of surgery. Tensioning of the capsule in the midrange can potentially overtighten and constrain the joint, limiting rotation. In extreme cases, this can lead to posterior subluxation of the humeral head and arthritis.

Thermal capsular modification is a relatively new method of treating capsular laxity associated with glenohumeral instability. Laser energy and radiofrequency energy (monopolar and bipolar) are the available treatment modalities. The disruption of the hydrogen bonds in the capsule by either photostimulation (laser) or electrostimulation (radiofrequency) leads to a structural change, transforming the extended crystalline conformation of the molecules into a contracted amorphous random coil conformation that is more extendable. Results depend on the orientation and density of the collagen fibrils in the shoulder capsule. The proteoglycan content varies within the capsule, being highest in the anterior and superior capsule and lowest in the posterior inferior region. This gradient leads to viscoelastic stiffening, as the collagen fibers are "uncrimped" during tension. This may explain why some regions of the shoulder capsule are more responsive to thermal treatment than others. Early success of clinical applications has led to a wide use of thermal capsular modification technique. In one clinical study, a holmium: yttrium-aluminum-garnet (Ho:YAG) laser at a nonablative level was applied to the anterior capsule under arthroscopic guidance in patients with glenohumeral instability but without capsulolabral detachment or full-thickness rotator cuff tears. The laser energy shrank the joint capsule, stabilizing the shoulder in most patients. In animal experiments using rabbits or sheep, laser energy at nonablative levels significantly altered joint capsule length and its mechanical properties. Although nonablative laser and radiofrequency treatments appear to decrease capsular laxity, almost no information is available regarding how the process of repair and long-term healing may affect the biologic and mechanical properties of capsular tissue in humans and animals. Moreover, the indications for thermal capsulorrhaphy are poorly defined, and clinical outcomes have not been superior to those resulting from conventional stabilization procedures. Prospective clinical studies are needed to determine the safety and efficacy of these methods.

Lesions of the Rotator Cuff

An age-related attrition of the tendons of the rotator cuff makes this a weak link when a dislocation occurs in patients older than age 40 years. This is why a rotator cuff tear is not uncommonly associated with a traumatic anterior dislocation in a patient older than age 40 years. This has been described as the "posterior mechanism of dislocation." In younger individuals, especially in athletes with acquired capsular laxity, eccentric load on the maximally contracted rotator cuff may explain partial-thickness tears.

Fatigue or Weakness of the Scapular Rotators

Clinical and radiographic studies have demonstrated abnormal scapulothoracic motion in patients with glenohumeral instability, and electromyographic analysis has shown that the serratus anterior and trapezius fatigue with repetitive overhead motions such as throwing and swimming. It is not clear if scapulothoracic dysfunction is a cause or a result of shoulder instability, but it is reasonable to assume that if the scapular rotators are too weak to position the glenoid effectively, to provide a stable platform for the humeral head, instability may result.

Annotated Bibliography

Static Stability Factors

Boileau P, Walch G: The three-dimensional geometry of the proximal humerus: Implications for surgical technique and prosthetic design. *J Bone Joint Surg Br* 1997; 79:857-865.

This three-dimensional analysis of 65 humeri used a micron precision probe linked to a computer to determine the dimensions and orientation of the articular surface of the humeral head.

Boileau P, Walch G: Normal and pathological anatomy of the glenoid: Effects on the design, preparation and fixation of the glenoid component, in Walch G, Boileau P (eds): *Shoulder Arthroplasty.* Berlin, Germany, Springer, 1999, pp 127-140.

This three-dimensional analysis of 34 glenoid cavities used a micron precision probe linked to a computer to determine the dimensions and the orientation of the articular glenoid surface.

Gerber C, Lambert SM: Allograft reconstruction of segmental defects of the humeral head for the treatment of chronic locked posterior dislocation of the shoulder. *J Bone Joint Surg Am* 1996;78:376-382.

This clinical study demonstrates the value of restoration of the humeral head anatomy using allograft bone in chronic locked posterior dislocations.

Lazarus MD, Sidles JA, Harryman DT, Matsen FA: Effect of a chondral-labral defect on glenoid concavity and glenohumeral stability: A cadaveric model. *J Bone Joint Surg Am* 1996;78:94-102.

This article describes the stability ratio as the ratio between the maximum dislocating force that can be stabilized in a given direction and the load compressing the head in the glenoid.

McMahon PJ, Debski RE, Thompson WO, Warner JJ, Fu FH, Woo SL: Shoulder muscle forces and tendon excursions during glenohumeral abduction in the scapular plane. *J Shoulder Elbow Surg* 1995;4:199-208.

Using a dynamic shoulder testing apparatus, the authors determined that humeral head translation on the glenoid was less than 2 mm under their testing conditions and that the joint behaved kinematically as a ball-and-socket.

Soslowsky LJ, Malicky DM, Blasier RB: Active and passive factors in inferior glenohumeral stabilization: A biomechanical model. *J Shoulder Elbow Surg* 1997;6:371-379.

Various ligament cuts and applied rotator cuff forces were examined to determine the effect of individual components of the rotator cuff, glenohumeral ligaments, and capsule in preventing inferior translation. The coracohumeral and the interior glenohumeral ligaments as well as the supraspinatus and the biceps were found to be the most significant restraints to inferior translation.

Dynamic Stability Factors

Apreleva M, Hasselman CT, Debski RE, Fu FH, Woo SL, Warner JJ: A dynamic analysis of the glenohumeral motion after simulated capsulolabral injury: A cadaver model. *J Bone Joint Surg Am* 1998;80:474-480.

Nine cadaveric entire upper extremities were used in a dynamic shoulder-testing apparatus to evaluate the effects of varying degrees of capsulolabral injury on the kinematics of the glenohumeral joint. No increase in anterior or posterior translation was observed during abduction of the arm in the scapular plane after simulation of a large Bankart lesion.

Blasier RB, Soslowsky LJ, Malicky DM, Palmer ML: Posterior glenohumeral subluxation: Active and passive stabilization in a biomechanical model. *J Bone Joint Surg Am* 1997;79:433-440.

This cadaveric study examined the role of the glenohumeral and coracohumeral ligaments as well as the forces provided by the rotator cuff muscles, the long head of the biceps, the deltoid, and the pectoralis muscles in the stabilization of the glenohumeral joint in the posterior direction in eight shoulder specimens.

Lee SB, Kim KJ, O'Driscoll SW, Morrey BF, An KN: Dynamic glenohumeral stability provided by the rotator cuff muscles in the mid-range and end-range of motion: A study in cadavera. *J Bone Joint Surg Am* 2000;82:849-857.

A dynamic testing apparatus was used in this cadaveric study to determine the dynamic stability index. This index relates the shear load that can be resisted by the reaction of the compressive force component of the muscle through the concavity-compression mechanism and a second shear force of the muscle in the anterioposterior direction. The higher the index, the greater the stability in the anterior direction.

Pagnani MJ, Deng XH, Warren RF, Torzilli PA, O'Brien SJ: Role of the long head of the biceps brachii in glenohumeral stability: A biomechanical study in cadavera. *J Shoulder Elbow Surg* 1996;5:255-262.

This study, using cadaver models, showed that application of force to the biceps creates compressive load and helps to stabilize the glenohumeral joint. This effect is more pronounced in the lower and middle ranges of elevation and is affected by humeral rotation.

Warner JJ, Lephart S, Fu FH: The role of proprioception in pathoetiology of shoulder instability. *Clin Orthop* 1996;330:35-39.

The authors evaluated proprioception in individuals with normal shoulders, unstable shoulders, and after surgical stabilization by assessing the threshold to detection of passive motion and the ability to passively reposition the arm in space. In normal shoulders, there was no difference between the dominant and nondominant shoulder; unstable shoulders had a decreased proprioceptive ability.

Yamaguchi K, Riew KD, Galatz LM, Syme JA, Neviaser RJ: Biceps activity during shoulder motion: An electromyographic analysis. *Clin Orthop* 1997;336:122-129.

This electromyographic study showed that in all ranges of active motion the supraspinatus develops 20% to 50% of maximum contraction, whereas the biceps brachii shows only minimal activity. No increase of activity was showed in the biceps in patients with rotator cuff tears.

The Effect of Structural Lesions on Instability

Gerber A, Warner JJP: Thermal capsulorrhaphy to treat shoulder instability. *Clin Orthop*, in press.

This article reviews basic science information and clinical experience with thermal capsulorrhaphy in the treatment of glenohumeral instability.

Gerber C, Nyffeler RW: Abstract: Pathology of dislocated Bankart fracture: Experimental and clinical aspects. *J Bone Joint Surg Br* 1999;81(suppl 2):133-134.

This article presents an experimental analysis of the influence of fragment size in relation to glenohumeral instability. It also presents the clinical outcome in 22 patients after reconstruction of the anteroinferior glenoid with bone graft.

Classic Bibliography

Bigliani LU, Pollock RG, Soslowsky LJ, Flatow EL, Pawluk RJ, Mow VC: Tensile properties of the inferior glenohumeral ligament. *J Orthop Res* 1992;10:187-197.

Cooper DE, Arnoczky SP, O'Brien SJ, Warren RF, DiCarlo E, Allen AA: Anatomy, histology, and vascularity of the glenoid labrum: An anatomical study. *J Bone Joint Surg Am* 1992;74:46-52.

Harryman DT, Sidles JA, Clark JM, McQuade KJ, Gibb TD, Matsen FA: Translation of the humeral head on the glenoid with passive glenohumeral motion. *J Bone Joint Surg Am* 1990;72:1334-1343.

Harryman DT, Sidles JA, Harris SL, Matsen FA: The role of the rotator interval capsule in passive motion and stability of the shoulder. *J Bone Joint Surg Am* 1992;74:53-66.

Kumar VP, Balasubramaniam P: The role of atmospheric pressure in stabilizing the shoulder: An experimental study. *J Bone Joint Surg Br* 1985;67:719-721.

Lippit SB, Vanderhooft JE, Harris SL, et al: Glenohumeral stability from concavity-compromise: A quantitative analysis. *J Shoulder Elbow Surg* 1993;2:27-35.

O'Brien SJ, Neves MC, Arnoczky SP, et al: The anatomy and histology of the inferior glenohumeral ligament complex of the shoulder. *Am J Sports Med* 1990;18:449-456.

Turkel SJ, Panio MW, Marshall JL, Girgis FG: Stabilizing mechanisms preventing anterior dislocation of the glenohumeral joint. *J Bone Joint Surg Am* 1981;63:1208-1217.

Warner JJ, Deng XH, Warren RF, Torzilli PA: Static capsuloligamentous restraints to superior-inferior translation of the glenohumeral joint. *Am J Sports Med* 1992;20:675-685.

Warner JJ, Micheli LJ, Arslanian LE, Kennedy J, Kennedy R: Scapulothoracic motion in normal shoulders and shoulders with glenohumeral instability and impingement syndrome: A study using Moiré topographic analysis. *Clin Orthop* 1992;285:191-199.

Chapter 3

Basic Science of the Rotator Cuff

Paul S. Robinson, MS

Paul R. Reynolds, MD

Louis J. Soslowsky, PhD

Introduction

The deep muscles about the shoulder have long been known collectively as the rotator cuff because of their anatomic locations and their function in shoulder motion. However, the rotator cuff provides much more to the shoulder than simply motion. The gross and histologic anatomy of the rotator cuff, including detailed treatments of the vascularity and organization of the layers of the tendon complex, has been well described in the literature. More recently, the focus has shifted to the biomechanical and biochemical environments of the shoulder. Changes in these areas have been studied in normal shoulders as well as in aging shoulders and those with pathologic conditions. The emergence of appropriate animal models has enabled researchers to address the causation of tendinopathies rather than being limited to descriptions of existing pathologies. Continued research on both living and cadaveric tissue has further described the many changes that occur with tendinopathy using gross, histologic, biomechanical, molecular biologic, and biochemical analyses. These methodologies help researchers to identify the structural and mechanical properties that are associated with normal and injured tissue.

Anatomy

The description of the gross anatomy of the rotator cuff has remained constant. Briefly, the four musculotendinous units that comprise the rotator cuff are the subscapularis anteriorly, the supraspinatus superiorly, and the infraspinatus and the teres minor posteriorly (Fig. 1). These musculotendinous units envelop approximately 75% of the glenohumeral articulation. Clinical dysfunction can occur in any of the tendons but most frequently occurs in the supraspinatus tendon alone or with involvement of one or more of the other tendons. One primary reason for this clinical finding is believed to be the relationship of the supraspinatus tendon to the coracoacromial arch. This tendon must glide beneath a bony outlet through all planes of humeral elevation. The vascularity of this tendon has also been investigated as a significant etiologic factor. Furthermore, the mechanical loading of the tendon has been evaluated. Investigators have reexamined the gross anatomy and described a distinct anterior and posterior portion of the supraspinatus tendon. The anterior portion has a significantly larger physiologic cross-sectional area, making it better suited to withstand greater mechanical loads.

The microstructure of the rotator cuff has been described as a five-layer complex because the tendons of the rotator cuff coalesce near their insertions onto the humeral head. The thickness of the terminal 2 cm of the rotator cuff complex ranges from 9 to 12 mm.

The coracoacromial arch, formed by the coracoacromial ligament and coracoid anteriorly and the acromion posterosuperiorly, forms the outlet for the supraspinatus. The morphology of the acromion is well described and is often implicated in the etiology of bursal-sided cuff tears. Several series have associated the amount of bending ("hooking") of the anterolateral acromion with increased incidence of cuff tears. The dynamic outlet space (subacromial space) has recently been investigated with open MRI and shown to decrease maximally with a combination of abduction and internal rotation. This same technique has been used to demonstrate the centralizing effect of the rotator cuff by comparing the position of the humeral head during active motion with the position during passive motion (Fig. 2). Clinically, the acromial morphology is evaluated and classified based on the supraspinatus outlet view. This classification has been studied recently, and the potential for large interobserver and intraobserver variations has been noted. However, this classification system clearly remains the gold standard for evaluating acromial morphology and has been extremely useful for correlating such morphology with rotator cuff tears.

Biochemical Composition

The basic biochemical composition of tendons and ligaments can be characterized by using a variety of stan-

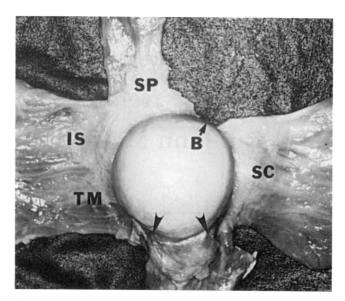

Figure 1 Anatomic view of the humeral head displaying the rotator cuff tendons. The rotator cuff encloses the humeral head articular surface except where the biceps tendon exits (B) and the capsule attaches (between arrows). SP = supraspinatus, SC = subscapularis, TM = teres minor, IS = infraspinatus. *(Reproduced with permission from Harryman DT, Clark JM Jr: Anatomy of the rotator cuff, in Burhead WZ Jr (ed): Rotator Cuff Disorders. Philadelphia, PA, Williams & Wilkins, 1996, pp 23-35.)*

dard assays. Type I collagen is dominant in rotator cuff tissue fibrils, as in most tendons, at approximately 85% of dry weight. Rotator cuff tendons also contain small amounts of type III collagen. Total collagen content in normal rotator cuff tissue does not change significantly with age, across genders, or along location in the supraspinatus tendon. While the total collagen content in the supraspinatus is the same as that in the neighboring biceps tendon, the distribution differs. The supraspinatus contains less type I collagen and more type III collagen than do tendons that are loaded only in tension, such as the biceps tendon.

With pathology, changes in this fibrillar structure are seen. Data obtained primarily from evaluation of cadaveric tissue and through assays performed on biopsy tissue from patients with rotator cuff disease show that the proportion of type III collagen increases with degeneration, tears, and tendinitis. In addition, fibrocytic activity in the form of tenocytes that stain positive for procollagen α1(I) and type III collagen has been found near tear edges. This finding suggests an intrinsic remodeling response of rotator cuff tendons; these markers may serve as indications of impending tendinitis or rupture. This information is a step toward completing the understanding of fibril formation and regulation within the rotator cuff.

Other important constituents of the extracellular matrix of the tendon are the tendon proteoglycans (PGs) and their associated glycosaminoglycans (GAGs). The amount and type of PGs and GAGs are thought to

be correlated with fibril regulation and tendon mechanical properties. Interestingly, the GAG content in rotator cuff tissue is 2.5 to 10 times higher than in the biceps tendon. Cadaver studies also revealed that GAG content does not differ among the three rotator cuff tendons within any individual. In these cadaver tendons, approximately 50% of all GAGs were hyaluronic acid, a much larger proportion than found in other tendons. The other rotator cuff GAGs were mostly chondroitin sulfate, with small amounts of dermatan sulfate; this is in contrast to the biceps tendon, which is primarily dermatan sulfate as is typical of tendons that are loaded only in tension. The level and type of GAGs in the rotator cuff are more typical of the fibrocartilage regions of other tendons, which further reflects the complex mechanical environment of the rotator cuff.

Of the fibril-associated PGs in the rotator cuff tendon, decorin is the most prevalent, followed by a large, aggrecanlike PG and biglycan. Small amounts of lumican and fibromodulin have also been found in the cuff. This is in contrast to the distal region of the biceps tendon, for example, in which decorin was the only PG observed in an analysis of adult cadavers with no history of shoulder problems. As with GAGs, the PG composition of the rotator cuff is like that of fibrocartilage, but the structure differs. Histologic staining has shown that these PGs exist in the loosely organized tissue between collagen bundles (Fig. 3). This finding demonstrates that PGs in the rotator cuff are found between collagen bundles and may play an important role in minimizing shear stresses between layers or in transferring mechanical loads across collagen bundles. In addition, they may play an important functional role in the multiaxial structure and loading of the rotator cuff. That GAG and PG composition correlates with loading environment is supported by studies in other tissues where the PG and GAG distributions become similar to that of the rotator cuff when tensile tendons are used to replace ligaments.

GAG content increases with pathology. Biopsy specimens of the supraspinatus in patients with tendinitis show increased levels of both chondroitin sulfate and dermatan sulfate. Preliminary studies have suggested that these specimens also show an increase in large, aggrecanlike PG and in biglycan, but not in decorin. These studies suggest that PGs are linked with supraspinatus pathology or its response to injury. Currently, advances are being made in localization studies of GAGs and PGs within biopsy tissue from surgery. This information will lead to an understanding of the changing roles of these extracellular matrix proteins in cuff pathology.

Cytokine activity precedes PG and collagen fiber changes in the timeline of healing. Granulation tissue

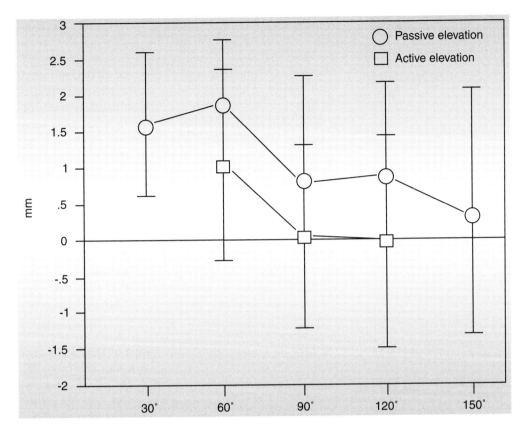

Figure 2 Position of the humeral head relative to the glenoid measured with open MRI during passive and active elevation. During passive elevation, a continuous inferior translation can be observed. Under muscle activity, the humeral head is translated inferiorly and centralized during elevation. *(Reproduced with permission from Graichen H, Stammberger T, Bonel H, Englmeier KH, Reiser M, Eckstein F: Glenohumeral translation during active and passive elevation of the shoulder: A 3D open-MRI study. J Biomech 2000;33:609-613.)*

surrounding tears in supraspinatus tendons harvested during surgery exhibits strong immunohistochemical staining of interleukin-1β, cathepsin D, and matrix metalloprotease-1 (Fig. 4). Researchers continue to try to localize these cytokines as they occur in healing and cuff formation to ascertain their role in either an intrinsic repair response or the propagation of tendon injury.

Biomechanical Models

The basic mechanical functions of the rotator cuff are to provide stability and aid in motion about the glenohumeral joint. While most of the forces required to create motion of the arm are provided by the larger superficial muscles such as the deltoid, the rotator cuff acts multiaxially during motion to maintain proper position of the humeral head within the glenoid. The biomechanical importance of the rotator cuff has been studied extensively through experimental and analytic models. In addition, basic science studies have quantified the material properties of the rotator cuff tendons, which helps both to understand the strength of these tissues and to develop models of the shoulder or the rotator cuff.

All the rotator cuff muscles are involved in most actions about the glenohumeral joint. They act to provide force couples, which are two muscles that act in the same direction but at different locations on the joint. This function provides joint loading without a moment around the joint center, leading to stability as well as limiting unwanted actions during shoulder motion. When one portion of a force couple is weakened or lost through injury or disease, abnormal mechanics result, leading to altered or lost shoulder function.

To study these mechanical actions, models are generated to determine joint forces and kinematics. One of the earliest was the classic model by Inman and associates that simplified the glenohumeral joint to three forces: cuff, deltoid, and limb weight. This study found that arm elevation requires forces on the order of body weight. Later, more complex studies have yielded similar results. Two types of models exist to study joint function: analytic, such as the one just mentioned, and experimental. Recent models of each type are presented in the following paragraphs.

Analytic Models

Analytic models are useful in studying mechanics based on known anatomy and properties and can be used to predict changes due to pathology or repair. Finite element models couple a mathematical model of anatomic geometry with average or "typical" mechanical properties of cuff components to simulate this portion of the glenohumeral joint. Mechanical effects of changes in geometry or properties can be studied computationally by altering the model parameters. These models can be very useful to simulate conditions such as weakening of tissue due to aging or tearing, trauma, or subacromial impingement.

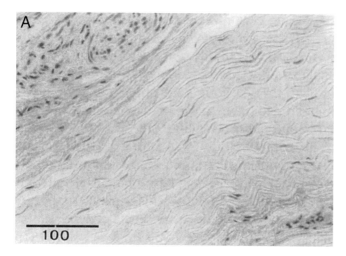

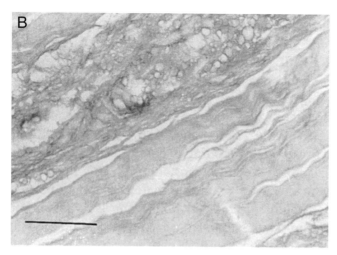

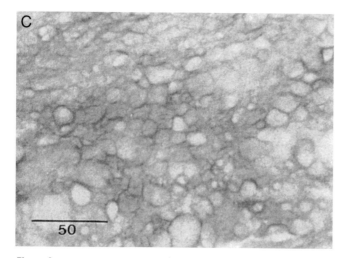

Figure 3 Histologic sections of infraspinatus tendon. **A,** Section stained with hematoxylin and eosin showing regions of loosely organized tissue between dense collagen bundles. **B,** Section stained with alcian blue, a marker for GAGs. Staining is found in regions of loosely organized tissue. **C,** Close-up view of B showing pattern of GAG staining around circles. *(Reproduced with permission from Berenson MC, Blevins FT, Plaas AH, Vogel KG: Proteoglycans of human rotator cuff tendons. J Orthop Res 1996;14:518-525.)*

Human Experimental Studies

In Vivo Studies

Human experimental studies are of two types: in vivo studies and in vitro cadaveric studies. In vivo studies include estimation of muscle forces by electromyography (EMG) during passive and active motion by a live subject. Generally, electrodes are placed on the surface or within a muscle belly. These electrodes measure the electrical activity of a muscle that corresponds to the physical activity of contracting and loading the joint. These data provide information on the intricacies of rotator cuff action and the onset of certain pathologies. For example, the infraspinatus is active at the same level throughout the range of rotation, while the supraspinatus and subscapularis have peaks of influence or activity during motion. This finding suggests that the infraspinatus plays a critical role as an overall stabilizer and controller of glenohumeral action, beyond that understood previously (Fig. 5).

EMG measurements taken during isometric strength tests in rotations about the glenohumeral joint have shown that all the rotator cuff muscles activate up to 0.25 s prior to motion, after which the muscle activations become motion specific. This finding provides physical evidence that the rotator cuff first provides joint stability and secondarily aids the other shoulder muscles in providing joint motion.

Other coupled EMG-strength studies have identified shoulder positions that isolate and maximize forces on selected rotator cuff components. The subscapularis is best isolated with the arm elevated 90° in the scapular plane in neutral rotation; the infraspinatus-teres minor complex is best isolated at 90° of elevation in the sagittal plane and half external rotation. These and future isolation studies will help determine optimum positions for clinical testing of rotator cuff injuries and rehabilitation.

In Vitro Cadaveric Studies

Cadaveric studies allow researchers to place known loads directly on rotator cuff and other shoulder tendons while measuring the resulting humeral motion. These studies recently have been used to demonstrate a decrease in the maximum amount of arm elevation when the rotator cuff is compromised. Also, the role of the supraspinatus in arm abduction has been evaluated; these results show that up to a 100% increase in middle deltoid force is required at the beginning of abduction when the supraspinatus is paralyzed. In addition, total rotator cuff paralysis reduces the maximum abduction angle to 18°.

In a cadaver model using fresh human shoulders with no gross or radiographic signs of pathology, the forces required on each muscle (rotator cuff and deltoid) to achieve glenohumeral elevation were quantified. The infraspinatus force continued to increase during elevation, while the forces in the other muscles decreased. These results agree with the in vivo EMG studies mentioned earlier.

Recent cadaveric experiments have identified the moment arms of cuff components through a range of shoulder positions. A cadaveric shoulder is moved through a specific motion, such as scapular-plane elevation, while tendon excursion is monitored with respect to joint angle. This approach allows calculation of moment arms of the cuff tendons about the humeral instantaneous center of rotation. Calculation of the moment arms allows determination of the extent to which forces generated in muscles translate to humeral motion. Moment arm calculations also isolate the contribution of each cuff component to specific motions and are necessary as inputs to many analytic models of both the cuff and entire shoulder girdle. Recent moment arm studies demonstrate that the subscapularis may be a more important elevator than previously believed and that the infraspinatus and supraspinatus are more efficient elevators in the coronal plane than in the sagittal or scapular planes.

Moment arm calculations can be combined with strength or EMG studies to calculate absolute forces and kinematic relationships about the glenohumeral joint. Such analysis quantifies average expected loads on cuff components during specific motions, which reveals that external rotations cause the highest force generation in the supraspinatus and infraspinatus, greater than the forces required for abduction. Thus, therapies or efforts to prevent cuff disease should focus on rotation as well as arm elevation.

Use of Models to Study Disease

The analytic and experimental models described here can be used to study disease and degeneration of the rotator cuff. In the past, models have defined or predicted the effects of paralysis, the role of the various cuff muscles in specific motions, the effect of different types and severity of cuff tears, and the results of clinical procedures such as acromioplasty. Recently, results of cadaveric studies have suggested that cuff tears must progress beyond a single tendon to significantly alter the joint reaction force and resultant reaction angle. This finding implies that other structures may sometimes compensate for the loss of part of one force couple. In the future, these studies may provide information on why some cuff tears early on are asymptomatic.

Knowledge of the structural and material properties of rotator cuff tissues is important in developing these models and also as an aid to understanding why and where certain pathologies develop. Such knowledge also helps in developing approaches to the repair and cre-

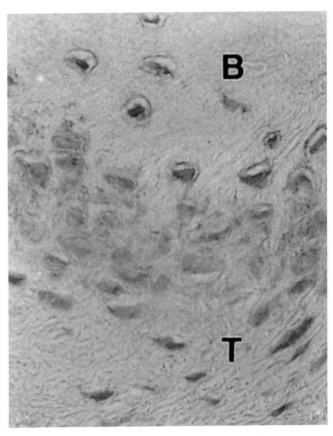

Figure 4 Photomicrograph showing positive (dark) staining for matrix metalloprotease-1 in granulation tissue of a torn supraspinatus insertion. T = tendon side, B = bone side. *(Reproduced with permission from Gotoh M, Hamada K, Yamakawa H, Tomonaga A, Inoue A, Fukuda H: Significance of granulation tissue in torn supraspinatus insertions: An immunohistochemical study with antibodies against interleukin-1beta, cathepsin D, and matrix metalloprotease-1. J Orthop Res 1997;15:33-39.)*

ation of suitable replacements for the rotator cuff. Past efforts have quantified the linear elastic properties of healthy rotator cuff constituents, focusing on the coracoacromial ligament and supraspinatus tendon because of their clinical importance. Recent research has focused on the tensile properties of the infraspinatus tendon. In a study isolating the infraspinatus from the teres minor tendon and sectioning the infraspinatus into four parts, tensile testing showed the superior and midinferior sections to be weaker than the midsuperior or inferior regions of the tendon. The relative weakness of the superior segment may help explain the progression of cuff tears into this region from the supraspinatus.

The previously discussed biochemical evidence that the supraspinatus undergoes compressive as well as tensile loading has turned interest to evaluation of the compressive properties of cuff components. The compressive stiffness of the supraspinatus is significantly higher on the bursal side than on the articular side. The compressive stiffness is also greater 10 mm proximal to the bony insertion than at the insertion of points more proximal.

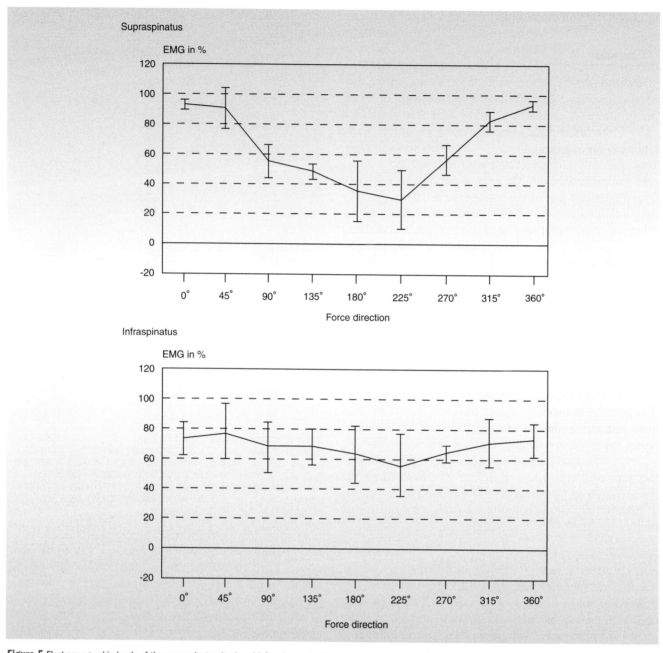

Figure 5 Electromyographic levels of the supraspinatus (top) and infraspinatus (bottom) compared with force direction measured in a plane perpendicular to the humerus with the arm in 90° of scapular abduction and the forearm horizontal. Note the variation in activity of the supraspinatus compared with the fairly consistent activity of the infraspinatus at all directions. Error bars represent 1 SD. *(Reproduced with permission from Arwert HJ, de Groot J, Van Woensel WW, Rozing PM: Electromyography of shoulder muscles in relation to force direction. J Shoulder Elbow Surg 1997;6:360-370.)*

Some recent studies have focused on the changes in rotator cuff properties attributable to differences in the mechanical environment of the tendon. The rotator cuff, like other soft tissues, exhibits viscoelasticity, where past history of use and the environment change the mechanical behavior. In a study on human cadaveric shoulders, the cross-sectional area was greater and the elastic modulus was lower in coracoacromial ligaments associated with rotator cuff tears compared with coracoacromial ligaments in healthy shoulders (Table 1 and Figure 6). Coracoacromial ligaments in shoulders with cuff tears also exhibit a greater decrease in the peak stress during cyclic testing but no difference in in situ ligament load when compared with coracoacromial ligaments in normal shoulders. These results indicate that the coracoacromial ligament clearly plays a role in rotator cuff degeneration but that tissue properties do not support the anecdotal observation of a "tighter" coracoacromial ligament in shoulders with pathologic rotator cuffs.

TABLE 1 | Material Properties of the Coracoacromial Ligament

Measurement	Shoulders With Rotator Cuff Tears (n = 10)	Normal Shoulders (n = 10)
Failure stress* (MPa)	25.3 ± 8.7	46.9 ± 30.7
Total specimen failure strain (%)	28.3 ± 8.6	23.7 ± 9.5
Ligamentous failure strain (%)	5.1 ± 1.2	5.6 ± 1.7
Total specimen modulus* (MPa)	120.3 ± 38.9	291.6 ± 154
Ligamentous modulus† (MPa)	658.4 ± 261.3	1174.4 ± 437.7

*$P < 0.0005$

†$P < 0.05$

(Reproduced with permission from Soslowsky LJ, An CH, Johnston SP, Carpenter JE: Geometric and mechanical properties of the coracoacromial ligament and their relationship to rotator cuff disease. Clin Orthop 1994;304:10-17.)

Other current investigations attempt to quantify in vivo strain within various rotator cuff tissues during motion. These studies will help determine the most likely locations where a tear will initiate by providing a visual representation of the extremes of tissue strains. Preliminary studies have suggested that strain is not uniform throughout the cuff tissues during loading as would be expected. Future studies include the noninvasive measurement of two- and three-dimensional strains within cuff tendons using MRI.

Injury

Musculoskeletal conditions represent the most frequent reason for office visits to physicians, at nearly 100 million annually. Of these, shoulder pain represents the third most common musculoskeletal complaint, after back and knee pain. It ranks as second only to low back pain in terms of work-related injuries and remains a large source of occupational illness as well as overall decreased productivity. Injury to the supraspinatus tendon of the shoulder is one of the most common disorders of the soft tissues of the musculoskeletal system. The incidence of rotator cuff disease, which has been implicated largely as an overuse-related injury, increases with each decade of life after the second. Injuries range from various degrees of tendinopathy to full-thickness rotator cuff tears and may very well represent the same disease process at different stages.

The pathogenesis of rotator cuff disease is typically divided into two mechanisms of injury, intrinsic and extrinsic, and previous studies have addressed the etiology of these two mechanisms. Intrinsic injuries originate within the tendon from direct tendon overload, intrinsic degeneration, or other insult. Overuse is considered a type of intrinsic tendon injury caused by submaximal repetitive loading. Extrinsic injuries are caused by compression against surrounding structures, specifically the

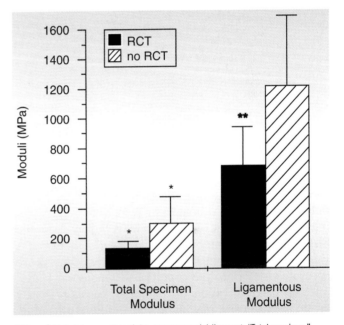

Figure 6 Material properties of the coracoacromial ligament. "Total specimen" denotes entire bone-ligament-bone preparation of coracoacromial ligament. "Ligamentous" denotes properties calculated from local ligament strain as measured optically. RCT = ligaments from shoulders with rotator cuff tears; no RCT = ligaments from normal shoulders. In both cases, the ligaments from shoulders with cuff tears had significantly lower moduli than those from shoulders without tears. Asterisk denotes $P < 0.0005$; double asterisk denotes $P < 0.05$. *(Reproduced with permission from Soslowsky LJ, An CH, Johnston SP, Carpenter JE: Geometric and mechanical properties of the coracoacromial ligament and their relationship to rotator cuff disease. Clin Orthop 1994;304:10-17.)*

coracoacromial arch and, as more recent studies have revealed, the posterosuperior glenolabral complex, causing internal impingement.

Intrinsic Injury Mechanisms

Intrinsically caused conditions can be traumatic, reactive, or degenerative. Traumatic failures usually occur in younger patients and involve a bony avulsion. Reactive-

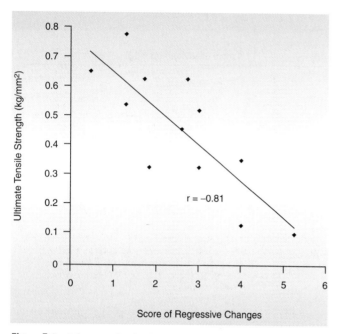

Figure 7 Graph from a study using 55 cadaver shoulders depicting the negative correlation between the histologic score of regressive changes and ultimate tensile strength in the supraspinatus tendon. *(Reproduced with permission from Sano H, Uhthoff HK, Backman DS, et al: Structural disorders at the insertion of the supraspinatus tendon: Relation to tensile strength. J Bone Joint Surg Br 1998;80: 720-725.)*

type cuff failures include calcifying tendinitis, which has been described as intratendinous calcific deposits that cause swelling within the subacromial space. Degenerative failures encompass the most frequent causes of failure in the cuff. Although the term tendinitis, implying an inflammation of the tendon, is widely used, the histopathology available offers no real evidence of a significant inflammatory response. A term that more accurately describes the condition is tendinosis. Under microscopic observation, the pathology occurs primarily at the insertion site, making the condition a true enthesopathy. Regardless of the nomenclature for the disease process, the degenerative changes that have been described include disruption and thinning of fascicles, formation of granulation tissue, dystrophic calcifications, disorganization of collagen fibers, abnormalities of the tidemark, and changes in cellularity.

Using a cadaver model, investigators have recently attempted to correlate the degree of degenerative changes present in the supraspinatus tendon with its tensile strength. One group came to two important conclusions regarding the site of the failure and the ultimate tensile stress. There were two areas of failure, at the insertion and at the midsubstance. The histologic score of degeneration used by these investigators was significantly higher in the insertion failure group. There was a negative correlation between the amount of degeneration and the ultimate tensile stress. In other words, the absence of degenerative changes preferentially led to midsubstance tears that failed

at higher loads. The ultimate tensile strength of the supraspinatus decreases significantly with a higher score of regressive changes (a histologic marker of degeneration) at the insertion (Fig. 7).

Another study compared the width of the sulcus (defined as the distance between the edge of the articular cartilage and the tendon insertion of the supraspinatus) and a score of regressive changes. The authors also noted a negative correlation between the score of regressive changes and the ultimate tensile strength. In addition, they noted a relationship between the width of the sulcus and the tensile properties. As the width of the sulcus increased, the tensile properties of the tendon decreased. This result may be useful clinically, as the sulcus width can be observed arthroscopically. The authors also found no correlation between age and score of regressive changes. Both studies contributed concrete information about the existing condition of the tendon and how degenerative changes may serve as stress risers, resulting in failure at lower loads. Contrary to previous studies that noted failure at the critical zone using gross evaluation, most specimens in this study failed at the insertion site when examined microscopically. This finding correlates well with the location of degenerative changes, which represent the biomechanical weak link in the bone-tendon complex.

Extrinsic Injury Mechanisms

Extrinsic causes of rotator cuff injury are best known as subacromial impingement lesions. This syndrome has been well described and often studied. The source of compression can either be bone or soft tissue. The acromion is notorious for its role in impingement, and its morphology has been characterized and is known to be a cause of outlet narrowing. In addition, narrowing of the outlet can result from osteophytes that arise from the acromion or acromioclavicular joint. The soft-tissue structures that are implicated in the impingement syndrome include the subacromial bursa and the coracoacromial ligament.

The bursa represents another potential source of compression, although the literature most likely misrepresents its true relationship to rotator cuff pathology. In the past, the bursa was believed to be involved with the inflammatory response of "tendinitis," either as a possible causal agent of cuff disease or the primary disease. Recent histologic evaluation of bursal reactions in rotator cuff tears shows lack of true inflammatory reaction. The bursal changes were localized and secondary to the underlying tendinopathy. In addition, the bursa appears to be part of the healing response, as a direct correlation was found between the degree of perivascular new collagen and type III collagen expression. Consequently, bursal reactions were noted to be worst with large rotator cuff tears in which there is a large amount of type

III collagen around the damaged tendon. Bursal tissue from sites distant to the rotator cuff tear did not have the same response as tissue from the lesion, indicating that the bursal reaction is confined to the tendon lesion.

Several studies have investigated the coracoacromial ligament as part of the impinging complex of the outlet. In some patients, the ligament has calcifications about its acromial insertion, thereby altering the properties of the native ligament. A recent study noted that patients with rotator cuff tears had a greater amount of nervous tissue distribution in the lateral one third of the ligament than did patients with anterior instability. This may indicate that the coracoacromial ligament plays a role in the pain recognition mechanism associated with rotator cuff disease. Another study noted decreases in the material properties of the lateral band of the ligament corresponding to histologic changes seen in the same area. This correlation suggests a role in the pathogenesis of tendinopathy and tears, although it is unclear if these changes represent causes or effects of rotator cuff pathology. Both studies indicate that the lateral band of the ligament plays an important role in the pathogenesis of cuff disease.

Another form of extrinsic trauma that has recently received attention is the concept of internal impingement (Fig. 8). This condition was originally described in throwing athletes with increased glenohumeral joint motion who reported persistent shoulder pain. The clinical findings include articular-sided rotator cuff injury, posterosuperior labral fraying, and bony changes at the same position on the glenoid. The pathokinematics of this condition can be described as the arm moves into abduction and maximal external rotation such as in the late cocking phase of throwing. The humeral head runs out of articulating surface, and the articular side of the cuff makes contact with the posterosuperior glenoid. The greater tuberosity compresses the cuff against the glenolabral complex. Most commonly it involves the posterior aspect of the supraspinatus or the superior portion of the infraspinatus. This is further aggravated by increased anterior translation, which can result from laxity in the anterior capsule and the inferior glenohumeral ligament, and as the secondary restraints of the glenohumeral joint fatigue with repetitive throwing. As a result, impingement of the articular side of the cuff occurs. A potential risk factor that was identified in one series was decreased retroversion of the humeral head.

To delineate the stress environment in the supraspinatus using biphasic material properties, one research group created a two-dimensional finite element model based on measurements from one specimen. Previous work had focused on mutually exclusive causal mechanisms: articular-sided lesions as the result of intrinsic causes, and bursal-sided lesions as the result of an extrinsic cause. By simulating the loading environment of the

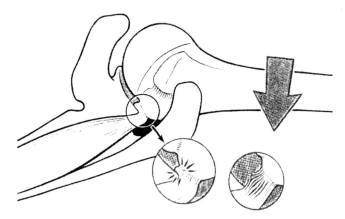

Figure 8 Schematic representation of internal impingement between the posterior edge of the glenoid and the articular surface of the supraspinatus and infraspinatus tendons. *(Reproduced with permission from Walch G, Boileau P, Noel E, Donell ST: Impingement of the deep surface of the supraspinatus tendon on the posterosuperior glenoid rim: An arthroscopic study. J Shoulder Elbow Surg 1992;1:238-245.)*

tendon, the authors hoped to explain the clinical presence of the articular-sided lesion. Two conditions were modeled, one with no impingement and one with impingement on the bursal side producing a 1-mm indentation on the bursal surface. The results demonstrated high stress concentration at the critical zone as defined by Codman. Interestingly, the model calculated high stresses on both surfaces.

Animal Studies

Neither cadaveric nor patient-based studies can address questions related to the etiology and pathogenesis of rotator cuff disease. Therefore, an essential component in the study of the disease was the development of an animal model, where factors believed to be important in the etiology of the condition could be prescribed and their effect quantitatively monitored and evaluated over time.

The Rat Model

After investigation of more than 30 different animals to determine their appropriateness according to a checklist of criteria, the rat has been identified as the most appropriate animal model, excluding primates, for such studies. Two very important features are present in the rat shoulder model. The rat has a prominent supraspinatus tendon that inserts on the greater tuberosity of the proximal humerus. The rat also has a bony arch composed of the coracoid, clavicle, and acromion. The supraspinatus tendon passes under this bony outlet in a repetitive fashion during forward locomotion, similar to the action in the human shoulder, where the tendon must pass under the coracoacromial arch during forward elevation (Fig. 9). Researchers have used this model to test hypotheses regarding the etiology of rotator cuff tendinosis and the process of rotator cuff tears (Fig. 10). One weakness associated

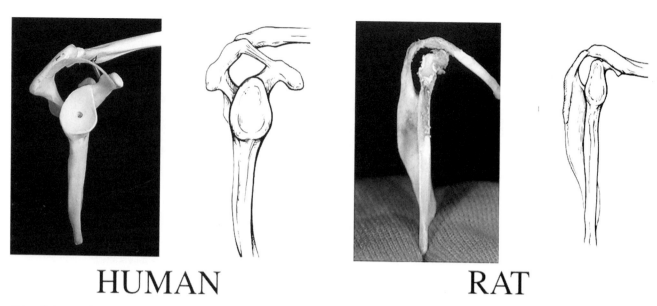

Figure 9 Features of the rat shoulder model. Photographs and schematics of human and rat right shoulders from a lateral, or "outlet," view with the humerus removed. Both have a similar enclosed bony outlet through which the supraspinatus must pass.

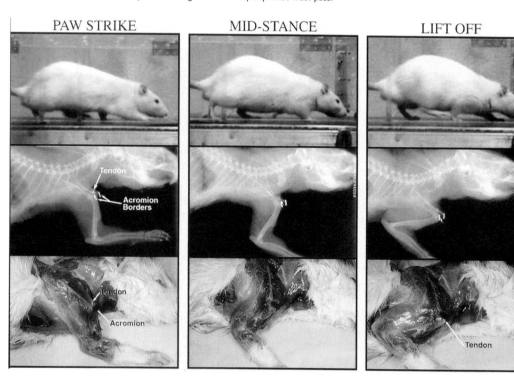

Figure 10 Video frames, radiographs, and anatomic dissections of the rat in three positions achieved during treadmill running depicting the motion of the supraspinatus underneath the acromial arch. At paw strike, the supraspinatus tendon (denoted by radiopaque markers) can be seen in both the radiographs and dissection photographs to lie behind or caudal to the acromion. (The borders are denoted by radiopaque markers.) At midstance, the tendon lies directly below the acromion. At lift-off, it can be seen in front of or cranial to the acromion. *(Reproduced with permission from Soslowsky LJ, Carpenter JE, DeBano CM, Banerji I, Moalli MR: Development and use of an animal model for investigations on rotator cuff disease. J Shoulder Elbow Surg 1996;5:383-392.)*

with almost all animal models is that they are quadrupeds, so all their limbs are weight bearing. While the human shoulder is not a weight-bearing joint, it is a significant load-bearing joint, so the loading environment is not too dissimilar from that of a weight-bearing extremity. The rat model is therefore an imperfect but useful model for studying certain questions about the human shoulder.

Tendon Healing

To assess the healing capacity of the rat supraspinatus tendon compared with human tendon healing, a tendon

defect was created and then evaluated at several points in time. One study group was treated with in situ freezing of the adjacent tissue to model a tendon with an intrinsically reduced capacity to heal. There were no significant differences in histologic and mechanical properties between the normal tendon group and the tendon group that was frozen in situ. Although the later time points showed improvement in both structural (histologic properties) and functional (increased load to failure and tissue modulus) parameters, the values remained one order of magnitude below control (uninjured) tendons. This result indicates

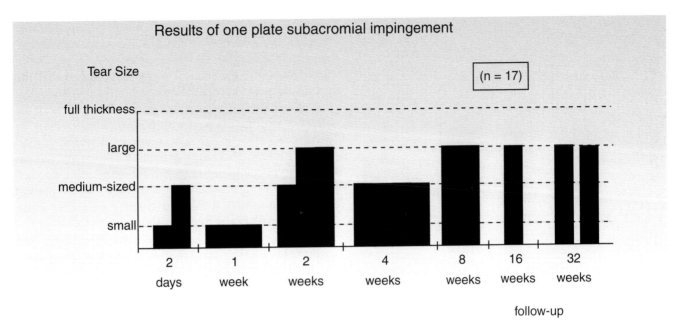

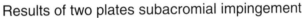

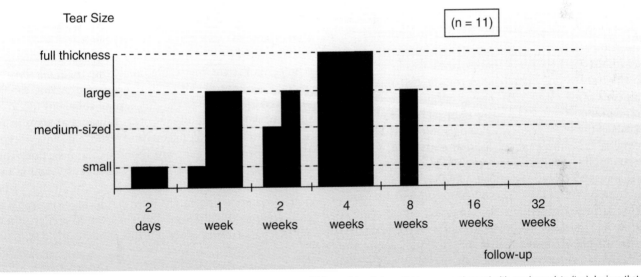

Figure 11 Rotator cuff tears of rats with experimental subacromial impingement with bony plates. Only partial tears were observed with one bony plate (top). Lesions that occurred from two bony plates included three full-thickness tears (bottom). All partial tears were localized on the bursal side of the infraspinatus tendon. No articular side or intratendinous lesions occurred. *(Reproduced with permission from Schneeberger AG, Nyffeler RW, Gerber C: Structural changes of the rotator cuff caused by experimental subacromial impingement in the rat.* J Shoulder Elbow Surg *1998;7:375-380.)*

that the tendon has an active but inadequate healing response. Despite the fact that studies of human biopsy specimens demonstrate histologic evidence of significant proliferation of reparative tissues at the tendon edges, human rotator cuff tendons do not appear to heal in any significant manner, which correlates well with the findings of the rat rotator cuff tear model. Knowing that the healing responses in rat and human tendons are similar means that the rat model is useful for investigating the mechanisms of failure in the healing process and finding ways to improve the healing response of the native tendon.

Intrinsic and Extrinsic Injury Models

To study individual injury mechanisms, a model of each injury was created. The intrinsic injury was created with a collagenase injection, a method that has been used previously, particularly in studies of equine tendon injury. The extrinsic injury was created with an Achilles tendon allograft to simulate an impingement lesion. Each model produced recognizable histologic changes as compared in control specimens. The tissues remained the same histologically or began to improve after several weeks of healing, indicating that the response of

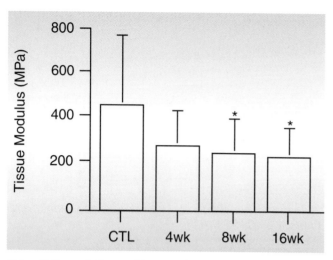

Figure 12 Changes in tissue modulus across time in supraspinatus tendons of rats undergoing an overuse protocol. Asterisk denotes statistically significant difference compared with control group, *P* < 0.05. Error bars denote 1 SD. *(Reproduced with permission from Soslowsky LJ, Thomopoulos S, Tun S, et al: Overuse activity injures the supraspinatus tendon in an animal model: A histologic and biomechanical study. J Shoulder Elbow Surg 2000;9:79-84.)*

the tissue to injury was beginning to have some positive effects. However, neither of these mechanisms alone appears to be responsible for persistent tendinosis.

Another research group created an impingement model to test the hypothesis that extrinsic lesions contribute to the etiology of bursal-sided rotator cuff tears. Bony implants of two sizes were placed on the undersurface of the acromial spine. Rats were then sacrificed at various points in time to assess evidence of cuff tears. Bursal-sided tears in the infraspinatus tendon existed in every experimentally created subacromial lesion. The size of the implants obliterated the subacromial space and indented the tendon of interest. These results support the notion that extrinsic factors are the primary etiologic agent for bursal-sided tears, whereas articular-sided tears have other primary causes. Additional research is currently being done with this and other impingement models that reproduce the outlet narrowing as seen in humans to further assess the effects of extrinsic mechanisms in the development of tendinosis (Fig. 11).

Overuse Injury Model
Overuse has long been suspected as an etiologic factor in rotator cuff disease. To test this mechanism independently, an experiment using rats running in a treadmill was performed (Fig. 12). The effects of overuse were compared with normal cage activity. The histologic changes produced were similar to those in the intrinsic and extrinsic injury models and were consistent with human biopsy studies. In addition, over the course of the experiment, the cross-sectional area significantly increased and the mechanical

properties significantly decreased. It is to be expected that changes in physiologic demands will produce remodeling, ultimately enhancing the tissue properties. However, the decrease in the mechanical properties implies that the process is most likely pathologic rather than physiologic.

Another study compared the effect of overuse with the effect of overuse coupled with intrinsic tendon injury or extrinsic tendon compression on the development of rotator cuff injury. This study evaluated histologic changes (increase in cellularity, collagen disorganization, and cell morphology), cross-sectional area, and biomechanical changes (maximal stress and tissue moduli). Overuse combined with either injury model produced a higher histologic score and decreased mechanical strength than overuse alone. The combination of overuse and injury (either intrinsic or extrinsic) results in more severe injury than does overuse alone. Clearly, more research is needed to investigate etiologic factors associated with rotator cuff tendinosis. Many studies have been conducted using the existing rat model to test intrinsic, extrinsic, overuse, and combination-type injuries.

Other Animal Models
Larger animal models are currently being investigated as well. Surgically created tears have been repaired in sheep with generally varying results, likely due to an inability to adequately control postoperative loading. A dog model was used to investigate the differential collagens found in the supraspinatus tendon. It was found that significant amounts of type III collagens and lesser amounts of type II and type V collagens are found at the insertion. This contrasts with the primarily type I collagens found in the tendon proper. The authors hypothesized that this variation in composition might play a role in supraspinatus pathology, as the different collagens would confer different mechanical properties. Further study is needed.

Summary
The tendons and muscles of the rotator cuff are essential to shoulder motion and stability. The basic anatomy and mechanics of the cuff have been investigated in depth. Current efforts focus on achieving this same level of understanding of the rotator cuff on the tissue, ultrastructural, cellular, and molecular levels. Biomechanical, biochemical, and histologic assays are being used on tissues from cadaver models, surgical biopsies, and animal models to help better identify the pathology of the rotator cuff and the mechanisms involved in its injury and repair. As a result, significant and fundamental advancements are expected in these areas over the next few years.

Annotated Bibliography

Arwert HJ, de Groot J, Van Woensel WW, Rozing PM: Electromyography of shoulder muscles in relation to force direction. *J Shoulder Elbow Surg* 1997;6:360-370.

The EMG level of 14 shoulder muscles was related to force direction during active motion about the shoulder by live subjects. The principal action of each muscle was identified.

Berenson MC, Blevins FT, Plaas AH, Vogel KG: Proteoglycans of human rotator cuff tendons. *J Orthop Res* 1996;14:518-525.

Grossly normal rotator cuff and biceps tendons procured from adult cadavers with no history of shoulder problems showed that GAG and PG content in the rotator cuff tendons was much different than in the distal biceps.

Carpenter JE, Flanagan CL, Thomopoulos S, Yian EH, Soslowsky LJ: The effects of overuse combined with intrinsic or extrinsic alterations in an animal model of rotator cuff tendinosis. *Am J Sports Med* 1998;26:801-807.

A rat model was used to evaluate overuse and overuse combined with intrinsic tendon injury or extrinsic tendon compression in the development of rotator cuff injury. Damage to the rotator cuff was caused by all three injury mechanisms.

Gerber C, Schneeberger AG, Perren SM, Nyffeler RW: Experimental rotator cuff repair: A preliminary study. *J Bone Joint Surg Am* 1999;81:1281-1290.

In an in vivo sheep study, a modified Mason-Allen stitch with a bone augmentation plate was found to be superior to a simple stitch through a transosseous tunnel. Lack of postoperative protection resulted in a high rate of failure.

Gotoh M, Hamada K, Yamakawa H, Tomonaga A, Inoue A, Fukuda H: Significance of granulation tissue in torn supraspinatus insertions: An immunohistochemical study with antibodies against interleukin-1beta, cathepsin D, and matrix metalloprotease-1. *J Orthop Res* 1997;15:33-39.

Comparison of torn supraspinatus tendons obtained during surgery with grossly normal cadaveric supraspinatus tendons showed strong immunoreactivity for interleukin-1β, cathepsin D, and matrix metalloprotease-1 among the torn tendons only, mostly between the osteochondral margin of the enthesis and granulation tissue.

Hamada K, Tomonaga A, Gotoh M, Yamakawa H, Fukuda H: Intrinsic healing capacity and tearing process of torn supraspinatus tendons: In situ hybridization study of α1(I) procollagen mRNA. *J Orthop Res* 1997;15:24-32.

In situ hybridization was performed on tissue sections from torn and normal supraspinatus biopsy specimens. Significant increases in labeled tenocytes and undifferentiated mesenchymal cells around tear locations suggested an intrinsic healing response.

Ishii H, Brunet JA, Welsh RP, Uhthoff HK: "Bursal reactions" in rotator cuff tearing, the impingement syndrome, and calcifying tendinitis. *J Shoulder Elbow Surg* 1997;6:131-136.

In subacromial bursal biopsies from patients with rotator cuff tears, impingement syndrome, or calcifying tendinitis, the intensity of bursal reaction correlated with degree of formation of both perivascular and type III collagen. Bursal reactions were localized to tendon lesions.

Lee SB, Nakajima T, Luo ZP, Zobitz ME, Chang YW, An KN: The bursal and articular sides of the supraspinatus tendon have a different compressive stiffness. *Clin Biomech* 2000;15:241-247.

Indentation tests at 15 bursal- and articular-side locations on cadaveric supraspinatus tendons revealed a higher compressive stiffness on the bursal surface. On both sides, the compressive stiffness was nonhomogenous and maximum at 10 mm proximal to the insertion.

Sano H, Uhthoff HK, Backman DS, et al: Structural disorders at the insertion of the supraspinatus tendon: Relation to tensile strength. *J Bone Joint Surg Br* 1998;80:720-725.

Cadaver supraspinatus tendons and attachments were judged histologically for regressive changes, measured to determine sulcus width, and tested mechanically. Ultimate tensile strength was negatively correlated with sulcus width and regressive changes.

Schneeberger AG, Nyffeler RW, Gerber C: Structural changes of the rotator cuff caused by experimental subacromial impingement in the rat. *J Shoulder Elbow Surg* 1998;7:375-380.

Subacromial impingement of the infraspinatus tendon was experimentally created in a rat model causing various degrees of controlled bursal-sided tears.

Soslowsky LJ, An CH, DeBano CM, Carpenter JE: Coracoacromial ligament: In situ load and viscoelastic properties in rotator cuff disease. *Clin Orthop* 1996;330:40-44.

Coracoacromial ligaments from normal cadaveric shoulders and those with rotator cuff tears were evaluated biomechanically. While in situ loads were present, no difference of in situ load was observed between groups. Ligaments associated with cuff tears showed a decrease in peak stress during cyclic loading.

Soslowsky LJ, Carpenter JE, DeBano CM, Banerji I, Moalli MR: Development and use of an animal model for investigations on rotator cuff disease. *J Shoulder Elbow Surg* 1996;5:383-392.

Using a set of anatomic and functional criteria, various animal models were evaluated for their appropriateness in studying rotator cuff disease. The rat was selected as the most acceptable because of the anatomic relationship between the supraspinatus tendon and an adjacent bony outlet.

Soslowsky LJ, Thomopoulos S, Tun S, et al: Overuse activity injures the supraspinatus tendon in an animal model: A histologic and biomechanical study. *J Shoulder Elbow Surg* 2000;9:79-84.

The effects of an overuse regimen on the supraspinatus tendon were evaluated in a rat running model. Over time, the tendon had marked increases in cellularity, decreases in fiber orientation, and a decreased tissue modulus reflective of an injured tendon.

Classic Bibliography

Inman VT, Saunders JB, Abbott LC: Observation on the function of the shoulder joint. *J Bone Joint Surg Am* 1944;26:1-30.

Riley GP, Harrall RL, Constant CR, Chard MD, Cawston TE, Hazleman BL: Glycosaminoglycans of human rotator cuff tendons: Changes with age and in chronic rotator cuff tendinitis. *Ann Rheum Dis* 1994;53:367-376.

Walch G, Boileau P, Noel E, Donell ST: Impingement of the deep surface of the supraspinatus tendon on the posterosuperior glenoid rim: An arthroscopic study. *J Shoulder Elbow Surg* 1992;1:238-245.

Chapter 4

Shoulder Kinematics and Kinesiology

Michael L. Pearl, MD

Karyn A. Wong, PT

Introduction

The shoulder functions to position the hand in space by moving the arm with respect to the thorax. Describing shoulder motion and measuring the accompanying forces are challenging tasks. Three skeletal segments (the clavicle, scapula, and humerus) move in three dimensions across three articulations (the sternoclavicular, acromioclavicular, and glenohumeral joints). The scapulothoracic articulation adds additional constraints and stability to the shoulder complex.

Kinematics is the study of motion without regard to forces; kinesiology refers to the broader study of all aspects of motion, including the underlying muscle forces. The current understanding of shoulder kinematics and kinesiology comes from both in vivo and in vitro sources.

In vivo study of shoulder motion poses significant difficulties. Localizing skeletal segments such as the scapula, with its irregular shape and subcutaneous position, impedes an accurate description of motion. Measuring the tension of individual muscles is not possible in vivo, and efforts to indirectly calculate moment arms are compromised when the position of the skeletal segments is uncertain. In vitro analysis does allow for relatively precise localization of the individual skeletal segments and study of the mechanical properties of ligament, bone, and muscle, but it provides only an approximation of the in vivo reality for both the normal and pathologic states.

Description of Shoulder Positions

The mathematical description of shoulder motion poses no difficulty for biomechanical researchers. Several internally consistent systems are available for the description of rigid bodies (skeletal segments) moving with respect to each other. The greatest impediment to progress in measuring shoulder motion is the lack of defined reference axes for the involved skeletal segments and a nomenclature that has at least some application in the clinical setting.

Ideally, both laboratory and clinical measurements of motion should be based on the same reference axes for the thorax, scapula, and humerus. These reference axes would be reproducible, accessible in vivo, and consistent with three-dimensional motion analysis. This would allow one study to be compared with another regardless of the nomenclature adopted. For the thorax and scapula, examples of reference axes that meet these criteria exist in both the clinical literature and that of biomechanical modeling (Fig. 1).

Various systems of nomenclature have been used to identify the position of one skeletal segment relative to another, but they all describe the plane of elevation, the angle of elevation, and the rotational orientation of the arm (Fig. 2). The clinical conventions for describing positions with respect to the coronal and sagittal planes remain consistent as representative positions within the range of motion (ROM). Even the more rigorous sys-

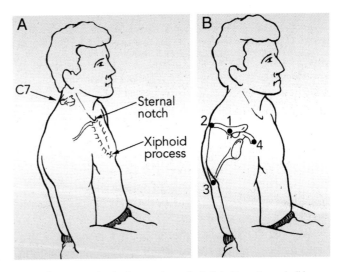

Figure 1 Landmarks for the thorax and scapula. **A,** Palpable and reproducible landmarks for the thorax are the C7 spinous process, the sternal notch, the xiphoid process, and, if needed, the spinous process of T8. **B,** Landmarks for the scapula include (1) the posterior corner of the acromion, (2) the junction of the scapular spine at the medial border of the scapula, (3) the inferior angle of the scapula, and (4) the tip of the coracoid process.

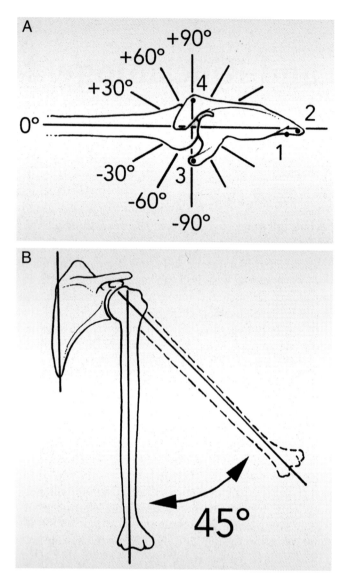

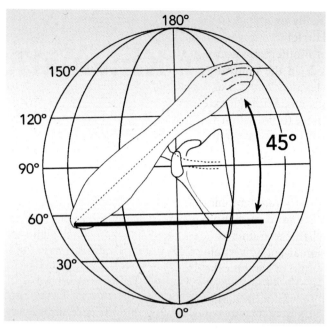

Figure 3 Global diagram based on scapular coordinate system showing rotation (45°) referenced to the latitude. *(Reproduced with permission from Pearl ML, Jackins S, Lippitt SB, Sidles JA, Matsen FA III: Humeroscapular positions in a shoulder range-of-motion examination. J Shoulder Elbow Surg 1992;1:296-305.)*

Figure 2 Planes and angles of elevation. **A,** Planes of elevation for a scapular-based coordinate system are shown from a superior view. **B,** The angle of elevation is shown with respect to a scapular reference. *(Reproduced with permission from Pearl ML, Jackins S, Lippitt SB, Sidles JA, Matsen FA III: Humeroscapular positions in a shoulder range-of-motion examination. J Shoulder Elbow Surg 1992;1: 296-305.)*

tems for describing humerothoracic and humeroscapular positions encounter problems, however, as points of singularity make the description of rotational orientation difficult, or a sequence of movements reveals the nonadditive nature of rigid body rotations, as exemplified by Codman's Paradox.

A global diagram like the one shown in Figure 3 provides the least ambiguous description of shoulder motion. Planes of elevation are analogous to lines of longitude, and angles of elevation to lines of latitude. Rotational orientation can be expressed graphically by an arrow or some similar symbol. In addition, advances in three-dimensional computer graphics technology greatly facili-

tate the visual presentation of data relating to complex motion patterns.

Normal Shoulder Motion

In a study of humerothoracic positions using electromagnetic tracking technology with percutaneous pins rigidly fixed to the scapulae and humeri of eight middle-aged men, active elevation averaged 148° (+/- 11°). Normal elevation is commonly considered to be in the range of 180°, but this study suggests that when referenced to the thorax, the arm rarely achieves this degree of elevation. The study found that most activities that take place in front of the body, such as eating and hair combing, including maximum elevation, occurred in a plane about 60° anterior to the coronal plane.

Elevation

A study of humeroscapular positions in normal subjects undergoing ROM examination found that maximum elevation of the arm usually occurs with the humerus in the plane of the scapula, at an angle of humeroscapular elevation of about 90°. A cadaver study found that the humerus could be maximally elevated in a plane 23° anterior to the scapular plane to a humeroscapular angle of 120°. This finding does not imply, however, that this is the optimum strategy of humeroscapular elevation an individual should use when trying to reach maximally overhead (maximum humerothoracic elevation). Humeroscapular relationships were also notable in several other common positions. When the arm was at the side in the neutral position, the humerus was already elevated 25° and externally rotated 47° relative to the scapula. With full external rotation, the forearm actually came to lie within the scapular plane. With the arm at 90° of coronal-plane humerothoracic elevation (abduction) and in external rotation, the humerus is 20° to 30° behind the plane of the scapula at 50° to 60° of humeroscapular elevation.

Early radiographic studies of arm elevation identified a 2:1 ratio of glenohumeral to scapulothoracic motion when the humerus is elevated in the coronal plane. A similar analysis of elevation in the scapular plane found a ratio of 5:4 after the first 30° of elevation. Similar studies carried out by other researchers found slight variations on these earlier observations. It has become customary to refer to elevation in a plane 30° to 40° anterior to the coronal plane as scapular plane elevation. However, the scapula is a highly mobile reference point. The plane of the scapula not only moves with arm elevation but also inclines forward early in motion, clearly a different direction than that of the intended elevation.

The relative motion between the scapulothoracic interface and the glenohumeral joint has been referred to as the humeroscapular (glenohumeral) rhythm. The ratios of 2:1 and 5:4 are commonly accepted as representing the ratio of glenohumeral motion to scapulothoracic motion, but these values are clearly only a limited reflection of the scapulothoracic and humeroscapular combinations possible to achieve a given humerothoracic position. These ratios are based on two-dimensional radiographic projections of angular rotations taken at discrete positions of elevation, whereas the arm moves in three dimensions, and for positions other than elevation, much of this motion is under voluntary control. More recently, an in vivo three-dimensional study found that for a given individual, the scapulothoracic and humeroscapular postures were much the same whether the shoulder was loaded (weight on the wrist) or unloaded. This consistency may allow a three-dimensional definition of shoulder rhythm, at least with respect to arm elevation.

Axial Rotation

The relative contributions of scapulothoracic and humeroscapular motion to axial rotation have not been studied. In looking at humerothoracic (combined scapulothoracic and humeroscapular) motion, a study of seven young adult men found that the range of axial rotation of the upper arm depends strongly on the position of the arm (plane and angle of elevation) and varies among individuals (average range, 94° to 157°).

Authors have disagreed about the amount and type of motion of the humeral head that occurs on the glenoid. Early authors described rolling, sliding, and spinning movements of the humeral head, suggesting that normal shoulder motion requires translations at the glenohumeral joint. Electromagnetic tracking technology and the most recent radiographic studies have convincingly demonstrated that the humeral head remains centered on the glenoid for movements within the midrange (when the ligaments are not under tension). When the position of the glenohumeral joint extends beyond this range (when soft-tissue tension develops), the humeral head begins to translate in a direction away from the tight tissue. This mechanism is referred to as capsular constraint.

A novel method for applying coupled moments to the distal humerus using compressed nitrogen, thereby removing factors other than the joint capsule and articular surface contact that may affect glenohumeral translations, also demonstrates the principle of capsular constraint. A study of seven cadaver specimens in both passive and simulated active modes found that translations during the active mode were consistent with descriptions in the literature and the existence of ball-and-socket joint kinematics. Passive movements displayed greater translations than active movements, but these translations appeared to be related to increased ROM because they were not apparent when the specimens were kept within the range observed in the active modes. The extent to which the normal glenohumeral joint in vivo remains centered during passive motion remains in question. Counterbalancing the forces that would otherwise displace the center of rotation, whether they are external or internal, is clearly one of the primary functions of the rotator cuff.

Muscle Function

Muscle function of the shoulder is at least as complex as the description of its motion. The tension generated by a muscle is a combination of active and passive elements. The active contribution is proportional to the cross-sectional area of the muscle and is greatest when the muscle is at its resting length; the passive contribution is secondary to the elastic properties of the muscle and is greatest when the muscle is in maximum extension. The function of a muscle with respect to any joint depends on the position of the skeletal components, its distance from the center of rotation of the joint, and the external and internal forces acting at the time of muscle contraction.

The tools currently used to study muscle function about the shoulder include electromyography (EMG),

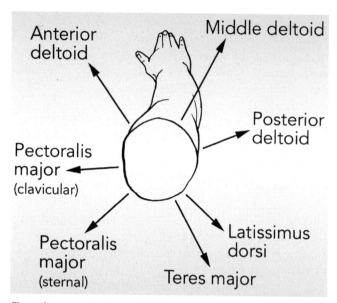

Figure 4 Direction of action of prime movers of the shoulder with the arm elevated about 90° between the sagittal and coronal planes as determined electromyographically. Diagram should be viewed as if the observer is looking down the shaft of the right arm. *(Reproduced with permission from Pearl ML, Perry J, Torburn L, Gordon LH: An electromyographic analysis of the shoulder during cones and planes of arm motion. Clin Orthop 1992;284:116-127.)*

dynamic testing devices that simulate muscle forces in cadaveric shoulders, theoretical analysis of increasingly sophisticated mathematical models, and careful clinical observation of patients with known anatomic deficits. Of these, only EMG reflects the activation of a muscle in vivo. EMG is extremely useful for measuring the timing of muscle activation within a given movement. If the kinematics of the movement and the position and motion of the skeletal segments are known precisely, the function of the muscle becomes apparent. EMG has limitations, however. Surface electrodes may inadvertently reflect muscle activity from adjacent muscles, while intramuscular electrodes sample from only a portion of the muscle. In addition, the relationship of signal intensity to force production is not linear when muscles change length (signals diminish at extended lengths and increase at shortened ones). Conclusions with respect to the force generated by the muscle, therefore, must be made carefully.

The Prime Movers

For the most part, the prime movers of the shoulder (the deltoid, pectoralis, latissimus dorsi, and teres major muscles) function in ways predictable from their line of pull (Fig. 4). An EMG study of five normal volunteers making conical arm movements demonstrated the directional nature of shoulder muscle activation. Even for movements along a curved path, muscle recruitment was consistent with the instantaneous vector at any

given point in the motion. A large part of the versatility of the shoulder in moving the arm stems from the functional anatomy that makes this multidirectional motion possible. The prime movers of the arm drape over the shoulder, creating the potential for infinite lines of pull that nearly complete a 360° arc.

An analogous study compared the direction of force intended by study subjects with EMG activity, looking at positions of the suspended arm elevated 90° in the sagittal and scapular planes. This study defined two important parameters of muscle activity to be considered in EMG analysis. The principal action of a muscle is the force direction in which the EMG activity of a specific muscle is maximal. This parameter was compared with the mechanical action, which was defined as the force vector of a specific muscle based on a mechanical analysis of the line of pull of the muscle. The mechanical action in this study was determined for each muscle with respect to each joint (acromioclavicular, sternoclavicular, and glenohumeral). Most of the prime movers crossing the glenohumeral joint were maximally active in mechanically favorable directions. The exception was the teres major, for which the mechanical action was inclined 20° more inferiorly than the principal action. The latissimus dorsi was in agreement with its mechanical action at the sternoclavicular joint. The trapezius and serratus anterior were active in upward and outward movements and would best be identified as stabilizers of the scapula.

The Rotator Cuff

The rotator cuff participates in shoulder motion in multiple ways and often serves more than one function simultaneously. The muscles themselves can act as prime movers if their line of action is consistent with the intended direction of motion. They can act as stabilizers by creating compressive forces that hold the humeral head on the glenoid and shear forces that are antagonistic to other forces that would otherwise displace the centered position of the humeral head. This aspect is discussed in greater detail in chapter 2. In addition, they function to impart axial rotation to the humerus. The interplay between this latter aspect of rotator cuff function and that of the larger prime movers creates a musculoskeletal system capable of moving the arm in nearly any direction with any combination of axial rotation.

Rotator Cuff as Elevator and Prime Mover

A cadaver study of 10 specimens that evaluated tendon excursions to calculate muscle moment arms in different humeroscapular positions demonstrated that rotator cuff muscles may contribute to elevation, depending on the rotational position of the arm. The exception was the teres minor, for which the line of action was always below the center of rotation. Different positions of the arm alter the orientation of the muscles. In external rotation, the upper fibers of the subscapularis sit atop the humeral head and contribute to elevation. In internal rotation, the line of pull of the infraspinatus contributes to elevation. This study found that at 0° of elevation, the supraspinatus had a greater moment arm for elevation than did the deltoid. Its anterior portion contributed to internal rotation, but with elevation, it became a weak external rotator. At greater than 60° of abduction, the infraspinatus no longer had a significant external rotational moment arm, leaving the teres minor as the predominant external rotator.

Another cadaveric study evaluated shoulder muscle moment arms during horizontal motion and elevation in the sagittal, scapular, and coronal planes. The middle and anterior deltoids were found to have the largest moment arms for elevation, each more than twice that of the supraspinatus. The supraspinatus was an important elevator early in the motion, with its moment arm decreasing with increasing elevation. In contrast to the earlier study, this study found the moment arm of the supraspinatus at the beginning of elevation was equal to, not greater than, that of the anterior and middle deltoids. The pectoralis major was more than twice as efficient in horizontally flexing the humerus than was the anterior deltoid. The posterior deltoid, infraspinatus, supraspinatus, and teres minor were the primary movers for horizontal extension.

Another cadaveric study looked specifically at the relative contributions of the supraspinatus and deltoid to elevation. The study examined simulated middle deltoid and supraspinatus forces in the following ratios: 1:1, 2:3, 3:2, and zero supraspinatus force. With greater middle deltoid force, less supraspinatus force was required to achieve full abduction. Simulated supraspinatus paralysis (zero force) required the greatest middle deltoid activity to elevate the humerus, especially early in the motion, from 15° to 45°. Humeral head translations were less than 2 mm for all combinations, displaying ball-and-socket kinematics even in the case of supraspinatus paralysis.

Rotator Cuff as Rotator

A study of external and internal rotation compared torque production and EMG activity with the arm in five basic humerothoracic positions: dependent, 45° and 90° of elevation in the scapular plane, and 90° of elevation in the sagittal and coronal planes. Full internal, neutral, half external, and full external axial rotation were studied in each of these basic positions. The most torque was generated in the frontal and scapular planes. No position distinguished the teres minor and infraspinatus activity. The position that best recruited both of these muscles was half external rotation in 90° of forward ele-

vation. No position isolated the supraspinatus. Of the positions tested, neutral rotation at 90° of elevation in the scapular plane best isolated the subscapularis.

Recent biomechanical models have evaluated earlier assumptions and compared new ways of predicting muscle moments and forces with those used previously. A study of 12 cadaveric specimens using the tendon excursion method looked at elevation and rotation in three positions of the arm: neutral, 90° of scapular elevation with the forearm horizontal, and the same position with 30° of external rotation. This model predicted the highest rotator cuff forces during internal rotation (for the subscapularis) and external rotation (for the infraspinatus, teres minor, and supraspinatus) and suggested that models studying abduction and elevation of the arm may underestimate the potential loads on the rotator cuff. A subsequent study compared the origin-insertion and the tendon excursion methods for determining moment arms. The origin-insertion method gave higher rotator cuff muscle force estimates (predicted lower moment arms) than methods using the slope of the tendon excursion versus joint angle relationship. Predicting muscle forces by applying Monte Carlo simulation methods to an EMG-driven model has been evaluated. The results suggest that this may have application for better correlation of EMG data and estimating muscle forces.

Correlation of EMG and Clinical Examination of the Rotator Cuff

EMG has been used in conjunction with common manual muscle tests to find optimal selective positions for examining rotator cuff muscles. Identifying a selective position for testing a specific muscle involves recognizing its primary action and placing the arm in a position that makes it difficult for other muscles with a similar action to participate. The findings from these studies, along with those gained from detailed examinations of patients with known anatomic and neurologic deficits, not only provide useful clinical tests but also clarify the function of individual muscles of the arm in specific positions (Fig. 5).

An EMG study of 29 isometric challenges to the arm tested the utility of the lift-off test, with and without force, and every combination of elevation and rotation in the scapular plane at elevations of 0°, 45°, and 90° and rotations of –45°, 0°, and +45°. The selective positions identified for the various rotator cuff muscles were as follows: for the supraspinatus, 90° of scapular plane elevation, +45° of rotation (the "full can test"); for the infraspinatus, 0° of elevation, –45° of rotation; and for the subscapularis, the lift-off test with force.

In a detailed clinical study of 100 consecutive patients with rotator cuff symptomatology, three tests were used to evaluate specific rotator cuff function: external rotation

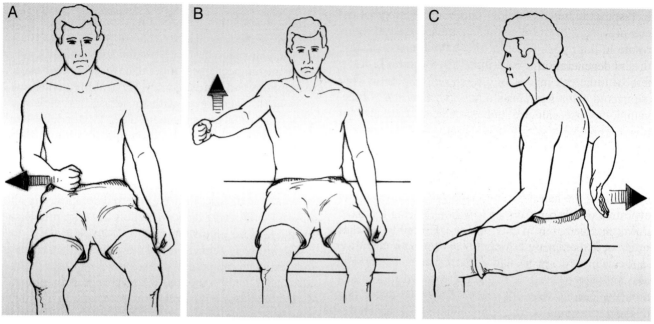

Figure 5 Clinically useful positions for testing. **A,** Infraspinatus **B,** Supraspinatus **C,** Subscapularis.

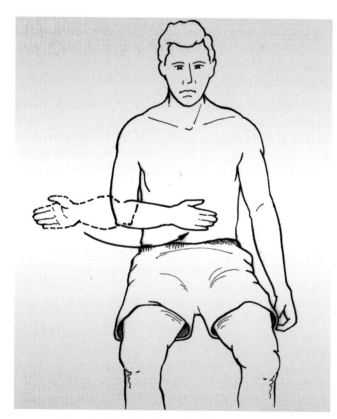

Figure 6 The ERLS for infraspinatus dysfunction. Patient has no ability to actively maintain external rotation with the arm by the side.

lag sign (ERLS) (Fig. 6), drop sign, and internal rotation lag sign (IRLS). The ERLS and drop signs had a 100% positive predictive value for a tear of the posterosuperior rotator cuff. The IRLS was more sensitive and equally

specific to the lift-off test, and it had a positive predictive value of 97% for a tear of the subscapularis.

Another clinical study that looked specifically for ways of distinguishing the supraspinatus examined arm elevation strength manually in external and internal rotation (full can and empty can tests) and compared these findings to MRI findings of rotator cuff tears. Both tests were sensitive (86% and 89%, respectively) and specific (74% and 68%, respectively) for supraspinatus tears. The empty can test was more painful, suggesting that the externally rotated position (full can) may be more useful in the clinical setting. An EMG study of normal shoulders with a similar purpose compared a position of external rotation (Blackburn position) to one of internal rotation (Jobe position). The study concluded that both positions result in significant supraspinatus activation, but neither is selective.

A study of 54 patients with tears involving the supraspinatus and infraspinatus distinguished the clinical function and testing of the infraspinatus and teres minor. This study compared findings on physical examination to CT arthrography graded according to the classification system of Goutallier. Patients were divided into three groups. Group I compared 13 patients with no active ability to externally rotate either with the arm at the side or in elevation. These patients showed degeneration of the infraspinatus and teres minor of at least stage 3 or stage 4. Group II compared 12 patients with no active ability to externally rotate with the arm by the side but capable of doing so with the arm elevated. These patients showed stage 3 or stage 4 degeneration of the infraspinatus but none of the teres minor. Group III comprised 29 patients with the ability to externally rotate in both positions. These patients showed stage 2 or less degeneration of the infraspinatus and stage 1 or less of the teres minor. Teres minor dysfunction was associated with a positive hornblower's sign, or the inability to externally rotate the arm in an elevated positive hornblower's sign, or the inability to externally rotate the arm in a elevated position (Fig. 7).

A study specifically looking at the lift-off test confirmed the selective activation of the subscapularis and found that placing the hand in the midlumbar region was more evocative of subscapularis activity than placing the hand lower, in the region of the buttocks. However, another study of 15 subjects, including five subjects who also underwent subscapular nerve blocks and two patients who had surgically confirmed subscapularis tears, was less convincing. In the normal subjects, marked EMG activity was noted from the latissimus dorsi and teres major (40% to 85% maximal voluntary contraction) in addition to the subscapularis. Subjects who underwent subscapular nerve blocks could do most versions of the lift-off test despite electrical silence of the subscapularis. Similarly, the two patients with subscapularis tears were also able to perform most versions of the test.

The ability to place the arm in selective positions that distinguish one muscle function from others is not limited to rotator cuff muscles. A report studied five patients with axillary nerve palsies after traumatic anterior dislocation of the shoulder for the ability to extend the arm. The inability to achieve posterior humerothoracic elevation, also called the "swallow tail sign," is a good test for posterior deltoid function (Fig. 8).

The Biceps

EMG studies of biceps function at the shoulder have produced somewhat conflicting results. One study of the biceps, brachioradialis, and supraspinatus looked at elevation in multiple planes in both internal and external rotation. Forty-four shoulders were tested, 14 with documented cuff tears. Subjects wore a fixed elbow brace in neutral and 100° of flexion. The arm was unweighted. No significant activity was noted during any shoulder motion. This study concluded that the biceps does not function significantly at the shoulder.

Another EMG study of 11 normal men tested isometric shoulder elevation in 24 different positions of flexion and abduction, with and without internal and external rotation. Tests were done with the elbow in a brace at either 0° or 90° of flexion and neutral rotation. In this study, the biceps was active, more active in external rotation than internal, but not significantly different in elbow flexion than in extension. The difference

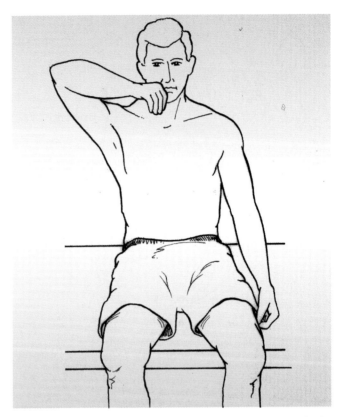

Figure 7 The "hornblower's sign, " or inability to achieve active external rotation in elevation, reflects dysfunction of the teres minor.

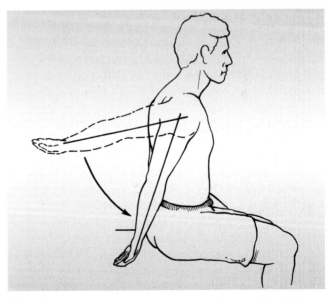

Figure 8 Ability to actively extend the arm posterior to the plane of the body is a function of the posterior deltoid. Deficiency of this muscle produces the "swallow tail sign," the inability to achieve posterior elevation.

between these studies may be the force production required of the subjects during testing.

Another EMG study compared 40 patients with full-thickness rotator cuff tears with 40 normal individuals, looking at scapular-plane elevation with the elbow ex-

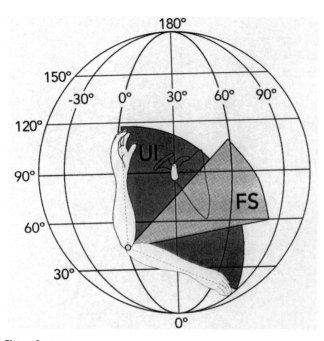

Figure 9 Global diagram of the humeroscapular coordinate system showing arcs of humeral rotation with the arm at 45° of elevation in the scapular plane, comparing the uninvolved (UI) shoulder to the frozen shoulder (FS). On average, patients showed a glenohumeral arc that was 31% that of the normal side. *(Reproduced with permission from Harryman D: Frozen shoulder, in Matsen FA III, Rockwood C (eds): The Shoulder, ed 2. Philadelphia, PA, WB Saunders, 1998.)*

tended and the forearm pronated. Tests were repeated with the addition of a 1-kg weight to the wrist. Some of the patients with cuff pain received a lidocaine injection if pain was an issue. Normal subjects did not recruit the biceps with arm elevation, but 14 of the 40 patients with cuff tears did. The authors suggest that the biceps plays a supplemental role in shoulders with rotator cuff tears.

Kinematics of Clinical Conditions

Rotator Cuff Tears and Instability

A better understanding of normal shoulder motion has directed attention to the study of patients with known anatomic derangement. Examples of strength deficits secondary to lost muscle function were cited earlier. The extent to which clinical conditions affect normal kinematics and range of motion is also of interest. A radiographic study of scapular-plane elevation compared 15 patients with stage 2 impingement and 20 patients with rotator cuff tears with 12 individuals with normal shoulders. Superior translation of the humeral head and increased scapulothoracic motion were noted in both patient groups. No significant difference was noted between the impingement and rotator cuff tear groups in the amount of superior translation of the humeral head.

Another radiographic study examined similar kinematic variables in the scapular plane and in the horizontal plane, both preoperatively and postoperatively.

Eighteen patients with confirmed traumatic anterior instability and 15 patients with cuff tears were compared with 6 normal control subjects. Seven of the 18 patients with instability and all of the patients with cuff tears demonstrated superior translation of the humeral head on the glenoid. In the horizontal plane, 14 of the 18 patients with instability and none of the patients with cuff tears demonstrated abnormal anterior translation of the humeral head on the glenoid. Both groups demonstrated abnormal scapulothoracic motion when compared with the controls. Two years after surgery, 12 of the patients with instability and 14 of the patients with cuff tears, all with abnormal kinematics preoperatively, were reevaluated; except for two of the patients with cuff tears, all were found to have normal kinematics in both planes. Scapulothoracic kinematics remained abnormal for the patients with instability but normalized for the patients with cuff tears.

Yet another radiographic study of patients with MRI-documented rotator cuff tears compared scapular-plane elevation in symptomatic and asymptomatic patients with normal control subjects. Both rotator cuff tear groups showed progressive superior translation of the humeral head on the glenoid with increasing arm elevation. The normal group maintained a constant center of rotation with respect to the glenoid center line. This study concluded that abnormal kinematics do not necessarily lead to symptoms.

Stiffness

Stiffness develops as a result of a variety of causes, most of which emanate from the glenohumeral joint. In vivo and in vitro methods for measuring motion specifically at this joint are, therefore, important. Clinical experience suggests that these conditions can nearly obliterate glenohumeral motion, but little information is available that quantifies the extent to which this is true. A study of frozen shoulders at the time of presentation evaluated the arc of glenohumeral motion possible with the humerus positioned at 45° of scapular-plane elevation and found that motion in the frozen shoulder was restricted to 31% of that of the normal side (95% confidence interval, 50% that of the normal side) (Fig. 9). Quantifying the arc of glenohumeral motion in this manner may be useful in developing an objective definition of frozen shoulder and also providing a reference point to assess the effectiveness of treatment.

In arthritis, the anatomy and motion of the articular surfaces are altered. Treatment of advanced cases includes prosthetic replacement. A cadaveric study of glenohumeral motion found that altering the dimensions of the humeral articular surface significantly affected the kinematics. Increasing humeral head thickness by 5 mm diminished the glenohumeral range by 30° to 40° and resulted in obligate translation at the glenohumeral joint earlier in ROM. Others have estimated a similar reduction in ROM by decreasing humeral head thickness by the same amount on the basis of loss of joint excursion. Additionally, research using several commonly available prosthetic systems has found it difficult to recreate the anatomy within this range. The press-fit systems analyzed all tended to position the prosthetic humeral head superiorly and laterally relative to its original anatomy. A theoretical analysis based on an established shoulder model found that superior and lateral displacement of the articular surface significantly diminished the lever arms of the shoulder abductors.

Kinesiology of Sports

EMG combined with high-speed cinematography has been used to study a number of athletic activities. The overhand baseball throw has been the most extensively studied. More recently, muscle firing patterns during the windmill softball pitch were studied in 10 collegiate-level female softball pitchers. The kinematics of the windmill pitch were found to be markedly different from that of the overhand throw. The majority of arm motion was nearly in the plane of the body. At ball release, the arm simultaneously contacted the lateral hip and thigh, decelerating the arm. EMG shows teres minor function to be distinct from that of the infraspinatus, with the former becoming active as the arm elevates above the horizontal position.

In another study, the serving and spike motions of 15 professional or collegiate-level volleyball players were examined. The movements are similar, but the spike involves a jumping motion. Both are analogous to the throwing motion, but instead of ball release, the volleyball motions, like the tennis serve, involve ball impact, which begins a deceleration phase. Follow-through was defined to begin when the arm was perpendicular to the body. During the cocking phase, the infraspinatus and teres minor are both active. In acceleration, however, these muscles are used differently; the activity of the teres minor remains high, whereas that of the infraspinatus declines.

Rehabilitation

Passive ROM is an important part of many postoperative rehabilitation programs. This is especially true for the supraspinatus in rotator cuff surgery. A study of 10

normal subjects looked at seven modes of exercise: continuous passive motion (CPM), pulley, pendulum, self-assisted bar raise using contralateral arm power, self-assisted internal and external rotation, therapist-assisted scapular-plane elevation, and therapist-assisted internal and external rotation. For all muscle groups tested, the pulley showed more activity than the CPM machine. The supraspinatus muscle in pulley exercises averaged 17.6% of maximal activity and 8.7% for self-assisted bar raise, compared with 5% for the CPM machine. These findings contradict the notion that many so-called passive exercises do not involve activation of the rotator cuff muscles.

Summary

The description of shoulder motion requires above all a clear definition of reference axes for the involved skeletal segments. Rotational positions can be represented in a variety of ways but are most clearly presented graphically. Humerothoracic elevation in the normal adult man usually averages about 150° when referenced to the thorax. In this position the humerus is elevated about 90° in the plane of the scapula. In the normal shoulder, the humeral head remains centered on the glenoid through the mid range of motion and only begins to translate when the ligaments and capsule come under tension. The prime movers of the shoulder are used in ways consistent with their mechanical line of action. The muscles of the rotator cuff serve multiple functions, often simultaneously, acting as prime movers, stabilizers, and axial rotators of the arm. The directional nature of the prime movers may be exploited to selectively test for specific deficits of rotator cuff function. Abnormal kinematics may be associated with these deficits but are not always symptomatic.

Annotated Bibliography

Description of Shoulder Positions

Meskers CG, van der Helm FC, Rozendaal LA, Rozing PM: In vivo estimation of the glenohumeral joint rotation center from scapular bony landmarks by linear regression. *J Biomech* 1998;31:93-96.

Five bony landmarks from 36 cadaveric scapulae were digitized and related to the projected joint center of rotation. A regression procedure was then applied to determine the joint center of rotation in 10 volunteers for tracking the arm with an electromagnetic tracking device with 6° of freedom.

Normal Shoulder Motion

de Groot JH, van Woensel W, van der Helm FC: Effect of different arm loads on the position of the scapula in abduction postures. *Clin Biomech* 1999;14:309-314.

This study identifies a consistency of shoulder postures that can be defined as the three-dimensional shoulder rhythm. This rhythm appears not to be significantly affected by the level of external gravitational load.

Novotny JE, Nichols CE, Beynnon BD: Normal kinematics of the unconstrained glenohumeral joint under coupled moment loads. *J Shoulder Elbow Surg* 1998;7: 629-639.

The authors developed a novel testing mechanism to apply unconstrained, coupled moments to the distal humerus using compressed nitrogen. For adduction-abduction and flexion-extension, the humeral head translates in a direction consistent with the concept of capsular constraint.

Muscle Function

Arwert HJ, de Groot J, Van Woensel WW, Rozing PM: Electromyography of shoulder muscles in relation to force direction. *J Shoulder Elbow Surg* 1997;6:360-370.

This EMG study defined two important parameters of muscle activity: the principal action of a muscle is the direction of maximal EMG activity, and the mechanical action is the direction of the mechanical line of pull of the muscle. Most prime movers were maximally active in mechanically favorable directions.

Hertel R, Ballmer FT, Lambert SM, Gerber C: Lag signs in the diagnosis of rotator cuff rupture. *J Shoulder Elbow Surg* 1996;5:307-313.

This study reports on the clinical examination of 100 consecutive patients with rotator cuff symptomatology evaluated with three tests: ERLS, drop sign, and IRLS. The ERLS and drop sign had a 100% positive predictive value for a tear of the posterosuperior rotator cuff. The IRLS was more sensitive and equally specific to the lift-off test and had a positive predictive value of 97% for a tear of the subscapularis.

Hertel R, Lambert SM, Ballmer FT: The deltoid extension lag sign for diagnosis and grading of axillary nerve palsy. *J Shoulder Elbow Surg* 1998;7:97-99.

In this report, five patients with axillary nerve palsies after traumatic anterior dislocation of the shoulder were studied for the ability to extend the arm. The inability to achieve posterior elevation was shown to be a good test for posterior deltoid function.

Kido T, Itoi E, Konno N, Sano A, Urayama M, Sato K: Electromyographic activities of the biceps during arm elevation in shoulders with rotator cuff tears. *Acta Orthop Scand* 1998;69:575-579.

This EMG study of the biceps in 40 patients with full-thickness rotator cuff tears and 40 normal control subjects found that normal subjects did not recruit the biceps with arm elevation while 14 of the 40 patients with cuff tears did.

Kuechle DK, Newman SR, Itoi E, Morrey BF, An KN: Shoulder muscle moment arms during horizontal flexion and elevation. *J Shoulder Elbow Surg* 1997;6: 429-439.

This study used the tendon-excursion/joint-displacement technique to calculate instantaneous shoulder muscle moment arms during horizontal flexion and elevation in multiple planes. The middle and anterior deltoids were found to have the largest elevator moment arms, each more than twice that of the supraspinatus. The supraspinatus was more important as an elevator early in the motion.

Lee SB, Kim KJ, O'Driscoll SW, Morrey BF, An KN: Dynamic glenohumeral stability provided by the rotator cuff muscles in the mid-range and end-range of motion: A study in cadavera. *J Bone Joint Surg Am* 2000;82:849-857.

Ten cadaveric shoulders were studied, comparing the dynamic stability afforded by the rotator cuff muscles in the apprehension position of anterior instability with the stability afforded in the midrange. In both mid- and end-range positions, the rotator cuff muscles were confirmed to be primarily compressors, as the compressive components were far greater than the shear components regardless of humeral rotation.

Stefko JM, Jobe FW, VanderWilde RS, Carden E, Pink M: Electromyographic and nerve block analysis of the subscapularis liftoff test. *J Shoulder Elbow Surg* 1997;6: 347-355.

Fifteen subjects underwent EMG during four versions of the lift-off test. Five subjects that underwent subscapular nerve blocks and two patients with surgically confirmed subscapularis tears were also studied. Marked EMG activity was noted from the latissimus dorsi and teres major in normal subjects. Subjects that received nerve blocks and the two patients with tears could perform most versions of the lift-off test.

Walch G, Boulahia A, Calderone S, Robinson AH: The 'dropping' and 'hornblower's' signs in evaluation of rotator-cuff tears. *J Bone Joint Surg Br* 1998;80:624-628.

Fifty-four patients with combined tears of the supraspinatus and infraspinatus had CT arthrography graded according to the classification system of Goutallier. Hornblower's sign was strongly associated with degeneration of the teres minor. The drop sign (loss of active external rotation with the arm at the side) was strongly associated with degeneration of the infraspinatus.

Yamaguchi K, Riew KD, Galatz LM, Syme JA, Neviaser RJ: Biceps activity during shoulder motion: An electromyographic analysis. *Clin Orthop* 1997;336:122-129.

In this EMG study of the biceps, brachioradialis, and supraspinatus, 44 shoulders were tested, 14 with documented cuff tears. No significant biceps activity was noted during shoulder motion.

Kinematics of Clinical Conditions

de Leest O, Rozing PM, Rozendaal LA, van der Helm FC: Influence of glenohumeral prosthesis geometry and placement on shoulder muscle forces. *Clin Orthop* 1996; 330:222-233.

This theoretical analysis of the shoulder model showed the effect of altering various anatomic parameters. Displacing the humeral head laterally and superiorly in relation to the humeral shaft was found to be most problematic. Displacements in this direction diminished the size of the lever arms of the main shoulder abductors.

Paletta GA, Warner JJ, Warren RF, Deutsch A, Altchek DW: Shoulder kinematics with two-plane x-ray evaluation in patients with anterior instability or rotator cuff tearing. *J Shoulder Elbow Surg* 1997;6:516-527.

In this radiographic study of scapular- and horizontal-plane kinematics in patients with anterior instability and other patients with rotator cuff tears, both groups demonstrated abnormal glenohumeral kinematics and scapulothoracic motion in comparison to the controls. Two years after surgery, all but two of the patients with cuff tears were found to have normal kinematics.

Pearl ML, Kurutz S: Geometric analysis of commonly used prosthetic systems for proximal humeral replacement. *J Bone Joint Surg Am* 1999;81:660-671.

This computer optimization study compared the coronal-plane anatomy of 21 cadaveric specimens to the geometry of four press-fit prosthetic systems. The mismatch between prosthetic systems studied and normal anatomy obligated a superior and lateral displacement of the center of rotation and articular surface.

Yamaguchi K, Sher JS, Andersen WK, et al: Glenohumeral motion in patients with rotator cuff tears: A comparison of asymptomatic and symptomatic shoulders. *J Shoulder Elbow Surg* 2000;9:6-11.

This radiographic study looked at scapular-plane elevation in both symptomatic and asymptomatic MRI-documented cuff tears. Both rotator cuff tear groups showed progressive superior translation of the humeral head in contrast to the normal group.

Kinesiology of Sports

Maffet MW, Jobe FW, Pink MM, Brault J, Mathiyakom W: Shoulder muscle firing patterns during the windmill softball pitch. *Am J Sports Med* 1997;25:369-374.

In this EMG and high-speed cinematographic study of 10 collegiate-level female softball pitchers, kinematics showed arm motion nearly in the plane of the body, with ball release simultaneous with the arm contacting the lateral hip and thigh, which decelerated the arm. Electromyographically, the teres minor distinguished itself from the infraspinatus, which becomes active as the arm elevates above the horizontal position.

Rokito AS, Jobe FW, Pink MM, Perry J, Brault J: Electromyographic analysis of shoulder function during the volleyball serve and spike. *J Shoulder Elbow Surg* 1998; 7:256-263.

This study examines the serving and spike motions of 15 professional or collegiate-level athletes. The movements are similar, but the spike involves a jumping motion; both are analogous to the throwing motion. During the cocking phase, the infraspinatus and teres minor are both active. In acceleration, these muscles are used differently; activity of the teres minor remains high, whereas the activity of the infraspinatus declines.

Classic Bibliography

Inman VT, Saunders JB dec M, Abbott LC: Observations on the function of the shoulder joint. *J Bone Joint Surg Am* 1944;26:1-30.

Otis JC, Jiang CC, Wickiewicz TL, Peterson MG, Warren RF, Santner TJ: Changes in the moment arms on the rotator cuff and deltoid muscles with abduction and rotation. *J Bone Joint Surg Am* 1994;76:667-676.

Pearl ML, Jackins S, Lippitt SB, Sidles JA, Matsen FA III: Humeroscapular positions in a shoulder range-of-motion examination. *J Shoulder Elbow Surg* 1992;1: 296-305.

Pearl ML, Perry J, Torburn L, Gordon LH: An electromyographic analysis of the shoulder during cones and planes of arm motion. *Clin Orthop* 1992;284: 116-127.

Pearl ML, Sidles JA, Lippitt SB, Harryman DT II, Matsen FA III: Codman's paradox: Sixty years later. *J Shoulder Elbow Surg* 1992;1:113-118.

Chapter 5

Basic Science Considerations in Glenohumeral Arthroplasty and Proximal Humeral Fractures

Brian D. Cameron, MD

Matthew L. Ramsey, MD

Gerald R. Williams, Jr, MD

Glenohumeral Anatomy

The goal of glenohumeral arthroplasty, as for any prosthetic reconstruction, is to recreate normal anatomy as much as possible. This requires a working knowledge of the important anatomic parameters of the glenohumeral joint. Relevant glenohumeral anatomic relationships include humeral head size and shape, humeral head position (ie, offset, retroversion, and height), humeral neck-shaft angle, glenoid size and shape, glenoid offset, and lateral glenohumeral offset.

Humeral Head Size and Shape

The thickness (or neck length) and radius of curvature of the articular segment define the size and surface arc of the humeral head (Fig. 1). The average radius of curvature of the humeral head is 24 mm and the average thickness of the humeral head is 19 mm. The radius of curvature and thickness correlate with humeral shaft length and patient size, but the ratio of thickness to radius of curvature is fairly constant at 0.7 to 0.9, regardless of patient height or shaft size. Although the size of the humeral head varies widely, most (85%) fall within eight fixed combinations of radius of curvature and thickness (Table 1). Combinations consisting of a large radius but small thickness, or small radius and large thickness, are not common in normal shoulders. The central 80% of the articular surface is spherical in both the coronal and axial planes, whereas the peripheral 20% is elliptical, with the axial radius of curvature approximately 2 mm smaller than that of the coronal plane.

Humeral Head Offset, Retroversion, and Height

The center of rotation of the humeral head is not coincident with the axis of the humeral shaft. Rather, the axis of the humeral shaft (or orthopaedic axis) is 7 to 9 mm lateral (in the coronal plane) and 2 to 4 mm ante-

rior (in the axial plane) to the center of rotation of the humeral head (Fig. 2). Alternatively stated, the geometric center of the humeral head is eccentrically located, or offset, in relation to the axis of the humeral canal. Humeral retroversion averages 29.8° (range, 10° to 55°). The superior articular surface of the humeral head usually lies 8 to 10 mm superior to the highest point of the greater tuberosity (Fig. 1, *A*).

Humeral Neck-Shaft Angle

The neck-shaft angle is the angle subtended by the central axis of the humeral shaft and the base of the articular segment. Although the average neck-shaft angle is 40° to 45°, it varies widely, from 30° to 55°. There is also a direct correlation between head size and neck-shaft angle (ie, larger humeral heads exhibit larger neck-shaft angles).

TABLE 1	Humeral Head Sizes*		
Radius of curvature (mm)	Thickness (mm)		
	15-17	18-20	21-24
19-20	10	3	2
21-22	7	18	3
23-24	0	9	18
25-26	0	8	14
27-28	0	0	4

* Numbers inside box comprise the eight fixed combinations of humeral head radius of curvature and thickness

(Reproduced with permission from Iannotti JP, Gabriel JP, Schneck SL, Evans BG, Misea S: The normal glenohumeral relationships: An anatomical study of one hundred and forty shoulders. J Bone Joint Surg Am 1992;74:491-500.)

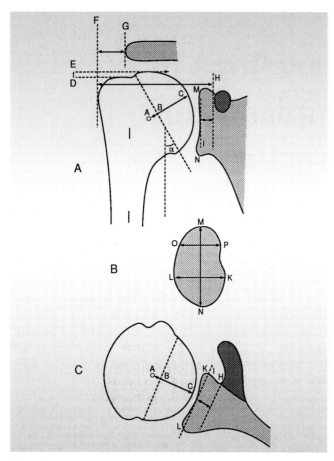

Figure 1 A and **B,** Glenohumeral relationships. Radius of curvature of humeral head (A to C); thickness of humeral head (B to C); glenoid offset (H to I); joint line (M to N, or K to L); lateral glenohumeral offset (F to H); acromial to greater tuberosity distance (F to G); superior articular surface to greater tuberosity distance (D to E). **C,** Superoinferior and anteroposterior dimensions of the glenoid. *(Reproduced with permission from Iannotti JP, Gabriel JP, Schneck SL, Evans BG, Misra S: The normal glenohumeral relationships: An anatomical study of one hundred and forty shoulders. J Bone Joint Surg Am 1992;74:491-500.)*

Glenoid Size and Shape

The articular surface of the glenoid has a pear-shaped appearance (Fig. 1, *C*), being wider in the inferior anteroposterior dimension (mean, 29 mm) than the superior anteroposterior dimension (mean, 23 mm). The average superoinferior dimension of the glenoid is 39 mm. The size and shape of the normal glenoid is closely correlated with the size (radius of curvature) of the humeral head.

The articular cartilage is thin at the center of the glenoid and increases in thickness toward the periphery. The subchondral bone of the glenoid is relatively flat. Therefore, the radius of curvature of the articular surface is smaller than the radius of the subchondral bone and more closely resembles the humeral head radius. The relationship between the humeral head radius and the glenoid radius shows significant individual variation. However, on average, the humeral head radius of curvature is within 2 mm of the glenoid radius.

Glenoid Offset

The deepest portion of the glenoid articular surface lies within 5 mm of the lateral base of the coracoid process. This glenoid offset is relatively constant regardless of patient size, humeral head size, or humeral shaft size. The distance between the lateral base of the coracoid process and the glenoid articular surface determines the location of the glenohumeral joint line (Fig. 1, *A*). Glenoid erosion in arthritic glenohumeral joints may complicate identifying the exact location of the joint line during prosthetic arthroplasty, but under these circumstances the joint line may also be located at the medial one third of the distance from the middle of the coracoid base to the middle of the humeral canal.

Lateral Glenohumeral Offset

The distance from the joint line to the greater tuberosity (insertion of the rotator cuff) determines the normal soft-tissue tension and the moment arm of the deltoid and rotator cuff muscles. This distance in the normal shoulder is called the lateral glenohumeral offset. Pathologic conditions that result in cartilage loss (glenohumeral arthritis) will distort (medialize) the joint line. Therefore, the lateral glenohumeral offset is best defined from the lateral base of the coracoid to the lateral margin of the greater tuberosity (Fig. 1, *A*). The lateral glenohumeral offset averages 54 to 57 mm (range, 43 to 68 mm).

The distance from the lateral edge of the acromion to the lateral extent of the greater tuberosity (Fig. 1, *A*) correlates with the lateral glenohumeral offset and averages 17 mm (range, 15 to 21 mm). This distance is easily measured intraoperatively. Both the lateral glenohumeral offset and the distance from the greater tuberosity to the acromion are directly related to the size of the humeral head and the height of the individual.

Biomechanics of the Glenohumeral Joint

Forward elevation in the scapular plane consists of glenohumeral motion and scapulothoracic motion in a ratio of 2:1, respectively. The first 30° of elevation is primarily glenohumeral, while the remaining glenohumeral and scapulothoracic contributions are nearly equal, with a ratio of 5:4. The humeral head translates superiorly less than 2 to 3 mm during elevation of the arm.

The glenohumeral joint does not bear as much weight as do the lower extremity joints. However, as the arm is elevated with the elbow extended, a substantial lever arm is created. The maximum joint reactive force of 89% of body weight occurs at 90° of abduction. This decreases to 40% of body weight at 60° and 150° of abduction. The addition of a 5-kg weight to the arm abducted to 90° results in a joint reaction force that is

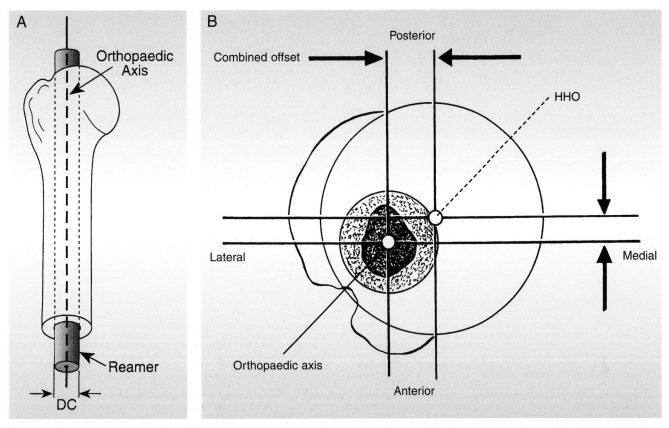

Figure 2 A, The intramedullary canal defines the orthopaedic axis of the humerus. DC = Diameter of the canal. *(Reproduced with permission from Matsen FA III, Lippitt SB, Sidles JA, Harryman DT II: Smoothness, in Practical Evaluation and Management of the Shoulder. Philadelphia, PA, WB Saunders, 1994, pp 151-219.)* **B,** The humeral head offset defines the center of rotation of the humeral head and is posterior and medial to the central axis of the intramedullary canal. *(Reproduced with permission from Boileau P, Walch G: The three-dimensional geometry of the proximal humerus: Implications for surgical technique and prosthetic design. J Bone Joint Surg Br 1997;79:857-865.)*

2.5 times body weight. The direction of the joint force changes with respect to shoulder abduction. At the side, the force is directed inferiorly. A superior shear force is seen at 60° of abduction; this changes to a compressive force at 90° and returns to an inferiorly directed shear force at 150° of abduction. The high shear forces occurring between 30° and 60° of abduction may account for the high rate of glenoid loosening in the absence of a functional rotator cuff and with the use of constrained glenoid components.

Articular Conformity

The humeral articular surface is of uniform thickness throughout, while the glenoid articular cartilage is thicker peripherally than at the center. The labrum extends the arc of the glenoid and deepens the socket, but it does not change the radius of curvature. Articular conformity, or congruence, is determined by the difference between the radius of curvature of the glenoid and that of the humerus (Fig. 3). A less congruent joint is one in which the radius of curvature is greater in the glenoid than in the humeral head. In the normal shoulder, the radius of curvature of the humeral head is not more than 2 to 3 mm smaller than that of the glenoid.

Articular Constraint

Articular constraint, defined as the ability of the joint to resist dislocation, is a function of wall height, or glenoid depth, and is independent of articular conformity (Fig. 3). Glenoid depth essentially refers to the amount of the humeral head that is covered by the glenoid and labrum. The normal glenoid is more constrained (has greater depth) in the superoinferior direction than in the anteroposterior direction (9 mm compared to 5 mm). Because the amount of the humeral head covered by the glenoid in the coronal (ie, superoinferior) plane is 60% and in the axial (ie, anteroposterior) plane is 46%, overall the glenoid covers 28% of the humeral articular cartilage.

As the humeral head rotates through any given plane, the articular surfaces remain in contact until the humeral head runs out of articular cartilage and the capsule and rotator cuff impinge on the labrum and the rim of the glenoid (internal glenoid impingement). In the coronal plane, the humeral head arc of 159° is covered by 96° of glenoid, leaving 63° uncovered and available for motion before contact occurs between nonarticular structures. In the transverse plane, 160° of humeral arc is covered by 74° of glenoid, leaving 86° uncovered and available for motion. In obligate exter-

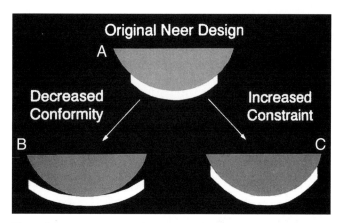

Figure 3 Conformity refers to the difference between the humeral head radius of curvature and the glenoid radius. Glenoid B is less conforming than is glenoid A. Constraint is determined by glenoid wall height (depth) and is independent of conformity. Glenoid C has a greater wall height than either A or B and is therefore more constrained. Two articulations may demonstrate identical conformity but different constraint. *(Reproduced with permission from Iannotti JP, Williams GR: Biomechanics of the glenohumeral joint: Influence on shoulder arthroplasty, in Disorders of the Shoulder: Diagnosis and Management. Philadelphia, PA, Lippincott-Williams & Wilkins, 1999, pp 471-483.)*

nal rotation of the humeral head during elevation, additional humeral cartilage is available to articulate with the glenoid, allowing 160° of abduction.

Glenohumeral Translations

The humerus can be moved on the glenoid by either active or passive joint positioning. During active joint positioning, coordinated contraction of the deltoid, rotator cuff, scapular rotators, and other shoulder muscles results in glenohumeral motion. The compressive effect of the rotator cuff muscles resists translation of the humeral head and encourages rotational motion. Consequently, humeral head translations during active joint positioning are small (approximately 2 mm in the superoinferior and anteroposterior directions) and are determined by articular surface conformity and rotator cuff muscular forces. The center of rotation is within 1 to 3 mm of the geometric center of the humeral head. Joints with a larger radial mismatch experience more humeral translation.

The range of rotational motion during passive joint positioning is larger than that during active joint positioning and is associated with greater humeral translation. Anteroposterior and superoinferior passive translations are four times higher and two times higher than active translations, respectively. This humeral translation is obligate in nature, independent of conformity, and related to tightening of the capsular ligaments (wrap length). Large passive translations are observed at the end range of motion and occur in a direction opposite to the portion of the capsule that becomes taut. For example, passive external rotation of the abducted arm tightens the anterior band of the inferior

glenohumeral ligament and leads to obligate posterior translation of the humeral head.

Active and passive translations over the midrange of glenohumeral motion, when capsular tension is less important, are nearly equal (Fig. 4, *A*). In the midrange of active or passive motion, the humeral head translates from 0 to 2 mm. At the end range of motion, capsular tightening occurs and humeral head translations may approach 10 to 12 mm (Fig. 4, *B*).

Glenohumeral Arthroplasty

Humeral Component

Selection of a humeral head size requires a combination of humeral head radius of curvature and head thickness that maximizes the humeral surface area available for contact. Most humeral heads can be reconstructed to within 2 mm of their native dimensions using eight fixed combinations of radius of curvature and thickness. Important relationships to consider when selecting head size include joint line positioning, lateral glenohumeral offset, and the distance from the lateral acromial edge to the lateral extent of the greater tuberosity.

Oversizing the humeral head will increase the lateral glenohumeral offset. Although the moment arm of the deltoid and rotator cuff will increase, excessive tightening of the soft-tissue envelope (overstuffing the joint) will result in decreased range of motion or subscapularis rupture. Overstuffing the joint will also lead to earlier obligate translation of the humeral head on the prosthetic glenoid. A head with an extremely long neck relative to the radius of curvature will have the same result.

Undersizing the humeral head will shorten the lateral humeral offset and weaken the deltoid and rotator cuff by decreasing the moment arm (Fig. 5). Excessive laxity in this setting also may lead to instability. A head size that is too small will also decrease the available humeral surface area and will result in internal impingement of the proximal humerus and rotator cuff on the glenoid at the end range of motion, resulting in limited range of motion. A 5-mm reduction in humeral head thickness results in a 24° loss of coronal plane rotation from an original coronal humeral arc of 63° (Fig. 6). Appropriate offset can usually be achieved by selecting a head size that places the lateral margin of the greater tuberosity approximately 1.5 to 2 cm lateral to the lateral margin of the acromion.

Humeral head modularity offers some advantages by increasing the available number of humeral head sizes without a concomitant increase in humeral stems. Modularity also facilitates revision arthroplasty by allowing removal of the head without removing the stem. Disadvantages include dissociation of the humeral head from the stem and the potential loss of articular surface area.

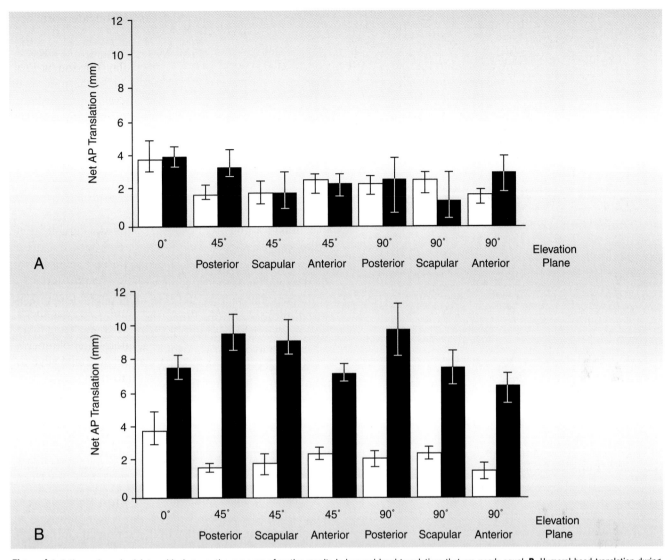

Figure 4 A, Active and passive joint positioning over the same arc of motion results in humeral head translations that are nearly equal. **B,** Humeral head translation during active joint positioning averages 1 to 2 mm (open bars). With passive joint positioning, humeral head translation is significantly greater (shaded bars). *(Reproduced with permission from Iannotti JP, Williams GR: Total shoulder arthroplasty: Factors influencing prosthetic design. Orthop Clin North Am 1998;29:377-391.)*

Humeral head dissociation is a function of many factors, including taper surface geometry and taper interface quality. The presence of even small amounts of fluid or blood in the taper interface can decrease the uncoupling force in a reverse Morse taper by 50% to 66%.

Loss of articular surface area can occur with some modular humeral designs that incorporate a large gap between the modular humeral head and the stem collar (Fig. 7). A thick collar also may result in substantial loss of articular surface area. When intra-articular space is lost to nonarticular design features, the reduction in humeral surface area leads to a substantial loss of full articular contact area. The range of motion available before contact occurs between nonarticular portions of the humerus and glenoid (ie, internal glenoid impingement) is also limited.

Placement of the humeral head on the cut surface of the humeral metaphysis is important in determining soft-tissue balance and maximizing the arc of glenohumeral rotation. Optimal prosthetic design and placement of the humeral head require an understanding of humeral head offset and the distance from the greater tuberosity to the humeral head. The superior surface of the prosthetic head should be 8 to 10 mm above the top of the greater tuberosity. The prosthetic humeral head should cover the cut surface of the humeral metaphysis without overhanging the anterior or posterior bone edge. In some patients, the axis of rotation of the humeral head is offset with respect to the intramedullary canal. The prosthetic head must then be similarly offset. This can be accomplished in one of two ways. Newer prosthetic designs currently allow the prosthetic humeral head to be placed eccentrically with respect to the humeral stem. If this design feature is not available, the prosthetic stem may be undersized and

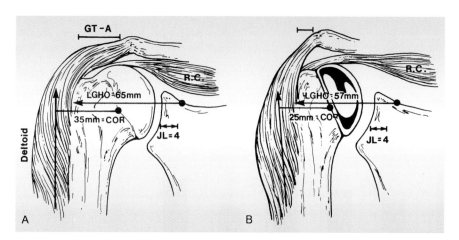

Figure 5 **A,** Normal lateral glenohumeral offset (LGHO). **B,** Undersizing the humeral head results in shortening of the LGHO, and weakening of the deltoid and rotator cuff by decreasing the moment arm. GT-A = Distance from the greater tuberosity to the acromion. COR = Center of rotation. JL=4 = Joint line to the base of the coracoid = 4 mm. RC=rotator cuff. *(Reproduced with permission from Iannotti JP, Williams GR: Total shoulder arthroplasty: Factors influencing prosthetic design. Orthop Clin North Am 1998;29:377-391.)*

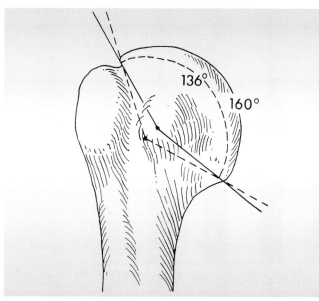

Figure 6 Effect of using a short humeral head prosthesis. Shortening the head by 5 mm reduces the coronal surface arc of the head from 160° to 136°. This leaves only 40° uncovered by the glenoid and available for motion and shortens the lever arm by 5 mm. *(Reproduced with permission from Jobe CM, Iannotti JP: Limits imposed on glenohumeral motion by joint geometry. J Shoulder Elbow Surg 1995;4:281-285.)*

the prosthetic head and stem together may be cemented eccentrically relative to the intramedullary canal.

Humeral head malposition can cause several complications, depending on the direction and magnitude of the malposition. An anteriorly placed prosthetic head may overhang anteriorly and place undue tension on the subscapularis. The uncovered posterior portion of the metaphyseal cut surface may impinge on the posterosuperior glenoid when the arm is placed in abduction and external rotation. This results in decreased range of motion and may increase the risk of glenoid loosening. Inferior malposition of the humeral head will leave the greater tuberosity relatively prominent, increasing the risk of impingement against the acromion.

Neck-Shaft Angle

Some current prosthetic systems feature a variable neck-shaft angle. Once the surgeon removes the humeral head at the articular margin, the neck-shaft angle can be measured intraoperatively. When the measurement falls between sizes, the smaller neck-shaft angle should be selected to avoid varus positioning of the stem.

Fixed neck-shaft angle designs allow anatomic placement of the humeral head only when the neck-shaft angle of the prosthesis exactly matches that of the native humerus. Altering the humeral head radius of curvature, thickness, or offset cannot compensate for a nonanatomic neck-shaft angle. Efforts to do so will change the head volume and place the head in a nonanatomic location.

Varus stem alignment will occur when the neck-shaft angle of the prosthesis is fixed and is less than that of the native humerus (Fig. 8). In this setting, the prosthetic humeral head will be placed inferiorly and medially. The joint will be overstuffed as the center of rotation of the humeral head is shifted medially and the lateral humeral offset is increased. Downsizing the humeral head to avoid overstuffing decreases the humeral articular surface area and allows for internal impingement of the components. This contact results in decreased range of motion and may increase the risk of glenoid loosening. Furthermore, a varus cut will place the humeral head too low relative to the greater tuberosity. A prominent greater tuberosity will impinge on the acromion during abduction and will impinge on the posterosuperior glenoid during abduction and external rotation. Increasing the head size in an effort to restore the relationship of the humeral articular surface above the greater tuberosity will further overstuff the joint. Use of an offset taper will allow superior offset of the humeral head and improve the situation but will still not result in anatomic placement of the humeral head.

Valgus stem alignment results when the prosthetic neck-shaft angle is fixed and is greater than that of the

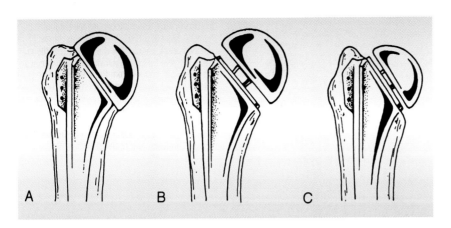

Figure 7 **A,** A humeral prosthesis that rests flush on the humeral metaphysis and matches the neck-shaft angle of the native humerus offers an anatomic reconstruction that maximizes the surface area available for contact with the glenoid. **B,** A modular prosthesis with a large gap between the head and collar will diminish the surface contact area, predispose to internal component impingement, and overstuff the joint. **C,** Undersizing the head to account for the gap will not only worsen the potential for internal impingement but will also leave the greater tuberosity prominent. *(Reproduced with permission from Iannotti JP, Williams GR: Total shoulder arthroplasty: Factors influencing prosthetic design.* Orthop Clin North Am *1998;29:377-391.)*

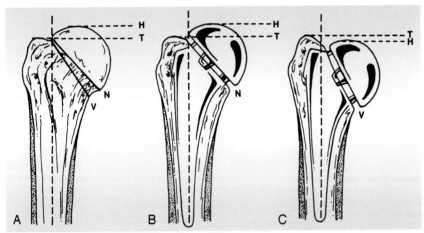

Figure 8 **A,** The distance from the superior articular surface of the humerus (H) to the greater tuberosity (T) is affected by the humeral osteotomy (N = normal, V = varus). **B,** The prosthetic neck-shaft angle is equal to the normal neck-shaft angle, restoring the normal height of the humeral head. **C,** A varus osteotomy cut will lead to inferior malposition of the humeral head and a decreased distance from the greater tuberosity to the head. *(Reproduced with permission from Iannotti JP, Williams GR: Total shoulder arthroplasty: Factors influencing prosthetic design.* Orthop Clin North Am *1998;29:377-391.)*

native humerus. The prosthetic head will be placed superiorly and laterally. Intra-articular space is occupied not only by the prosthetic head but also by the volume of the remaining natural head.

Fixation

The rate of clinical (symptomatic) loosening and failure is low (1% to 2%) for both cemented and cementless humeral components. Early experience with cementless humeral stems revealed a very low rate of symptomatic or radiographic loosening, especially in the absence of a glenoid component. More recent experience has demonstrated a tendency for implants with a low proximal profile to subside radiographically. The clinical significance of this subsidence is not clear. As data from larger follow-up studies become available, aseptic humeral loosening may play an increasing role in the failure and revision rates for total shoulder arthroplasty. Radiolucent lines are frequently noted around humeral stems, but their significance is not completely understood. Cementless humeral stems have a higher rate of radiolucent lines (up to 70%) and subsidence (49% to 53%) than do cemented stems (less than 15% and less than 1%, respectively). Paralleling the experience with total hip and knee arthroplasty, a recent report clearly demonstrates that polyethylene particulate-induced osteolysis contributed

to aseptic clinical loosening of a cementless humeral stem.

The mode of fixation affects the placement of the humeral stem and, potentially, the humeral head. Press-fit stems are designed to have distal circumferential endosteal contact. Press fitting of a prosthesis with a fixed neck-shaft angle eliminates all but two of the six degrees of freedom for humeral component placement. The two variables under the surgeon's control are the height and the stem version. Prosthetic version should attempt to reproduce the normal degree of humeral version. Because humeral version is variable, the superior and posterior rotator cuff insertion should be visualized and palpated prior to humeral head resection to avoid inadvertent cuff injury. Increased retroversion may lead to posterior instability or rotator cuff injury, while increased anteversion may lead to loss of external rotation. Improper version will directly affect stability and range of motion but will have little effect on the lateral glenohumeral offset and soft-tissue tensioning. Altering the humeral version changes the lateral glenohumeral offset by only up to 2 mm.

The requisites for bone ingrowth and stability are not completely understood but probably include maximizing bone contact, minimizing micromotion, and optimizing pore size. Press-fit fixation may not be appropriate

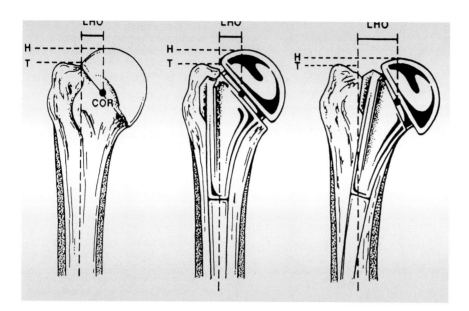

Figure 9 Varus stem positioning will medialize the humeral head and increase the lateral glenohumeral offset, overstuffing the joint. The humeral head will also be inferiorly malpositioned, decreasing the distance from the greater tuberosity to the head. LHO = lateral humeral offset; H = top of the humeral articular surface; T = top of the greater tuberosity; COR = center of rotation. *(Reproduced from Iannotti JP, Williams GR: Total shoulder arthroplasty: Factors influencing prosthetic design. Orthop Clin North Am 1998;29:377-391.)*

in the presence of poor bone quality, inadequate metaphyseal bony support, or a loose fitting canal, which precludes rotational stability of the stem. Impaction grafting techniques may extend the indications for cementless humeral fixation under these circumstances.

The surgeon controls six degrees of freedom in the placement of a cemented stem: medial/lateral positioning, anterior/posterior positioning, varus/valgus alignment (coronal rotation), sagittal (anteroposterior) rotation, proximal/distal positioning (height), and axial rotation (version). If the trial components exhibit inferior malposition of the head, the joint will be overstuffed and the greater tuberosity will be prominent. The surgeon may choose to correct this by undersizing the stem and cementing the final prosthesis superiorly and laterally to restore proper height and lateral glenohumeral offset. Alternatively, the stem may be cemented in the canal and an offset humeral head design used to place the head in a more anatomic position. Varus malposition of the stem (Fig. 9) will medialize the humeral head and increase the lateral humeral offset, resulting in overstuffing of the joint.

Modern cementing techniques such as pulsatile lavage of the canal, drying and packing of the canal, use of a cement restrictor, retrograde filling, vacuum mixing, and cement pressurization have been developed based on experience with total hip and knee arthroplasty. Certain precautions need to be observed, however. Excessive pressurization may cause humeral fracture. Moreover, revision of a solidly cemented humeral stem may be extremely difficult. Recent studies have indicated that cementing proximally without cementing distally may yield similar initial failure strengths. There is currently no consensus on the ideal humeral cementing technique. The merits of modern hip and knee

cementing techniques must be balanced against the lower glenohumeral joint stresses and the potential for humeral fracture during pressurization or revision.

Glenoid Component

Size and Shape
The size and shape of the prosthetic glenoid and the corresponding size of the humeral head will affect the potential for contact between the nonarticular portion of the proximal humerus (greater tuberosity, rotator cuff) and the glenoid. An oval-shaped glenoid may allow earlier contact between the glenoid rim and the non-articular portions of the proximal humerus. A pear-shaped glenoid component with a smaller superior anteroposterior dimension will allow a larger arc of motion before internal component impingement occurs. Factors that predispose to component impingement include decreased humeral surface area (small head size), increased anteroposterior dimension of the glenoid component, nonanatomic (ie, anterior) humeral head placement, and an oval-shaped glenoid.

Ideally, the prosthetic glenoid should have circumferential osseous support. An oval-shaped glenoid component risks overhanging the anterosuperior and posterosuperior margins of the bony glenoid. Humeral head contact with these unsupported portions of the component potentially creates a bending moment at the rim, leading to increased glenoid wear and higher stresses at the point of fixation. If an oval component is used, the size should be chosen in an effort to minimize anterior and posterior overhang of the superior portion of the component.

Asymmetric posterior glenoid erosion is usually associated with osteoarthritis and affects outcomes of hemiarthroplasty as well as total shoulder arthroplasty. Outcome following hemiarthroplasty is correlated with the presence of asymmetric glenoid wear. Hemiarthroplasty for osteoarthritis with an intact rotator cuff yields satisfactory results in 86% of patients with concentric wear of the glenoid. In contrast, hemiarthroplasty in the presence of nonconcentric bone loss (ie, posterior glenoid erosion) results in satisfactory results up to 63% of the time.

Glenoid component failure may be associated with inadequate support of the glenoid component. Concentric reaming provides better osseous support for the glenoid component than other forms of glenoid preparation (curetting, burring). Asymmetric reaming (lowering the high side) of an incongruent glenoid is performed to provide a concentric surface. This strategy is preferred for small to moderate defects (ie, less than 25% to 30%). The glenoid component may tolerate a noncontained defect of up to 33% provided that the remaining bone has been concentrically reamed to provide osseous support that matches the radius of curvature of the glenoid component. Larger noncontained defects can be compensated for with an augmented component or bone graft. Methylmethacrylate is not a good bone substitute in this situation because noncontained cement has been shown to fail under cyclic loading, leading to cement fracture, loss of component support, and failure of the glenoid component.

Although the studies for metal-backed tibial polyethylene components indicate that a thickness of at least 8 mm is required to optimize wear characteristics, the optimal thickness of glenoid polyethylene is not known. A thick glenoid component will lateralize the joint line and theoretically weaken the moment arm of the deltoid and rotator cuff musculature. However, maintaining adequate polyethylene thickness to optimize wear characteristics also is important. A minimum of 4 mm of polyethylene seems desirable. Metal backing adds to this thickness and may require additional reaming to prevent joint overstuffing.

The most physiologic distribution of stress at the component-bone interface is obtained with preservation of the subchondral bone, concentric reaming of the glenoid, and the use of a cemented all-polyethylene glenoid component. A metal-backed glenoid will either decrease available polyethylene thickness or increase lateral humeral offset. Cementing of metal-backed components was originally thought to increase the pullout strength of the glenoid components. However, finite-element analysis demonstrated that metal-backed components produce high nonphysiologic stresses at the fixation interface. This was commensurate with reported clinical results in one series in which half of the clinical glenoid failures occurred in cemented metal-backed glenoids. Some of the early results of cementless tissue ingrowth and press-fit glenoid prostheses have been encouraging, while others demonstrate high failure rates. The potential for increased polyethylene wear rates and dissociation of the polyethylene liner from the metal back have slowed the acceptance of currently available metal-backed designs. The use of alternate bearing surfaces such as metal-on-metal or ceramic-on-ceramic has not been reported at this time. However, early experience with these surfaces in hip and knee arthroplasty may lead to indications for their use in shoulder arthroplasty.

The literature currently supports the use of a cemented all-polyethylene component but is not clear regarding component design. The stair-step and wedge designs tend to provide a more natural stress distribution when compared with keel designs. Among pegged designs, a component with multiple small pegs seems to preserve more bone stock and provides greater resistance to shear forces at the bone-cement interface. Angled-stem designs produce higher stresses inferiorly than do perpendicular stem designs. A recent study using photoelastic plastic demonstrated a more favorable glenoid stress distribution pattern with the pegged design than with the keeled component, with normal and posteriorly directed forces.

Kinematics

Humeral head translation in the normal shoulder is accommodated by elastic deformation of the articular glenoid cartilage and labrum. Unfortunately, polyethylene does not possess the same reversible loading characteristics as do articular cartilage and labrum. Therefore, in a prosthetic shoulder with conforming radii of curvature, any humeral head translation must be accompanied by either glenoid component rim loading or polyethylene cold flow. Rim loading of the glenoid component may result in asymmetric peripheral deformation, increased wear, or glenoid loosening. Conversely, nonconforming articular surfaces allow humeral head translation without rim loading; the amount of translation allowed before rim loading is determined by the degree of nonconformity. However, prosthetic radial mismatch has the theoretical disadvantage of increased wear because of decreased contact area and increased point contact forces (Fig. 10).

After prosthetic arthroplasty, as in the normal joint, humeral head translations are small (less than 2 mm) with active joint positioning. Passive translations are large (5 to 9 mm) and are independent of conformity. The ideal amount of articular mismatch is unknown. However, kinematic studies in a cadaver model demonstrated that a radial mismatch of 3 to 4 mm reproduces the humeral head translation seen in the normal, unreconstructed cadaver shoulder.

Articular conformity also affects the strain characteristics at the fixation interface. As the humeral head translates across the glenoid, compressive strain at the keel is maximum when the humeral head is over the center of the glenoid. Tensile keel strain is maximum when the humeral head is over the opposite glenoid

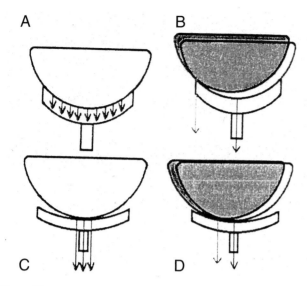

Figure 10 A, A conforming articulation will have an even distribution of contact stresses over the entire glenoid surface. **B,** Translation of the humeral head in a perfectly conforming joint will lead to immediate rim loading. **C,** Prosthetic radial mismatch leads to decreased contact area and increased point contact forces. **D,** In a nonconforming articulation, humeral translation can occur prior to rim loading. *(Reproduced with permission from Flatow EL: Prosthetic design considerations in total shoulder arthroplasty. Semin Arthroplasty 1995;6:233-244.)*

rim. In conforming joints, maximum tensile strain at the keel during rim loading is increased. In nonconforming joints, the maximum compressive strain when the head is centered is increased.

Stability of a prosthetic joint is directly related to wall height rather than conformity. The force required to dislocate the humeral head is the function of constraint (wall height or glenoid depth) and is independent of joint conformity. Changes in the conformity will affect the amount of translation allowed prior to dislocation, but nonconforming prosthetic designs are not at increased risk of dislocating when compared with conforming joints.

Radiolucent Line and Glenoid Loosening

In light of the experience with total hip arthroplasty, a worrisome prospect is the high rate of radiographic lucent lines around the glenoid at the bone-cement interface. Radiolucent lines are seen in up to 69% of radiographs taken in the recovery room. The lines probably represent blood, which eventually develops into nonmineralized fibrous tissue containing numerous histiocytes. A review of the current literature reveals evidence of radiolucent lines in 26% to 100% of glenoid components, with revision rates ranging from 0% to 12.5%. The overall revision rate for the glenoid component (3.2%) is nearly twice that for humeral head arthroplasty (1.8%). A recent long-term follow-up study demonstrated lucent lines in 84% of glenoid components. Progressive radiographic loosening, which occurred in 44% of glenoid components, was associated with a significant increase in pain. Revision was required in 5.6% of patients. Although the presence of

radiolucent lines is not tantamount to impending clinical failure, the prospect of increased glenoid failure rates with longer follow-up is worrisome. Survival analysis for total shoulder arthroplasty is about 95% at 10 years and 84% at 15 years.

No rigid criteria currently exist to evaluate loosening of the glenoid or humeral components. According to recent studies, radiographic analysis has been performed based on methods described for total hip arthroplasty (seven humeral zones, three glenoid zones, width and length of lucency, evidence of subsidence). Progression of a lucency or a complete radiolucent line wider than 1 mm is suggestive of humeral component loosening, while subsidence of the glenoid component, fracture of either the cement or component, or lucency at the cement-prosthesis interface is indicative of glenoid component loosening.

Clinical failure of the glenoid is the primary complication of total shoulder arthroplasty and accounts for 30% of complications. Glenoid component failure rates are increased in certain settings. Rotator cuff deficiency (tear) or dysfunction (as seen in rheumatoid arthritis) is associated with an increased prevalence of glenoid component loosening. In the absence of a functional rotator cuff, the humeral joint reaction force is not directed into the glenoid. Rather, the muscle imbalances between a dysfunctional rotator cuff and a strong deltoid create a dynamic instability that directs the humeral head proximally toward the superior rim of the glenoid. This eccentric loading then contributes to glenoid loosening through the "rocking horse" effect.

Results of Prosthetic Arthroplasty

In most studies, reliable pain relief has been reported following both total shoulder arthroplasty and hemiarthroplasty. A recent prospective study confirmed the assertion of authors of previous studies that glenoid resurfacing provides more reliable pain relief and functional improvement than does hemiarthroplasty. A retrospective review of patients with glenohumeral osteoarthritis who were treated with hemiarthroplasty found that pain had substantially increased in more than 50% of patients after 10 years. Glenoid resurfacing was required in 26% of these patients and provided excellent relief of symptoms.

Poorer results are noted among patients younger than 50 years who undergo either hemiarthroplasty or total shoulder arthroplasty. Long-term pain relief and improvement of motion were reported in a published series. However, half of the patients had an unsatisfactory score according to the rating system. Progressive erosion of the glenoid was seen in 68% of patients undergoing hemiarthroplasty. In an effort to avert these complications, humeral head replacement has been combined with biologic resurfacing (fascia lata or anterior capsule) of the glenoid. Short-term follow-up has revealed good to excellent results in all patients, with no progression of glenoid erosion.

Functional restoration is dependent on the integrity of the deltoid and rotator cuff, as well as the preoperative diagnosis. Total shoulder arthroplasty provides more reliable pain relief and improvement in function in patients with osteoarthritis and an intact rotator cuff. Management of arthritis in patients with a deficient rotator cuff remains controversial. Most authors recommend hemiarthroplasty alone to avoid the risk of glenoid loosening. Others recommend total shoulder arthroplasty, citing better pain relief with the use of a glenoid component.

Constrained prostheses were designed to provide a fulcrum through which the deltoid could drive the shoulder. Component loosening and fracture, dissociation, and periprosthetic fracture have led clinicians to abandon fixed fulcrum devices. There has been revived interest, particularly in Europe, in the use of a constrained prosthesis for the treatment of cuff tear arthropathy among patients with a functioning deltoid. The constrained prosthesis boasts a reverse ball-and-socket joint with the center of rotation deep within the scapula. This medialization of the center of rotation decreases the moment at the prosthetic anchoring. Good short-term results (after 2 years) have been reported in a series of 14 patients who received this implant.

Proximal Humeral Fractures

Blood Supply to the Humeral Head

Multiple vessels contribute to the vascular anatomy of the humeral head. The ascending branch of the anterior humeral circumflex artery is the primary blood supply to the proximal humerus, via the intraosseous continuation of the arcuate artery. The artery continues posteromedially after penetrating the humeral head. A rich extraosseous anastomotic system exists among the anterior humeral circumflex, posterior humeral circumflex, thoracoacromial, subscapular, suprascapular, and profunda brachii arteries. The final common pathway is provided by the anterior lateral branch of the anterior humeral circumflex artery. An intraosseous anastomosis consisting of the anterior humeral circumflex, large metaphyseal arteries that traverse the fused growth plate, and a contribution from the posterior humeral circumflex artery supplies the posterior portion of the greater tuberosity and the posteromedial aspect of the humeral head. Perfusion of the humeral head may persist through this anastomosis despite ligation of the anterior humeral circumflex artery.

Osteonecrosis

Knowledge of the vascular anatomy may be helpful in predicting the risk of osteonecrosis following four-part proximal humerus fractures. The reported rate of osteonecrosis associated with these complex fractures varies from 20% to 100% and relates to the severity of the injury as well as the characteristics of the fracture. Four-part fracture-dislocations have an associated osteonecrosis rate approaching 100%, while valgus-impacted four-part fractures have an osteonecrosis rate of about 20%. In the latter setting, humeral head perfusion may persist through the posteromedial vessels when the head fragment has a soft-tissue (periosteal) attachment to the medial neck.

Surgical Considerations

Nonsurgical treatment of four-part fractures results in functional impairment when associated with residual displacement. Limited open reduction and minimal internal fixation yields a high rate of satisfactory results (75%). Only patients with a malreduction of the fracture have poorer outcomes than those who undergo hemiarthroplasty. Recently, closed reduction and percutaneous pinning of four-part fractures has been advocated in an attempt to avoid jeopardizing the tenuous blood supply to the fragments. The valgus-impacted fracture appears to be more amenable to this technique because the medial portion of the head retains a periosteal hinge that facilitates reduction of the head fragment. Again, functional results are dependent on the quality of the reduction, with an associated osteonecrosis rate of about 10%.

Hemiarthroplasty is performed in most cases of four-part fracture-dislocations, significantly displaced four-part fractures, and in some three-part fractures with extremely poor bone quality. Careful attention should be directed at maintaining appropriate height (8 to 10 mm) of the prosthetic articular surface above the greater tuberosity, appropriate retroversion, and secure fixation of the tuberosities to the humeral shaft. The current results of hemiarthroplasty for proximal humerus fractures are inferior to the results of prosthetic replacement for glenohumeral osteoarthritis.

Annotated Bibliography

Glenohumeral Anatomy

Pearl ML, Volk AG: Coronal plane geometry of the proximal humerus relevant to prosthetic arthroplasty. *J Shoulder Elbow Surg* 1996;5:320-326.

This study measures proximal humeral anatomy in relation to the surgically reamed canal. The coronal humeral head offset was found to be 9.7 mm medial to the intramedullary axis. Prosthetic systems with fixed geometry may produce nonanatomic alterations that have biomechanical consequences.

Biomechanics of the Glenohumeral Joint

Karduna AR, Williams GR, Iannotti JP, Williams JL: Total shoulder arthroplasty biomechanics: A study of the forces and strains at the glenoid component. *J Biomech Eng* 1998;120:92-99.

This cadaveric study examined the effect of glenohumeral conformity and loading patterns on the strains measured at the glenoid keel. The maximum compressive strain is seen when the head is in the center of the glenoid. These strains become tensile as the head is translated toward the rim. Conforming joints develop peak tensile strains 50% greater than those at nonconforming joints.

Karduna AR, Williams GR, Williams JL, Iannotti JP: Kinematics of the glenohumeral joint: Influences of muscle forces, ligamentous constraints, and articular geometry. *J Orthop Res* 1996;14:986-993.

Active and passive translation and rotation were studied in cadaveric glenohumeral joints. Active joint positioning resulted in minimal humeral head translation. Passive positioning over the same range of rotation resulted in similar translations. However, large translations were observed at the extremes of motion during passive positioning. Joint conformity and muscle forces play a role in controlling translations during active motion, while capsular constraint (ligament wrap length) is more important during passive motion.

Karduna AR, Williams GR, Williams JL, Iannotti JP: Glenohumeral joint translations before and after total shoulder arthroplasty: A study in cadavera. *J Bone Joint Surg Am* 1997;79:1166-1174.

Seven cadaveric humeri were studied to determine the patterns of translation in natural and reconstructed joints. Glenohumeral translations during active motion depend on articular conformity. Active translations of the natural joint were most similar to those of the reconstructed joints that had a radial mismatch of 4 mm.

Glenohumeral Arthroplasty

Gartsman GM, Roddey TS, Hammerman SM: Shoulder arthroplasty with or without resurfacing of the glenoid in patients who have osteoarthritis. *J Bone Joint Surg Am* 2000;82:26-34.

Fifty-one shoulders with glenohumeral osteoarthritis were entered into a randomized, prospective study of hemiarthroplasty versus total shoulder arthroplasty. Total shoulder arthroplasty provided superior pain relief. Three patients with a hemiarthroplasty required revision total shoulder arthroplasty.

Karduna AR, Williams GR, Williams JL, Iannotti JP: Joint stability after total shoulder arthroplasty in a cadaver model. *J Shoulder Elbow Surg* 1997;6:506-511.

Prosthetic components were placed in seven cadaveric glenohumeral joints. Variations in joint conformity affected the amount of translation prior to dislocation but did not affect the force required for joint dislocation. Joint stability is directly related to constraint (wall height or glenoid depth) and is independent of joint conformity.

Levine WN, Djurasovic M, Glasson JM, Pollock RG, Flatow EL, Bigliani LU: Hemiarthroplasty for glenohumeral osteoarthritis: Results correlated to degree of glenoid wear. *J Shoulder Elbow Surg* 1997;6:449-454.

The outcome of hemiarthroplasty in 31 patients correlated with the nature of glenoid wear. Patients with concentric erosion had 86% satisfactory results, compared with 63% satisfactory results with nonconcentric wear. Hemiarthroplasty should be reserved for patients with a concentric glenoid, which affords a better fulcrum for motion.

Norris BL, Lachiewicz PF: Modern cement technique and the survivorship of total shoulder arthroplasty. *Clin Orthop* 1996;328:76-85.

The so-called "modern cement" technique was used during 38 Neer II total shoulder arthroplasties in 35 patients with a preoperative diagnosis of osteoarthritis, osteonecrosis, rheumatoid arthritis, or posttraumatic arthritis. Patients were followed for a mean of 5 years (range, 2 to 9.5 years). At the most recent follow-up, 36 shoulders had no or slight pain with activity. The authors concluded that long-term survival of cemented total shoulder arthroplasty components can be improved with meticulous attention to cement technique.

Sperling JW, Cofield RH, Rowland CM: Neer hemiarthroplasty and Neer total shoulder arthroplasty in patients fifty years old or less: Long-term results. *J Bone Joint Surg Am* 1998;80:464-473.

Seventy-four hemiarthroplasties and thirty-four total shoulder arthroplasties were performed in patients younger than 50 years old and followed for a minimum of 5 years. Erosion of the glenoid was found in 46 (68%) of the hemiarthroplasties. Both procedures provided long-term pain relief and functional improvement. However, nearly half of the patients reported an unsatisfactory result according to their rating system.

Torchia ME, Cofield RH, Settergren CR: Total shoulder arthroplasty with the Neer prosthesis: Long-term results. *J Shoulder Elbow Surg* 1997;6:495-505.

Eighty-nine Neer total shoulder replacements were followed for a minimum of 5 years. Radiolucent lines were demonstrated in 84% of patients. Progressive loosening occurred in 44% of patients and was associated with pain; 5.6% of these patients required revision. Subsidence of the humeral component was noted in 49% of press-fit stems and in none of the cemented stems.

Proximal Humeral Fractures

Resch H, Povacz P, Frohlich R, Wambacher M: Percutaneous fixation of three- and four-part fractures of the proximal humerus. *J Bone Joint Surg Br* 1997;79:295-300.

    The authors report that untreated three- and four-part proximal humeral fractures have a poor functional outcome, and the risk for osteonecrosis is increased with open surgery. Percutaneous reduction and fixation was performed on nine patients with three-part fractures and 18 patients with four-part fractures. Average follow-up was at 24 months. Good to very good functional results were achieved in the patients with three-part fractures. Good radiologic results were seen in the patients with four-part fractures; osteonecrosis developed in 11% of patients with four-part fractures.

Classic Bibliography

Ballmer FT, Lippitt SB, Romeo AA, Matsen FA III: Total shoulder arthroplasty: Some considerations related to glenoid surface contact. *J Shoulder Elbow Surg* 1994;3:299-306.

Ballmer FT, Sidles JA, Lippitt SB, Matsen FA III: Humeral head prosthetic arthroplasty: Surgically relevant geometric considerations. *J Shoulder Elbow Surg* 1993;2:296-304.

Burkhead WZ Jr, Hutton KS: Biologic resurfacing of the glenoid with hemiarthroplasty of the shoulder. *J Shoulder Elbow Surg* 1995;4:263-270.

Cofield RH, Frankle MA, Zuckerman JD: Humeral head replacement for glenohumeral arthritis. *Semin Arthroplasty* 1995;6:214-221.

Collins D, Tencer A, Sidles J, Matsen F III: Edge displacement and deformation of glenoid components in response to eccentric loading: The effect of preparation of the glenoid bone. *J Bone Joint Surg Am* 1992;74:501-507.

Franklin JL, Barrett WP, Jackins SE, Matsen FA III: Glenoid loosening in total shoulder arthroplasty: Association with rotator cuff deficiency. *J Arthroplasty* 1988;3:39-46.

Friedman RJ, LaBerge M, Dooley RL, O'Hara AL: Finite element modeling of the glenoid component: Effect of design parameters on stress distribution. *J Shoulder Elbow Surg* 1992;1:261-270.

Grammont PM, Baulot E: Delta shoulder prosthesis for rotator cuff rupture. *Orthopedics* 1993;16:65-68.

Harryman DT II, Sidles JA, Clark JM, McQuade KJ, Gibb TD, Matsen FA III: Translation of the humeral head on the glenoid with passive glenohumeral motion. *J Bone Joint Surg Am* 1990;72:1334-1343.

Harryman DT II, Sidles JA, Harris SL, Lippitt SB, Matsen FA III: The effect of articular conformity and the size of the humeral head component on laxity and motion after glenohumeral arthroplasty: A study in cadavera. *J Bone Joint Surg Am* 1995;77:555-563.

Iannotti JP, Gabriel JP, Schneck SL, Evans BG, Misra S: The normal glenohumeral relationships: An anatomical study of one hundred and forty shoulders. *J Bone Joint Surg Am* 1992;74:491-500.

Jacobson SR, Mallon WJ: The glenohumeral offset ratio: A radiographic study. *J Shoulder Elbow Surg* 1993;2:141-146.

Jobe CM, Iannotti JP: Limits imposed on glenohumeral motion by joint geometry. *J Shoulder Elbow Surg* 1995;4:281-285.

Lippitt SB, Vanderhooft JE, Harris SL, et al: Glenohumeral stability from concavity-compression: A quantitative analysis. *J Shoulder Elbow Surg* 1993;2:27-35.

O'Driscoll SW, Wright TW, Cofield RH: Abstract: Radiographic analysis of the glenoid component in total shoulder arthroplasty. *J Bone Joint Surg Br* 1991;73(suppl 2):105-106.

Pearl ML, Volk AG: Retroversion of the proximal humerus in relationship to prosthetic replacement arthroplasty. *J Shoulder Elbow Surg* 1995;4:286-289.

Poppen NK, Walker PS: Normal and abnormal motion of the shoulder. *J Bone Joint Surg Am* 1976;58:195-201.

Section 2

Instability and Athletic Injuries

Section Editor:
Michael A. Wirth, MD

Glenohumeral Instability: Classification, Clinical Assessment, and Imaging

Kirk L. Jensen, MD

Charles A. Rockwood, Jr, MD

Introduction

The glenohumeral joint is unique in its ability to allow a wide range of motion while maintaining a consistent and stable relationship between the humeral head and glenoid. This balance of stability and motion is maintained through an interaction of static and dynamic factors. Instability of the glenohumeral joint occurs when this interaction is disrupted or when stabilizing components are injured. The diagnosis and treatment of glenohumeral instability can be improved by a thorough understanding of the pathophysiology and clinical presentation of the condition. Imaging studies can be used to confirm the clinical diagnosis and to guide treatment protocols.

Pathophysiology of Instability

Glenohumeral stability is a complex interaction between static and dynamic factors that involve the strength and coordination of the rotator cuff and periscapular muscles, the integrity of the capsuloligamentous complex, and the glenoid labrum articular surface. Glenohumeral interactive factors contributing to stability include concavity-compression, adhesion-cohesion, and finite joint volume. The diagnosis and management of symptomatic instability of the glenohumeral joint, which can occur as a result of disruption of any of these interactions, has received much attention in the last 25 years.

Glenohumeral stability while at rest results from an interaction of mechanisms including adhesion-cohesion, the glenoid suction cup, and limited joint volume. In the midrange of motion, glenohumeral stability occurs if the net humeral joint reaction force (the combined force of the rotator cuff and scapular muscles) is directed within the effective glenoid. At the extremes of motion, ligamentous glenohumeral stabilization has been shown to occur via a checkrein effect. Anatomic studies of the three anterior glenohumeral ligaments have revealed variations in the respective size and number of interposing recesses of the ligaments. Embryologic examination revealed that most anterior capsules inserted directly into the labrum and only one fourth inserted into the scapular neck.

The superior glenohumeral ligament is noted to be the most consistent capsular ligament; combined with the rotator interval and coracohumeral ligament, it forms the anterosuperior complex. When the anterosuperior complex comes under tension, posterior and inferior displacement is diminished. Although the superior glenohumeral ligament and coracohumeral ligament are under tension with external rotation in adduction, the middle glenohumeral ligament comes under tension with external rotation when the arm is abducted to 45°. In more than one third of shoulders, the middle glenohumeral ligament is poorly defined or absent.

With greater degrees of shoulder abduction, the inferior glenohumeral ligament and inferior capsular sling tighten and provide static stabilization. Static properties of the glenohumeral ligaments include resting length, strength, and elasticity and can be affected by biochemical factors, anatomic factors, disease, age, and surgery. Excessive ligamentous shortening has been shown to produce obligate glenohumeral translations: anterior humeral translation at the extremes of flexion, and cross-body abduction and posterior humeral translation at the extremes of extension and external rotation.

Glenoid concavity is a static factor of stability. The concavity is formed by a combination of underlying bone and overlying cartilage and labrum. The effective glenoid arc may be compromised by congenital deficiency, traumatic lesions (glenoid rim fracture), or wear. Altered glenoid version has also been shown to be present in shoulders with both recurrent anterior and recurrent posterior instability. Isolated labral deficiency has not been shown in cadaver studies to be sufficient to allow glenohumeral dislocation without associated injury to the capsule. Therefore, a traumatic anterior dislocation of the shoulder requires both an injury to the anterior portion of the glenohumeral joint and an injury (osseous, ligamentous, or tendinous) to the posterior portion of the joint.

The circle concept of joint stability, which considers the shoulder capsule between the glenoid and humeral head as a circle, should be kept in mind while evaluating both acute and recurrent glenohumeral subluxation or dislocation. For instability to occur in one direction, there must be damage to both sides of the capsule. Arthroscopic examination of the acute traumatic anterior dislocation has revealed anterior labral detachment, anterior capsular tearing or detachment, and capsular detachment from the humeral neck. Thus, recurrent instability may result from either glenoid or humeral glenohumeral ligament detachment with or without ligament deformation. Proprioceptive receptors are present in the glenoid labrum and glenohumeral ligaments. Individuals with generalized joint laxity have been shown to have less acute proprioception and altered muscle activation. Glenohumeral joint motion and position sense have also been shown to be compromised in patients with traumatic anterior instability and can be restored following surgical reconstruction.

The clinical assessment of glenohumeral instability requires a thorough understanding of the mechanisms involved. Recurrent shoulder subluxation or dislocation can result from various factors, ranging from neuromuscular imbalance to a combination of abnormal anatomy on opposite sides of the joint. Identifying disrupted stabilizing factors, both static and dynamic, is critical in developing a treatment plan that can successfully restore glenohumeral stability through a rehabilitation program or surgical reconstruction.

Classification of Glenohumeral Joint Instability

Glenohumeral instability is classified according to a number of factors, including voluntary versus involuntary subluxation or dislocation, traumatic versus atraumatic injury, direction of instability, and degree of instability. Some classification schemes have incorporated clinical presentation with treatment: TUBS (Traumatic Unidirectional Bankart Surgery) and AMBRI (Atraumatic Multidirectional Bilateral Rehabilitation Inferior capsular shift).

Clinical Assessment

Clinical glenohumeral instability can be categorized according to the circumstances of its presentation, its degree, and its direction. A meticulous history and physical examination are both essential in evaluating the patient with suspected glenohumeral instability.

Glenohumeral instability is considered acute when seen in the first days after onset and recurrent if dislocation, subluxation, or both have occurred on multiple occasions. Instability can result from a single traumatic event that

can alter the integrity of the humeral head or glenoid osseous structure, tear the rotator cuff tendons, injure the glenoid labrum, or stretch and detach the glenohumeral capsule. However, glenohumeral instability can also result from repetitive microtrauma to the capsular ligaments.

Acute Dislocation

Examination following an acute traumatic event should accurately confirm the degree and direction of instability. The neurovascular status of the affected extremity should be evaluated and documented prior to attempted reduction.

The patient with an acute anterior dislocation will report moderate or severe pain and will have loss of the normal shoulder contour, with posterior squaring and anterior swelling or fullness. The patient may be supporting the arm in slight abduction and external rotation. Adduction and internal rotation are usually limited.

A patient with an acute posterior dislocation may have minimal or moderate pain, and the problem frequently is misdiagnosed in a muscular or obese patient. The patient usually holds the affected arm to the side in an adducted, internally rotated position. In the thin patient, the coracoid process will be prominent and a posterior fullness will be noted. The patient usually has limited external rotation of the shoulder and limited elevation of the arm.

Recurrent Instability

Both shoulders are inspected for muscular atrophy or surgical scars. Viewed from behind, bilateral symmetric motion is assessed with attention to glenohumeral rhythm and scapulothoracic motion. The sternoclavicular and acromioclavicular joints are palpated, as well as the subacromial space. Subacromial crepitus and posterior cuff tenderness may be present in the overhead athlete with transient subluxation. Active and passive motion of both shoulders are assessed and recorded. External rotation is assessed with the elbow at the side and with the elbow at 90° of abduction. Posterior capsular contracture will result in a loss of internal rotation, which is detected through examination in two ways: (1) by measuring how high on the spine the patient can reach with his or her thumb and comparing that with the height reached by the contralateral hand; or (2) by internally rotating the arm with the shoulder in 90° of abduction. Overhead athletes usually demonstrate a slightly asymmetric examination, with increased muscle mass and an increase in external rotation on the dominant side.

The rotator cuff is evaluated routinely to identify rotator tendon injury or deinnervation. An acute dislocation rarely results in an injury to the suprascapular nerve and commonly causes tearing of the infraspinatus and supraspinatus tendons in patients older than age 45 years. Patients with subtle anteroinferior subluxation may have posterior rotator cuff pain and weakness; a history of years of overhead sporting activities is common. Therefore, assessing external rotator strength, lag testing in 90° of shoulder abduction, and supraspinatus tendon testing should be routine. Subscapularis tendon integrity also is evaluated by resistance testing in maximum internal rotation, using the lumbar lift-off or abdominal press test.

Superior shoulder pain has been associated with underlying glenohumeral instability in overhead athletes younger than age 40 years. Therefore, impingement testing also should be performed routinely as part of the instability examination, just as instability testing should be performed routinely when investigating superior shoulder pain in the overhead athlete. The Neer test is performed as follows: the examiner supports the posterior scapula, then brings the internally rotated arm into full forward flexion. A positive sign is pain elicited as the greater tuberosity and the superior cuff come into contact with the overlying coracoacromial arch. The Hawkins test is performed by internally rotating the affected arm in 90° of abduction and flexion. The painful arc test is another useful impingement test and is performed by externally rotating the affected arm while in 90° of abduction. The subacromial pain elicited by these tests is usually adjacent to the anterolateral acromion and is accompanied by crepitus. These tests also may generate pain referred from underlying glenohumeral instability. An injection of 10 mL of Xylocaine into the subacromial bursa, followed by retesting, can help differentiate subacromial pain from other pain sources, such as glenohumeral instability.

Voluntary instability should be evaluated routinely by asking if the patient can subluxate or dislocate at will. The direction and degree of instability can be determined by observation and by palpation of the scapula and humerus as the shoulder is translated and reduced. Common patterns of voluntary instability include posterior instability, demonstrated by the patient bringing the internally rotated arm across the chest, causing the humeral head to subluxate posteriorly; inferior instability, demonstrated as the patient attempts to lift an object; and anterior instability, demonstrated as the patient elevates the arm in a posterior plane with spontaneous reduction on return of the arm to the coronal plane.

Glenohumeral Laxity Tests

Tests for laxity are to be performed with the patient relaxed or anesthetized; the affected shoulder is compared to the opposite shoulder. The purpose of these tests is to assess capsuloligamentous laxity, reproduce mechan-

ical symptoms, and determine the degree and direction of laxity. It should be pointed out that many athletes such as gymnasts and swimmers have stable asymptomatic shoulders even though they exhibit substantial laxity.

The anterior and posterior drawer tests assess the anterior and posterior translation of the humeral head in the midrange position. Capsular laxity, joint volume, and glenoid concavity are tested. The technique requires the examiner to stabilize the shoulder girdle by grasping the clavicle and scapular spine with one hand. The other hand first compresses the humeral head into the glenoid fossa, then pushes the humeral head anteriorly to the limit, and then pulls the humeral head posteriorly to the limit. Significant findings would include a translation greater than the opposite shoulder, translation over the glenoid rim, or a grinding or painful popping on translation that may indicate a labral tear or detachment.

The sulcus test evaluates the inferior translation of the humeral head with the arm at the side in a neutral and in an externally rotated position. The anatomic mechanisms tested include capsular laxity, joint volume, glenoid concavity, and the integrity of the rotator interval (the superior glenohumeral ligament and coracohumeral ligament). The shoulder is stabilized by one of the examiner's hands, and the tested arm is at the side in an adducted position. The examiner centers the humeral head with a mild compressive force, then applies a downward force to the arm and palpates the gap between the acromion and the humeral head. This sequence is then repeated with the arm in external rotation. Significant findings include an increased inferior translation on the affected side compared to the opposite side, which indicates the presence of inferior joint laxity, and increased inferior translation below the glenoid rim, which demonstrates diminished glenoid concavity and inferior joint laxity. Laxity or incompetence of the rotator interval is revealed when performing the sulcus test with the arm in external rotation does not abolish or lessen a sulcus sign that appeared when the test was performed with the arm in internal rotation.

The push-pull test evaluates the posterior translation of the humeral head in the midrange position. It assesses posterior glenoid concavity, the integrity of the posterior labrum, and joint volume. The patient is placed in a supine position with the scapula supported by the examination table; the arm of the affected shoulder is held by the examiner in 90° of abduction and 30° of flexion. The wrist is then pulled up by one hand, while the other hand pushes posteriorly on the proximal humerus. Significant findings would include a greater posterior translation, a popping or grinding associated with the posterior translation, or a posterior dislocation with palpable relocation. This test usually demonstrates 50% posterior humeral head translation in a normal, relaxed shoulder.

Glenohumeral Instability Tests

These tests evaluate the ability of the shoulder to maintain stability when the ligamentous restraints are placed under tension.

The apprehension and crank tests assess the continuity of the anteroinferior glenohumeral ligament complex and the integrity of its labral attachment. The middle glenohumeral ligament can be evaluated with the shoulder in 45° of abduction, and the anteroinferior glenohumeral ligament is evaluated with the shoulder in 90° of abduction. Both tests can be performed similarly. The patient is seated, and the examiner's hand stabilizes the shoulder by grasping the superior aspect of the shoulder with the middle finger on the coracoid, the index finger on the anterior aspect of the humeral head, and the thumb directed posteriorly. The forearm of the tested shoulder is then externally rotated and extended in varying degrees of abduction. Significant findings include the sensation of impending subluxation or dislocation, restriction of external rotation because of apprehension, or pain located posteriorly with the shoulder externally rotated and extended. To detect subluxation, the examiner can use the stabilizing hand to apply an anteriorly directed force to the posterior aspect of the humeral head.

The relocation test is performed with the patient in a supine position, usually following the apprehension test. The tested shoulder is positioned in 90° of abduction and neutral rotation. The scapula is supported and the shoulder is externally rotated until symptoms are produced. The examiner then applies a posteriorly directed force to the anterior aspect of the humeral head. Alleviation of symptoms with this maneuver suggests the presence of anterior instability. Recent clinical investigation of the relocation test suggests that pain from rotator cuff pathology is a confounding factor and that the accuracy of the relocation test is greater than 80% only when symptoms of apprehension are relieved.

The jerk test is a posterior apprehension test and is performed with the patient sitting or in a supine position. The arm is flexed forward to 90° and internally rotated. The examiner stabilizes the scapula, axially loads the humerus in a posterior direction, and then moves the arm across the body. A sudden jerk indicates that the humeral head has slid off the glenoid posteriorly; when the arm is returned to the original position, a second jerk may be observed, indicating reduction of the humeral head into the glenoid.

Imaging

Imaging studies can be used to confirm clinical diagnosis and guide glenohumeral instability treatment protocols. Following completion of a detailed history and physical examination, radiographic evaluation is required for diagnosis and the detection of commonly associated pathology such as glenoid or proximal humeral fractures. In the acute setting, the glenohumeral joint is evaluated by the trauma series that consists of three orthogonal views (true AP, transscapular lateral, and axillary lateral). In some trauma settings, the axillary lateral view cannot be obtained, so an apical oblique view is used to confirm the direction of dislocation.

In atraumatic instability, plain radiographs rarely show bony pathology. Occasionally, radiographs may suggest factors underlying the atraumatic instability, such as a hypoplastic glenoid or posteriorly inclined glenoid. Rarely, radiographs may reveal translation of the humeral head with respect to the glenoid. Stress radiographs and arthrography are not useful in the diagnosis of atraumatic instability.

Plain radiographs are useful to provide confirmation of traumatic glenohumeral instability. Humeral head changes, such as indentation or impaction of the posterior aspect of the humeral head from contact with the anterior inferior glenoid, are best seen on the Stryker notch view. Standard radiographs also may reveal a fracture of the glenoid rim, erosion of the glenoid rim, a periosteal reaction to a ligamentous avulsion at the glenoid rim, or new bone formation at the glenoid rim. Identification of these glenoid rim changes is helped by special views that are modifications of the axillary view.

Special Views

Additional radiographic views can be used to delineate bony pathology associated with acute or chronic recurrent instability. The apical oblique view is a true AP view of the glenohumeral joint with a 45° caudal tilt of the x-ray beam. The West Point axillary view is obtained with the patient in a prone position with the x-ray beam centered at the axilla and directed 25° downward from the horizontal and 25° medially.

Magnetic Resonance Imaging

MRI without intra-articular contrast may be useful in limited situations. Rotator cuff pathology or associated bony changes (Hills-Sachs lesion) can be identified with routine MRI. The ability to accurately detect glenoid labral pathology has been shown to be limited in several studies. Authors of one arthroscopic study that compared MRI and clinical examination reported that MRI had a sensitivity of 59% and specificity of 85%. Physical examination was shown to be more accurate in predicting glenoid labral tears. In another report it was noted that only 21% of labral abnormalities could be categorized, and the authors suggested that MRI did not provide useful preoperative information regarding the integrity of the capsular labral complex.

Magnetic Resonance Arthrography

MR arthrography has been used to evaluate both labral pathology and joint volume. Reported diagnostic sensitivities have ranged from 85% to 90% and specificities from 88% to 93%. The addition of the abduction and external rotation (ABER) position has been shown to increase the sensitivity of MR arthrography in revealing tears of the anterior glenoid labrum. In one study conventional axial MR arthrograms were compared with oblique axial MR arthrograms in the ABER position. The latter were found to be significantly more sensitive in revealing anterior glenoid labral tears ($P = .005$). Saline MR arthrography has also been performed with a reported sensitivity of 89%. MR arthrography has been shown prospectively to be superior to CT arthrography in the evaluation of superior labral pathology.

Summary

Successful management of glenohumeral instability requires an accurate diagnosis and appropriate treatment. The clinical history and physical examination of the patient with glenohumeral instability most often will provide the correct diagnosis. Radiographic examination of the acutely injured shoulder is crucial for initiating proper treatment; it is also helpful when assessing the chronic or recurrently unstable shoulder. Routine MRI of the unstable shoulder has limited usefulness, whereas MR arthrography can provide helpful information regarding labral pathology.

Annotated Bibliography

Classification of Glenohumeral Joint Instability

Bigliani LU, Newton PM, Steinmann SP, Connor PM, McIlveen SJ: Glenoid rim lesions associated with recurrent anterior dislocation of the shoulder. *Am J Sports Med* 1998;26:41-45.

The authors reviewed 25 shoulders with recurrent instability and associated anterior glenoid rim lesions. Lesions were classified into three types and were detected by plain radiographs (19 shoulders) or supplemental CT arthrograms (12 shoulders) or both. The authors concluded that recurrent anterior dislocations with associated glenoid rim lesions can be treated by suturing the fracture fragment or capsule or both to the glenoid rim and addressing associated capsular laxity.

Habermeyer P, Gleyze P, Rickert M: Evolution of lesions of the labrum-ligament complex in posttraumatic anterior shoulder instability: A prospective study. *J Shoulder Elbow Surg* 1999;8:66-74.

The authors present an evolution of labral-ligament complex findings prospectively observed in 91 consecutive patients.

This progressive theory of anatomic lesions classifies arthroscopic anatomic findings and correlates them with chronicity in an attempt to explain a pathophysiologic mechanism. Clinical treatments and outcomes are not discussed, as this study simply provides a useful theory of intra-articular findings in anteroinferior shoulder instability.

Maruyama K, Sano S, Saito K, Yamaguchi Y: Trauma-instability-voluntarism classification for glenohumeral instability. *J Shoulder Elbow Surg* 1995;4:194-198.

The authors' classification is composed of three main factors: level of trauma, direction, and voluntarism. The study does not provide correlation with treatment plans.

Silliman JF, Hawkins RJ: Classification and physical diagnosis of instability of the shoulder. *Clin Orthop* 1993;291:7-19.

The authors propose a useful classification scheme based on volition, direction, cause, frequency, and degree of instability. Identification of subtle forms of glenohumeral instability is highlighted.

Speer KP, Deng X, Borrero S, Torzilli PA, Altchek DA, Warren RF: Biomechanical evaluation of a simulated Bankart lesion. *J Bone Joint Surg Am* 1994;76:1819-1826.

The authors review the results of ligament sectioning studies and define the circle concept of glenohumeral stability. This biomechanical study reports that a Bankart lesion alone was insufficient under the conditions used to allow sufficient translation for dislocation.

Clinical Assessment

Faber KJ, Homa K, Hawkins RJ: Translation of the glenohumeral joint in patients with anterior instability: Awake examination versus examination with the patient under anesthesia. *J Shoulder Elbow Surg* 1999;8:320-323.

The authors evaluated bilateral shoulder translation in 50 patients, both while awake and under general anesthesia, who had a clinical diagnosis of traumatic anterior instability. The authors concluded that clinical translation testing was helpful; however, side-to-side differences were negligible while patients were awake and more apparent during examination under anesthesia (EUA). EUA was thought to provide useful information to confirm direction and degree of instability.

Levy AS, Lintner S, Kenter K, Speer KP: Intra- and interobserver reproducibility of the shoulder laxity examination. *Am J Sports Med* 1999;27:460-463.

The authors evaluated the inter- and intraobserver reproducibility of clinical examination of glenohumeral laxity in the unanesthetized shoulder. Forty-three asymptomatic shoulders underwent bilateral shoulder laxity examination initially and again after 3 months. Overall intraobserver reproducibility of examination was 46%. The data demonstrated that the laxity examination of the unanesthetized shoulder is not easily reproducible in either intra- or interobserver comparison. The authors recommend caution when determining diagnosis and treatment based on this examination.

Oliashirazi A, Mansat P, Cofield RH, Rowland CM: Examination under anesthesia for evaluation of anterior shoulder instability. *Am J Sports Med* 1999;27:464-468.

The authors evaluated 30 patients with unilateral, traumatic recurrent anterior instability by EUA of both shoulders. There were significant side-to-side differences in humeral head translation, depending on arm rotation. The authors concluded that assessing humeral head translation by EUA should be expanded to include the anteroinferior and posteroinferior directions, and the tests should be done with the arm in varying degrees of rotation.

Speer KP, Hannafin JA, Altchek DW, Warren RF: An evaluation of the shoulder relocation test. *Am J Sports Med* 1994;22:177-183.

The authors evaluated the sensitivity, specificity, negative and positive predictive values, and accuracy of the shoulder relocation test in 100 patients who underwent shoulder surgery. The only positive responses for apprehension were in the anterior instability group, of which 63% had apprehension with 90°/90° alone and 74% had apprehension when an anterior humeral force was applied.

Imaging

Allmann KH, Uhl M, Gufler H, et al: Cine-MR imaging of the shoulder. *Acta Radiol* 1997;38:1043-1046.

This article presents cine-MRI and its proposed advantages.

Beltran J, Bencardino J, Mellado J, Rosenberg ZS, Irish RD: MR arthrography of the shoulder: Variants and pitfalls. *Radiographics* 1997;17:1403-1415.

This is an excellent review of the usefulness and limitations of MR arthrography.

Palmer WE, Caslowitz PL: Anterior shoulder instability: Diagnostic criteria determined from prospective analysis of 121 MR arthrograms. *Radiology* 1995;197:819-825.

The authors concluded that MR arthrography was accurate in defining anteroinferior labral pathology but was not useful in delineating capsular abnormalities.

Sanders TG, Morrison WB, Miller MD: Imaging techniques for the evaluation of glenohumeral instability. *Am J Sports Med* 2000;28:414-434.

The authors have provided a useful review of current imaging techniques available for evaluation of glenohumeral instability.

Sher JS, Iannotti JP, Williams GR, et al: The effect of shoulder magnetic resonance imaging on clinical decision making. *J Shoulder Elbow Surg* 1998;7:205-209.

One hundred cases were prospectively evaluated to determine the impact of MRI on clinical decision making. Each was analyzed for changes in the clinical diagnosis or treatment. A change of either the primary diagnosis or type of treatment (surgical versus nonsurgical) was observed in 29% of glenohumeral instability cases (4 of 14).

Classic Bibliography

Bahr R, Craig EV, Engebretsen L: The clinical presentation of shoulder instability including on field management. *Clin Sports Med* 1995;14:761-776.

Cofield RH, Nessler JP, Weinstabl R: Diagnosis of shoulder instability by examination under anesthesia. *Clin Orthop* 1993;291:45-53.

Garth WP Jr, Slappey CE, Ochs CW: Roentgenographic demonstration of instability of the shoulder: The apical oblique projection: A technical note. *J Bone Joint Surg Am* 1984;66:1450-1453.

Iannotti JP, Zlatkin MB, Esterhai JL, Kressel HY, Dalinka MK, Spindler KP: Magnetic resonance imaging of the shoulder: Sensitivity, specificity, and predictive value. *J Bone Joint Surg Am* 1991;73:17-29.

Jahnke AH Jr, Petersen SA, Neumann C, Steinbach L, Morgan F: A prospective comparison of computerized arthrotomography and magnetic resonance imaging of the glenohumeral joint. *Am J Sports Med* 1992;20:695-701.

Palmer WE, Caslowitz PL, Chew FS: MR arthrography of the shoulder: Normal intraarticular structures and common abnormalities. *AJR Am J Roentgenol* 1995;164:141-146.

Chapter 7

Acute and Chronic Dislocations of the Shoulder

Mark D. Lazarus, MD

Acute Anterior Dislocations

Most orthopaedists have developed their own algorithms for the management of acute anterior glenohumeral dislocations. Information gained from several recent studies may convince surgeons to alter their established protocols, however.

Pathology

For the humeral head to escape the glenoid fossa, the soft-tissue restraint must be disrupted. The location of the disruption depends on several factors, the most important of which is the age of the patient. In older patients, the more common lesion is a tear of the rotator cuff, the "posterior mechanism" of dislocation, with or without labral pathology. However, in patients younger than age 40 years, the predominant finding is a tear of the anteroinferior glenoid labrum (Bankart tear). The arthroscopic findings in 63 patients who sustained an initial anterior dislocation were described in a recent study. All patients were younger than 24 years of age. Sixty-one of the 63 patients (97%) had an avulsion of the anteroinferior glenoid labrum with no evidence of intracapsular injury. Fourteen of the 63 (22%) had an associated osseous lesion of the glenoid rim. In addition, there were six superior labral tears, two of which included the biceps origin. There were no full-thickness rotator cuff tears.

The pathology that occurs at the time of initial dislocation may be the most important variable in determining the risk of recurrence. In an arthroscopic study of 45 patients who sustained an initial dislocation, Bankart tears were found in most patients. These patients also had gross instability on examination under anesthesia. Six of 45 patients had interstitial capsular injury with no evidence of labral avulsion; these shoulders were found to be stable on examination under anesthesia.

Natural History

Treatment decisions need to be based not only on the effectiveness of a particular modality but also on the natural history of the disease process. Multiple studies have addressed the ultimate outcome of the patient who sustains a first-time traumatic dislocation. The risk of recurrence after initial dislocation has been reported to be as high as 95% for patients younger than 20 years of age, with recurrence ranging from 50% to 75% for patients younger than 25 years of age. A recent study reported a 10-year follow-up of 245 patients (247 shoulders) who sustained an initial dislocation at age 40 years or younger. The patient group was markedly heterogeneous, including various levels of inciting trauma (if any) and 32 shoulders that sustained greater tuberosity fractures during dislocation. Of the 247 shoulders, 52% sustained no further dislocations, while 23% required later surgical stabilization. For patients younger than 25 years of age, the risk of recurrence was greater than 60%, with the recurrence rate rapidly decreasing with initial dislocation after 25 years of age.

Although various rates of recurrence have been reported, it is clear that the risk is extremely high and that it is strongly inversely related to the age of the patient at the time of initial dislocation (Fig. 1). Treatment should therefore be based on the patient's age.

Patient Presentation/Evaluation

Diagnosis of an anterior glenohumeral dislocation is usually straightforward. The history most often includes an eccentric load applied to the hand while the arm is outstretched, such as contact with an opponent's hand during a volleyball spike or basketball block, reaching out into abduction to grab a passing runner, or a backward fall onto an outstretched hand. Typically, at presentation, the patient is leaning forward with the humerus in slight abduction, flexion, and internal rotation. Unless the patient is exceptionally muscular or obese, the humeral head can be palpated anteriorly, and there will be a palpable and visible deficiency under the acromion posteriorly. Many patients present after the dislocation has reduced spontaneously, however, and the diagnosis may not be evident. Key clues include the mechanism of injury, the patient reporting a "pop" at the moment of injury or pain that was relieved after a "pop," or a history of a "dead arm" event, such as

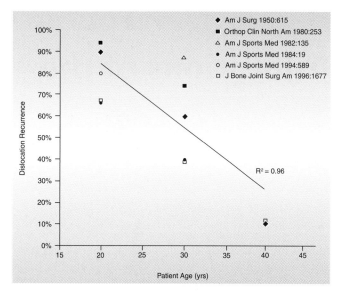

Figure 1 Graph of results of selected studies over several decades showing a high rate of instability recurrence in initial dislocations that occur before age 25 years. The rate of recurrence decreases dramatically with increasing age.

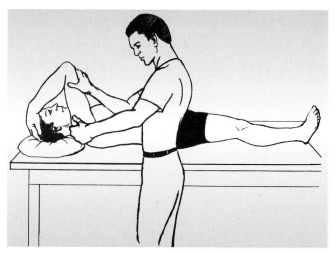

Figure 2 A gentle and effective method of reduction involves the patient actively placing the hand on top of the head, leaving the surgeon with both hands free to perform the reduction.

the arm dropping or becoming flail when placed in the abducted and externally rotated position. During examination, the patient will display prominent guarding against combined abduction and external rotation.

The initial evaluation should include a thorough neurovascular examination. Most patients with a glenohumeral dislocation can still provide some resistance with the posterior and middle deltoids and the biceps, ruling out the more common neurapraxias. Pulses, warmth, and capillary refill should be compared with the contralateral extremity, although symmetry does not completely exclude axillary artery injury.

The radiographic assessment, which is usually completed prior to orthopaedic consultation, is most likely to consist of a single oblique view of the shoulder. If there are no associated injuries that require additional imaging, the surgeon should reduce the shoulder before ordering further radiographs. If radiographs cannot be taken at the time of presentation (as in the case of an on-field injury), a gentle attempt at reduction prior to radiographic evaluation is appropriate.

Management

Reduction

Many reduction techniques have been described in the literature. Adequate patient relaxation and analgesia are more important than the particular technique, however. An intravenous sedative and anxiolytic such as midazolam is helpful. Several authors have reported the successful use of intra-articular lidocaine for anesthetic. An 18-gauge spinal needle is inserted into the joint posteriorly. Entrance

into the glenohumeral space is easily confirmed by aspiration of the hemarthrosis. Approximately 15 to 20 mL of 1% lidocaine will provide adequate analgesia, and the patient can then usually cooperate with the reduction efforts. The patient should lie supine and slowly lift the hand on the affected side to the top of the head. This puts the humerus in a reduction position and permits the surgeon to have both hands free. The surgeon can then immobilize the scapula with one hand while gently distracting the humerus and lifting the humeral head back into the glenoid with the other hand (Fig. 2). Normal humeroscapular relationships and smooth glenohumeral rotation confirms that the reduction was successful. A postreduction neurovascular check is necessary.

Imaging

Once reduction has been successfully achieved, the patient typically experiences dramatic relief of discomfort. Having been sedated and locally anesthetized, the patient can easily undergo a more thorough radiologic evaluation, including a true glenohumeral AP in internal and external humeral rotation, an axillary lateral, and, if a glenoid rim defect is suspected, an apical oblique (Garth) view (Fig. 3). The surgeon may need to position the patient and hold the arm, but a few minutes of time spent obtaining quality radiographs with the patient in this cooperative state is time well spent. If the radiographic assessment suggests an osseous Bankart lesion that involves more than 25% to 30% of the glenoid width, CT is necessary (Fig. 4).

Postreduction Immobilization

Only a simple sling is necessary for postreduction immobilization. A sling with strap padding usually is better tolerated than a shoulder immobilizer. The duration of immobilization is debatable, but several investi-

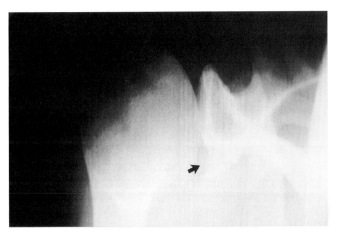

Figure 3 Garth apical oblique view demonstrating an obvious large osseous Bankart lesion (*arrow*).

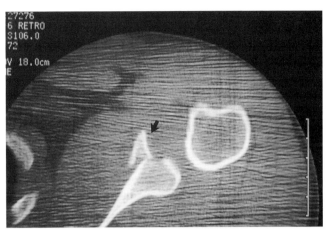

Figure 4 CT scan after an acute, traumatic, initial anterior dislocation. Notice the large, displaced anterior glenoid rim fracture (*arrow*), which required open reduction and internal fixation.

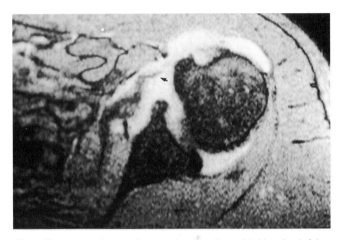

Figure 5 Traumatic subscapularis rupture (*arrow*) and associated long head of the biceps subluxation after an acute anterior dislocation.

gators have demonstrated that it has no bearing on the recurrence rate. The sling is typically continued for up to 3 weeks, but absolutely no longer.

Postimmobilization Assessment

Repeat examination is necessary when immobilization is discontinued. Range of motion should be assessed; often, appreciable tightening of the shoulder, particularly in external rotation in the unelevated position, will be apparent. External rotation that is greater than on the contralateral side suggests a possible subscapularis rupture. Although testing will be limited because of patient guarding, rotator cuff function should be assessed, particularly in patients older than age 40 years. Several studies have demonstrated the high incidence of rotator cuff pathology in this age group. Particular attention should be paid to the subscapularis, even in younger individuals. A lumbar lift-off test as described by Gerber has been shown to be an accurate predictor of subscapularis integrity and can usually be performed at the 3-week postdislocation visit. If examination yields evidence of a rotator cuff tear, particularly a subscapularis rupture, MRI is required (Fig. 5). Otherwise, MRI has limited use. A prospective study analyzed the accuracy of a subacute MRI scan to identify a labral tear in patients with a first-time traumatic dislocation. Only 15 of 22 arthroscopically confirmed labral tears were diagnosed using MRI. Deltoid or rotator cuff weakness without other clinical evidence of cuff tear should be evaluated by electromyography.

Exercise Therapy

At 3 weeks postdislocation, the patient is started on a home exercise program of gentle supine self-passive forward elevation and external rotation stretching, with an external rotation limit of 40°. An overdoor pulley is also used to assist in forward elevation range. A scapular strengthening and posture program is begun next. Pendulum exercises should be avoided because they promote

anteroinferior translation of the humeral head and encourage poor scapular mechanics. Contact athletics and heavy lifting are restricted. Aerobic conditioning is encouraged.

At 6 weeks postdislocation, formal, supervised therapy is prescribed. Passive stretching is used to correct any residual contracture. Rotator cuff and scapular strengthening is the mainstay of the program (Fig. 6). Activities using devices that promote normal humeroscapular rhythm, such as pulleys, upper body ergometers, and body blades, are instituted. Athletes can attempt to return to their sport during midseason. Prophylactic taping or use of a protective harness is controversial but may provide proprioceptive feedback that helps avoid extreme abduction and external rotation.

The final stage in the rehabilitation program is begun at 12 weeks postdislocation. In this phase, sport-specific exercises are started. Plyometrics (ie, exercises that use short, sudden motions) are used to assist athletes in returning to their sport. For some heavy laborers, work hardening for overhead lifting may be necessary.

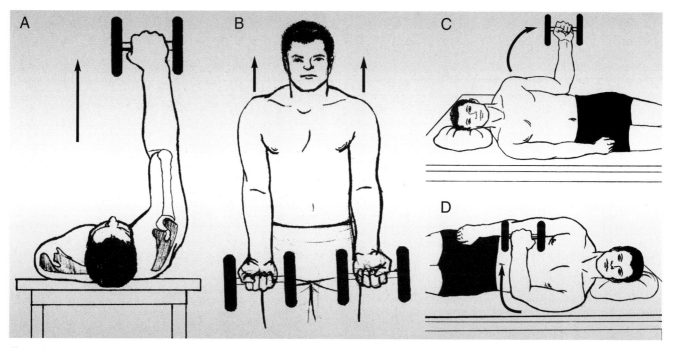

Figure 6 Home exercises for the patient who sustained a traumatic dislocation. **A,** Patient lies supine and presses weight toward ceiling. The scapula should follow the humerus in a "press plus" position. **B,** Patient stands with arms unelevated. A weight is used in each hand. Patient shrugs shoulders, concentrating on scapular symmetry. **C,** Patient lies on contralateral side and externally rotates against gravity. **D,** Patient lies on affected side and internally rotates against resistance.

The role of exercise therapy in preventing recurrence is controversial. Two studies involving students at military academies, which are highly compliant patient populations, demonstrated success rates of approximately 75% after involving individuals with initial dislocations in a coordinated therapy program. Whether these results would also be achieved in a more general population followed over a longer period of time is unclear. In one study, it was demonstrated that only 16% of patients who had sustained a traumatic subluxation decreased their risk of recurrence with exercise therapy.

Surgical Intervention

Surgical intervention for a patient with an initial dislocation has become more accepted in recent years. In theory, these patients have a better-defined pathology and healthier tissue, making them prime candidates for surgical repair, particularly with arthroscopic techniques. In a prospective study among students at the United States Military Academy at West Point, comparing the results of nonsurgical management and arthroscopic repair in patients with initial dislocations, the recurrence rate in this high-demand patient population was 80% in the nonsurgical group and 14% in the surgical group. More recently, another group of investigators randomized patients younger than 30 years with initial dislocations into two groups: those treated with immobilization and rehabilitation and those treated with arthroscopic Bankart repair. At a follow-up of 33 months, those who had undergone arthroscopic stabilization had a

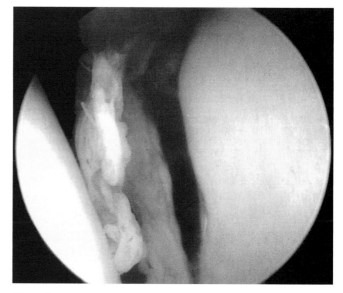

Figure 7 Arthroscopic evaluation after an initial anterior dislocation. The labrum is robust tissue that has not retracted medially and is in excellent position for arthroscopic repair.

recurrence rate of 15.9%, compared with 47% in the nonsurgical group. Although it is sometimes difficult to compare the reported results of different arthroscopic repair techniques, these data suggest that arthroscopic Bankart repair may be most advantageous if done after the initial dislocation, prior to the development of the pathologic changes of recurrent instability.

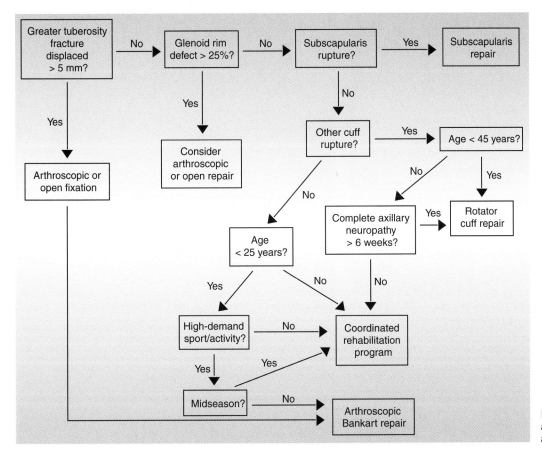

Figure 8 Algorithm for the management of first-time traumatic anterior dislocations.

The technique of arthroscopic Bankart repair for first-time dislocations is similar to, but easier than, that performed for recurrent instability. Usually, the labral tissue is of excellent quality and requires little mobilization from the scapular neck. Although the issue of intracapsular injury in recurrent instability is still debated, for Bankart repair after a single dislocation it is clear that excellent results can be obtained by repair of the Bankart lesion alone, without any associated capsular tightening procedures. However, a natural inferior displacement of the capsulolabral complex occurs even with a simple Bankart tear. Therefore, although formal capsular shift is not necessary in this patient population, the anteroinferior labrum must be "shifted" back to its anatomic position prior to repair to bone (Fig. 7).

Treatment Algorithm
Although each surgeon must develop his or her own algorithm for treating patients who sustain first-time dislocations (Fig. 8), that approach should be based on current science, taking into account the patient's age, activity level, and goals. Several important points should be included in any protocol. An associated greater tuberosity fracture displaced more than 5 mm requires reduction and fixation; particularly in younger patients,

concomitant arthroscopic Bankart repair should be considered. A technique for arthroscopic fixation of the tuberosity has been described that is extremely useful in the case of combined Bankart and tuberosity repair (Fig. 9). Surgical treatment of a traumatic subscapularis rupture should be undertaken as soon as possible to try to limit musculotendinous retraction. If the patient is younger than 45 years of age, participates in an occupation or sport with high physical demands, and has sustained a full-thickness rotator cuff tear as a direct result of the dislocation, surgical treatment probably should include rotator cuff repair and repair of the Bankart lesion, if present. For the older patient with both a large, full-thickness rotator cuff tear and axillary neuropathy, strong consideration should be given to rotator cuff repair if deltoid function does not return substantially after 6 to 12 weeks. For a competitive athlete younger than 25 years of age, arthroscopic Bankart repair should be strongly considered in the off-season. Finally, for any patient younger than 25 years of age who sustains a first-time dislocation, the advantages and disadvantages of immediate arthroscopic Bankart repair should be discussed, and this treatment should be offered as a viable option. Open Bankart repair also may be an option, but because no significant difference in surgical ease or out-

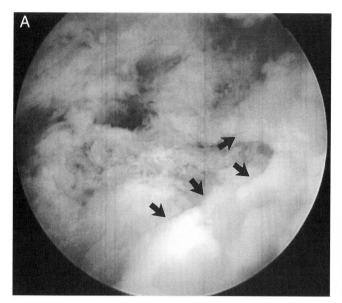
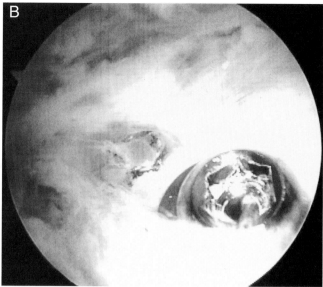

Figure 9 A, Subacromial bursoscopy demonstrates a displaced greater tuberosity fracture that occurred with an initial anterior dislocation (*arrows*). **B,** At the time of arthroscopic Bankart repair, the fracture can be effectively managed arthroscopically by reduction and percutaneous placement of 4.0-mm cannulated screws.

come between early and late open Bankart repair has been demonstrated, arthroscopic repair is probably indicated for first-time dislocations.

Acute Posterior Dislocation

Several facts about posterior dislocation are significant. First, it is an uncommon injury, comprising less than 5% of all dislocations. Second, the rate of misdiagnosis is approximately 50%. Finally, advances in radiography have not decreased the rate of misdiagnosis.

These facts indicate that to avoid misdiagnosis, posterior dislocation should be suspected in certain circumstances. For example, most posterior dislocations are associated with seizures, such as those seen in alcoholism or associated with electroshock therapy. In these seizures, the strong internal rotators and adductors of the shoulder overpower the external rotators, creating a posteriorly directed vector on the humeral head. A blow to the anterior shoulder can also result in a posterior dislocation, although this mechanism rarely causes a true fixed dislocation. Although certain sporting activities (such as playing the position of offensive lineman in football) are associated with recurrent posterior instability, fixed posterior dislocations are rare in this group.

In a study of 73 shoulders with posterior dislocations or fracture-dislocations, a seizure was the most common cause of injury. Of the 56 dislocations not associated with a fracture or with an isolated tuberosity fracture, 21 were acute. Of the chronic cases, 52% were initially misdiagnosed.

Patient Presentation/Evaluation

The hallmark examination finding in the patient with a posterior glenohumeral dislocation is the lack of passive external rotation. The patient will present with the arm held in adduction and internal rotation. Usually, it is impossible to achieve any passive external rotation. In the absence of obesity or significant muscular development, an abnormal contour of the shoulder, with a diffuse posterior prominence and a very prominent coracoid process, is readily apparent. When large amounts of soft tissue obscure these body contours, however, a fixed internal rotation contracture and the mechanism of injury may be the only clues to the presence of a posterior dislocation. Extreme diligence is required in the radiologic examination in this patient population.

Obtaining quality radiographs when a posterior dislocation is suspected is of prime importance. Even a good AP view of the shoulder may not reveal the dislocation, although occasionally the classic "light bulb sign" is apparent, indicating a humeral head in fixed internal rotation (Fig. 10). The best radiographic view is the axillary lateral, which will clearly demonstrate a posterior dislocation and any associated articular impression fracture. This view also best reveals the integrity of the lesser tuberosity. If the history and examination are consistent with a posterior dislocation and a quality axillary radiograph cannot be obtained, CT is necessary.

Management

With acute presentation, reduction of an uncomplicated posterior glenohumeral dislocation is often surprisingly

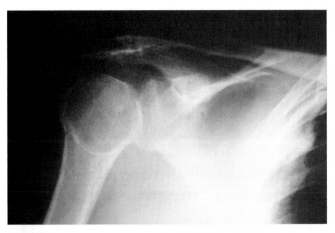

Figure 10 Radiograph showing the classic "light bulb sign," which is consistent with the internal rotation contracture of a posterior dislocation.

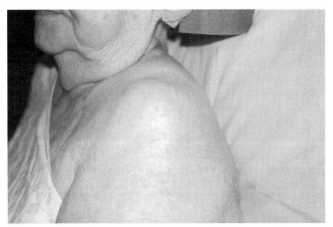

Figure 11 Photograph of a 76-year-old woman with a 6-week-old anterior dislocation after a fall onto an outstretched hand. Note the anterior prominence.

easy. Generous use of intravenous sedation and muscle relaxant is helpful. With the patient supine, in-line traction is applied until the humeral head can be manually placed back into the glenoid fossa. Gentle internal rotation during the application of traction is sometimes helpful. For a stable, cooperative patient, reduction can sometimes be accomplished with the patient in the sitting position, using a maneuver similar to a posterior drawer test.

Once reduction has been achieved, range of motion should be tested to ascertain the stable arc. Most patients can be treated with either simple sling immobilization or a neutral-position sling, which places the arm in a position of less tension on the posterior capsule. This immobilization is used for 4 weeks. For a shoulder with a very limited stable arc, a "gunslinger brace" similar to that often recommended after open capsular shift is used for 6 weeks. Following immobilization, an active therapy program is begun, concentrating on rotator cuff strengthening, scapular strengthening, and humeroscapular balance. As opposed to the anterior capsular tightening that often occurs with lengthy immobilization following an initial, acute anterior dislocation, significant motion restriction rarely develops after a posterior dislocation, and range-of-motion exercises are usually unnecessary.

Surgical treatment is indicated for irreducible dislocations. A large, anteromedial humeral head defect (McLaughlin lesion) that is locked on the posterior glenoid rim indicates the possibility of a difficult closed reduction. An initial attempt at closed reduction should be made with the patient under general anesthesia. If this fails, open reduction should be performed through a deltopectoral approach. If a large, anteromedial humeral head defect is present, the anterior approach facilitates reconstruction by transfer of the subscapularis insertion (McLaughlin procedure) or lesser tuberosity (Neer modification) into the lesion, rendering the defect extra-articular. Postoperative

immobilization and rehabilitation are similar to that following closed reduction, including restriction against resisted internal rotation for 6 weeks.

Acute Inferior Dislocation/Luxatio Erecta

Acute inferior dislocations are extremely uncommon. The most notorious of these injuries is luxatio erecta, which is associated with high-velocity trauma in which a hyperabduction force is applied to the arm and the humeral head is levered out of the glenoid inferiorly. The patient presents with the arm locked in an abducted position. Various authors have described the severe soft-tissue disruption that accompanies this injury, including capsular and cuff avulsions. In one study, an anecdotal report on 19 shoulders with this injury, all of the shoulders studied had some degree of brachial plexus symptoms and vascular compromise prior to reduction. Acute treatment consists of reduction by traction and countertraction, often requiring general anesthesia, followed by neurovascular observation and appropriate management. Further shoulder reconstruction depends on the degree of soft-tissue disruption, and MRI is helpful in defining cuff integrity.

Chronic Anterior Dislocations

The exact definition of when a dislocation becomes "chronic" is unclear, but a dislocation that persists for several days should be managed differently than an acute one. These injuries are most common in the elderly or in those with cognitive impairment, multiple trauma, or alcohol-related conditions. Often, the patient has discovered the problem secondary to functional limitations and presents with little discomfort. Examination reveals an obvious palpable and sometimes visible prominence anteriorly (Fig. 11) and limited motion.

Management can be extremely challenging; absolute recommendations do not exist. In general, gentle closed

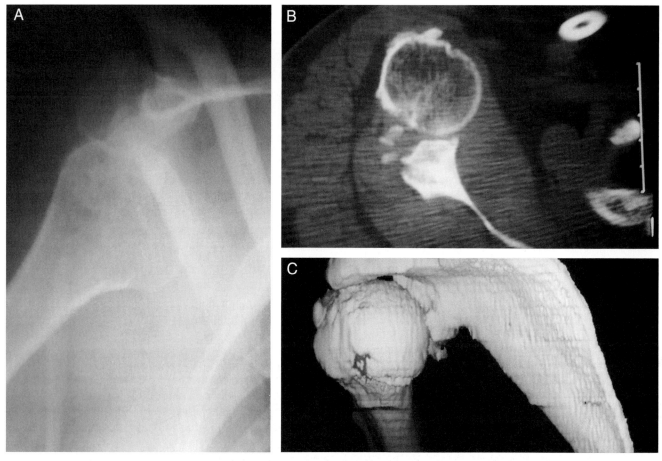

Figure 12 Chronic anterior glenohumeral dislocation. **A,** AP radiograph. **B,** CT scan better delineating the anterior glenoid rim. **C,** Three-dimensional reconstruction further defining the anterior glenoid involvement.

reduction should be tried in patients who present within 3 weeks of injury. This maneuver must be performed in a controlled situation with sufficient sedation and relaxation to avoid humeral fracture or neurovascular injury. Therefore, general anesthesia is usually required.

For dislocations present longer than 4 weeks or those that do not reduce with a gentle attempt at closed reduction, the surgeon must decide between more aggressive surgical intervention and benign neglect. For the nondominant shoulder in a low-demand, elderly, debilitated patient, benign neglect should be considered. Most patients of this activity level will be able to use the arm to assist in the activities of daily living. If function is severely limited, surgical intervention can be considered at a later date. However, benign neglect is contraindicated in the presence of neurovascular compromise. If open reduction is chosen, a preoperative CT scan is necessary to assess the size of the Hill-Sachs humeral head defect or the presence of an anterior glenoid deficiency, and three-dimensional reconstructions may be helpful (Fig. 12). An anterior deltopectoral approach is used for open reduction. Depending on the length of time from injury, the anterior scar formation can be extensive, and scar release and subscapularis mobilization may be necessary. If the dislocation has been present for several months, a Z-plasty of the subscapularis tendon may be needed to achieve reduction. For a Hill-Sachs lesion that includes 20% to 40% of the humeral head, an attempt to render the lesion extra-articular is important. Surgical choices include transfer of the greater tuberosity into the defect, a humeral rotational osteotomy, or grafting of the defect with an osteochondral allograft (Fig. 13). If the lesion comprises more than 40% of the head, a humeral hemiarthroplasty is necessary. The best management for an anterior glenoid rim deficiency in conjunction with a chronic dislocation is unclear. However, if the defect involves more than 30% of the glenoid, strong consideration should be given to bone grafting of the glenoid or total shoulder arthroplasty, depending on patient age, activity level, and humeral-side management.

There are several important facts about the management of this injury that can be gleaned from the literature. The largest published series involved 44 shoulders and in half of these, an associated fracture on either the humeral or scapular side was present. Closed reduction was successful in one third of the patients but in only one in which the dislocation was present for more than 4 weeks. In another study, 10 of 17 patients with chronic anterior dislocations were treated surgically, 9 by shoulder arthroplasty. The technique required extensive mobilization of anterior soft tissues, but the results were excellent or satisfactory in all patients.

Chronic Posterior Dislocations

A few important articles in the literature are helpful in the management of chronic posterior dislocations, and a management algorithm can be formulated (Fig. 14). One study reported on 41 shoulders with posterior dislocation. As discussed previously, misdiagnosis was common and was a principal cause of resultant chronic injury for most patients. Several treatment strategies were tried, with success rates as follows: closed reduction, 6 of 12; McLaughlin procedure, 4 of 9; modified McLaughlin procedure, 4 of 4; hemiarthroplasty, 6 of 9; and total shoulder arthroplasty, 9 of 10.

A 1998 study reported on posterior dislocations or fracture-dislocations of 73 shoulders in 66 patients. Of these, 42 were chronic and presented at an average of

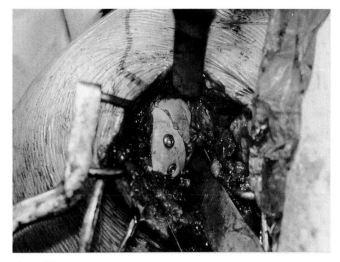

Figure 13 Reconstruction of a large Hill-Sachs lesion with an osteochondral allograft.

23.6 months after injury, very consistent with the typical time of misdiagnosis found in the literature. Surgical management was similar to the techniques used in the first study. Patients addressed within 2 years of injury fared better than those treated after 2 years. The key variables in determining treatment type were the size of

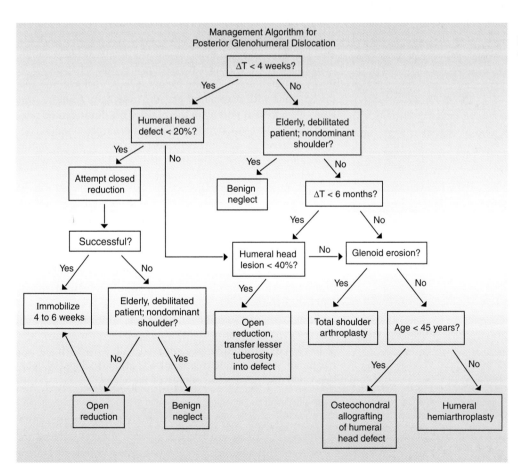

Figure 14 Management algorithm for posterior glenohumeral dislocation. ΔT = time from injury.

the anteromedial humeral head defect (McLaughlin lesion) and the time from injury.

In a third study, the results of filling the McLaughlin lesion with an osteochondral allograft in four patients with chronic posterior dislocations were reported. The size of the defect ranged from 40% to 55% of the humeral head. All grafts incorporated. Although at follow-up all four patients either had evidence of some

graft collapse or osteonecrosis of the humeral head, all patients were stable; three of the four patients had good function with little pain.

Using the principles outlined in the literature, a reasonable treatment algorithm for the management of posterior glenohumeral dislocation can be formulated (Fig. 14). As suggested by the authors of the 1998 study, principles are based on the time from injury and the size of the McLaughlin lesion, which is best identified on a CT scan (Fig. 15). Given the rarity of this injury and the lack of large treatment series, this protocol should be considered a guide only.

Annotated Bibliography

Acute Dislocation

Gartsman GM, Taverna E, Hammerman SM: Arthroscopic treatment of acute traumatic anterior glenohumeral dislocation and greater tuberosity fracture. *Arthroscopy* 1999;15:648-650.

This case report and technique article describes the successful use of the arthroscope to perform Bankart repair and reduction and fixation of a displaced greater tuberosity fracture.

Hovelius L, Augustini BG, Fredin H, Johansson O, Norlin R, Thorling J: Primary anterior dislocation of the shoulder in young patients: A ten-year prospective study. *J Bone Joint Surg Am* 1996;78:1677-1684.

This 10-year follow-up study reported on 245 patients younger than 40 years who sustained primary anterior shoulder dislocations. Although the group was somewhat mixed in terms of diagnosis, including "spontaneous" dislocations and dislocations with associated greater tuberosity fracture, the study is important purely on the basis of the duration and percentage of follow-up. Important conclusions were a high recurrence rate, which was inversely correlated with age at initial dislocation; a rate of dislocation arthropathy of 20%, which was unrelated to surgical treatment or number of recurrences; and a lack of effect of initial treatment on recurrence rate.

Kirkley A, Griffin S, Richards C, Miniaci A, Mohtadi N: Prospective randomized clinical trial comparing the effectiveness of immediate arthroscopic stabilization versus immobilization and rehabilitation in first traumatic anterior dislocations of the shoulder. *Arthroscopy* 1999;15:507-514.

Immediate arthroscopic stabilization after initial dislocation resulted in a rate of redislocation of 15.9% at an average follow-up of 33 months as compared with 47% for exercise treatment. Arthroscopic treatment was also associated with an improved disease-specific quality of life index.

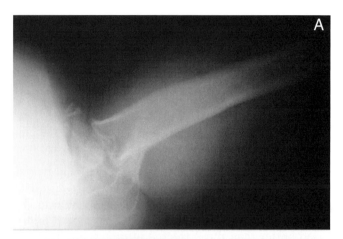

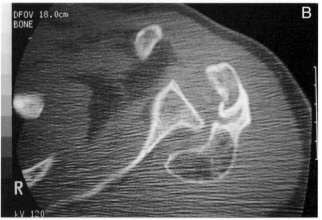

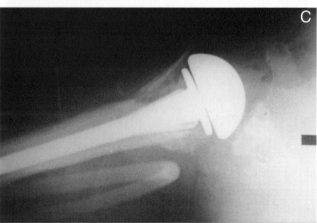

Figure 15 Posterior glenohumeral dislocation. **A,** Axillary radiograph. **B,** CT scan of the same patient, further defining the humeral head defect (McLaughlin lesion). **C,** Radiograph of the shoulder following effective total shoulder arthroplasty.

Matsen III FA, Thomas SC, Rockwood Jr CA, Wirth MA: Glenohumeral instability, in Rockwood CA Jr, Matsen FA III, Wirth MA, Harryman DT II (eds): *The Shoulder*, ed 2. Philadelphia, PA, WB Saunders, 1998.

This chapter provides an excellent review of the management of acute and chronic glenohumeral dislocations. In addition, the chapter includes a report by Rockwood and Wirth on a series of 19 shoulders with luxatio erecta injuries.

Taylor DC, Arciero RA: Pathologic changes associated with shoulder dislocations: Arthroscopic and physical examination findings in first-time, traumatic anterior dislocations. *Am J Sports Med* 1997;25:306-311.

This study reported the arthroscopic findings in 63 patients who sustained a first-time traumatic dislocation. Sixty-one of 63 patients (97%) were found to have a Bankart tear. Six patients had superior labral tears, two of which involved the biceps origin. A concurrent group of nonsurgically treated patients had a recurrence rate of 90%.

Wintzell G, Haglund-Åkerlind Y, Nowak J, Larsson S: Arthroscopic lavage compared with nonoperative treatment for traumatic primary anterior shoulder dislocation: A 2-year follow-up of a prospective randomized study. *J Shoulder Elbow Surg* 1999;8:399-402.

This study prospectively compared the results of nonsurgical treatment and arthroscopic lavage after first-time traumatic dislocation in 30 patients. All arthroscopic patients were found to have a Bankart tear. At 2-year follow-up, the recurrence rate in the nonsurgical group was 60%, while that in the surgical group was 20%.

Chronic Dislocation

Checchia SL, Santos PD, Miyazaki AN: Surgical treatment of acute and chronic posterior fracture-dislocation of the shoulder. *J Shoulder Elbow Surg* 1998;7:53-65.

This large retrospective review of 73 shoulders with acute or chronic posterior dislocation or fracture-dislocation provides treatment guides based on outcomes. Surgical outcome was best when intervention was applied within 2 years of dislocation. Shoulder arthroplasty was particularly successful but was also found to be technically challenging.

Gerber C, Lambert SM: Allograft reconstruction of segmental defects of the humeral head for the treatment of chronic locked posterior dislocation of the shoulder. *J Bone Joint Surg Am* 1996;78:376-382.

This study reported results of allograft filling of the anteromedial humeral head defect in four patients with chronic posterior dislocation. All four patients were stable and three had a good functional outcome, despite signs of either slight graft collapse or osteonecrosis of the humeral head.

Classic Bibliography

Arciero RA, Wheeler JH, Ryan JB, McBride JT: Arthroscopic Bankart repair versus nonoperative treatment for acute, initial anterior shoulder dislocations. *Am J Sports Med* 1994;22:589-594.

Baker CL, Uribe JW, Whitman C: Arthroscopic evaluation of acute initial anterior shoulder dislocations. *Am J Sports Med* 1990;18:25-28.

Burkhead WZ Jr, Rockwood CA Jr: Treatment of instability of the shoulder with an exercise program. *J Bone Joint Surg Am* 1992;74:890-896.

Flatow EL, Miller SR, Neer CS II: Chronic anterior dislocation of the shoulder. *J Shoulder Elbow Surg* 1993; 2:2-10.

Hawkins RJ, Neer CS II, Pianta RM, Mendoza FX: Locked posterior dislocation of the shoulder. *J Bone Joint Surg Am* 1987;69:9-18.

Matthews DE, Roberts T: Intraarticular lidocaine versus intravenous analgesic for reduction of acute anterior shoulder dislocations: A prospective randomized study. *Am J Sports Med* 1995;23:54-58.

Rowe CR, Zarins B: Chronic unreduced dislocations of the shoulder. *J Bone Joint Surg Am* 1982;64:494-505.

Suder PA, Frich LH, Hougaard K, Lundorf E, Wulff Jakobsen B: Magnetic resonance imaging evaluation of capsulolabral tears after traumatic primary anterior shoulder dislocation: A prospective comparison with arthroscopy of 25 cases. *J Shoulder Elbow Surg* 1995; 4:419-428.

Chapter 8

Recurrent Anterior Shoulder Instability

Stephen S. Burkhart, MD

Introduction

Recurrent anterior shoulder instability is the most dramatic manifestation of a traumatic anterior glenohumeral dislocation. Since ancient times, physicians have recognized the often extreme functional impairment created by recurrent anterior shoulder instability and have worked to develop surgical techniques that would restore stability. The degree of anterior instability can be quite variable, ranging from frank dislocations to minor subluxations to symptomatic microinstability patterns. Regardless of the degree of instability, symptoms are attributable to specific mechanical abnormalities. The mechanical abnormalities will vary from patient to patient, and therefore the job of the orthopaedic surgeon is to recognize and correct the mechanical aberrations specific to the individual.

Classification

This chapter focuses only on traumatic recurrent anterior instability. For this type of instability to occur, a disruption of the anteroinferior labroligamentous complex must be present. Most often, these disruptions occur as soft-tissue avulsions from the glenoid (soft-tissue Bankart lesions or Perthes lesions) or as combined bone–soft-tissue avulsions from the glenoid (bony Bankart lesions). A less common cause of instability is interstitial failure of the glenohumeral ligaments. The least common cause of anterior instability is humeral avulsion of the glenohumeral ligaments (HAGL lesion). Although one study found a 9.3% incidence of HAGL lesions in patients with recurrent instability, most studies have reported a much lower incidence. Even so, the surgeon must be particularly alert for the possibility of a HAGL lesion in a patient who sustains an anterior dislocation as the result of a significant traumatic event, especially in the absence of a Bankart lesion.

Evaluation

A thorough evaluation of the patient begins with the history and physical examination. Injury to the extremity typically occurs in the abducted externally rotated position. Such an injury can strip the labrum from the anterior glenoid, causing a Bankart lesion. Furthermore, as the humerus comes to rest in the dislocated position at the anteroinferior aspect of the glenoid, compressive forces can produce an impression defect in the humeral head (Hill-Sachs lesion) or a fracture of the glenoid (inverted-pear glenoid) (Fig. 1). The orientation of the humeral defect depends on the position of the shoulder when the compressive force is applied, and the angle of the Hill-Sachs lesion relative to the humeral shaft can be quite variable. The angle of some Hill-Sachs lesions, called engaging Hill-Sachs lesions, is such that they will engage the anterior glenoid in a parallel fashion when the shoulder is in abduction and external rotation (Fig. 2). Other Hill-Sachs lesions, called nonengaging Hill-Sachs lesions, will not engage the glenoid when the arm is in abduction and external rotation (Fig. 3). In patients with recurrent anterior dislocations, the bone defects potentially become larger with each dislocation. Certain sports may predispose the athlete to unique bone injury patterns. For example, ball carriers in rugby have a high incidence of bony Bankart lesions, probably because these injuries are usually sustained when an athlete stiff-arms an opponent with the arm in midabduction and extension. An axial load applied to the arm in this position may produce edge loading at the front of the glenoid, causing a bony Bankart lesion.

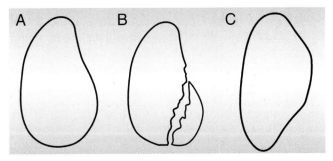

Figure 1 Normal and abnormal configurations of the glenoid. **A,** The normal shape of the glenoid is that of a pear, larger below than above. **B,** A bony Bankart lesion can create an inverted-pear configuration. **C,** A compression Bankart lesion can also create an inverted pear configuration.

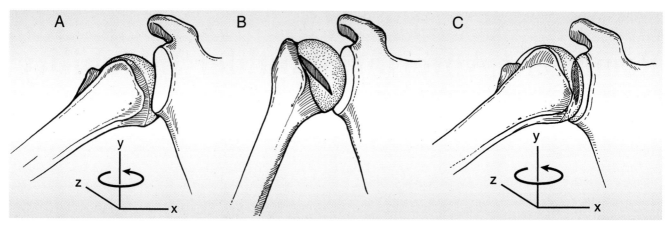

Figure 2 The engaging Hill-Sachs lesion. In a functional position of abduction and external rotation, the long axis of the Hill-Sachs lesion is parallel to the anterior glenoid and engages its anterior corner. **A,** Creation of lesion with the arm in abduction and external rotation. **B,** Orientation of Hill-Sachs lesion. **C,** Engagement of Hill-Sachs lesion in functional position of abduction and external rotation. The orthogonal three-dimensional Cartesian coordinate system is represented by xyz.

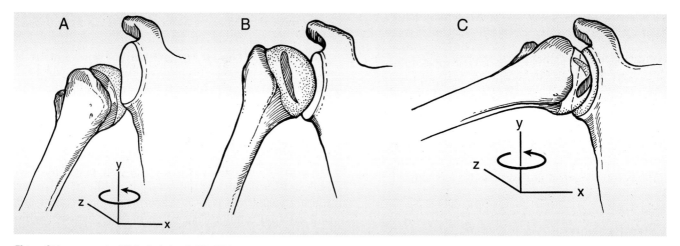

Figure 3 The nonengaging Hill-Sachs lesion. **A,** This Hill-Sachs lesion was created with the arm at the side and in some extension and will engage only with the arm at the side with external rotation and extension, which is not a functional position. **B,** Orientation of the Hill-Sachs lesion. **C,** In a functional position of abduction and external rotation, the Hill-Sachs lesion is diagonal to the anterior margin of the glenoid and does not engage. The orthogonal three-dimensional Cartesian coordinate system is represented by xyz.

Recurrent instability is less likely to develop in patients older than age 40 years who sustain a first-time dislocation than in younger patients. However, these older patients are at greater risk of sustaining a concomitant rotator cuff tear or nerve injury. One study suggests that patients older than age 40 years who have significant pain and weakness for more than 3 weeks postinjury should undergo an MRI study or arthrogram to rule out a rotator cuff tear.

Patients older than age 40 years are also at higher risk for sustaining a subscapularis tendon tear at the time of a traumatic anterior dislocation. In patients who do sustain such a tear, recurrent instability is common.

Physical Examination

The examination for shoulder instability constitutes only one part of the general shoulder examination. The patient also must be examined for generalized ligamen-

tous laxity, and a neurovascular evaluation must be carefully done. If, as is usually the case, some arc of pain-free motion exists, strength testing is indicated to evaluate for the possibility of a rotator cuff tear.

Specific provocative tests for anterior instability include the apprehension test, the relocation test, and the load-and-shift test. Athletes who participate in sports that involve overhead throwing and who have no history of frank dislocation will sometimes experience pain with these provocative maneuvers, but not apprehension. Apprehension in the provocative position of abduction and external rotation is the hallmark of anterior instability.

Radiographs and Other Imaging Studies

Radiographs and other imaging studies comprise an important part of the evaluation of the unstable shoulder. The West Point view is useful for visualizing bony

Bankart lesions, whereas the Stryker notch view reliably profiles the Hill-Sachs lesion. Magnetic resonance arthrography has been shown to be superior to plain MRI in identifying anterior labral pathology.

Examination Under Anesthesia

After general anesthesia has been administered and the patient's muscles are relaxed, an examination under anesthesia (EUA) is carried out with the patient in the supine or the lateral position. The examiner applies anterior and posterior forces to the proximal humerus at varying degrees of abduction. The examiner can feel the increased anterior excursion of the humeral head under load in the patient with anterior instability. Increased anterior excursion under load at greater degrees of abduction (ie, 45° and greater) indicates disruption of the sling effect of the inferior glenohumeral ligament.

Arthroscopic Evaluation

Following EUA, arthroscopic evaluation can provide the surgeon with additional useful information. Arthroscopy can be performed with the patient in either the beach chair position or the lateral position. The Bankart lesion can be easily visualized. Anterior labroligamentous periosteal sleeve avulsion (ALPSA) lesions, in which the labroligamentous soft-tissue sleeve has healed in a medialized position on the glenoid neck, can be identified (Fig. 4). Superior labrum anterior and posterior (SLAP) lesions can be diagnosed with confidence by arthroscopy; these lesions are very difficult to diagnose in any other way, even with MRI. The size of a bony Bankart lesion can be measured arthroscopically with a calibrated probe. The diameter of the inferior glenoid can be compared with that of the superior glenoid to determine whether an inverted-pear configuration exists. By taking the arm out of traction and moving it into a position of combined abduction and external rotation while maintaining an arthroscopic view, the surgeon can observe the dynamic relationship of the Hill-Sachs lesion to the anterior glenoid to determine if the patient has an engaging or nonengaging Hill-Sachs lesion. The drive-through sign, in which the arthroscope can be "driven through" the glenohumeral articulation from superior to inferior with minimal resistance, is generally indicative of anterior instability. However, the drive-through sign can also be present with isolated SLAP lesions as a result of anterior pseudolaxity caused by superior labral disruption. Repair of the labral pathology, including the Bankart or SLAP lesion, will usually eliminate the drive-through sign. In arthroscopic repairs of anterior instability, elimination of the drive-through sign can be taken as the end point for correction.

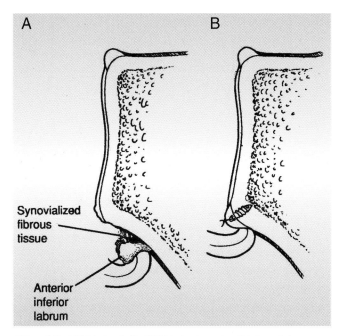

Figure 4 The ALPSA lesion. **A,** The ALPSA lesion is one in which the anterior labroligamentous soft-tissue sleeve has healed in a medialized position on the glenoid neck. **B,** Repair of anterior instability in a patient with an ALPSA lesion requires that the soft-tissue sleeve be mobilized adequately to allow it to be anatomically repaired to the "corner" of the anterior glenoid. *(Reproduced with permission from Neviaser TJ: The anterior labroligamentous periosteal sleeve avulsion lesion: A cause of anterior instability of the shoulder. Arthroscopy 1993;9:17-21.)*

Another dynamic arthroscopic test is the peel-back test for pathologic SLAP lesions. In this test, the shoulder is brought into 70° to 90° of abduction; it is then slowly externally rotated while the biceps–superior labrum complex is observed arthroscopically. In type 2 SLAP lesions with loss of a firm anchor for the biceps root and posterosuperior labrum, the biceps–superior labrum complex will peel back over the edge of the glenoid as the arm is externally rotated. A positive peel-back test, which is caused by the effect of the biceps vector shift as the biceps twists at its base, occurs when the loose, unanchored labrum rolls over the edge of the glenoid.

Additional pathologies can be identified arthroscopically, including HAGL lesions, subscapularis tears, rotator cuff tears, posterior labral lesions, and loose bodies.

Treatment

Arthroscopic Versus Open Repair

Arthroscopic Bankart repairs remain controversial, primarily because of reports of high recurrence rates, which range up to 70% for transglenoid repairs. However, a critical analysis of the literature reveals that the recurrence rate is quite variable and can be very low, even with transglenoid repairs. Among arthroscopic repairs, the best results have been reported with suture anchor techniques. A recent series of arthroscopic suture anchor

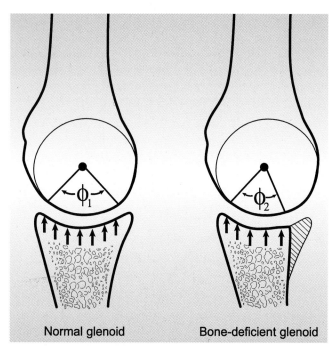

Normal glenoid | Bone-deficient glenoid

Figure 5 Glenoid bone loss shortens the "safe arc" through which the glenoid can resist axial forces. $\emptyset_2$ (bone-deficient condition) is less than $\emptyset_1$ (normal glenoid).

repairs has reported excellent results, with a recurrence rate of only 7% in an athletic population.

The best results for arthroscopic procedures are reported for those that emphasize repair of the capsulolabral tissue to the corner or even the face of the glenoid rather than in a medial position. This is not surprising given that a fairly common pattern of medialized capsulolabral healing, the ALPSA lesion, has been associated with recurrent anterior dislocation. Repairing the capsule in a medial position, which is the position of an ALPSA lesion, would be expected to lead to a high recurrence rate. Indeed, because many of the techniques of arthroscopic staple capsulorrhaphy or transglenoid labral repair do place the labrum in this position, a fairly high failure rate is to be expected.

In contrast, the classic open Bankart repair uses transosseous tunnels for suture that exit onto the face of the glenoid and automatically lateralize the capsulolabral repair. Suture anchor repairs, both open and arthroscopic, that lateralize the labrum have been shown to give excellent results. For a straightforward Bankart lesion without significant bone deficiency, some reports in the literature indicate that both open and arthroscopic Bankart repairs give equally good results.

Bone Deficiency: Implications for Treatment

A recent study of 194 consecutive arthroscopic Bankart repairs performed with suture anchors analyzed two subgroups of patients: 173 patients without significant

bone defects, and 21 patients with significant bone defects. Significant bone defects were defined as: (1) glenoid bone deficiency with an inverted pear configuration, and (2) proximal humeral bone deficiency in the form of an engaging Hill-Sachs lesion. The group of 173 patients without significant bone defects experienced seven recurrences, for a 4% recurrence rate. The group of 21 patients with significant bone defects experienced 14 recurrences, for a 67% recurrence rate. The study subjects included 101 contact athletes. Contact athletes without significant bone defects experienced a 6.5% recurrence rate, whereas those with significant bone defects experienced an 89% recurrence rate. Patients with these significant bone defects should not be considered candidates for arthroscopic instability repair.

Treatment of a significant glenoid bone defect requires a bone graft to extend the articular arc of the glenoid (Fig. 5). The graft may be either a large coracoid graft (Latarjet procedure) or a large iliac graft. Allograft bone is not recommended unless there is no satisfactory donor site for an autogenous graft.

An engaging Hill-Sachs lesion can be treated by capsular plication to restrict external rotation, thereby preventing engagement of the lesion. Alternatively, if the Hill-Sachs lesion exists in combination with an inverted pear-shaped glenoid that requires glenoid bone grafting, the lengthened glenoid articular arc created by the bone graft will usually be sufficient to prevent engagement of the Hill-Sachs lesion.

Arthroscopic Repair

As stated earlier, the surgeon should not attempt arthroscopic instability repairs in patients with significant bone defects. In patients without significant bone defects, however, results can be quite good, with recurrence rates of only 4% to 7%, if close attention is paid to important details of surgical technique.

In general, suture anchor repairs yield the best results of the arthroscopic repairs, with lower recurrence rates than transglenoid repairs, staple repairs, and polyglycolic acid tack repairs. The suture anchors must be placed on the corner of the anterior glenoid or even a couple of millimeters onto the articular face of the glenoid to incorporate the labroligamentous sleeve as a prolongation of the glenoid concavity. The surgeon must attempt to achieve a proximal shift of the labrum to the anchor to help reduce capsular redundancy, particularly in the axillary recess. Knot security and loop security will ensure tight apposition of soft tissues to bone.

A recent study reported success with isolated rotator interval closure in patients with anterior instability and increased sulcus signs. However, none of these patients had Bankart lesions, and many did not have a history of trauma that initiated their symptoms. If a patient still has a positive drive-through sign after an arthroscopic Bankart repair, the surgeon should consider doing a rotator interval closure to augment the Bankart repair.

Capsular reduction by radiothermal shrinkage has been proposed as an adjunct to arthroscopic Bankart repair. However, no clinical series currently suggest that the addition of radiothermal shrinkage improves the results of arthroscopic Bankart repair.

In performing rotator interval closure or adjunctive capsular reduction by plication or radiothermal shrinkage, the surgeon must be careful not to overtighten the shoulder. The goal of surgery is stability, not stiffness.

Open Repair

Most recent reports of open instability repairs emphasize anatomic approaches. The most common procedure is one variation or another of the Bankart repair. The use of suture anchors in place of transosseous tunnels simplifies and expedites the surgical technique. As with arthroscopic approaches, rotator interval closure is probably not necessary in patients with traumatic anterior instability who have Bankart lesions.

Bone deficiency must be recognized and properly addressed. Anteroinferior glenoid deficiency involving more than 25% of the inferior glenoid diameter can be successfully restored by means of a coracoid bone graft (Latarjet procedure) or an iliac crest bone graft. For an engaging Hill-Sachs lesion, a capsular shift procedure to restrict external rotation can prevent the lesion from engaging. For a massive Hill-Sachs lesion involving more than 40% of the articular arc of the humerus, the surgeon must consider allografting the humeral head defect to restore the articular arc or a humeral head replacement.

Complications

The most frequently reported complication after either open arthroscopic or instability surgery is recurrent instability. Although failure rates up to 70% have been reported for transglenoid repairs, this technique is seldom performed at the present time. The high recurrence rates seem to have less to do with whether the procedure was done open or arthroscopically than with medialization of the repair. For example, the early arthroscopic procedures (staple capsulorrhaphy and transglenoid repair) tended to medialize the repair, and the recurrence rates were often unacceptably high. In a similar fashion, the open Dutoit staple capsulorrhaphy medialized the capsulolabral complex to create a surgically produced ALPSA lesion. Not surprisingly, long-term follow-up of

this open stabilization procedure revealed an unacceptable recurrence rate of 22%. An operation based on an ill-conceived principle (in this case, medialization of the capsuloligamentous complex) will give poor results whether it is done open or arthroscopically.

Subscapularis tendon failure following open repair has been reported. Subscapularis tendon rupture can be diagnosed by means of the lift-off test or the belly-press test. Meticulous attention to a stable repair of the subscapularis is essential in order to prevent this complication. An irreparable subscapularis tear may require a pectoralis major transfer.

Loss of motion can occur after instability repairs. Most often, the loss is small and inconsequential, but patients will occasionally develop capsular contractures with marked loss of motion, necessitating open or arthroscopic capsular release. Long-standing anterior capsular contracture will produce repetitive posterior shear stresses that can contribute to articular degeneration. This process has been labeled "capsulorrhaphy arthropathy."

Annotated Bibliography
Classification

Bokor DJ, Conboy VB, Olson C: Anterior instability of the glenohumeral joint with humeral avulsion of the glenohumeral ligament: A review of 41 cases. *J Bone Joint Surg Br* 1999;81:93-96.

The authors report the largest series by far of HAGL lesions in contact athletes. They make the compelling point that if a patient undergoes a traumatic anterior dislocation and arthroscopic examination does not reveal a Bankart lesion, the surgeon must have a high suspicion for a HAGL lesion.

Field LD, Warren RF, O'Brien SJ, Altchek DW, Wickiewicz TL: Isolated closure of rotator interval defects for shoulder instability. *Am J Sports Med* 1995;23:557-563.

The authors report their generally good results of isolated rotator interval closure in anterior shoulder instability. Despite a diagnosis of anterior instability, these patients had no Bankart lesions and had positive sulcus signs. Extrapolation of these results to a population of patients with traumatic instability and Bankart lesions is problematic.

Flatow EL, Warner JJP: Instability of the shoulder: Complex problems and failed repairs. Part I: Relevant biomechanics, multidirectional instability, and severe glenoid loss. *Instr Course Lect* 1998;47:97-112.

This instructional course explains the biomechanics of instability and discusses ways in which mechanical factors must be considered in undertaking instability repairs, particularly those with bone loss.

Wolf EM, Cheng JC, Dickson K: Humeral avulsion of the glenohumeral ligaments as a cause of anterior shoulder instability. *Arthroscopy* 1995;11:600-607.

The authors describe the HAGL lesion as a cause of anterior instability. This diagnosis, though rare, must be kept in mind by the surgeon, particularly in the case of the traumatic anterior dislocation in the absence of a Bankart lesion.

Evaluation

Burkhart SS, De Beer JF: Traumatic glenohumeral bone defects and their relationship to failure of arthroscopic Bankart repairs: Significance of the inverted-pear glenoid and the humeral engaging Hill-Sachs lesion. *Arthroscopy* 2000;16:677-694.

The authors present 194 consecutive arthroscopic Bankart repairs performed using a suture anchor technique, analyzed at an average follow-up of 27 months. They recognize the important contribution to recurrent instability of two types of significant bone defects: the inverted-pear glenoid and the humeral engaging Hill-Sachs lesion. The 173 patients without significant bone defects sustained a 4% recurrence rate. The 21 patients with significant bone defects sustained a 67% recurrence rate. The authors emphasize the importance of restoring the bony anatomy and conclude that arthroscopic Bankart repairs should not be performed in patients with the aforementioned significant bone defects.

Treatment

Allain J, Goutallier D, Glorion C: Long-term results of the Latarjet procedure for the treatment of anterior instability of the shoulder. *J Bone Joint Surg Am* 1998; 80:841-852.

The Latarjet procedure, using a large coracoid bone graft, was performed on 95 shoulders, 58 of which were retrospectively reviewed at an average follow-up of 14.3 years. There were no recurrent dislocations. At final follow-up, 34 shoulders had osteoarthritis of some degree, but it was mild (grade 1) in 25 shoulders. Placement of the coracoid graft lateral to the glenoid articular margin correlated with the higher degrees of osteoarthritis.

Bacilla P, Field LD, Savoie FH III: Arthroscopic Bankart repair in a high demand patient population. *Arthroscopy* 1997;13:51-60.

Arthroscopic anterior shoulder stabilization using a suture anchor technique was performed on 40 patients with an average age of 18 years. Average follow-up was 30 months. A 7% rate of recurrent dislocation or subluxation was found, a rate that compares favorably with the gold standard open Bankart procedure.

Wirth MA, Blatter G, Rockwood CA Jr: The capsular imbrication procedure for recurrent anterior instability of the shoulder. *J Bone Joint Surg Am* 1996;78:246-259.

A follow-up of 142 shoulders at an average of 5 years is presented. The traumatic group had a 3% recurrence rate, whereas the atraumatic group had a 6% recurrence rate. This procedure combines a Bankart repair with capsular imbrication, and the authors recommend it for anterior instability regardless of the etiology.

Complications

Bigliani LU, Newton PM, Steinmann SP, Connor PM, McIlveen SJ: Glenoid rim lesions associated with recurrent anterior dislocation of the shoulder. *Am J Sports Med* 1998;26:41-45.

The authors report on 25 shoulders with anterior instability in association with glenoid rim lesions. At an average follow-up of 30 months, there was a 12% rate of recurrent dislocation. The authors point out the worse prognosis for recurrent instability in this group of patients, and they advise coracoid bone graft if the rim fracture fragment comprises 25% or more of the glenoid diameter.

Lazarus MD, Harryman DT II: Complications of open anterior stabilization of the shoulder. *J Am Acad Orthop Surg* 2000;8:122-132.

Complications of glenohumeral instability surgery are discussed, along with innovative ways of salvaging shoulders with such complications.

Roberts SN, Taylor DE, Brown JN, Hayes MG, Saies A: Open and arthroscopic techniques for the treatment of traumatic anterior shoulder instability in Australian Rules football players. *J Shoulder Elbow Surg* 1999; 8:403-409.

This study compares three types of repair: arthroscopic transglenoid repair, arthroscopic biodegradable tack repair, and open Bankart/capsular shift repair. The recurrence rates were 70% for arthroscopic transglenoid repair, 38% for arthroscopic tack repair, and 30% for open repair. Even with open repair, the recurrence rate (30%) in this high-risk group was at a level that is generally considered unacceptable.

Classic Bibliography

Bankart ASB: Recurrent or habitual dislocation of the shoulder-joint. *BMJ* 1923;2:1132-1133.

Hawkins RJ, Angelo RL: Glenohumeral osteoarthrosis: A late complication of the Putti-Platt repair. *J Bone Joint Surg Am* 1990;72:1193-1197.

Levine WN, Richmond JC, Donaldson WR: Use of the suture anchor in open Bankart reconstruction: A follow-up report. *Am J Sports Med* 1994;22:723-726.

Lusardi DA, Wirth MA, Wurtz D, Rockwood CA Jr: Loss of external rotation following anterior capsulor-rhaphy of the shoulder. *J Bone Joint Surg Am* 1993; 75:1185-1192.

Morgan CD, Bodenstab AB: Arthroscopic Bankart suture repair: Technique and early results. *Arthroscopy* 1987;3:111-122.

Neviaser TJ: The anterior labroligamentous periosteal sleeve avulsion lesion: A cause of anterior instability of the shoulder. *Arthroscopy* 1993;9:17-21.

O'Driscoll SW, Evans DC: Long-term results of staple capsulorrhaphy for anterior instability of the shoulder. *J Bone Joint Surg Am* 1993;75:249-258.

Rowe CR, Patel D, Southmayd WW: The Bankart procedure: A long-term end-result study. *J Bone Joint Surg Am* 1978;60:1-16.

Thomas SC, Matsen FA III: An approach to the repair of avulsion of the glenohumeral ligaments in the management of traumatic anterior glenohumeral instability. *J Bone Joint Surg Am* 1989;71:506-513.

Chapter 9

Multidirectional and Posterior Shoulder Instability

Thomas A. Joseph, MD

John J. Brems, MD

Introduction

This chapter presents current concepts related to posterior and multidirectional instabilities of the shoulder. Although posterior instability may occur in isolation, it can also be a component of multidirectional instability (MDI), and several common features exist between the two conditions. The information presented reflects knowledge gained over the past 5 years in the basic science of instability as well as a discussion of clinical studies and evolving treatment options.

Multidirectional Instability

Neer and Foster first outlined a detailed description and management algorithm for MDI of the shoulder in 1980. Since that time, MDI has become a more widely appreciated clinical entity and remains a focus of continued investigation. Neer and Foster distinguished MDI from the more commonly recognized forms of anterior and posterior instability. They described the often subtle presentation of MDI and emphasized the problems that might be encountered when traditional unidirectional repairs are used to treat this condition. The surgical treatment Neer and Foster proposed, the inferior capsular shift procedure, has withstood the test of time, producing uniformly good results over the short and intermediate terms.

Despite an increased awareness of MDI and continuous progress in shoulder instability research, understanding of this disorder remains incomplete. Patient presentations are quite variable. In addition, MDI still lacks a universal definition in the orthopaedic literature. Because of these ambiguities, the diagnosis of MDI is somewhat subjective, with the current tendency being to overdiagnose this once-overlooked, complex condition.

Definition and Classification

MDI has been defined by various authors both simply, as "global instability" or "instability in more than one direction," and in more complex terms, as part of classification systems with multiple subtypes. The most appropriate and comprehensive description of MDI defines it as global shoulder laxity (anterior, posterior, and inferior) that is associated with the concurrent reproduction of symptoms inferiorly and in at least one other direction. Additionally, most symptoms are experienced in the midrange of glenohumeral motion, resulting in frequent limitations in activities of daily living. The patient usually avoids extremes of motion because of significant apprehension.

Several classification systems have been proposed for shoulder instability; some incorporate MDI, and others attempt to subclassify the disorder. The Atraumatic Multidirectional Bilateral Rehabilitation Inferior capsular shift/Traumatic Unidirectional Bankart lesion Surgery (AMBRI/TUBS) classification is a popular means of categorizing instability patterns because of its simplicity.

In classifying MDI with regard to etiology, the condition can be thought of as being either congenital, acquired, or posttraumatic. Congenital, or primary, MDI occurs in patients with inherited ligamentous laxity. This includes connective tissue disorders such as Ehlers-Danlos or Marfan's syndrome, as well as milder forms of generalized ligamentous laxity. Patients with specific collagen-related diseases tend to present at a younger age and are more likely to be refractory to surgical treatment. A positive family history is frequently seen. Acquired MDI arises from repetitive microtrauma to the shoulder and is commonly seen in swimmers, weight lifters, gymnasts, and athletes who participate in throwing or racquet sports. These individuals may or may not have some degree of underlying laxity and are sometimes described as having secondary MDI. Although MDI is commonly thought of as being purely atraumatic, this is a misconception. Previously asymptomatic patients with underlying laxity quite commonly become symptomatic after a single traumatic event. These traumatic insults are often relatively minor, and when dislocation occurs, it is usually self-reduced. A Bankart lesion can occur in this setting and must be addressed along with the underlying patholaxity. Because patients with MDI present with substantial variations in history, physical findings, and degree of trauma, MDI may be regarded as a continuum rather than as a discrete entity.

The primary direction of the instability is another important consideration when classifying the disorder. Inferior capsular redundancy and rotator interval lesions are considered the hallmark lesions of MDI, making inferior instability a universal finding in patients with MDI. Combined anteroinferior or posteroinferior instability patterns are most common but occasionally instability exists in all three directions. In his original study, Neer separated his patients into three groups based on the direction of instability and the degree of instability: those with anterior and inferior dislocation with posterior subluxation; those with posterior and inferior dislocation with anterior subluxation; and those with dislocation in all three directions. Many patients present with varying degrees of subluxation but do not experience frank dislocation.

Further considerations are the duration of symptoms, either acute or chronic, and any history of volitional instability. Volitional instability includes both voluntary dislocators with psychiatric histories or secondary gain issues and habitual and positional dislocators. The distinction between these types of volitional instability is important and is described in more detail in the section on posterior instability.

Etiology

The etiology of MDI is thought to be multifactorial, with current theories focusing on structural or anatomic abnormalities, biochemical abnormalities, and neuromuscular mechanisms. In the normal shoulder, glenohumeral stability is maintained by an intricate balance of static and dynamic mechanisms. The capsuloligamentous restraints in the shoulder are generally thought of as checkreins that impart stability at various extremes of motion. The functions of individual static restraints have been delineated by several excellent basic science studies and have been outlined in chapter 2. Within the midrange of glenohumeral motion, the precise centering of the humeral head on the glenoid by the rotator cuff muscles is achieved by a mechanism known as concavity-compression. Recurrent instability results in deconditioning of the dynamic stabilizers and ineffective concavity-compression. Labral detachment can further compromise concavity-compression, as an intact labrum deepens the glenoid by 50% and contributes to 20% of the stability ratio in the inferior and posteroinferior directions.

The two anatomic lesions consistently associated with MDI are a redundant inferior capsular pouch and deficiency of the rotator interval tissue. The rotator interval

is the triangular space separating the anterior edge of the supraspinatus from the superior edge of the subscapularis; it is normally bridged by capsule (rotator interval capsule). Anatomically, the rotator interval includes the underlying superior glenohumeral ligament and is reinforced by the overlying coracohumeral ligament. Cadaveric sectioning studies have demonstrated the importance of these structures in resisting inferior and posterior displacement of the humeral head, with the superior glenohumeral ligament being the primary biomechanical restraint to inferior subluxation in the adducted arm. In patients with MDI, the rotator interval capsule is consistently characterized by the presence of either a discrete cleft or insubstantial, attenuated tissue. Defects in the rotator interval capsule disrupt the negative intra-articular pressure that exists in the normal shoulder and may further contribute to instability in this respect.

The inferior glenohumeral ligament complex functions as the primary restraint to inferior translation in the progressively abducted arm. In this same position, the anterior and posterior bands reciprocally tighten with rotation, imparting anterior stability when the arm is externally rotated and posterior stability when the arm is internally rotated. A capacious inferior pouch could therefore easily contribute to instability in all three directions.

The search continues for a consistent biochemical explanation for capsular laxity. Several basic science studies have found no difference between the quantity or type of collagen in shoulders of patients with MDI and that of normal control subjects. Collagen fibril diameter and cross-linking are properties that are directly related to tensile strength. A recent study comparing shoulder capsular tissue from patients with MDI, from patients with unidirectional (anterior) instability, and from normal control subjects made several unique observations. The capsular tissues from both instability groups demonstrated more stable and reducible collagen cross-links, greater mean collagen fibril diameter, higher cysteine concentration, and a higher density of elastin than did the normal samples. Whether these differences are factors predisposing to laxity or responses to repetitive stretch injury remains undetermined. Skin samples taken from these same patients revealed significantly smaller mean collagen fibril diameter in patients with MDI than in those with unidirectional (anterior) instability, suggesting a possible underlying connective tissue abnormality. The clinical observation that some patients with MDI experience poor wound healing and/or keloid formation supports this idea.

The following four observations support the idea of an underlying neuromuscular mechanism for MDI: (1) Many patients with MDI in one shoulder have an equal or greater amount of laxity in the contralateral, asymptomatic shoulder. (2) Symptoms occur within the mid-range of glenohumeral movements, where capsuloligamentous restraints remain lax. (3) Patients with MDI have been shown to have altered glenohumeral and scapulothoracic rhythm. (4) Mechanoreceptors have been identified in shoulder joint capsule, and proprioceptive deficits have been demonstrated both in patients with anterior instability and, more recently, in patients with MDI. In both groups, these deficits were shown to be reversible by surgical stabilization.

Clinical Presentation

History

Correctly diagnosing MDI requires a high index of suspicion and sharp clinical acumen. Patients may present with a variety of symptoms including pain; instability; looseness; weakness; paresthesias; fatigue; popping, clicking, or grinding; difficulty throwing, lifting, or sleeping; or "dead arm syndrome." In the absence of a documented dislocation, a chief complaint of pain sometimes overshadows subtle instability and can result in misdiagnosis. In addition, apprehension often complicates the examination. For these reasons, the value of multiple physical examinations, performed at different times, cannot be overemphasized. Patients should be questioned specifically about provocative arm positions because this can provide important clues to the primary direction of instability. Discomfort or "traction paresthesias" associated with carrying objects at the side are classic symptoms of inferior instability. Patients with anterior instability often will experience difficulty reaching overhead or sleeping with the arms overhead. Symptoms that occur when the arms are in a position of forward flexion, such as when bench pressing or pushing open doors, can signify posterior instability. Patients also should be asked whether they can voluntarily demonstrate what happens to their shoulder.

The incidence of MDI peaks in the second and third decades of life, with most patients younger than 35 years of age. A subset of preadolescent patients also has been recognized. These children appear to experience a higher incidence of voluntary subluxation, and pain is typically absent. Most authors caution against surgical intervention in the preadolescent population because the natural history of instability in this age group is favorable. This condition should not be confused with traumatic anterior dislocation in children, which carries a poor prognosis. There is also a significantly increased incidence of shoulder laxity in normal asymptomatic adolescents, with one study showing a 57% incidence in boys and a 48% incidence in girls. The role of physical therapy in the young patient is somewhat controversial because outcomes depend greatly on having the maturity to participate reliably in the therapy. Some surgeons recommend limiting treatment to reassurance and observation in this population of patients.

Some disagreement currently exists regarding the incidence of shoulder instability relative to gender. A comprehensive review of the literature on MDI reveals an approximately equal number of affected male and female patients. Although at least two studies have demonstrated a higher incidence of shoulder laxity in females than in males, a recent review article disputed any gender differences for MDI, stressing that laxity is not synonymous with instability.

Physical Examination

The physical examination for instability should include an evaluation of the cervical spine and of scapulothoracic mechanics in addition to a complete shoulder examination. This first step is visual inspection of the shoulder girdle from both the front and the back to evaluate for shoulder asymmetry, scapular winging, atrophy, and previous incisions. Squaring of the shoulder, in contrast to the normal rounded deltoid contour, is a common finding with inferior instability. Signs of generalized ligamentous laxity have been reported in 19% to 75% of patients undergoing surgery for MDI. These signs include hyperextension of the elbows and metacarpophalangeal joints, genu recurvatum, patellar subluxation, and the ability to abduct the thumb to reach the ipsilateral forearm. The acromioclavicular and sternoclavicular joints are frequently overlooked during this examination. Subluxation at either joint can be easily misinterpreted, by patients and physicians alike, as being glenohumeral. The same holds true for the scapulothoracic articulation, which can generate a variety of mechanical symptoms. Some patients will present with an "instability complex," wherein one or more of these joints is affected.

Instability tests should be performed first on the asymptomatic shoulder to enhance patient confidence and relaxation. Most patients with MDI will have increased passive range of motion of the shoulder joint. As with translation, if these findings are not accompanied by symptoms, they are not considered pathologic. Inferior instability is assessed first by applying downward traction on the arm at the side (sulcus test). As previously discussed, this assesses the integrity of the rotator interval structures. The degree of subluxation is graded based on the acromiohumeral distance. With the patient still in the seated position, the arm is then abducted 90°, and with the forearm in neutral rotation, a downward force is applied to the lateral brachium. Inferior translation in this position reflects redundancy of the inferior capsule. Anterior and posterior instability may be assessed with the patient in either the seated or supine position. Better patient relaxation and reproducibility can be obtained with the supine load-and-shift test. This test should be performed with the arm in approximately 20° of abduction, in the plane of the scapula. Application of a slight compressive load along the humeral axis centers the humeral head on the glenoid before it is translated. This maneuver helps to minimize errors caused by translating an already subluxated humeral head into a reduced position. Apprehension and relocation tests can be used to help confirm or rule out suspected anterior or posterior instability. Impingement tests are commonly positive in patients with MDI; a distinction should be made between maneuvers that produce pain and maneuvers that result in apprehension.

Radiographic Studies

All patients suspected of having shoulder instability require plain radiographs. A routine series includes AP, true AP, and axillary or West Point views. These studies will be normal in most patients with MDI. Osseous pathology is occasionally present, and it is important to routinely look for humeral head defects (Hill-Sachs and reverse Hill-Sachs lesions), traumatic glenoid changes (bony Bankart lesions, erosions, and rounding), and inherent architectural abnormalities such as hypoplasia or retroversion. Stress radiographs or arthrograms have not been found to be helpful or necessary in making a diagnosis of MDI.

CT is indicated to more accurately assess the osseous anatomy if a suspected abnormality such as increased glenoid retroversion is noted on plain radiographs. With the addition of a contrast medium, capsulolabral detachments can be accurately identified. More work is currently being done with MRI, which has replaced CT in many centers. In the absence of a suspected bony abnormality, a traumatic history, or confusing mechanical symptoms, these additional studies are not warranted.

Treatment

Nonsurgical Management

Nonsurgical management remains the first line of treatment for MDI. Current physical therapy programs, which are aimed at strengthening and retraining the rotator cuff muscles and scapular stabilizers, produce functional improvement in most patients. The most successful nonsurgical program reported satisfactory results in 29 of 33 shoulders (88%) with MDI. A more recent retrospective study tracing the natural history of nonsurgical treatment produced less optimal results, with 20 of 59 patients (33.9%) eventually requiring surgery. Of the 39 patients who did not undergo surgical treatment, 19 (48.7%) had persistent symptoms.

The fundamentals of a good rehabilitation plan include patient education, activity modification, and a supervised conditioning program lasting at least 3 to

6 months. From a basic science standpoint, the goals of shoulder rehabilitation are to restore effective concavity-compression through strengthening, identify and correct any abnormal muscle firing patterns, and improve deficient proprioceptive function. A brief period of immobilization, along with anti-inflammatory medications or a mild analgesic, may be used prior to starting formal physical therapy. The exercise program consists of two phases. Phase I includes progressive resistance exercises focusing on strengthening the rotator cuff, deltoid, and scapular stabilizers. They are performed with the arm below 90° of abduction to avoid the aggravating effects of secondary impingement. After 10 to 12 weeks, phase II begins, with an emphasis on proprioceptive training and the correction of any aberrant glenohumeral or scapulothoracic mechanics. Most patients who respond to physical therapy show some benefit within the first 3 months.

Surgical Management

Open Techniques Patients who fail to respond to 3 to 6 months of nonsurgical treatment are considered candidates for surgical intervention. The most time-honored surgical procedure remains the inferior capsular shift, which has given uniformly good results over short and intermediate periods and has begun to yield reports after longer follow-up. A recent clinical review with an 8.3-year mean follow-up reported 85% satisfactory outcomes in a group of 34 shoulders. Recurrent instability occurred in nine shoulders (25%) overall, six of which had a history of voluntary instability. Nineteen patients were assessed 3.5 years and again 11 years after surgery. There was no deterioration in stability or functional outcome score, leading the authors to conclude that the repair maintained its integrity over time. Radiologic examination showed a posterolateral defect in the humeral head in 9 of 14 shoulders (64%) treated with a posterior or combined approach. This is a previously unreported finding. Possible causative factors include subclinical anterior instability caused by an excessively tightened posterior capsule, growth disturbance to the epiphysis in young patients, and ischemic changes related to disruption of the posterior humeral circumflex artery.

The technical aspects of the inferior capsular shift and its modifications have been well described. The procedure may be performed through an anterior or posterior approach, depending on the direction of primary instability. An approach from the most unstable side allows for direct imbrication and reinforcement while simultaneously shifting to reduce global capsular laxity. One drawback to the posterior approach is the thin and pliable nature of the posterior capsule. Therefore, soft-tissue reconstructions for global instability may be performed through an anterior approach. The robust anterior capsular tissues provide for a more secure repair, and appropriate posterior capsular tensioning can be achieved with a generous capsular shift. An anterior incision also facilitates closure of the rotator interval and allows for simultaneous repair of any unexpected anterior Bankart lesion. Surgeon preference determines whether a humeral- or glenoid-based shift is performed; each has certain advantages. To avoid excessive tightening in a medial to lateral direction, the shift is performed with the arm in 30° of abduction, 40° of external rotation, and 10° of flexion.

Traditional postoperative care consists of 6 weeks of immobilization in a shoulder spica cast. The cast can be molded and split ahead of time to facilitate application in the operating room. Comparable results have been reported using commercial braces or slings. A recent report describes an accelerated rehabilitation program in a group of patients treated with an inferior capsular shift augmented with suture anchors. Restricted range-of-motion and isometric strengthening exercises were initiated within the first week, and immobilization was limited to the use of a sling for 2 weeks. At 12 to 30 months follow-up, range of motion and isokinetic strength were near normal in all subjects, and instability had not recurred. The use of a shoulder spica cast should be considered in most cases, while acknowledging that rehabilitation needs must be individualized.

Authors of both Japanese and American studies report success with isolated closure of rotator interval defects in patients who had findings consistent with MDI. Adequate stability was achieved by closure of the defect without further surgery.

Arthroscopic Techniques The arthroscopic treatment of shoulder instability is arguably one of the most significant technical advances in orthopaedics. These techniques have been greeted with cautious enthusiasm because although early results appear encouraging, the long-term results and sequelae remain unknown. Recent advances in arthroscopic stabilization for MDI include knot-tying techniques (imbrication, plication, and shifting) and the use of thermal energy in the so-called capsular shrinkage procedure. The potential advantages of these minimally invasive techniques include lower surgical morbidity, improved cosmesis, shorter hospital stays, quicker recovery, and improved range of motion. Direct visualization of the joint improves diagnostic accuracy and can help guide surgical planning.

A rapid evolution in shoulder arthroscopy has occurred since the first edition of this text was published in 1997. Initially, higher failure rates were reported in association with the arthroscopic treatment of anterior instability, but results now being reported parallel those obtained with open techniques. Application of this technology has been extended to the more severe forms of instability (posterior and multidirectional), and excellent results are being reported by select groups with long-standing experience in this area. The earliest reports of arthroscopic treatment of MDI involved the use of transglenoid sutures similar to those described for arthroscopic Bankart repairs. A retrospective review of 25 patients with MDI and no previous shoulder surgery yielded 88% satisfactory results at an average follow-up of 60 months, with preservation of motion achieved in all but one patient. A high (56%) incidence of concomitant Bankart lesions was seen. The described technique involves releasing the anteroinferior capsule from the glenoid with a shaver, then shifting the tissues superiorly to an abraded glenoid rim. The sutures are then passed through a drill hole in the glenoid and tied posteriorly. A variation of this technique has been described using an anterior transglenoid repair coupled with a posterior capsular advancement. A good or excellent result was obtained in 95% of these patients, with only 1 of 19 patients experiencing a recurrence. These techniques have not been widely adopted because of their technical difficulty and concerns about suprascapular nerve injury.

Capsular shrinkage procedures have received far more attention over the past 5 years and have largely supplanted the aforementioned arthroscopic techniques. Using thermal energy delivered arthroscopically via a laser or radiofrequency probe, capsular tissues are altered morphologically. The acronyms LACS (Laser Assisted Capsular Shift) and ETAC (Electrothermally Assisted Capsulorrhaphy) have been coined to represent laser and radiofrequency delivery systems, respectively. Regardless of the mode of delivery, the effects on tissue are essentially the same. Heat is applied directly to shrink the tissue and decrease capsular volume. The effect on tissue depends on many variables, including temperature, duration of exposure, depth of penetration, and the proximity of the probe tip to the target tissue. These effects also appear to be patient dependent, with different shoulders experiencing noticeably different results despite the use of consistent technique and thermal settings.

Regardless of the thermal device used, the technique is similar. For global instability, the probe is inserted through an anterior working portal, and the posterior band of the inferior glenohumeral ligament is addressed first. The inferior capsule is then shrunk, working from posterior to anterior in a controlled fashion. The anterior band of the inferior glenohumeral ligament is then treated, along with the middle glenohumeral ligament when present. The portals are then changed; a posterior working portal is established to provide access to the remainder of the posterior capsule. It has become common practice to also address the rotator interval capsule either with heat shrinkage or by reapproximating the defect with arthroscopically placed sutures. The anterior portal can be shrunk thermally as well so that it does not contribute to any preexisting interval defect. The thermal probe can be used in a paintbrush, grid, or spot-weld fashion when treating the capsular tissues; it has not been determined which of these techniques is most effective. Four to 6 weeks of postoperative immobilization is routine for MDI; however, care following thermal capsulorrhaphy still needs to be refined.

Several animal and cadaveric studies have provided useful information regarding the effects of thermal energy on capsular tissue. More recently, intraoperative human tissue samples have been studied biomechanically and histologically. The resulting understanding of the basic science of thermal techniques has helped guide clinical applications. It should be kept in mind, however, most of these studies involve animal or cadaveric tissue, and the long-term effects in vivo are completely unknown.

The exact mechanism by which thermal techniques impart stability remains uncertain. Although intuition would suggest a mechanical tightening effect, postoperative histologic and MRI findings have demonstrated capsular thickening caused by cicatrix formation and increased collagen deposition. This may serve to reinforce weakened restraints. In addition, studies have demonstrated improvements in proprioception as early as 9 weeks following thermal capsulorrhaphy. The tightening effect achieved with thermal capsulorrhaphy may restore normal capsular tension such that mechanoreceptors can again function properly.

Encouraging short-term results are presently being reported for both laser and electrothermal techniques. In general, results of MDI treatment have not been as predictable as those for anterior and microinstabilities. Prior stabilization surgery, multiple recurrent dislocations, and participation in contact sports appear to be risk factors for poor outcome with thermal capsulorrhaphy. It is hoped that future clinical trials will help distinguish which subgroups of patients with MDI can expect the best results with capsular shrinkage.

Summary of MDI Management

The diagnosis of MDI rests upon a sound history and physical examination. Physicians must be consistent in their use of the diagnosis so that proper treatment can be executed and consistent cohorts compared in the orthopaedic literature. Although most patients will respond to a well-regimented rehabilitation program, predictable results have been obtained with the inferior capsular shift procedure and its modifications in those who remain symptomatic following nonsurgical treatment. These results have remained consistent over time and have not been associated with the high incidence of postcapsulorrhaphy arthropathy seen with other stabilization procedures. Arthroscopic techniques offer a less invasive means of achieving stability in these patients,

and encouraging results are being reported over the short term. As with any new procedure, caution must be exercised until data from longer follow-up are available.

Posterior Instability

Posterior instability may occur in isolation or as part of bidirectional or multidirectional instability. When it exists in isolation, symptoms are usually mild and can be easily overlooked or misdiagnosed. A high percentage of affected patients are athletes who participate in activities that repetitively stress the posterior capsule (Table 1). In most cases, a well-designed physical therapy program will provide enough symptomatic relief that surgical intervention can be avoided. Historically, high failure rates have been associated with the surgical treatment of posterior instability, and multiple procedures have been described. Distinct structural abnormalities such as excessive glenoid or humeral head retroversion can be contributing factors and may warrant corrective osteotomy.

Definition and Classification

As with MDI, many confounding variables complicate classifying posterior instability in a simple and reliable fashion. One such variable is voluntary instability, which is present in some form in a substantial percentage of patients with posterior instability. The term "voluntary dislocator" carries negative connotations because it implies possible underlying personality disorders and high failure rates with surgical treatment. Some authors list "voluntary dislocation" as a contraindication to surgical treatment. The presence of voluntary instability certainly complicates the care of affected patients; however, those who are truly disabled but without psychiatric illness or secondary gain issues may be helped by surgery.

Recurrent posterior subluxation is classified into voluntary and involuntary subtypes, with a further distinction made between habitual and positional dislocators. Habitual instability refers to dislocation or subluxation that occurs as a result of underlying neuromuscular imbalance: abnormal muscle contraction and relaxation patterns result in the simultaneous activation and suppression of the two halves of a force couple causing subluxation. Many habitual dislocators have underlying psychiatric problems and will continue to dislocate despite attempts at surgical stabilization. However, even involuntary habitual dislocators can be refractory to surgical measures. Therefore, biofeedback and muscular retraining must be incorporated into the rehabilitation efforts of such patients.

A positional dislocator is a patient who is able to demonstrate instability by placing the arm in a position of risk. These patients do not have underlying psychiatric illness or secondary gain issues, and ordinarily they would avoid such provocative maneuvers. Although physical therapy remains the first-line treatment, in this group of patients, surgical intervention has yielded acceptable results. In recent retrospective review, 92% of 24 patients with voluntary posterior instability but no overt psychiatric condition subjectively rated the results good or excellent following posterior-inferior capsular shift. Recurrent instability occurred in six patients (23%).

Etiology

In many ways the etiology of posterior instability is similar to that of MDI, with multiple contributing factors possible. The same classifications used for MDI (congenital, acquired, and posttraumatic) can be applied to posterior instability to better understand the etiology and to direct appropriate treatment. Congenital instability can be a result of inherited ligamentous laxity as well as of abnormal scapulohumeral anatomy. Osseous architectural findings such as excessive glenoid or humeral retroversion and glenoid hypoplasia have been described in association with posterior instability. Although rare, these structural changes can be a reason for failure when soft-tissue reconstructions alone are performed. A purely atraumatic history of isolated posterior instability should prompt a search for an underlying inherited ligamentous or osseous cause.

In athletes, acquired symptoms usually can be linked to some repetitive stress to the posterior capsule such as the axially applied load experienced in bench pressing, boxing, and gymnastics. Offensive linemen in football risk injury by this same mechanism because many of their maneuvers involve impact loading with the arms locked in front of the body. A second mechanism of injury common among athletes involves tractional stretching caused by muscular pull and momentum. This occurs in swimmers, in pitchers (during the follow-through phase of throwing), and with backhand strokes in racquet sports. The lead arm of batters and golfers can also experience a posterior joint reactive force. A similar mechanism has been described recently in archers.

The most common traumatic cause of posterior instability is a fall or a blow to the arm while in the "at-risk" position (forward flexion, adduction, and internal rotation). This mechanism also has been associated with a high incidence of posterior labral detachment. In a recent report of posterior labral injury in contact athletes, nine patients were found on arthroscopic examination to have posterior labral detachment without instability. The authors hypothesized that the shear force that results from impact loading with the arms in front of the body can result in posterior labral detachment without capsular injury. All nine athletes responded to arthroscopic reattachment and returned to

TABLE 1	Specific Athletic Activities Associated With Posterior Instability
Activity	**Motion**
Weight lifting	Bench press, push-ups
Pitching	Follow-through phase
Swimming	Butterfly and freestyle strokes
Boxing	Axial load with punching
Gymnastics	Parallel bars, rings
Racquet sports	Backhand strokes
Batting	Motions of lead arm
Golf	Motions of lead arm
Football	Offensive lineman maneuvers
Archery	Motions of both arms
Volleyball	Follow-through phase of serve

contact sports. There have been numerous other reports of posterior capsulolabral injury (reverse Bankart lesions) in patients with posterior instability. The exact contribution of the posterior labrum to posterior stability is not well defined, but it is in general less significant than its anterior counterpart.

Clinical Presentation

Patients with posterior instability most frequently present with pain rather than instability per se. In athletes, symptoms are usually mild and occur during or after activities that stress the glenohumeral joint. Injuries with underlying anatomic or posttraumatic causes may be more severely debilitating. It is not uncommon for patients with habitual posterior dislocation to be completely free of pain.

Physical Examination

As described previously for MDI, attention should first be directed to the unaffected shoulder, and repeat examinations may be needed. The classic provocative arm position for posterior instability is one of forward flexion, adduction, and internal rotation. Taking the arm out of adduction and internal rotation relaxes the posterior capsule. Subluxation or discomfort with a stress test performed in either position is suggestive of posterior instability. In addition, the examiner should stabilize the scapula and gently extend the patient's arm in the horizontal plane while the affected shoulder is in a subluxated position; a palpable clunk constitutes a positive relocation test. Patients may also have tenderness to palpation of the posterior joint line. Translation is assessed in the seated or supine position with the load-and-shift test. Posterior translation of 50% or less can be considered normal. The patient's reaction to the translation provides more important information than the magnitude of displacement.

Nonsurgical Treatment

The principles of nonsurgical treatment for posterior instability are similar to those presented for MDI. It is important that provocative maneuvers and any abnormal scapulothoracic rhythms be considered before prescribing a nonspecific exercise program. Provocative maneuvers will identify those arm positions that must be avoided during the rehabilitation process. Electromyographic evaluation of patients with voluntary posterior subluxation has revealed two different muscle activation patterns, each requiring a specific program of biofeedback and strengthening. Selective muscle contraction may occur anteriorly, pushing the humeral head backward, or posteriorly, causing a backward pull. Depending on the underlying mechanism, subluxation may occur either in the classic position of forward flexion, adduction, and internal rotation or in abduction and external rotation. Recognition of these patterns is critical to designing a proper rehabilitation plan.

Most traditional nonsurgical protocols for posterior instability have focused on strengthening the posterior deltoid, infraspinatus, and teres minor. More contemporary approaches incorporate biofeedback, muscle retraining, and proprioceptive exercises. Scapular winging, which is commonly seen in patients with posterior instability, usually results from the inhibition of scapular stabilizers. Therapeutic efforts aimed at correcting scapulothoracic mechanics will improve the dynamic effects of concavity-compression at the glenohumeral joint. Using such principles, most patients will experience enough symptomatic relief to return to athletic activity, although certain exercises and predisposing activities should be discouraged indefinitely.

Surgical Treatment

Open Techniques

The fact that many different surgical procedures have been proposed over the years to address posterior instability testifies to the current poor understanding of this condition. Because various anatomic abnormalities may exist, no single procedure has proved to be universally effective. Failure rates as high as 50% have been reported. In general, procedures can be separated into those addressing the soft tissues and those involving bone. Table 2 lists the many proposed surgical options, including those of historical interest but not in current use.

Soft-tissue abnormalities are the predominant cause of posterior instability. Soft-tissue procedures may be used alone or in combination with bony procedures. As with MDI, a posterior capsular shift to treat posterior instability that includes an inferior or global component may be performed through either an anterior or posterior approach. The posterior capsule is much thinner than the anterior tissues, with an average thickness of 1.5 mm. For this reason as well as those mentioned in the section on MDI, an anterior approach is preferred whenever possible.

When posterior instability occurs in isolation and without an identifiable osseous cause, a patulous posterior capsule or capsulolabral deficiency is usually responsible. Posterior capsulorrhaphy through a posterior approach can be combined with a capsulolabral repair or augmented with a bone block if necessary. The use of staples has fallen out of favor because of high failure rates and complications. As an alternative, a posterior capsulotendinous tensioning procedure in which the posterior capsule and the overlying infraspinatus are shortened in a medial to lateral fashion without a circumferential shift has been described. In one recent report, 13 of 14 patients were satisfied with their results at 44 months average follow-up. None of the patients experienced a recurrence.

Several studies have demonstrated increased glenoid retroversion in patients with posterior instability. Glenoid hypoplasia or flatness, which can theoretically compromise the glenohumeral stability ratio, has also been implicated as a cause of diminished glenoid concavity. One approach to dealing with this fundamental deficit is to increase the depth of the glenoid by performing an opening wedge osteotomy (or glenoplasty) in an attempt to increase the mechanical stability of the glenohumeral joint. This procedure has been done for years, based on theory and clinical observations of improvement in an acceptable number of patients. Recently, a study in cadaveric models confirmed that posteroinferior glenoplasty changes the effective glenoid shape and improves stability. Glenoid depth increased from 3.8 ± 0.6 mm to 7.0 ± 1.8 mm. The center of the humeral head shifted an average of 2.2 mm anteriorly and 1.8 mm superiorly. Posteroinferior glenoid slope increased from 0.55 ± 0.07 to 0.83 ± 0.12. The result was an increase of more than 70% in the tangential force that can be resisted before dislocation. Earlier studies have shown that scapular inclination contributes to inferior glenohumeral stability as well, possibly by a cam effect that tightens the superior capsule.

Despite an established scientific basis and the reasonable short-term results obtained with glenoid osteotomy, several complications are unique to this procedure. Glenohumeral arthritis, iatrogenic anterior instability, coracoid impingement, intra-articular fracture, and osteonecrosis have all been reported. In a recent series, 17 patients with atraumatic posterior instability were followed after glenoid osteotomy at an average follow-up of 5 years, 81% were rated as good or excellent, and only 12.5% had experienced a recurrence. Postoperative degenerative changes were seen radiographically in 25% of the patients. To be considered for glenoid osteotomy, patients should have radiographically measurable retroversion that exceeds –7° to –10°. An average retroversion angle of about –4° has been established using normal control subjects.

Humeral osteotomy has also been proposed as a means of treating posterior instability. An external rotation osteotomy is indicated when symptoms are exacerbated by internal rotation. There are limited reports of this technique in the orthopaedic literature.

Arthroscopic Techniques

Within the past 5 years, three arthroscopic techniques have emerged for the treatment of posterior instability. They are the capsular shift, capsulolabral augmentation, and thermal capsulorrhaphy.

The arthroscopic posterior capsular shift entails releasing the capsulolabral structures from the posterior glenoid and freshening the glenoid neck with a burr. Multiple sutures passed arthroscopically through the ligamentous tissue are then brought out through a supraclavicular portal and are tied down over the clavicle or scapular spine. Because this technique is glenoid based, it may be used without modification in patients with posterior Bankart lesions. At follow-up of 2 years or more, authors have reported a 25% overall recurrence rate in 20 patients using this technique. This is consistent with recurrence rates using open techniques.

The capsulolabral augmentation procedure is a scientifically based operation that aims to enhance glenolabral concavity while simultaneously reducing capsular laxity. In laboratory studies, capsulolabral augmentation was shown to increase glenoid depth and increase resistance to translational displacement of the humeral head. Arthroscopic capsulolabral augmentation resulted in improved functional outcomes in a large percentage of 41 patients with posteroinferior instability. Although some residual instability was noted in 41% of the patients, 86% had improved stability on physical examination, and 84% stated that they would have the procedure performed again. The authors report an 83% incidence of arthroscopically observable pathologic lesions affecting the posteroinferior glenolabral concavity in this group of patients. In 78% of the cases, a traumatic injury could be identified by history. Four patterns were described: Bankart-type detachment (12%), chondral or labral erosion (17%), synovial or capsular stripping (22%), and labral split or flap tear (32%).

Thermal techniques (laser and radiofrequency) are also being applied to treat posterior instability. Short-term results rivaling those of open techniques have been reported. When using arthroscopy as a diagnostic tool, the

TABLE 2	Surgical Procedures for Posterior Instability	
Soft Tissue	**Bony**
Posterior capsulorrhaphy	Glenoid osteotomy
Inferior capsular shift (anterior/posterior)	Posterior bone block
Infraspinatus advancement	Humeral osteotomy
Posterior Bankart repair	
Staple capsulorrhaphy*	
Biceps tendon transfer*	
Subscapularis transfer*	
Posterior capsulolabral augmentation[†]	
Posteroinferior capsular shift[†]	
Thermal capsulorrhaphy[†]	

*Procedures that are of historical interest but are not currently used
[†]Denotes arthroscopic procedure

surgeon should perform a complete surgical inventory to evaluate all areas of potential anatomic aberration. Arthroscopic treatment should attempt to restore normal anatomic relationships. Capsular shrinkage should be directed at posterior capsule retensioning in cases of isolated posterior instability and circumferential retensioning in cases of global instability. Early experience has shown that the thin, frequently attenuated posterior capsular tissues are less responsive to thermal shrinkage than are the anterior tissues. In addition, they are more susceptible to ablation and necrosis. Some surgeons have reported that observable posterior capsular tensioning can be achieved with thermal treatment of the anterior and inferior tissues without risking further injury to the already compromised posterior capsule. This technique relies on the "circle" concept of shoulder instability, which suggests that increased translation may result from injury to one side of the capsule, whereas dislocation requires injury to both sides of the joint. Biomechanical studies support a secondary role for the superior glenohumeral ligament and rotator interval capsule in resisting posterior translation. The restraining effects of the inferior glenohumeral ligament complex in preventing posterior displacement of the humeral head have also been demonstrated for the elevated, internally rotated arm. The thermal modification of these tissues alone could theoretically impart enough posterior stability to achieve the desired clinical effect.

In cases of posterior instability, the arm must be immobilized in a neutral or slightly externally rotated position postoperatively. Placing the arm in an internally rotated position in a sling risks early stretching of the posterior capsule. Most surgeons advocate at least 3 or 4 weeks of immobilization following thermal capsulorrhaphy for posterior instability.

Summary

The advancements achieved in the treatment of posterior instability over the past several years can be attributed to improved recognition of alterations in functional anatomy. Laboratory research has better defined the roles of specific structures, resulting in a more anatomic treatment approach. Arthroscopy has evolved from a purely diagnostic tool into a therapeutic means of potentially achieving the same results as open procedures by using minimally invasive techniques.

Posterior and multidirectional instability of the shoulder pose challenges to the treating physician in terms of both diagnosis and treatment. With these instability patterns, it is important to first pursue nonsurgical treatment options because many patients respond to neuromuscular conditioning. In addition, symptoms are frequently related to specific athletic endeavors, and changes in lifestyle often affect the degree of symptoms experienced. In refractory cases, good results have been achieved with various surgical procedures; however, outcomes have in general been less predictable than those achieved with anterior instability operations. There appears to be a current trend toward arthroscopic intervention, and early results have been promising.

Annotated Bibliography

Multidirectional Instability

Anderson K, Warren RF, Altchek DW, Craig EV, O'Brien SJ: Risk factors for early failure after thermal capsulorrhaphy. *Am J Sports Med* 2002;30:103-107.

Of 106 patients treated with thermal capsulorrhaphy for a variety of shoulder instability patterns, 15 failures were identified. Statistically significant risk factors for early failure included a history of previous operations and multiple recurrent dislocations.

Brown GA, Tan JL, Kirkley A: The lax shoulder in females: Issues, answers, but many more questions. *Clin Orthop* 2000;372:110-122.

A comprehensive review of data related to shoulder instability reveals that there are no conclusive data supporting a higher incidence of shoulder laxity or instability in females compared to males. An up-to-date review of MDI is included.

Hamada K, Fukuda H, Nakajima T, Yamada N: The inferior capsular shift operation for instability of the shoulder: Long-term results in 34 shoulders. *J Bone Joint Surg Br* 1999;81:218-225.

The authors report long-term results (mean follow-up of 8.3 years) in 26 patients (34 shoulders) treated with inferior capsular shift for MDI. Anterior and posterior approaches were used, both alone and in combination. Thirty of 34 shoulders (88%) had a satisfactory subjective outcome. Nine of 34 shoulders (26%) experienced recurrent instability, all of which occurred within the first 3 years postoperatively. These results suggest that the inferior capsular shift procedure holds up over time.

Hawkins RJ, Schutte JP, Janda DH, Huckell GH: Translation of the glenohumeral joint with the patient under anesthesia. *J Shoulder Elbow Surg* 1996;5:286-292.

This study compares radiographically assessed humeral translation in anesthetized patients with anterior instability, MDI, and a control group. Although on average, statistically significant increased translation occurred anteriorly and inferiorly in patients with anterior instability and in all three directions in those with MDI, considerable overlap was seen among all three groups. This work supports the concept that translation alone is not a reliable indicator of instability.

McIntyre LF, Caspari RB, Savoie FH III: The arthroscopic treatment of multidirectional shoulder instability: Two-year results of a multiple suture technique. *Arthroscopy* 1997;13:418-425.

Nineteen patients with MDI and no history of previous shoulder surgery underwent arthroscopic capsular shift using an anterior transglenoid suturing technique coupled with a posterior capsular advancement. A good or excellent result was reported in 18 of 19 patients (95%) based on the Athletic Shoulder Outcome Rating Scale. These early results compare favorably with those obtained with open techniques.

Nixon RT Jr, Lindenfeld TN: Early rehabilitation after a modified inferior capsular shift procedure for multidirectional instability of the shoulder. *Orthopedics* 1998; 21:441-445.

Sixteen patients with MDI were treated with an inferior capsular shift procedure augmented with suture anchors. An accelerated rehabilitation program following 2 weeks of immobilization in a sling is described. Range of motion and isokinetic strength were near normal in all subjects tested. No patient experienced recurrent instability postoperatively.

Rodeo SA, Suzuki K, Yamauchi M, Bhargava M, Warren RF: Analysis of collagen and elastic fibers in shoulder capsule in patients with shoulder instability. *Am J Sports Med* 1998;26:634-643.

Increases in collagen cross-links, collagen fibril diameters, cysteine content, and elastin content were demonstrated in unstable shoulders (unidirectional and MDI) compared with stable shoulders from a control group. No significant differences existed between shoulders with unidirectional instability and those with MDI. Significantly smaller mean collagen fibril diameters were found in skin samples taken from patients with MDI compared with those of the unidirectional instability group.

Schenk TJ, Brems JJ: Multidirectional instability of the shoulder: Pathophysiology, diagnosis, and management. *J Am Acad Orthop Surg* 1998;6:65-72.

This article provides a concise review of the subject, including classification, etiology, pathophysiology, and diagnosis of the condition. A contemporary approach to managing MDI is also presented.

Treacy SH, Savoie FH III, Field LD: Arthroscopic treatment of multidirectional instability. *J Shoulder Elbow Surg* 1999;8:345-350.

A retrospective analysis of 25 patients treated for MDI with an arthroscopic capsular shift performed with a transglenoid technique is presented. Twenty-two of 25 patients (88%) received a satisfactory rating according to the Neer system. Recurrent instability occurred in 3 of 25 shoulders (12%). Preservation of motion was achieved in all but one patient.

Posterior Instability

Antoniou J, Harryman DT II: Arthroscopic posterior capsular repair. *Clin Sports Med* 2000;19:101-114.

This review article highlights the technical details of arthroscopic posterior capsular repair and presents a summary of early results using various techniques.

Bigliani LU, Pollock RG, McIlveen SJ, Endrizzi DP, Flatow EL: Shift of the posteroinferior aspect of the capsule for recurrent posterior glenohumeral instability. *J Bone Joint Surg Am* 1995;77:1011-1020.

Thirty-five shoulders (34 patients) were treated with a posterior inferior capsular shift for recurrent instability. At follow-up averaging 5 years, 80% satisfactory results were obtained overall. In cases of primary repair, 23 of 24 shoulders (96%) were treated successfully.

Blasier RB, Soslowsky LJ, Malicky DM, Palmer ML: Posterior glenohumeral subluxation: Active and passive stabilization in a biomechanical model. *J Bone Joint Surg Am* 1997;79:433-430.

The contributions of various soft-tissue structures to stabilization of the glenohumeral joint in the posterior direction were evaluated through selective muscle and ligament cutting in a cadaveric model. In a position of 90° forward flexion, the subscapularis muscle contributed most to this subluxation force.

Fuchs B, Jost B, Gerber C: Posterior-inferior capsular shift for the treatment of recurrent, voluntary posterior subluxation of the shoulder. *J Bone Joint Surg Am* 2000;82:16-25.

Twenty-four patients (26 shoulders) with voluntary posterior subluxation in the absence of a psychiatric disorder were treated surgically with a posterior-inferior capsular shift. Satisfactory intermediate-term (average follow-up, 7.6 years) clinical outcomes were achieved in 24 of 26 patients (92% good or excellent subjective rating). Recurrent instability occurred in six patients (23%). They concluded that voluntary subluxation in the absence of a psychiatric disorder does not constitute a contraindication for surgical treatment in a disabled patient for whom conservative management has been unsuccessful.

Graichen H, Koydl P, Zichner L: Effectiveness of glenoid osteotomy in atraumatic posterior instability of the shoulder associated with excessive retroversion and flatness of the glenoid. *Int Orthop* 1999;23:95-99.

Glenoid osteotomy was performed in 17 patients with atraumatic posterior instability and excessive retroversion and flatness of the glenoid. At 5-year follow-up, there was a 12.5% recurrence rate, and 81% of the shoulders were rated as good or excellent. Twenty-five percent of the patients had degenerative changes of the glenohumeral joint on radiographs.

Harryman DT II, Duckworth DG: Abstract: The efficacy of capsulo-labral augmentation for managing pathologic findings and symptoms of primary posteroinferior instability. *J Shoulder Elbow Surg* 1998;7:314.

The authors review 41 patients with posteroinferior instability managed by arthroscopic capsulolabral augmentation. Eighty-three percent of the shoulders treated demonstrated observable pathologic lesions of the posteroinferior glenolabral concavity. These lesions are classified into four categories.

Hawkins RJ, Janda DH: Posterior instability of the glenohumeral joint: A technique of repair. *Am J Sports Med* 1996;24:275-278.

A posterior capsulotendinous tensioning procedure is described for the treatment of isolated posterior instability. At average follow-up of 44 months, 13 of 14 patients were satisfied with their outcomes, and no patient had a recurrence of posterior instability.

Mair SD, Zarzour RH, Speer KP: Posterior labral injury in contact athletes. *Am J Sports Med* 1998;26:753-758.

The authors describe nine cases of posterior labral detachment without instability in contact athletes. They propose that impact loading with the arms positioned in front of the body results in a shearing force to the posterior labrum and articular surface.

McIntyre LF, Caspari RB, Savoie FH III: The arthroscopic treatment of posterior shoulder instability: Two-year results of a multiple suture technique. *Arthroscopy* 1997;13:426-432.

Twenty shoulders in 19 patients were treated with an arthroscopic capsular shift for posterior shoulder instability. Twelve of 20 patients had posterior Bankart lesions and 10 had anterior Hill-Sachs lesions. At a minimum follow-up of 2 years, there was a 25% recurrence rate. Four of the five patients who experienced a recurrence had a voluntary component to their instability.

Metcalf MH, Duckworth DG, Lee SB, et al: Posteroinferior glenoplasty can change glenoid shape and increase the mechanical stability of the shoulder. *J Shoulder Elbow Surg* 1999;8:205-213.

In a cadaveric model, posteroinferior glenoplasty was shown to increase the mechanical stability of the glenohumeral joint by increasing posteroinferior glenoid depth and shifting the center of the humeral head to a more anterosuperior position.

Wirth MA, Groh GI, Rockwood CA Jr: Capsulorrhaphy through an anterior approach for the treatment of atraumatic posterior glenohumeral instability with multidirectional laxity of the shoulder. *J Bone Joint Surg Am* 1998;80:1570-1578.

The authors describe their results with a capsular reconstruction procedure performed through an anterior approach for posterior instability with multidirectional laxity. At a mean follow-up of 60 months, a good or excellent result was obtained in 9 of 10 patients.

Wolf EM, Eakin CL: Arthroscopic capsular plication for posterior shoulder instability. *Arthroscopy* 1998;14: 153-163.

Excellent results are reported in 12 of 14 patients (86%) treated with arthroscopic capsular plication for recurrent posterior instability. The technique is presented and discussed as a promising alternative to open surgery.

Classic Bibliography

Altchek DW, Warren RF, Skyhar MJ, Ortiz G: T-plasty modification of the Bankart procedure for multidirectional instability of the anterior and inferior types. *J Bone Joint Surg Am* 1991;73:105-112.

Burkhead WZ Jr, Rockwood CA Jr: Treatment of instability of the shoulder with an exercise program. *J Bone Joint Surg Am* 1992;74:890-896.

Cooper RA, Brems JJ: The inferior capsular-shift procedure for multidirectional instability of the shoulder. *J Bone Joint Surg Am* 1992;74:1516-1521.

Hawkins RJ, Koppert G, Johnston G: Recurrent posterior instability (subluxation) of the shoulder. *J Bone Joint Surg Am* 1984;66:169-174.

Huber H, Gerber C: Voluntary subluxation of the shoulder in children: A long-term follow-up study of 36 shoulders. *J Bone Joint Surg Br* 1994;76:118-122.

Hurley JA, Anderson TE, Dear W, Andrish JT, Bergfeld JA, Weiker GG: Posterior shoulder instability: Surgical versus conservative results with evaluation of glenoid version. *Am J Sports Med* 1992;20;396-400.

Neer CS II, Foster CR: Inferior capsular shift for involuntary inferior and multidirectional instability of the shoulder: A preliminary report. *J Bone Joint Surg Am* 1980;62:897-908.

Rowe CR, Pierce DS, Clark JG: Voluntary dislocation of the shoulder: A preliminary report on a clinical, electromyographic, and psychiatric study of twenty-six patients. *J Bone Joint Surg Am* 1973;55;445-460.

Rowe CR, Zarins B: Recurrent transient subluxation of the shoulder. *J Bone Joint Surg Am* 1981;63:863-872.

Surin V, Blader S, Markhede G, Sundholm K: Rotational osteotomy of the humerus for posterior instability of the shoulder. *J Bone Joint Surg Am* 1990;72:181-186.

Chapter 10

Arthroscopic Anterior Glenohumeral Ligament Reconstruction

Brian J. Cole, MD, MBA

Jon J.P. Warner, MD

Introduction

Arthroscopic reconstruction has become an accepted method of treatment for anterior shoulder instability. Although early reports indicated higher failure rates for arthroscopic methods than for traditional open stabilization techniques, arthroscopy has improved because of better understanding of pathology associated with instability, more careful patient selection, and advances in technology. Obvious contraindications to arthroscopic capsulolabral repair of instability are bony insufficiency of the glenoid from acute fracture or chronic erosion; a large Hill-Sachs lesion; capsular rupture, either within the midsubstance or at the insertion; and the presence of poor quality capsular tissue. If patients with these contradictions are screened out, the outcome of arthroscopic repair for recurrent anterior shoulder instability is equivalent to that for open repair.

The major advantages of arthroscopic repair over open repair of instability are lower morbidity and reduced pain, shorter surgical time, and improved cosmesis. Also, arthroscopy offers the opportunity to identify and treat concomitant pathology. Furthermore, some authors believe that patients experience an easier functional recovery and ultimately achieve better motion following arthroscopic reconstruction than with open repair.

Associated Pathoanatomy

Both static and dynamic factors maintain stability in the normal shoulder. With acute and chronic dislocation, soft-tissue failure usually involves static stabilizing elements such as the labrum, capsule, and ligaments. However, failure of dynamic stabilizers may also occur, including avulsion of the origin of the long head of the biceps (superior labrum anterior-posterior [SLAP] lesion) and rotator cuff tears. Careful preoperative assessment can help the surgeon anticipate the possible need to repair more than one structure. Not only is arthroscopic evaluation a very sensitive method of con-firming these concomitant injuries, but all of these pathologies can be treated arthroscopically.

The Labrum

Below the equator of the glenoid, the labrum is normally tightly approximated to the glenoid articular rim; any separation in this area is termed a Bankart lesion. This region of the glenoid labrum deepens the concavity of the glenoid and also acts as an anchoring point for the inferior glenohumeral ligament (IGHL) complex. Because the IGHL complex is the major static stabilizer when the shoulder is positioned in abduction and external rotation, a capsulolabral separation effectively disrupts the origin of this stabilizing structure. Furthermore, the normal stabilizing effect of the rotator cuff compressing the humeral head into the conforming glenoid socket is disrupted when the labrum is separated from the glenoid rim because the depth of the socket is decreased. A Bankart lesion is present in about 90% of all traumatic anterior shoulder dislocations.

Above the glenoid equator, the labral anatomy may be quite variable. Loose attachment below the biceps tendon (ie, a sublabral foramen) may be a normal anatomic variant.

Complete lesions of the superior labrum associated with destabilization of the biceps insertion, which Snyder has classified, may occur with shoulder instability. Both experimental and clinical studies have provided support for arthroscopic repair of these superior labral injuries when treating instability. Before undertaking such repairs, however, it is necessary to determine if the patient's anatomy is a normal variant or a true labral detachment. In general, a loosely attached superior labrum with a smooth cartilage transition is a normal variant and not a labral separation. True labral injury is associated with failure of the origin fibers of the superior labrum, cartilage injury at the margin of the labral attachment, and extension of a tear into the biceps tendon itself.

Capsular Laxity

Recurrent dislocations can also cause stretching of the glenohumeral capsule and ligaments. This plastic deformation results from repetitive loading. Identification of this stretch injury or laxity of the ligaments may be difficult, but it is necessary because failure to address this element of the instability when performing an arthroscopic repair may contribute to failure of the procedure. Indeed, the authors of some series have attributed the higher failure rates to this error.

New technology and techniques have made more reliable management of concomitant capsular laxity possible. Suture capsulorrhaphy and the use of thermal energy to shrink capsular tissue have been used successfully, but general experience with these techniques has not yet progressed to the point where their reliability is equivalent to that of open capsular shift techniques. This is why some surgeons choose an open capsular shift approach when capsular laxity is believed to be an important contributing factor. Other surgeons remain strong advocates of accomplishing both labral repair and management of capsular laxity by arthroscopic methods.

Actual macroscopic failure of the capsule within its substance or at the humeral insertion is not common but appears to constitute a relative contraindication to arthroscopic repair. In such cases, direct repair with capsule reinsertion or plication through an open approach appears to be more reliable than an arthroscopic approach.

Rotator Interval

Insufficiency of the region of the capsule known as the rotator interval has received attention recently because some failures of arthroscopic techniques have been attributed to this pathology. This interval lies within the anterior and superior capsular region, between the anterior border of the supraspinatus and the cranial border of the subscapularis tendon. Its major ligamentous components are the superior and middle glenohumeral ligaments, as well as the extra-articular coracohumeral ligament.

Studies have shown that the capsule may be open in the rotator interval, and its closure at the time of open instability repair has been recommended. Recent experience has demonstrated that if a patient has a large inferior drawer sign (sulcus sign) when the arm is in adduction and external rotation, the rotator interval region of the capsule is likely to be insufficient. This may represent either an injury or, more likely, a relative dysplasia of the ligaments of this region. In such cases, this area should be repaired by overlapping the capsule, either through an arthroscopic technique or an open technique.

Rotator Cuff Tears

The most common rotator cuff injury in younger patients is a partial-thickness undersurface tear of the supraspinatus. This injury usually results from eccentric loading of the tendon secondary to the recurrent instability. Full-thickness tears of the rotator cuff are usually seen in patients over the age of 40 years. A full-thickness tear should be suspected when weakness and pain persist 3 weeks after an anterior dislocation. In such cases, preoperative physical examination and imaging studies will discern the configuration of the tear. Generally, tears of the supraspinatus can be repaired arthroscopically, while significant tears of the subscapularis require an open approach.

Developments in Arthroscopic Labral Repair

Arthroscopic repair must be measured against a failure rate of generally less than 10% following open stabilization. Series are difficult to compare because the definitions of failure vary. Furthermore, many series of open repair have reported a low rate of return (less than 50%) to high-level sports after surgical repair. While no prospective randomized studies have compared arthroscopic and open repair, recent prospective reports of arthroscopic stabilization techniques have demonstrated failure rates as low as the best open repair series and also a high rate of return to sports activities.

Metallic Staples

Metallic staples were first introduced in 1982; subsequent reports demonstrated unacceptable recurrence rates as high as 33% with their use. Results generally improved, however, when postoperative immobilization was increased to 3 to 4 weeks. Even so, this technique has been largely abandoned because of its relatively high complication rate (between 5% and 10%), related principally to the hardware.

Transglenoid Sutures

Although transglenoid sutures were first introduced in 1987 as a two-pin transglenoid arthroscopic technique, later studies reported success rates of 90%. Other authors have reported variable experiences, with recurrence rates up to 60%. The authors of one series attributed their poor results to errors in patient selection because many of their patients demonstrated a large sulcus sign or had a concomitant bony Bankart lesion. The advantage of transglenoid suture repair compared with the staple technique is that it creates multiple points for fixation of the labrum. Furthermore, it allows the surgeon to address concomitant capsular laxity by shifting the capsule superiorly on the glenoid rim. The major disadvantage of this method is that it requires transscapular drilling, with the drill passing into the infraspinatus fossa in an orientation that places the suprascapular nerve at risk. The nerve could be injured either by the drill or by the sutures tied over the posterior infraspinatus fascia. Furthermore, loosening of the sutures over time is possible as the soft-tissue swelling decreases or the muscle of the infraspinatus atrophies. This would allow the capsulolabral repair to gap.

Cannulated Bioabsorbable Implants

First reported in 1991, the Suretac (Acufex Microsurgical, Norwood, MA) bioabsorbable (polyglycolic acid) device is a single-point transfixing implant for intra-articular labral repair. It was designed to avoid the risks presented by intra-articular metal staples, as well as to eliminate the need for transscapular drilling for suture repair. Initial enthusiasm was modified when recurrence rates of up to 21% were reported. Recent experience has suggested that the recurrence rate can decrease to less than 10% if treatment is limited to patients with an isolated Bankart lesion and no capsular injury. The disadvantages of this implant are its inability to address capsular laxity and a reported incidence of up to 6% of synovial reaction to the polyglyconate.

Suture Anchors

Using suture anchors with or without arthroscopically tied knots has become the most commonly used arthroscopic repair method and a preferred method of repair. This method, using metal anchor and knots tied with absorbable sutures, was first described in 1991. In 1994, the technique was modified with the use of permanent sutures. Although in the last 10 years several series have reported failure rates of up to 33%, recent comparative studies of arthroscopic repairs using suture anchors and open stabilization cite recurrence rates of less than 10% for arthroscopic methods. Unlike the transglenoid repair technique, suture anchor repair techniques allow knots to be tied in the joint arthroscopically, thus avoiding the need for a posterior incision. Furthermore, recent technology has allowed for suture repair using anchors without knots, thus eliminating knot tying.

Patient Selection

History

The history given by the patient can be of great value. For example, a patient who describes a sudden severe trauma sustained with the arm positioned in abduction and external rotation probably has a Bankart lesion. If, however, a patient with a dislocation reports minimal trauma, such as reaching overhead, then capsular laxity is likely to be the major pathology. Recurrent traumatic dislocations are likely to be associated with anterior glenoid rim erosion and a large Hill-Sachs lesion. Many patients who report only pain with the arm in a position of apprehension (abduction and external rotation) and no sense of instability may still be found to have a capsulolabral injury.

Patients older than age 40 years who sustain a dislocation should be suspected of having a concomitant rotator cuff tear. Patient age and activity level are important factors to consider when predicting the risk for recurrence without surgical intervention. Those younger than age 20 years or who participate in high-risk activities are at the highest risk for recurrence (approaching 90% to 95%).

Physical Examination

In evaluating a patient with a dislocation in the physician's office, the first step is to check for associated nerve injury. Careful motor and sensory evaluation should be directed at axillary nerve function. In addition, weakness in older patients may indicate a rotator cuff tear.

Provocative testing for instability may be performed when no documented dislocation has occurred and a question remains about the direction of instability. Both anterior and posterior apprehension tests are sensitive. The relocation maneuver will increase the specificity of the diagnosis of anterior instability.

Assessment of joint laxity may be difficult in an office setting because of patient muscle guarding in response to pain. Nevertheless, inferior laxity should be assessed. Although a positive sulcus sign does not necessarily indicate pathology, pain as a result of the maneuver suggests inferior instability. Furthermore, a large sulcus sign (ie, more than 2 cm) that persists when the adducted arm is externally rotated suggests insufficiency of the rotator interval capsular region.

Several tests have been described to confirm the presence of a SLAP lesion. The provocative O'Brien test has been found to be sensitive, but not specific. This maneuver is performed by having the patient resist downward pressure against the arm when the shoulder is positioned in adduction and internal rotation. If the patient experiences pain with this maneuver and if that pain is reduced when the shoulder is externally rotated, the test is positive, suggesting a SLAP lesion.

Radiographic Evaluation

Plain radiographic evaluation is useful as an initial screening tool to identify significant glenoid or humeral bone loss. In general, at least two orthogonal views are necessary. Several special imaging techniques increase accuracy for detecting bony Bankart and Hill-Sachs lesions. These include a West Point axillary view, an AP view with the shoulder in internal rotation, and a Stryker notch view.

Although MRI may not be required, it can be useful for three-dimensional clarification of capsuloligamentous and bony injury. When enhanced through the use of gadolinium dye, MRI is very accurate in confirming a Bankart lesion; it can also demonstrate a superior labral injury, the degree of bony injury, and associated rotator cuff injury. If significant bony loss of the glenoid or humeral head is suspected, CT may provide an even more definitive quantitative three-dimensional image of this deficiency.

Examination Under Anesthesia

Most often, the examination under anesthesia (EUA) supports the diagnosis established by the patient history and physical examination. Stability testing of the arm in the anterior, posterior, and inferior directions in different positions of abduction will help identify regions of labral or capsular pathology. For example, increased inferior translation with the arm adducted in external rotation may indicate the need to address capsular laxity and possibly the rotator interval.

Diagnostic Arthroscopy

A systematic evaluation of the glenohumeral joint will demonstrate concomitant pathology including, in order of decreasing frequency, anterior labral detachment, capsular injury, articular cartilage damage (glenoid or a Hill-Sachs lesion), SLAP lesions, and rotator cuff tears. The surgeon judges the quality and integrity of the anterior capsuloligamentous structures by observing these structures in different positions of arm rotation while probing and grasping. In general, when the shoulder is placed in abduction and external rotation, the inferior glenohumeral ligament should tighten while the humeral head remains in the glenoid. An anterior force can be applied to the humerus, causing the humeral head to move anteriorly on the glenoid. Although the humeral head may be observed to move to the anterior edge of the glenoid when the arm is in adduction, there should be no appreciable anterior translation when the shoulder is in abduction and external rotation. This mechanism is called the arthroscopic drawer test. In addition, an abnormal drive-through sign, in which the arthroscope passes easily from posterior to anterior and then into the axillary pouch, further delineates the extent of capsular laxity.

Surgical Indications

Some authors recommend treating young athletes with an initial anterior glenohumeral dislocation with immediate arthroscopic stabilization. This approach has the advantage that the surgeon works with optimal pathology with good-quality tissue and minimal collateral tissue damage. It is especially appropriate for patients who, despite immobilization, would be at high risk of recurrence without surgery. This approach must be considered on a case-by-case basis.

Patients with recurrent anterior instability despite physical therapy or activity modification are also candidates for surgical intervention. While the literature suggests higher failure rates following arthroscopic stabilization in athletes who participate in collision sports, attention to the entire spectrum of pathoanatomy identified at surgery is likely to lead to a satisfactory result. Whether these patients can be managed entirely by arthroscopic techniques depends on whether the labrum can be repaired arthroscopically as well as whether associated capsular laxity and rotator interval pathology can be adequately addressed with these techniques.

Surgical Reconstruction Using Suture Anchors

General Principles

The goals of surgery are to securely reattach the anterior-inferior labrum and reestablish the proper tension within the IGHL complex. Capsular laxity is addressed by a superior shift of the capsule, with or without the labrum, depending on the pathology. If capsulolabral suture repair does not address all of the capsular laxity, some surgeons supplement the repair with thermal capsulorrhaphy using radiofrequency probes. If insufficiency of the rotator interval region exists with persistent inferior laxity, then this region is also plicated. Finally, associated superior labral injuries are repaired as well. Rarely, midcapsular rupture or avulsion of the humeral insertion is found, possibly requiring conversion to open reconstruction.

Instrumentation

Arthroscopic repair requires a variety of instrumentation, including cannulas, cortical anchors, and suturing devices. The surgeon's choice of instrumentation is typically based on personal experience and familiarity with the various options.

Disposable cannulas are necessary to accommodate the instrumentation required for glenoid preparation, suture passage through soft tissue, and arthroscopic knot tying. Typically, 5- and 8-mm cannulas are used. A variety of cortical anchors are commercially available and have a pull-out strength that exceeds the ultimate failure strength of the suture, knot, and soft-tissue interface. Thus, the limiting factor is the security of the suture placement through the tissue and of the arthroscopic knot. Once the anchor has been placed in the tissue, the suture must be retrieved and placed through the capsule and ligaments. Several devices are available for this purpose: some pierce the ligaments and labrum and then retrieve the suture, whereas others permit a suture loop to be placed through the tissue so that the suture through the anchor can be shuttled back through the tissue and retrieved. The surgeon's preferred technique will determine the device used for this step of the procedure. A variety of knot pushers also are available. Some allow the individual suture limbs to be pushed away from each other, thus tensioning the knot. Others are simply straight pushers, which allow a sliding knot or a half hitch to be slid down a post. If a transfixing device such as the Suretac is used, then all of the required instrumentation is associated with the insertion of the device.

Preparation

Interscalene regional anesthesia, general anesthesia, or a combination of both may be used to decrease narcotic requirements and to aid in early postoperative pain relief. Arthroscopic glenohumeral ligament reconstruction is relatively fast, and the beach chair position facilitates efficient setup and may allow the patient to bypass the recovery room and be discharged after only a few hours. Furthermore, conversion to an open approach is easier when the patient is in the beach chair position than in the lateral decubitus position. Some surgeons prefer the lateral decubitus position, however, and find traction on the arm to be helpful.

EUA with side-to-side comparisons should be performed, documenting range of motion and the degree and direction of humeral head translation. Typically, translation anteriorly over the glenoid rim with (2+) or without (3+) spontaneous reduction is considered abnormal. Posterior translation of 2+ is usually considered normal and must be regarded in the context of other clinical factors. The sulcus between the inferolateral border of the acromion and the greater tuberosity is measured in centimeters. An inferior displacement force should be applied in different positions of rotation to evaluate capsular laxity and the rotator interval.

The patient may have a Bankart lesion even if translation does not appear to be significantly increased. Thus, results of the EUA should be correlated with the history and the preoperative examination.

Technique

The shoulder is prepared and draped in a sterile manner, and the bony landmarks are carefully marked. A standard posterior portal is established within the "soft spot," located approximately 2 cm medial to the lateral acromion and 2 cm inferior to the scapular spine. Two ante-

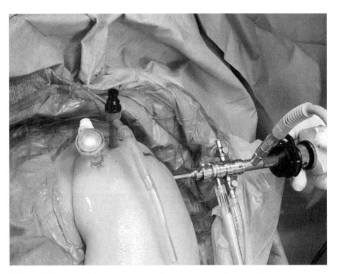

Figure 1 A beach chair setup for shoulder arthroscopy. Two anterior portals are established. An anterosuperior cannula (5.5-mm cannula) and an anteroinferior cannula (8-mm clear cannula) allow for easy passage of instrumentation and suture management.

rior portals (superior and inferior) are established using an outside-in technique with a spinal needle (Fig. 1). These function as utility portals for instrument passage, glenoid preparation, suture management, and knot tying. The anterior cannulas should be separated widely to allow easy access in the joint. Therefore, a 5- or 6-mm cannula is first placed in a vertical orientation so that it enters the joint just underneath the biceps tendon. This anterosuperior cannula is usually placed at a 90° angle to the arthroscope. The second cannula is 8 mm in diameter and should be placed as low as possible relative to the subscapularis tendon. Both portals are located and placed using an outside-in technique, using a spinal needle to first confirm orientation. The lower, larger cannula is usually placed 1 cm inferior and lateral to the palpable coracoid process so that it enters the joint just over the subscapularis tendon (Fig. 2). This usually allows the first anchor to be placed at the 5 o'clock position on the glenoid (all positions described are for a right shoulder).

A complete diagnostic arthroscopic examination is performed with the arthroscope placed in both the anterior and posterior portals. Special attention is paid to the rotator interval, superior labrum, rotator cuff, and articular cartilage, as well as reciprocal tightening of the glenohumeral ligaments, especially with the arm abducted and externally rotated. The labrum is evaluated circumferentially for signs of frank detachment or medial healing along the scapular neck. Detachment of the labrum with healing medially on the scapula may be difficult to recognize; it usually appears as a bare glenoid rim with the capsular attachment occurring medially. This condition results when repeated dislocations strip the capsulolabral attachment from its anatomic origin and push it medially

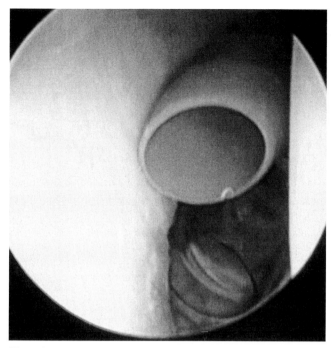

Figure 2 Arthroscopic view from the posterior portal of two anteriorly placed cannulas widely separated to minimize intra-articular crowding. An outside-in technique is used, with an 18-gauge spinal needle used to determine optimal placement. The anterosuperior cannula enters just lateral to the biceps tendon insertion. The anteroinferior cannula enters just proximal to the subscapularis tendon.

along the scapular neck. Recognizing this condition is important because the entire capsulolabral sleeve must be mobilized and returned to its anatomic insertion at the margin of the glenoid rim when the repair is performed.

Glenoid Preparation and Anchor Placement

The 30° arthroscope can be placed in the posterior viewing portal as well as in the anterosuperior portal; working instruments are placed in the anteroinferior portal. In some cases it is helpful to use a 70° scope to see over the glenoid rim while mobilizing the capsulolabral sleeve. The capsulolabral complex is mobilized off the glenoid neck inferiorly to the 6 o'clock position using electrocautery or a radiofrequency device. A periosteal elevator or knife rasp also may be useful. It is especially important to freely mobilize the capsulolabral sleeve so that it can be shifted superiorly and laterally to the glenoid rim. This often requires releasing it from the scapula until the muscle fibers of the subscapularis are visible. Although a motorized hooded burr may be used to decorticate the anterior and inferior glenoid neck, a motorized shaver may be sufficient. The abrasion of the juxta-articular scapula should be about 1 to 1.5 cm medial to the articular cartilage and should extend to the inferior glenoid (6 o'clock position) (Fig. 3).

Anchors are placed on the articular rim through the anteroinferior cannula at an angle of approximately 45°

to the frontal plane to avoid articular penetration and to minimize the risk of inadvertent medial placement along the scapular neck. Anchor placement is from inferior to superior, with the first anchor placed at approximately the 5 o'clock position. Suture passage and knot tying is performed prior to each subsequent anchor insertion. Anchor placement may be facilitated by a toothed or serrated guide that maintains the juxta-articular anchor position and by predrilling if necessary. The advantages of a metal screw-in anchor are that it can be removed and revised and most of these anchors are self-taping and require no predrilling, eliminating a step. Some surgeons, however, prefer push-in anchors, which are placed after predrilling. Tying sliding knots can be easier with plastic or absorbable anchors than with metal anchors. This is because the braided suture seems to slide more easily and less traumatically through the eyelet of a plastic or absorbable polymer anchor than through a metal eyelet.

An anchor technology that allows for suture repair without knots has been developed recently. This design permits the suture to be captured in the end of the anchor once the suture has been passed through the tissue. The anchor is then placed in a predrilled hole and impacted to a depth that pulls the capsulolabral tissue securely against the glenoid rim.

Following anchor placement, anchor security, suture slippage, and knot security are assessed. Most surgeons use No. 1 or No. 2 braided nonabsorbable suture material or prolonged braided, absorbable sutures because of their strength and handling properties, which allow for secure knots that do not slip.

Anterior Glenohumeral Reconstruction

After mobilization of the capsulolabral periosteal sleeve as described above, the first anchor is placed at the articular margin at least as low as the 5 o'clock position (Fig. 4, *A*). This first anchor is critical in establishing proper capsular tension. One limb of the suture from this anchor is retrieved through the superior cannula because it will be transported through the capsule with a device inserted through the inferior cannula. A crochet hook or other retrieving device can be used for this step (Fig. 4, *B*). The suture that comes out of the anchor should be transported on its inferior or medial surface, if possible, to prevent it from twisting on itself and permit easier tying of a sliding knot. A suture hook or piercing device is placed through the capsule medial and inferior to the lowest anchor so that the entire IGHL is shifted superiorly and laterally (Fig. 4, *C*). Pulling on the hook when it is in the tissue can confirm good shift of the IGHL. Tension also can be assessed using a soft-tissue grasper placed through the superior portal while pulling on the hook in the IGHL. As the labrum is included in this suture loop, it will be repaired when the capsule is shifted and repaired. Usually, the suture retrieval device is placed through the IGHL about 1 cm inferior and medial to the lowest anchor.

If a suture shuttle device or piercing device is used, then a shuttle relay is placed through the device and retrieved out of the superior cannula. Alternatively, a 2-0 monofilament suture can be placed through the device either as a loop or as a single strand (Fig. 4, *D*). If it is retrieved as a loop, it is used to shuttle the suture limb from the anchor back through the capsulolabral tissue. If it is a single strand, it is simply tied to the suture limb from the anchor, which is then shuttled through the tissue (Fig. 4, *E* and *F*). The shuttle relay device is used in the same manner. When transferring the suture, it is important to carefully observe the suture as it slides out of the superior cannula so that the suture is not inadvertently unloaded from the anchor. Placing a hemostat on the suture limb remaining within the anteroinferior cannula and observing the limb during transfer are the most effective ways to prevent such unloading from occurring.

The suture limb that exits the anterosuperior cannula is the suture that will ultimately pass through the soft tissue, and is the post suture because the sliding arthroscopic knot will move down this limb. It is important to choose this limb as the post because the knot will then sit on top of the tissue rather than underneath it.

The first step in knot tying is placing the knot pusher on each individual limb and passing it down into the joint to make sure there is no tangling or twisting of the suture limbs. Most surgeons prefer to tie a sliding knot first. This allows the knot to be securely placed, putting tension on the tissue. This may be a knot that does not lock, such as the Duncan loop (Fig. 5, *A*), or a self-locking knot, such as the Buntline half hitch. The knot is "set" by placing a hemostat between the two limbs just distal to the knot and eliminating the slack within the suture loops against the post (Fig. 5, *B*). Placing a knot pusher on the post limb to push the knot down the post while simultaneously pulling the knot into the joint minimizes suture trauma and reduces the risk for suture failure (Fig. 5, *C*). Next, several alternating half hitch nonsliding loops are advanced down the post, guided by the knot pusher. The first sliding knot is placed by simply pulling on the post and pushing on the knot; subsequent half hitches are pulled into the joint by placing the knot pusher just past the half hitch so that it pulls on the suture, bringing the knot down into the joint. The knot is then tightened by using a past-pointing technique with the knot pusher. Alternating the posts and the direction of each half hitch maximizes knot security. The ends are cut, leaving a 3-mm tail (Fig. 5, *D*). These steps are repeated for each subsequent anchor.

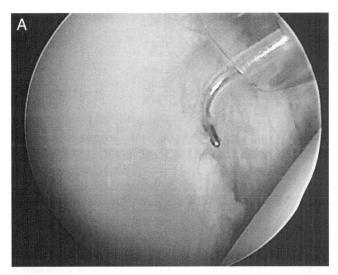

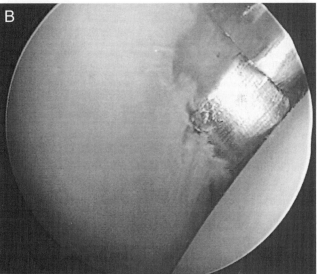

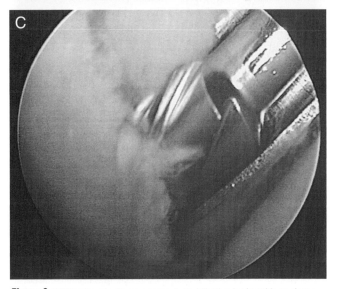

Figure 3 Mobilization of a Bankart lesion. **A,** Mobilization begins with an electrocautery device. **B,** A knife rasp is used to mobilize the periosteal sleeve. **C,** The rotary shaver or burr is used to decorticate the anterior and inferior glenoid neck to achieve a bleeding bed to optimize healing.

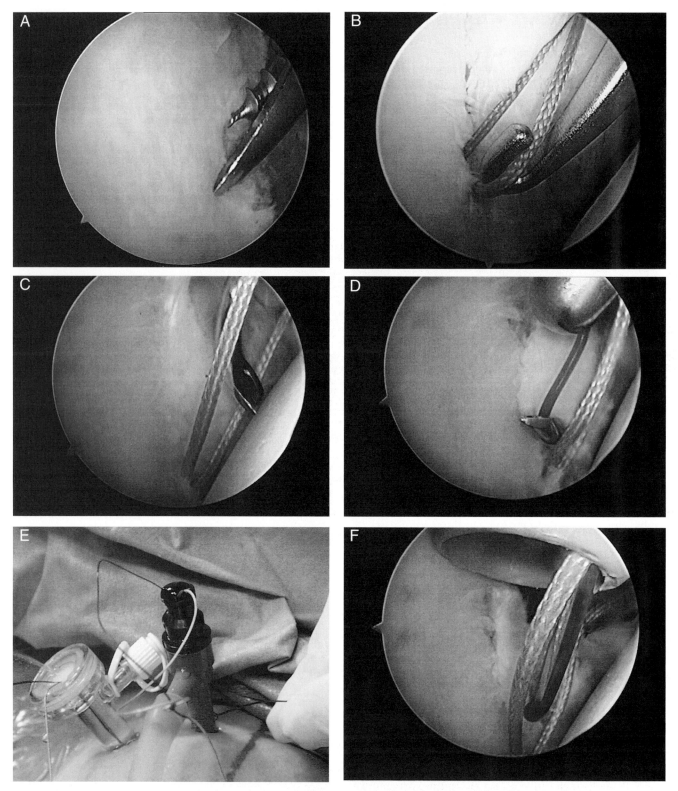

Figure 4 Anterior glenohumeral reconstruction. **A,** Anchor placement at the articular margin. **B,** A crochet hook is used through the anterosuperior cannula to retrieve the most inferior suture from within the anteroinferior cannula. **C,** A suture hook is placed through the anteroinferior cannula to penetrate the capsule and labrum medial and inferior to the anchor. **D,** A monofilament suture is advanced through the suture hook and retrieved with a retriever placed through the anterosuperior cannula. **E,** Outside the joint, the suture limb exiting the anterosuperior cannula is tied to the monofilament in preparation for shuttling this limb through the labrum and capsule. **F,** The superior suture limb and monofilament are pulled through the soft tissue into the anteroinferior cannula by pulling the free end of the monofilament shuttle that remains within the anteroinferior cannula.

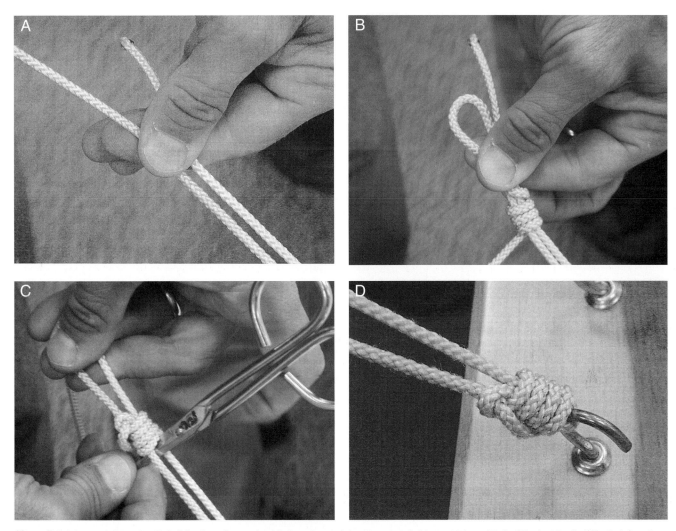

Figure 5 A, Arthroscopic knot tying. **B,** A sliding knot (Duncan loop) is formed around the suture post. **C,** A hemostat is used to "set" the knot to eliminate slack from the suture loops. The knot is advanced down the post by pulling the post and simultaneously pushing the knot with a knot pusher (not shown). **D,** Serial alternating half hitch nonsliding knots are subsequently passed over alternating posts to lock the knot. The suture limbs are cut, leaving a 3-mm tail.

Rotator Interval

If the shoulder demonstrates persistent inferior or inferior-posterior translation following repair of the inferior and middle glenohumeral ligament capsulolabral avulsion, some surgeons perform rotator interval closure. A curved suture hook is placed through the anterosuperior cannula or percutaneously through the portal without the cannula. Using No. 1 monofilament, the hook is advanced through the healthy tissue immediately adjacent to the supraspinatus tendon and then is advanced inferiorly through the tissue adjacent to the subscapularis tendon.

It can be difficult to grasp sufficient tissue with a single pass of the suture hook. An alternative method involves percutaneous placement of an inferiorly placed suture retriever to retrieve the suture after advancing the suture hook through the superior tissue only. In either case, the suture ends are retrieved through the anterior portal after removing the cannula and are secured using an arthro-

scopic sliding knot extra-articularly, anteriorly over the soft tissue. Alternatively, the sutures can be retrieved from within the subacromial space by viewing the space posteriorly from within and retrieving from a standard anterior portal and securing with an arthroscopic knot. Additional sutures are added as needed. Care must be taken to position the arm in external rotation and adduction during suture placement and tensioning.

Thermal Capsulorrhaphy

If translation and capsular laxity persist after the capsulolabral repair, some surgeons prefer to further tighten the capsule using thermal capsulorrhaphy. The acceptance of this technique is increasing, although peer-reviewed literature advocating its routine use is limited. Thermal capsulorrhaphy involves the thermal modification of collagen in capsular tissue, which has been shown experimentally, as well as in initial clinical experience, to reduce capsular lax-

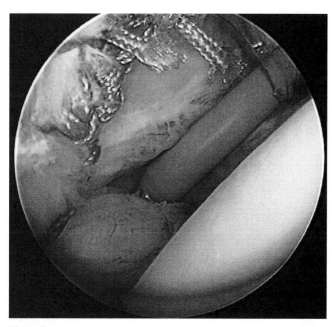

Figure 6 A monopolar radiofrequency device (Oratec Interventions, Menlo Park, CA) is used to further reduce capsular volume following an arthroscopic Bankart repair using suture anchors and nonabsorbable sutures. Care is taken to avoid thermal treatment near the suture line and weakening of this tissue.

ity. The application of heat in a range of 65°C to 70°C disrupts the heat-sensitive intra-molecular bonds in collagen, causing the molecular structure to change from an extended helical crystallinelike arrangement to a shortened random configuration. This results in a 20% to 30% shortening of the collagen molecules. The healing response includes inflammation with fibroblast infiltration followed by remodeling and restoration of histologic characteristics and biomechanical strength over a 6- to 12-week period. The degree of response, however, appears to vary among patients, so the extent of capsular shortening may also vary.

Thermal energy should be used only after all anchors have been placed and knots have been tied. Shrinking before suture placement increases the level of difficulty in assessing, approximating, and attaching the soft tissue to the glenoid rim. After suture repair, care is taken to avoid thermal treatment near the suture line because of the risk of soft-tissue weakening and failure. Either a monopolar or a bipolar radiofrequency device can be used. To date, no prospective randomized comparison of these devices has been performed. The technique used for thermal treatment of the capsule remains empiric; thermal energy can be applied to alternating regions of the capsule, creating a gridlike pattern and thus maintaining normal areas of tissue that may contribute to postoperative healing (Fig. 6).

Postoperative Rehabilitation

Rehabilitation after arthroscopic repair is identical to that following open reconstruction. Sling immobiliza-

tion is generally required for 4 to 6 weeks, depending on the surgical methods used and the instability pattern treated. Active and unrestricted range-of-motion exercises for the hand, wrist, and elbow should begin immediately following surgery, as should deltoid isometrics and gentle pendulum exercises. Some surgeons allow active forward elevation up to 120° after the first 2 to 3 weeks, as experimental studies have shown that this places little load on the capsulolabral region. At this point, external rotation up to 30° to 40° may be permitted as well, depending on the extent of repair. At 4 to 6 weeks, limits on rotation are gradually extended, and at 8 to 10 weeks, progressive resistive exercises are begun. The patient is allowed to resume sports participation at 18 to 36 weeks.

Summary

Arthroscopic stabilization for glenohumeral instability has evolved significantly over the last 15 to 20 years, with multiple techniques now available in carefully selected patients. Technological advances in arthroscopy and better understanding of the pathoanatomy associated with glenohumeral instability make it possible to duplicate the results of open stabilization techniques.

The arthroscopic suture anchor technique is advantageous because it most closely duplicates the traditional open Bankart repair. Several issues must be addressed to achieve optimal results. Patient selection is critical to the ultimate success of this procedure, as is appropriately addressing all pathology at the time of surgery. Capsular tension must be critically evaluated at the time of repair. Arthroscopic techniques should provide a convincing intraoperative examination of stability. Judicious use of adjuvant thermal capsulorrhaphy may address residual capsular laxity that might otherwise lead to failure; however, peer-reviewed literature on this method is still pending. Similarly, closing an open rotator interval may improve results.

Postoperative rehabilitation after arthroscopic repair is not significantly different from that after traditional open techniques. Premature return to activities that place stress on the reconstruction will likely result in early failure. Although no well-designed randomized prospective studies have compared the results of arthroscopic stabilization to that of a control group, several recent uncontrolled prospective studies confirm the efficacy of this technique. Surgeons are encouraged to practice the techniques described here in a continuing education setting prior to performing them in an operating room setting.

Annotated Bibliography

Associated Pathoanatomy

Cole BJ, Warner JJP: Anatomy, biomechanics, and patho-physiology of glenohumeral instability, in Iannotti JP, Williams GR Jr (eds): *Disorders of the Shoulder: Diagnosis and Management.* Philadelphia, PA, Lippincott-Williams & Wilkins, 1999, pp 207-232.

This comprehensive chapter presents an overview of the anatomy, biomechanics, and pathophysiology of glenohumeral instability.

Field LD, Warren RF, O'Brien SJ, Altchek DW, Wickiewicz TL: Isolated closure of rotator interval defects for shoulder instability. *Am J Sports Med* 1995;23:557-563.

In this study, 15 patients with isolated rotator interval defects underwent interval closure. All patients achieved good or excellent results at an average follow-up of 3.3 years using the American Shoulder and Elbow Surgeons and Rowe rating scales.

Hovelius L, Augustini BG, Fredin H, Johansson O, Norlin R, Thorling J: Primary anterior dislocation of the shoulder in young patients: A ten-year prospective study. *J Bone Joint Surg Am* 1996;78:1677-1684.

Risk factors for recurrent instability in 245 young patients at 10-year follow-up are reviewed. The type and duration of the initial treatment had no effect on the rate of recurrence. Twenty percent had at least mild arthritis at follow-up.

Kirkley A, Griffin S, Richards C, Miniaci A, Mohtadi N: Prospective randomized clinical trial comparing the effectiveness of immediate arthroscopic stabilization versus immobilization and rehabilitation in first traumatic anterior dislocations of the shoulder. *Arthroscopy* 1999;15:507-514.

Forty patients randomized to either 3 weeks of immobilization (n = 20) or arthroscopic stabilization (n = 20) were compared. At 24 months, 47% of the immobilized group and 16% of the surgical group had sustained redislocation (*P* = 0.03). Improvements in disease-specific quality of life measures were greater in the surgically treated group.

Lazarus MD, Sidles JA, Harryman DT III, Matsen FA III: Effect of a chondral-labral defect on glenoid concavity and glenohumeral stability: A cadaveric model. *J Bone Joint Surg Am* 1996;78:94-102.

Creation of a chondral-labral defect led to an 80% reduction in the height of the glenoid, with a concomitant reduction in the stability ratio of 65%.

Pagnani MJ, Deng XH, Warren RF, Torzilli PA, Altchek DW: Effect of lesions of the superior portion of the glenoid labrum on glenohumeral translation. *J Bone Joint Surg Am* 1995;77:1003-1010.

This biomechanical cadaver study establishes that increased anteroposterior translation occurs with concomitant SLAP lesions.

Pagnani MJ, Deng XH, Warren RF, Torzilli PA, O'Brien SJ: Role of the long head of the biceps brachii in glenohumeral stability: A biomechanical study in cadavera. *J Shoulder Elbow Surg* 1996;5:255-262.

This cadaver study demonstrated that the long head of the biceps tended to stabilize the joint anteriorly when the arm was internally rotated and served as a posterior stabilizer when the humerus was externally rotated.

Ticker JB, Bigliani LU, Soslowsky LJ, Pawluk RJ, Flatow EL, Mow VC: Inferior glenohumeral ligament: Geometric and strain-rate dependent properties. *J Shoulder Elbow Surg* 1996;5:269-279.

A biomechanical study of the IGHL demonstrating its viscoelastic behavior and strain rate–dependent properties during tensile testing.

Treacy SH, Field LD, Savoie FH: Rotator interval capsule closure: An arthroscopic technique. *Arthroscopy* 1997;13:103-106.

This article describes an all-arthroscopic technique using a suture retrieval device and a No. 1 Prolene suture passed through a spinal needle. Sutures are retrieved from within the subacromial space and tied arthroscopically from within the subacromial space.

Developments in Arthroscopic Labral Repair

Cole BJ, L'Insalata J, Irrgang J, Warner JJ: Comparison of arthroscopic and open anterior shoulder stabilization: A two to six-year follow-up study. *J Bone Joint Surg Am* 2000;82:1108-1114.

This study comparing arthroscopic and open stabilization in a high-demand population demonstrated a recurrence rate of 16% (6 of 37) in the group treated with arthroscopy using a biodegradable tack compared with 9% (2 of 22) in the group treated with open repair at an average follow-up of 52 and 55 months, respectively.

Cole BJ, Romeo AA, Warner JJP: The use of bioabsorbable implants to treat shoulder instability. *Tech Sports Med* 2000;8:197-205.

This article reviews indications, surgical technique, and results following the use of the Suretac device for the treatment of patients with recurrent traumatic anterior shoulder instability.

Cole BJ, Warner JJ: Arthroscopic versus open Bankart repair for traumatic anterior shoulder instability. *Clin Sports Med* 2000;19:19-48.

This is an overview of the basic science, indications, surgical techniques, and appropriate decision making regarding arthroscopic and open reconstruction in patients with traumatic anterior shoulder instability.

Gartsman GM, Roddey TS, Hammerman SM: Arthroscopic treatment of anterior-inferior glenohumeral instability: Two to five-year follow-up. *J Bone Joint Surg Am* 2000;82:991-1003.

This study followed 53 patients who underwent arthroscopic treatment for shoulder instability with an emphasis on addressing all associated pathology in addition to the Bankart lesions. Ninety-two percent (49 of 53) had a good or excellent result, with only four patients demonstrating recurrent instability after a minimum of 2 years.

Guanche CA, Quick DC, Sodergren KM, Buss DD: Arthroscopic versus open reconstruction of the shoulder in patients with isolated Bankart lesions. *Am J Sports Med* 1996;24:144-148.

Patients who elected to undergo arthroscopic suture stabilization had slightly higher failure rates than did patients who choose to undergo open stabilization (5 of 15 with recurrent subluxation or instability in the arthroscopic group compared to 1 of 12 with recurrent subluxation in the open group).

Higgins LD, Warner JJ: Arthroscopic Bankart repair: Operative technique and surgical pitfalls. *Clin Sports Med* 2000;19:49-62.

This is a well-illustrated review of the suture anchor technique using nonabsorbable sutures.

Laurencin CT, Stephens S, Warren RF, Altchek DW: Arthroscopic Bankart repair using a degradable tack: A follow-up study using optimized indications. *Clin Orthop* 1996;332:132-137.

A 10% recurrence rate occurred following procedures using a degradable tack in combination with refined selection criteria that included patients with traumatic instability, presence of a Bankart lesion, a robust IGHL, and minimal bony involvement of the glenoid.

Nottage WM, Lieurance RK: Arthroscopic knot tying techniques: Current concepts. *Arthroscopy* 1999;15:515-521.

This article is an excellent review of techniques for tying arthroscopic slip knots and nonsliding knots.

Shaffer BS, Tibone JE: Arthroscopic shoulder instability surgery: Complications. *Clin Sports Med* 1999;18:737-767.

This is a comprehensive review of the complications associated with the various techniques used to perform arthroscopic shoulder stabilization.

Speer KP, Warren RF, Pagnani M, Warner JJ: An arthroscopic technique for anterior stabilization of the shoulder with a bioabsorbable tack. *J Bone Joint Surg Am* 1996;78:1801-1807.

At an average follow-up of 42 months, 41 of 52 patients (79%) were asymptomatic, while in the other 11 patients (21%) surgical repair using a bioabsorbable tack has failed.

Steinbeck J, Jerosch J: Arthroscopic transglenoid stabilization versus open anchor suturing in traumatic anterior instability of the shoulder. *Am J Sports Med* 1998;26:373-378.

Sixty-two patients were prospectively observed (30 following transglenoid arthroscopic stabilization and 32 following open stabilization using suture anchors) at a mean follow-up of 36 and 40 months, respectively. Five patients (17%) in the arthroscopic group and two (6%) in the open repair group had sustained redislocations.

Torchia ME, Caspari RB, Asselmeier, MA, Beach WR, Gayari M: Arthroscopic transglenoid multiple suture repair: 2 to 8 year results in 150 shoulders. *Arthroscopy* 1997;13:609-619.

One hundred fifty-six arthroscopically performed transglenoid suture repairs were reviewed at a minimum follow-up of 2 years. Eleven (7.3%) had redislocated, and 14 (9.3%) had experienced at least one episode of recurrent subluxation. Patients older than 25 years and those without a Bankart lesion fared better.

Weber SC: Abstract: Arthroscopic suture anchor repair versus open Bankart repair in the management of traumatic anterior glenohumeral instability. *Arthroscopy* 1996;12:382.

This study found an 8% recurrence rate in 40 patients who chose arthroscopic stabilization with suture anchors compared with a 2% recurrence rate in 92 patients who chose open repair.

Patient Selection

Hintermann B, Gachter A: Arthroscopic findings after shoulder dislocation. *Am J Sports Med* 1995;23:545-551.

In 212 patients with documented shoulder dislocations, 87% (184) had anterior glenoid labral tears, 79% (168) had ventral capsular insufficiency, 68% (144) had Hill-Sachs lesions, 55% (116) had glenohumeral ligament insufficiency, 14% (30) had complete rotator cuff tears, 12% (26) had posterior labral tears, and 7% (14) had SLAP tears. The conclusions of this study are that multiple pathologic changes are associated with the unstable shoulder.

Sisto DJ, Cook DL: Intraoperative decision making in the treatment of shoulder instability. *Arthroscopy* 1998;14:389-394.

This article reviews decision making for arthroscopic versus open shoulder stabilization.

Surgical Reconstruction Using Suture Anchors

Bacilla P, Field LD, Savoie FH III: Arthroscopic Bankart repair in a high demand patient population. *Arthroscopy* 1997;13:51-60.

A prospective study of 40 consecutive high-demand patients treated with nonabsorbable sutures and anchors resulted in recurrent instability in 37 of 40 patients (93%) at an average follow-up of 30 months.

Belzer JP, Snyder SJ: Abstract: Arthroscopic capsulorrhaphy for traumatic anterior shoulder instability using suture anchors and nonabsorbable suture. *Arthroscopy* 1995;11:359.

At an average follow-up of 22 months, Rowe scores following suture anchor and nonabsorbable suture reconstruction were: 27 excellent, 5 good, 1 fair, and 4 poor (ie, recurrent instability).

Cohen B, Cole BJ, Romeo AA: Thermal capsulorrhaphy of the shoulder. *Oper Tech Orthop* 2001;11:38-45

This article reviews the basic principles of thermal capsulorrhaphy and gives succinct descriptions of surgical techniques useful in the treatment of all types of shoulder instability patterns.

O'Neill DB: Arthroscopic Bankart repair of anterior detachments of the glenoid labrum: A prospective study. *J Bone Joint Surg Am* 1999;81:1357-1366.

One author's experience with 41 patients undergoing transglenoid suture repair of anterior labral detachments led to restored stability in 39 of 41 patients (95%) at an average follow-up of 52 months.

Classic Bibliography

Bigliani LU, Pollock RG, Soslowsky LJ, Flatow EL, Pawluk RJ, Mow VC: Tensile properties of the inferior glenohumeral ligament. *J Orthop Res* 1992;10:187-197.

Snyder SJ, Wuh HCK: Arthroscopic evaluation and treatment of the rotator cuff superior labrum anterior posterior lesion. *Op Tech Orthop* 1991;1:212-213.

Speer KP, Deng X, Borrero S, Torzilli PA, Altchek DA, Warren RF: Biomechanical evaluation of a simulated Bankart lesion. *J Bone Joint Surg Am* 1994;76: 1819-1826.

Wolf EM: Arthroscopic capsulolabral repair using suture anchors. *Orthop Clin North Am* 1993;24:59-69.

Chapter 11

Athletic Injuries and the Throwing Athlete: Shoulder

Stephen Fealy, MD

David W. Altchek, MD

Introduction

The shoulder of a throwing athlete is subjected to significantly greater forces and tensile stresses than is the shoulder of the average patient. Through a combination of in vitro biomechanical studies, electromyographic (EMG) analysis, and clinical observation, a model of the throwing shoulder has been created. Of the well-known phases of throwing (Fig. 1), the early acceleration phase is where most injuries seem to manifest. It appears that proper shoulder mechanics during an overhead sports activity such as throwing requires the humeral head to remain relatively centered on the glenoid. The soft-tissue structures that stabilize the humeral head on the glenoid are the glenoid labrum, glenohumeral ligaments, capsule, rotator cuff muscle tendon units, and the shoulder girdle musculature. It is well documented that injury does occur to the labrum, capsule, and tendons of the rotator cuff and that these structures often are injured concurrently. The clinical syndromes that develop as a result of these injuries are internal impingement, internal impingement with anterior instability, and subacromial impingement.

Each phase of throwing is associated with different forces to the shoulder girdle that may produce injuries to the rotator cuff, glenoid labrum, and/or capsuloligamentous structures. During the pitching motion, the shoulder experiences a distractive force equivalent to the patient's body weight. The angular velocity of the shoulder during the late cocking and acceleration phases reaches 7,000°/s. The nature of throwing predisposes athletes to overuse injuries that may affect the shoulder, elbow, or wrist. The treatment of shoulder injuries in the overhead athlete does require special consideration because of the repetitive high loads the shoulder must bear in sports such as baseball, tennis, weight lifting, and volleyball. Injuries such as partial rotator cuff tears or labral tears, which often require only minimal treatment in the sedentary individual, will require thorough physical therapy and perhaps surgical repair in the overhead athlete. A generalized four-phase rehabilitation protocol for the throwing athlete has been developed. Athletes who are not able to return to throwing after 6 months of rehabilitation are considered clinical failures by the protocol criteria.

Advances in both MRI and ultrasound imaging as well as arthroscopic instrumentation and techniques have advanced the diagnosis and treatment of shoulder disorders in both the lay and athletic patient populations. The use of arthroscopy to perform repairs that formerly were performed through an open technique has been associated directly with a more rapid recovery, more rapid return to activities, and lower surgical and hospital costs.

History

Athletes frequently are willing to continue to play through pain, despite the fact that it affects their performance. During consultation, athletes routinely provide vague histories regarding the injury and its occurrence, and they tend to minimize the symptoms of the injury in an attempt to return to play sooner. Athletes who understand the risks associated with the throwing motion and overuse injuries often are willing to change their throwing mechanics to minimize injury.

History taking should include a detailed chronology of the patient's symptoms. The physician should understand the activities required by the position played by the athlete as well as where the shoulder hurts and during which phase of the throwing motion symptoms occur. Throwing athletes report pain in the front or in the back of the shoulder. Therefore, clinicians should be aware of the most common problems that present as anterior and posterior shoulder pain (Table 1).

Physical Examination

Examination of a thrower's shoulder reveals subtle differences from that of the nonthrower's shoulder. One study has shown that pitchers routinely have 8° more external rotation in the throwing arm than on the contralateral side, at the expense of internal rotation of the

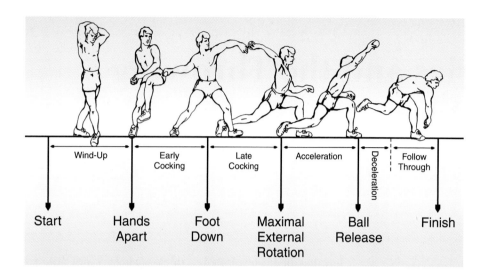

Figure 1 The six phases of throwing, shown here for the baseball pitch. From left to right, the phases are wind-up, early cocking, late cocking, acceleration, deceleration, and follow through. *(Reproduced with permission from DiGiovine NM, Jobe FW, Pink M, et al: An electromyographic analysis of the upper extremity in pitching. J Shoulder Elbow Surg 1992;1:15-25.)*

TABLE 1	Most Common Presenting Causes of Shoulder Pain

Anterior Shoulder Pain

Rotator cuff tendinitis

Anterior shoulder instability

Biceps tendinitis/subluxation

Anterior deltoid strain

Labral pathology (including biceps labral complex)

Posterior Shoulder Pain

Rotator cuff tendinitis

Posterior shoulder laxity

Posterior labral pathology

Posterior capsular tightness

Teres minor strain

Internal impingement

Quadrilateral space syndrome

Thrower's exostosis

Long thoracic nerve injury

Suprascapular nerve injury

Osteochondritis dissecans

throwing arm. Popular opinion has held that an increase in external rotation is the result of anterior capsular laxity, whereas a decrease in internal rotation is caused by posterior capsular tightness. Findings of an evaluation of this phenomenon with CT scans and physical examinations of 25 professional baseball pitchers and 25 nonthrowing participants recently were presented. Throwers were found to have an increase in humeral head retroversion relative to nonthrowers that corresponded to an increase in external rotation in the throwing arm. This study showed that there was a bony reason for the difference in increase in external rotation.

Physical examination should begin with a complete cervical spine examination and proceed with observation of the disrobed patient from both the front and the back. The shoulder and shoulder girdle should be evaluated with the patient sitting, standing, and supine. It is not uncommon for athletes to have overdevelopment of the shoulder girdle musculature and the humeral head of the throwing extremity. General posture and attitude of the shoulder girdle should be assessed. A gross inspection of the supraspinatus and infraspinatus fossae should be performed bilaterally. Significant atrophy of the infraspinatus fossa resulting from a suprascapular neuropathy at the spinoglenoid notch can frequently be picked up at this point.

The physician, observing the patient from behind, should assess scapulothoracic rhythm, particularly looking for abnormal scapular winging due to weakness of the scapular stabilizers. Patients should go through an active range of motion including forward elevation and abduction. Throwing athletes require a nearly full arc of motion in all planes to throw effectively. Scapular dyskinesias include but are not limited to changes in scapular elevation, changes in scapular retraction/protraction, and changes in muscle activity and synchrony.

Athletic injuries of the shoulder fall into two broad categories of microtrauma related to repetitive use and trauma caused by a sudden forceful event. Microtraumatic injuries to the shoulder from repetitive use include acromioclavicular joint osteolysis, injuries to the neurovascular structures about the shoulder, and glenohumeral instability. Sudden forceful events to the shoulder girdle often result in injuries to the glenoid labrum, rotator cuff, and glenohumeral ligaments.

Internal Impingement

Internal impingement is defined as abnormal contact between the rotator cuff undersurface and the glenoid margin, resulting in tearing of the rotator cuff and labrum. The actual incidence of these injuries is not known, but it appears that internal impingement is the most common shoulder injury in the throwing athlete. The cause of internal impingement has not been clearly documented. It has been postulated that the normal position of the humerus during the acceleration phase of throwing is to be aligned in the plane of the scapula and that shoulder girdle muscle fatigue that occurs during throwing allows the humerus to drift out of the scapular plane. This hyperangulation of the humerus stresses the anterior capsule and allows the undersurface of the rotator cuff to abut against the margin of the labrum (Fig. 2). Internal impingement is most likely caused by shoulder girdle muscle fatigue resulting from a lack of conditioning or overthrowing and/or anterior capsular stretch resulting in anterior instability. Patients commonly present with pain that is most frequently at the posterior joint line but may be anterior or anterolateral. One study found patients to have pain on full external rotation and 90° abduction. Two types of internal impingement have been observed.

Posterior internal impingement results in fraying or tearing of the undersurface of the infraspinatus and the posterior portion of the glenoid labrum. This injury is believed to occur during the maximal cocking or initial acceleration phase of throwing. Most posterosuperior rotator cuff tears probably are caused by internal impingement.

Superior internal impingement results in fraying or tearing of the anterior (supraspinatus) portion of the rotator cuff undersurface and the superior labrum. This injury is believed to occur during the midacceleration phase of throwing.

The pathomechanics of the shoulder that allow these injuries to occur have been the subject of debate. It is generally accepted that alteration from ideal throwing mechanics allows this abnormal contact between the cuff and labrum (Fig. 3). This alteration is believed, in the acute setting, to be caused by fatigue. As the humerus abducts horizontally, the fatigued athlete attempts to compensate and inadvertently increases external rotation. This increase allows impingement of the cuff undersurface against the glenoid margin. In chronic cases, anterior capsular stretch may occur. This stretch similarly allows the humerus to drift and again results in internal impingement.

Physical Examination

Pain during the throwing motion may be accompanied by a clicking sensation. Physical examination of patients with internal impingement reveals pain reproduced in the cocking phase at the posterior joint line. The patient may have a positive active compression test and may or may not have evidence of glenohumeral instability. Even though these patients frequently have no clinical evidence of instability, pain can be elicited during an

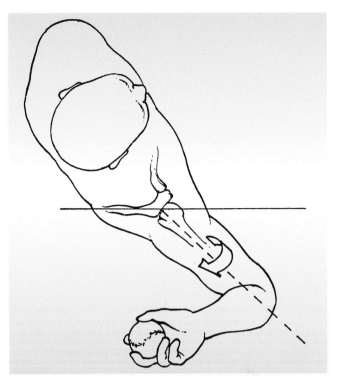

Figure 2 Hyperangulation of the humerus. *(Reproduced with permission from Jobe CM, Pink MM, Jobe FW, Shaffer B: Anterior shoulder instability, impingement, and rotator cuff tear, in Jobe FW, Pink MM, Glousman RE, Kvitne RS, Zemel NP (eds): Operative Techniques in Upper Extremity Sports Injuries. St Louis, MO, Mosby-Year Book, 1996, pp 164-177.)*

apprehension maneuver and relieved during a relocation test. The relocation test may be a sensitive means of diagnosing occult anterior instability that is contributing to rotator cuff disease.

Imaging

Radiographs of the patient with internal impingement should include AP, scapular-Y, axillary, and West Point views. The radiographs will show cystic and sclerotic changes in the greater tuberosity in nearly half of the patients with internal impingement. There will be evidence of rounding of the posterior glenoid rim in one third of patients. Bennett first observed posterior shoulder pain in throwing athletes and noted a bony exostosis on the posteroinferior glenoid rim that was seen on axillary plain films. MRI scans reveal partial undersurface rotator cuff tears and, often, a pathologic insertion of the supraspinatus tendon.

Arthroscopic Findings

In more than 80% of patients who are suspected clinically of having internal impingement, evidence of a partial undersurface rotator cuff tear is seen at arthroscopy (Fig. 4). Seventy percent of these patients have some element of posterosuperior glenoid labral detachment,

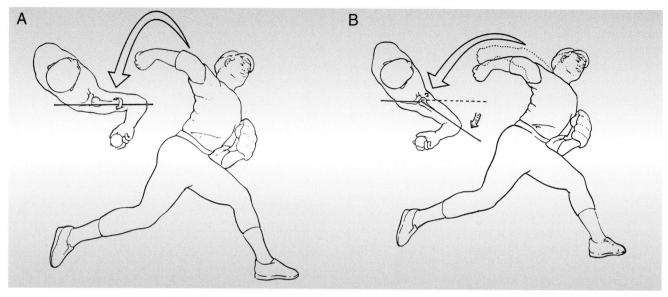

Figure 3 Pitching mechanics. **A,** Normal pitching mechanics from a side view and an overhead view. **B,** Pathologic pitching mechanics from a side view and an overhead view. *(Reproduced with permission from Jobe CM, Pink MM, Jobe FW, Shaffer B: Anterior shoulder instability, impingement, and rotator cuff tear, in Jobe FW, Pink MM, Glousman RE, Kvitne RS, Zemel NP (eds):* Operative Techniques in Upper Extremity Sports Injuries. *St Louis, MO, Mosby-Year Book, 1996, pp 164-177.)*

but more than 80% of patients have either a frayed or torn posterosuperior labrum that appears to be degenerative (Fig. 5). Synovitis and/or fraying of the long head of the biceps may be present. There is often an area of chondromalacia involving the posterosuperior glenoid rim under this frayed labral area. The authors of several studies noted that nearly half of patients with internal impingement have either an abrasion or fissure involving the posterosuperior glenoid cartilage. One study found that a posterior glenoid exostosis in the throwing athlete is consistent with the diagnosis of internal impingement. In 22 throwing athletes who had a posterior glenoid osteophyte, all but one of whom had an undersurface tear of the rotator cuff, débridement of the rotator cuff and labral tear and removal of the glenoid osteophyte were performed. At a mean follow-up of 6.3 years, 10 of the 18 patients available for evaluation (55%) had returned to premorbid levels of throwing. The authors of another recent study evaluated 1,232 skeletal shoulders. They noted characteristic osteophyte formation that interdigitated in a jigsaw-puzzle fashion on both the posterosuperior glenoid and superior humeral heads, which is suggestive of internal impingement. This was confirmed when the skeleton was put through a range of motion.

Arthroscopic evaluation of patients with internal impingement should include a thorough inspection involving internal and external rotation of the humerus to visualize the most posterior aspect of the humeral head and posterosuperior aspects of the undersurface of the rotator cuff. Evaluation of the glenohumeral joint during abduction and external rotation may reveal a kissing lesion between the rotator cuff and posterosuperior gle-

noid and labrum, which is evidenced if both structures are injured and directly in contact with each other. This kissing lesion has been implicated in the internal impingement peel-back phenomenon, whereby contact occurs between the undersurface of the rotator cuff and the labrum, resulting in continued delamination of the posterosuperior glenoid labrum and injury to the posterosuperior aspect of the glenoid rim (Fig. 6).

An arthroscopic study demonstrated that contact occurred between 90° and 150° of abduction between the 9 and 11 o'clock positions posteriorly on a right shoulder. These findings were reconfirmed in a study that used MRI to evaluate the throwing and nonthrowing shoulders of 10 throwing athletes. The authors noted that pathology of the rotator cuff and superior labrum was seen in the throwing shoulder but not the nonthrowing shoulder in each patient. Another study evaluated 105 consecutive patients who underwent shoulder arthroscopy. They found intraoperatively that contact between the rotator cuff and posterosuperior glenoid (with the arm in abduction and external rotation) occurred in a wide spectrum of diseases and was not limited to throwing athletes. In a recent evaluation of the shoulders in 41 professional throwing athletes, patients were examined arthroscopically with the shoulder in the position of the relocation test. All of these patients had either contact between the rotator cuff undersurface and the posterosuperior glenoid rim or osteochondral lesions when evaluated in this position. Undersurface cuff fraying was seen in 93% of patients, posterosuperior labral fraying in 88%, and anterior labral fraying in 36%.

Treatment

Treatment options in throwing athletes with internal impingement should include conservative therapy, arthroscopic débridement, and possibly open treatment involving capsulolabral repair. Initial nonsurgical measures for a patient with internal impingement include rest and anti-inflammatory agents followed by physical therapy. Once pain has remitted, dynamic stabilization rehabilitation with emphasis on the shoulder girdle, scapular, and rotator cuff musculature should be performed. Attempts at changing the throwing mechanics in the late cocking phase have proved successful. Throwers should try to avoid forceful external rotation and hyperextension in the late cocking phase.

Surgical treatment is considered if rehabilitation fails; it includes arthroscopic débridement of rotator cuff and labral injuries initially. Labral detachments and partial rotator cuff tears that extend through more than half the thickness of the total rotator cuff (Fig. 7) are repaired routinely. Arthroscopic capsulorrhaphy is performed when arthroscopic evidence of anterior capsular laxity is found. Arthroscopic capsular plication and thermal shrinkage techniques have been used with encouraging early results.

Suprascapular Neuropathy

Suprascapular neuropathy is an uncommon condition, but one that is seen in the throwing athlete and volleyball players. The suprascapular nerve is a mixed sensorimotor nerve without cutaneous branches. It is formed from nerve roots from C5 and C6 and occasionally involves the nerve root from C4, and it sends sensory branches to the glenohumeral joint, acromioclavicular joint, and subacromial space. The suprascapular nerve travels with the artery and vein until it passes through the suprascapular notch as the neurovascular bundle traverses above the transverse scapular ligament. The authors of an anatomic study of 79 cadaveric shoulders noted that the suprascapular notch formed a U shape in 77% of the specimens and a V shape in the remaining 23%. In 89% of the cadavers, these patterns were seen bilaterally. Twenty-three percent of the shoulders had either a partial or complete ossification of the suprascapular ligament, or multiple bands of the ligament were seen.

Direct compression of the suprascapular nerve results in supraspinatus and infraspinatus dysfunction. The nerve may be injured either through mass effect from a paralabral ganglion cyst or through being stretched. Ganglion cysts will appear as a low-intensity signal on T1 images and a high-intensity signal on T2 images. The suprascapular nerve is susceptible to compression proximally and distally. Ganglia emanating from labral cysts often are responsible for nerve compression. Patients

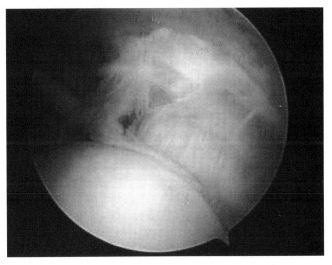

Figure 4 Arthroscopic evaluation of patients with internal impingement will frequently reveal undersurface partial-thickness tearing of the rotator cuff.

with suprascapular neuropathy present clinically with long histories involving weakness and a dull pain about the shoulder girdle. The authors of one study noted that 22 of 27 patients presented with pain directly over the suprascapular notch.

Patients with suprascapular neuropathy present with gross motor weakness that is out of proportion to their pain. Physical examination reveals a hollowness of the suprascapular and/or infrascapular fossae, depending on where nerve compression occurs. Gross motor weakness of either the supraspinatus or infraspinatus will be noted when compared with the contralateral side and can be confirmed with electrodiagnostic testing. When an anatomic etiology cannot be found, management should be nonsurgical because most patients will have a good to excellent result with physical therapy.

Proximal compression of the suprascapular nerve occurs at the suprascapular notch, where the nerve traverses underneath the transverse scapular ligament, which often becomes hypertrophied. Compression here produces weakness and atrophy of both the supraspinatus and infraspinatus. EMG and nerve conduction studies will confirm involvement of both muscle bellies.

The suprascapular nerve can be compressed distally at the lateral edge of the scapular spine as the terminal branches of the nerve innervate the infraspinatus muscle. Distal involvement of the nerve occurs at the spinoglenoid notch (Fig. 8). With distal compression, there will be wasting of only the infraspinatus muscle belly; the supraspinatus will be normal. Patients with distal suprascapular nerve compression will have, on average, a 22% loss in external rotation strength. This condition is unique to throwers. Dynamic involvement of the suprascapular nerve during the throwing motion has been demonstrated. In extreme abduction and external rotation (late cocking phase) of

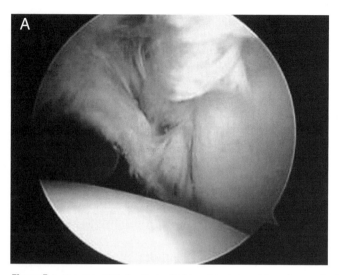

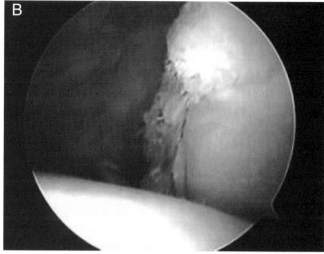

Figure 5 A, More than 80% of patients with internal impingement have degenerative fraying of the posterosuperior glenoid labrum. **B,** Degenerative labral fraying can be arthroscopically débrided back to a smooth labral rim posteriorly. Care must be taken to preserve the normal glenolabral attachment.

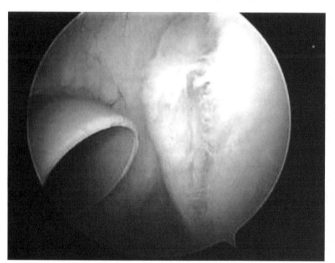

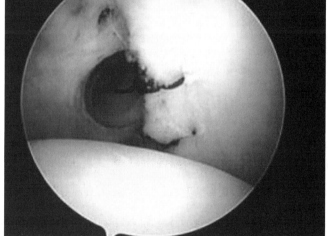

Figure 6 Arthroscopic evidence of the peel-back phenomenon in a professional baseball pitcher. Note that the posterosuperior labrum has been delaminated, or stripped away, from its original insertion on the glenoid.

Figure 7 Arthroscopic picture after repair of delaminated posterior labrum using Knotless Suture Anchor technique (Mitek Products Inc; Westwood, MA).

the shoulder, the medial tendinous margin between the infraspinatus and supraspinatus forcefully impinges against the scapular spine, thereby compressing the intervening infraspinatus branch of the suprascapular nerve. Patients with this condition will report pain when placed in this position. For patients with this clinical picture and confirmatory electrodiagnostic studies, a spinoglenoid notchplasty is an appropriate surgical procedure.

Outcomes

Electrodiagnostic studies have been recommended to help in diagnosing suprascapular neuropathy. One author reported that an increased latency on the affected side is consistent with nerve impairment and is indicative of entrapment of the suprascapular nerve; he recommended early surgical release of the suprascapu-

lar ligament before gross muscular atrophy. Authors in another study evaluated nonsurgical treatment of suprascapular neuropathy in 15 patients who were treated initially with physical therapy. Clinical diagnosis was made using electrodiagnostic studies in each case. Five patients had excellent results, seven had good results, and three required surgical intervention to treat the neuropathy. Of the three who had surgical intervention, one patient had a poor outcome, one had a good result, and one had an excellent result. Other authors recommended surgical decompression of the nerve through a posterior approach after failure of nonsurgical measures. They noted that motor function in the supraspinatus muscle improved in 87% of patients and that atrophy of the muscle improved in 81%. Motor weakness of the infraspinatus muscle improved in 71% of patients, and atrophy of the muscle resolved in 50%.

Spinoglenoid notchplasty was performed in five elite volleyball players who demonstrated isolated denervation of the infraspinatus muscle, which produced weakness and gross atrophy. All patients returned to the same or higher level of play within 8 months of the time of surgery. The authors of the study noted that in extreme abduction and external rotation of the shoulder, the medial tendinous margin between the infraspinatus and supraspinatus muscles impinged strongly against the lateral edge of the scapular spine and compressed the infraspinatus branch of the suprascapular nerve.

Instability in the Throwing Athlete

Treatment of patients with symptomatic glenohumeral instability is directed toward eliminating subtle pathologic humeral translation without compromising overall motion of the shoulder. Andrews, appropriately, has termed this problem the "throwers' paradox." Sports-specific laxity patterns among athletes have been determined. When evaluating a throwing athlete who is thought to have instability, the clinician should be able to distinguish the type and direction of the instability based on the clinical history. Instability in the throwing athlete, like that in the nonthrowing athlete, may be traumatic, atraumatic, or acquired.

On physical examination, it is essential to determine the position that creates apprehension in the patient because this information can implicate the specific anatomic structures that contribute to the glenohumeral instability. The primary anterior capsular restraint with the shoulder at 90° abduction and 0° of external rotation is the superior glenohumeral ligament. At 45° of external rotation and 90° of abduction, the middle glenohumeral ligament is responsible for stability, while the inferior glenohumeral ligament complex is the primary anterior capsular stabilizer at 90° of external rotation of the shoulder. The shoulder should be passively brought through an arc of motion and palpated for the presence of any distinguishable clunks or clicks that may represent torn labral pathology.

Management of glenohumeral instability in the throwing athlete with symptomatic laxity should focus on identifying the underlying pathology and then treating the patient with the goal of return to pain-free participation in sports. Initial treatment involves a nonsurgical protocol including rest followed by rehabilitation. Bracing is used occasionally to limit abduction and external rotation of the affected shoulder. After a period of rest and activity modification, protocols involving rotator cuff, periscapular, and large muscle (deltoid) strengthening are begun. Sport-specific drills and progression into throwing should take place in a functional stepwise fashion. Proprioceptive training involving taping also may be incorporated into the rehabilitation protocol. Throwing athletes are

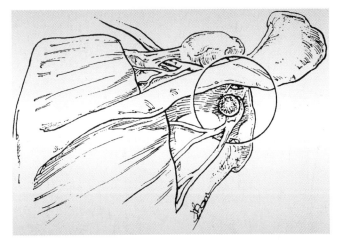

Figure 8 A ganglion cyst at the spinoglenoid notch with pressure on the suprascapular nerve. The cyst generally originates from the glenohumeral joint. *(Reproduced from McCluskey GM III, Dellaero DT: Special issues in athletes, in Norris TR (ed): Orthopaedic Knowledge Update: Shoulder and Elbow. Rosemont, IL, American Academy of Orthopaedic Surgeons, 1997, pp 101-110.)*

allowed to return to sports when they are pain free, have obtained a full range of motion, and have full strength. If patients continue to report symptomatic instability that limits their throwing, surgical intervention is considered.

Surgery on throwers with symptomatic laxity should repair injured structures, and treatment should follow a direction-based approach. Patients with anterior instability complain that the shoulder wants to slide out the front during late cocking and early acceleration phases. These patients may have an essential lesion involving anterior capsular laxity and, potentially, a Bankart lesion. Patients who undergo anterior stabilization procedures likely will experience a small loss of external rotation, but they routinely do well, with good to excellent results expected in more than 80% of patients. Patients with posterior laxity complain of pain and subluxation-type symptoms in the follow-through phase of throwing. They, too, will have gross capsular laxity and may or may not have a reverse Bankart lesion. Posterior glenohumeral laxity is less common than anterior laxity, and studies evaluating outcomes in these patients have grouped together various procedures and diagnoses. These studies have shown that treatment for posterior shoulder laxity produces good to excellent results in from 50% to 90% of patients. Patients with a traumatic multidirectional instability generally respond to a physician-directed rehabilitation program employing strengthening of the deltoid, rotator cuff, and scapular stabilizing musculature.

Open shoulder stabilization is the standard, but arthroscopic techniques are quickly developing and improving. Historically, the rate of recurrence after arthroscopic stabilization has been higher than 20%, whereas the rate of recurrence after open stabilization is lower than 10%. Arthroscopic stabilization procedures have used suture

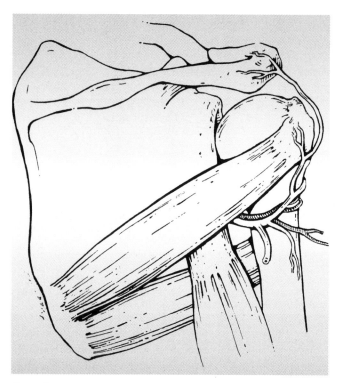

Figure 9 The quadrilateral space. Note the posterior humeral circumflex artery and axillary nerve traversing the interval. *(Reproduced with permission from Schneider K, Kasparyan NG, Altchek DW, Fantini GA, Weiland AJ: An aneurysm involving the axillary artery and its branch vessels in a major league baseball pitcher: A case report and review of the literature. Am J Sports Med 1999;27:370-375.)*

anchor techniques, bioabsorbable tack techniques, and, more recently, thermal stabilization. Arthroscopic stabilization often fails because of patient selection rather than surgical technique. Ideal candidates for an arthroscopic stabilization are patients with acute, unidirectional instability who have experienced fewer than three dislocations. Poor candidates for an arthroscopic stabilization procedure include patients who have chronic instability with subsequently poor tissues, no evidence of a Bankart lesion, and generalized laxity and those who are habitual dislocators.

New arthroscopic techniques for capsular shrinkage, including laser-assisted capsular shrinkage and thermal capsulorrhaphy, have been developed for the patient with subtle instability and glenohumeral laxity. Early studies are revealing acceptable short-term results, but complications, including glenohumeral stiffness, recurrent instability, and axillary nerve injury, have been reported.

Vascular Lesions in Throwing Athletes

Vascular pathologies in the upper extremity of a throwing athlete are rare. They include digital vessel thrombosis, proximal thrombosis with distal embolization, aneurysms, and vessel compression such as in thoracic outlet syndrome and quadrilateral space syndrome (QSS).

Vessel Aneurysms

Aneurysms of the subclavian artery, various portions of the axillary artery, and posterior humeral circumflex artery have been reported to occur in overhead athletes. Patients often relate a constellation of subtle signs and symptoms, but they generally report pain relating to ischemia. It is thought that aneurysms are related to repetitive trauma or impingement experienced during the throwing motion. The pectoralis minor muscle and humeral head have been implicated in vascular impingement of the axillary and circumflex vessels when the shoulder is in an abducted and externally rotated position. Wright called this phenomenon the hyperabduction syndrome. One study demonstrated that the axillary artery is compressed in more than 80% of arms when they are placed in the throwing position. However, less than 10% of patients demonstrate 50% stenosis of the vessel during this evaluation. This alteration in flow mechanics may create turbulent flow leading to the formation of thrombi, which in turn may embolize distally, leading to ischemic changes at remote sites. Intermittent vascular compression, arterial thrombosis, and frank aneurysms each may produce ischemic-type symptoms.

The diagnosis of a vascular aneurysm is challenging. Symptoms in these patients are activity related and frequently are long-standing. On physical examination, the extremity often appears normal, without any objective clinical findings. The extremity should be palpated for pulses and examined in both the neutral position and in the provocative position of hyperabduction and external rotation. Digits and nail beds should be inspected for evidence of emboli. Auscultation for the presence of a bruit should also be performed.

Digital ischemia due to an aneurysm that may be showering emboli distally causes pain, blanching, and numbness in the digits. Patients report an easily fatigued extremity that seems relatively heavy compared with the contralateral hand. Cold intolerance and hypersensitivity similar to reflex sympathetic dystrophy also may play a role in the clinical presentation despite the fact that the patient denies proximal symptoms. Other possible causes, including valvular heart disease, vasculitis, and cardiac arrhythmias, should be considered in the differential diagnosis. A chest radiograph should be ordered to rule out the presence of a cervical rib and the diagnosis of thoracic outlet syndrome. Several noninvasive tests often are required to confirm the diagnosis. Duplex Doppler scans, pulse volume recordings, photoplethysmography, and arteriograms are useful in establishing the correct diagnosis.

Treatment of vessel aneurysms includes rehabilitation and activity modification. In the case of the high-performance athlete, surgical reconstruction has yielded predictable results. Surgical options include segmental excision with primary anastomosis, patching, or bypass grafting.

Quadrilateral Space Syndrome

QSS was first described in 1983; it was associated with throwing athletes in 1986. QSS has an insidious onset of often vague posterior shoulder pain. Patients with QSS have pain poorly localized to the shoulder, paresthesias in a nondermatomal distribution, and discrete point tenderness in the quadrilateral space. Arteriograms show compression of the posterior humeral circumflex artery (PHCA) with abduction and external rotation of the affected shoulder. It is believed that symptoms result from compression of the axillary nerve and not compression of the PHCA. Investigators have noted that the neurovascular bundle frequently is compressed by fibrotic bands as it crosses through the quadrilateral space, but they were unable to identify these bands in cadaveric specimens, suggesting a physiologic rather than an anatomic cause of QSS.

The quadrilateral space is the area bordered superiorly by the teres minor, laterally by the humeral shaft, inferiorly by the teres major, and medially by the long head of the triceps (Fig. 9). The axillary nerve and the posterior humeral circumflex artery exit through the quadrilateral space. Symptoms including pain and paresthesias are increased with forward flexion and external rotation or abduction and external rotation. Discrete point tenderness is present over the quadrilateral space, generally near the insertion of the teres minor.

Physical examination of patients with QSS reveals signs and symptoms that are similar to those seen in thoracic outlet syndrome; differential diagnosis usually can be made on the basis of tenderness to palpation in the quadrilateral space. Similar to the hyperabduction maneuver diagnostic of thoracic outlet syndrome, holding the arm in the cocked position (abduction and external rotation) for 1 minute generally will reproduce symptoms associated with QSS. With the arm in this position, there may be a dampening of the radial pulse. Atrophy of the deltoid and/or teres minor may be seen in severe QSS or long-standing cases. Neurologic findings on examination are rare, and EMG studies of the deltoid and teres minor may be normal. Magnetic resonance angiography has been shown to be of little value in the diagnosis of QSS. Subclavian arteriography of the PHCA may reveal occlusion with abduction and external rotation of the affected arm, but this also has been demonstrated with normal control subjects. MRI may show evidence of atrophy of either the teres minor or deltoid muscle bellies. No specific tests confirm the diagnosis of QSS, which is made on the basis of excluding other pathologic entities.

Nonsurgical management is the standard treatment for throwers with QSS. Specific emphasis should be placed on stretching of the posterior capsule and teres minor. Surgical decompression of the quadrilateral space has been reported to provide relief of symptoms in patients who have failed nonsurgical treatment. In one study, 16 of 18 patients (89%) reported good or excellent results and two (11%) reported no change in symptoms following surgery.

Annotated Bibliography

Antoniadis G, Richter HP, Rath S, Braun V, Moese G: Suprascapular nerve entrapment: Experience with 28 cases. *J Neurosurg* 1996;85:1020-1025.

    The authors provide their experience and outcomes in treating patients with suprascapular nerve entrapment.

Bigliani LU, Codd TP, Connor PM, Levine WN, Littlefield MA, Hershon SJ: Shoulder motion and laxity in the professional baseball player. *Am J Sports Med* 1997;25:609-613.

    The authors studied 148 asymptomatic baseball players to assess range of motion and laxity. They found that pitchers had significantly greater forward elevation and external rotation and less internal rotation than position players. A sulcus sign was seen in 61% of dominant shoulders in pitchers, compared with 47% in position players.

De Maeseneer M, Jaovisidha S, Jacobson JA, et al: The Bennett lesion of the shoulder. *J Comput Assist Tomogr* 1998;22:31-34.

    The authors reviewed the imaging features and significance of the Bennett lesion, which is typically seen in baseball pitchers. They determined that associated labral and rotator cuff abnormalities should be suspected in patients with a diagnosed Bennett lesion.

Edelson G, Teitz C: Internal impingement in the shoulder. *J Shoulder Elbow Surg* 2000;9:308-315.

    The authors evaluated 1,232 skeletal specimens. They noted that internal impingement between the glenoid and humeral head may contribute to rotator cuff pathology.

Halbrecht JL, Tirman P, Atkin D: Internal impingement of the shoulder: Comparison of findings between the throwing and non-throwing shoulders of college baseball players. *Arthroscopy* 1999;15:253-258.

    In this study, the findings of gadolinium-enhanced MRI studies of throwing and nonthrowing shoulders in 10 college baseball athletes were evaluated and compared, then contrasted with clinical examination results. Three of 10 throwing shoulders had superior labral tears and adjacent paralabral cysts; four had abnormal signal change in the rotator cuff tendons. There was no correlation between positive MRI findings and the instability seen at the clinical examination.

Jobe CM, Pink MM, Jobe FW, Shaffer B: Anterior shoulder instability, impingement, and rotator cuff tear, in Jobe FW, Pink MM, Glousman RE, Kvitne RS, Zemel NP (eds): *Operative Techniques in Upper Extremity Sports Injuries.* St Louis, MO, Mosby-Year Book, 1996, pp 164-177.

The authors provide an excellent overview of the subject.

Kuhn JE, Bey MJ, Huston LJ, Blasier RB, Soslowsky LJ: Ligamentous restraints to external rotation of the humerus in the late-cocking phase of throwing: A cadaveric biomechanical investigation. *Am J Sports Med* 2000;28:200-205.

The authors used 20 cadaveric shoulders to determine ligamentous restraints to external rotation during the late cocking phase of throwing. Cutting the entire inferior glenohumeral ligament resulted in the greater increase in external rotation ($10.2° \pm 4.9°$). Sectioning the coracohumeral ligament also resulted in an increase in external rotation.

Lester B, Jeong GK, Weiland AJ, Wickiewicz TL: Quadrilateral space syndrome: Diagnosis, pathology, and treatment. *Am J Orthop* 1999;28:718-725.

The authors provide an excellent and thorough review of this relatively uncommon condition.

Martin SD, Warren RF, Martin TL, Kennedy K, O'Brien SJ, Wickiewicz TL: Suprascapular neuropathy: Results of non-operative treatment. *J Bone Joint Surg Am* 1997; 79:1159-1165.

In this retrospective review of the results of nonsurgical treatment in 15 patients with suprascapular neuropathy, diagnosis was confirmed with electrodiagnostic studies. Five patients had an excellent result; seven had good results. Three patients had surgical intervention with mixed results.

McFarland EG, Hsu CY, Neira C, O'Neil O: Internal impingement of the shoulder: A clinical and arthroscopic analysis. *J Shoulder Elbow Surg* 1999;8:458-460.

In this article, 105 patients undergoing shoulder arthroscopy were studied with the arm in abduction and external rotation until contact was made. Contact was made between the rotator cuff and glenoid rim at an average of 95° of abduction and 74° of external rotation in 85% of these patients. These findings were not limited to the throwing athlete. The authors' findings suggest that these factors may not be essential for the diagnosis of internal impingement.

Meister K: Internal impingement in the shoulder of the overhand athlete: Pathophysiology, diagnosis, and treatment. *Am J Orthop* 2000;29:433-438.

The authors review the mechanics, diagnosis, and treatment options for throwing athletes with internal impingement.

Meister K, Andrews JR, Batts J, Wilk K, Baumgarten T, Baumgartner T: Symptomatic thrower's exostosis: Arthroscopic evaluation and treatment. *Am J Sports Med* 1999;27:133-136.

The authors evaluate 22 patients who were throwing athletes with posterior glenoid osteophytes. Arthroscopy revealed undersurface tearing of the rotator cuff in all but one patient. Of those treated, 55% returned to their premorbid level of activity following débridement of the rotator cuff and labrum.

Paley KJ, Jobe FW, Pink MM, Kvitne RS, ElAttrache NS: Arthroscopic findings in the overhand throwing athlete: Evidence for posterior internal impingement of the rotator cuff. *Arthroscopy* 2000;16:35-40.

The authors note that with the arm in the position of the relocation test, 41 of 41 professional baseball players had contact between the rotator cuff undersurface and the posterosuperior glenoid rim or osteochondral lesions. Undersurface cuff fraying was seen in 93% of patients.

Post M: Diagnosis and treatment of suprascapular nerve entrapment. *Clin Orthop* 1999;368:92-100.

The author reports his experience in 39 patients who underwent a release of the suprascapular ligament for entrapment of the suprascapular nerve that was confirmed before surgery with abnormal electrodiagnostic findings. There were 27 excellent, 11 good, and one fair result.

Sandow MJ, Ilic J: Suprascapular nerve rotator cuff compression syndrome in volleyball players. *J Shoulder Elbow Surg* 1998;7:516-521.

The authors propose an alternative cause of infraspinatus weakness in volleyball players. They report on five patients in whom spinoglenoid notchplasty was performed. Correction of infraspinatus muscle wasting was seen in all patients.

Schneider K, Kasparyan NG, Altchek DW, Fantini GA, Weiland AJ: An aneurysm involving the axillary artery and its branch vessels in a major league baseball pitcher: A case report and review of the literature. *Am J Sports Med* 1999;27:370-375.

The authors report on baseball pitchers who are prone to aneurysms of the axillary artery and its branches, stating that the probable cause is from repetitive compression of or tension on blood vessels that is exacerbated by the pitching motion. Treatment varies based on the type and location of the lesion.

Ticker JB, Djurasovic M, Strauch RJ, et al: The incidence of ganglion cysts and other variations in anatomy along the course of the suprascapular nerve. *J Shoulder Elbow Surg* 1998;7:472-478.

The authors studied 79 shoulders from 41 cadavers to evaluate the morphologic characteristics of the suprascapular notch. Specimens also were evaluated for the presence of a ganglion cyst formation in the notch. A U-shaped notch was found in 77% of specimens, while a V-shaped notch was found in 23% of specimens; 89% of notches were the same bilaterally. One (1%) ganglion cyst was identified. Variations in the morphology of the superior transverse ligament also were noted.

Classic Bibliography

Altchek DW, Warren RF, Wickiewicz TL, Ortiz G: Arthroscopic labral debridement: A three-year follow-up study. *Am J Sports Med* 1992;20:702-706.

Andrews JR, Broussard TS, Carson WG: Arthroscopy of the shoulder in the management of partial tears of the rotator cuff: A preliminary report. *Arthroscopy* 1985;1:117-122.

Cahill BR, Palmer RE: Quadrilateral space syndrome. *J Hand Surg Am* 1983;8:65-69.

Jobe CM, Sidles J: Abstract: Evidence for a superior glenoid impingement upon the rotator cuff: Anatomic, kinesiologic, MRI, and arthroscopic findings, in Debeyre J, Duparc J, Patte D, et al (eds): *Fifth International Conference on Surgery of the Shoulder*. St Louis, MO, Mosby, 1993.

Lord JW Jr, Wright IS: Total claviculectomy for neurovascular compression in the thoracic outlet. *Surg Gynecol Obstet* 1993;176:609-612.

Montgomery WH, Jobe FW: Functional outcomes in athletes after modified anterior capsulolabral reconstruction. *Am J Sports Med* 1994;22:352-358.

Redler MR, Ruland LJ III, McCue FC III: Quadrilateral space syndrome in a throwing athlete. *Am J Sports Med* 1986;14:511-513.

Rohrer MJ, Cardullo PA, Pappas AM, Phillips DA, Wheeler HB: Axillary artery compression and thrombosis in throwing athletes. *J Vasc Surg* 1990;11:761-769.

Walch G, Boileau P, Noel E, Donell ST: Impingement of the deep surface of the supraspinatus tendon on the posterosuperior glenoid rim: An arthroscopic study. *J Shoulder Elbow Surg* 1992;1:238-245.

Chapter 12

Complications and Failures in Instability Repair

Patrick Hayes, MD

Yassamin Hazrati, MD

Evan L. Flatow, MD

Introduction

Glenohumeral instability encompasses a wide spectrum of clinical disorders. Surgical treatment of refractory instability is quite successful in general, but success rates vary depending on the nature of the instability, the surgical technique used, and the definition of success. Most definitions of successful surgery emphasize return to full function with preservation of motion and strength as well as elimination of the instability. Failures may be defined as recurrent or persistent instability or other complications (nerve injury, stiffness, or infection) encountered during or after surgical treatment. Persistent or recurrent instability can result from misdiagnosis of the instability, errors in selection of the appropriate surgical technique, technical problems at surgery and implant failure, inappropriate postoperative care, reinjury, or underlying biology. Misdiagnosis of underlying comorbidities, technical and rehabilitation errors, and perioperative complications can result in persistent postoperative pain, stiffness, arthritis, or other conditions that can compromise the final result. Success rates for reoperation for failed instability vary, depending on the reason for failure and whether the underlying pathology can be corrected at revision surgery.

Considerations in Choice of Treatment

Character of the Instability

Characterizing the patient's instability correctly and understanding how the instability impacts the patient's work and life are critical. Instability should be characterized by onset (traumatic, repetitive microtrauma, or insidious/atraumatic), direction (anterior, inferior, posterior, bidirectional, or multidirectional), magnitude (dislocation or subluxation), recurrence, chronicity, and volition. Subluxation is often amenable to rest and strengthening of the rotator cuff and periscapular musculature. Rehabilitation of throwing athletes should emphasize posterior capsular stretching and serratus anterior and rotator cuff

strengthening. Traumatic anterior dislocations in active patients younger than age 30 years frequently result in recurrent dislocations. Given the high rate of recurrence in this group, some authors recommend routine repair in young, first-time, traumatic, anterior dislocators to restore the anatomy acutely and decrease the chance of recurrence. One study prospectively randomized patients into two groups: those who underwent immediate arthroscopic stabilization and those treated with immobilization and rehabilitation. The immediate arthroscopic fixation group had sustained significantly fewer dislocations at 2 years, was capable of the same motion as was the nonsurgical group, and experienced an improvement in disease-specific quality of life on the Western Ontario Shoulder Instability Index.

Recurrent dislocations are not well treated with therapy alone. Recurrent traumatic anterior instability can be treated arthroscopically or with open procedures. One study attempted to define selection criteria for each technique based on examination under anesthesia and findings at arthroscopy. Arthroscopic repairs were offered to patients with ≤ 1 cm inferior translation, anterior translation over the glenoid rim, a Bankart lesion without a glenoid fracture, no capsular disruption, and discrete glenohumeral ligaments present on arthroscopy. Open repairs were used on patients with inferior translation ≥ 2 cm, a patulous or disrupted capsule, absence of discrete glenohumeral ligaments, or no Bankart lesion. Results were not significantly different, though patients with open repairs tended to have a lower rate of recurrence. Bidirectional and multidirectional instability (MDI) are initially best treated with physical therapy. Recently, 57 young, athletic patients with MDI were followed for 7 to 10 years. Those treated nonsurgically fared poorly. Response to nonsurgical treatment in this study usually occurred within the first 3 months. Surgically, MDI is best treated with procedures that address global capsular laxity as well as labral pathology. Bilateral and diffuse ligamentous laxity are clues to underlying "loose-jointed" anatomy and may influence the amount of capsular imbrication at surgery. Voluntary instability associated with an underlying psychiatric need to dislocate (as a way to obtain drugs or attention) has traditionally been thought of as doomed to failure. However, patients who can exhibit their instability reluctantly but voluntarily, have no underlying psychiatric disorders, and report pain and disability from their instability can be treated successfully with surgery. These patients are typically unstable posteriorly or posteroinferiorly, and open posterior capsular shift has been shown to be successful in treating this instability. A correct characterization of the instability is critical in the selection of treatment.

Surgical Selection

Incorrectly characterizing an instability may cause the surgeon to select the wrong procedure. The idealized poles of the pathologic spectrum are TUBS (Traumatic Unidirectional instability with a Bankart lesion best treated with Surgery) and AMBRI (Atraumatic Multidirectional instability that is Bilateral, responds to Rehabilitation and, as a last resort, Inferior capsular shift). It is critical to discern whether the instability is multidirectional or bidirectional or is closer to unidirectional, traumatic-onset instability. Treating bidirectional anteroinferior instability with an anterior capsular tightening procedure without capsular balancing may result in residual inferior instability. Although some investigators have reported disappointing results after surgery for MDI, one recently published series using Neer's inferior capsular shift achieved over 90% success at 2-year follow-up. Predominantly anterior instability that is approached from the anterior side and posterior instability approached from the posterior side allows preferential thickening, labral repair or reinforcement, and scarring on the side that is most unstable. This approach may also avoid fixed subluxation in the most symptomatic direction as is sometimes seen when posteroinferior instability is treated with an anterior approach. MDI has a high rate of failure after attempted arthroscopic reconstruction. An open shift is still the gold standard of treatment for MDI. Recent series report a high rate of failure for thermal capsulorrhaphy in treating MDI and multiple recurrent dislocations. The wrong diagnosis can lead to inappropriate procedures and persistent symptoms.

Patients with less severe instabilities may be good candidates for less invasive surgery. Patients with symptomatic subluxations but no history of dislocations may benefit from arthroscopic capsular tucks performed with sutures or capsular shrinkage performed with radiofrequency wands. There is no consensus at this time on which technique is better. In competitive baseball pitchers without frank dislocations but with painful subluxations or "dead arm syndrome," arthroscopic or minimally

open capsular imbrications have been reported to have good success. Success in this group must include not only a reduction in painful subluxation but also a high probability of return to competitive throwing. Procedures that significantly limit postoperative motion will end a pitcher's career and should not be used in this special population. Conversely, in contact athletes with no premium on overhead motion (eg, Australian Rules football players), open surgeries, which have been shown to be more reliable than arthroscopic procedures in eradicating instability, are indicated.

The current emphasis is on anatomic reconstructions. Subscapularis advancements such as the Putti-Platt and Magnuson-Stack procedures and coracoid transfers or musculotendinous slings such as the modified Bristow procedure are now less commonly performed than capsuloligamentous repairs and capsular imbrications or shifts, as required. Glenoid or humeral osteotomies are rarely indicated and should not be undertaken by the casual shoulder surgeon.

Technical Pitfalls

It is now understood that there is no single essential lesion that leads to recurrent instability. Stability results from a complex interplay of dynamic and various static restraints that must be evaluated and addressed appropriately at surgery. Characterizing instability by history and physical examination, imaging studies, and examination of the shoulder under anesthesia in various combinations of abduction, flexion, and rotation allows the surgeon to identify which parts of the capsule and labrum are contributing to the instability and need to be repaired or reconstructed.

Anatomic Concerns of the Labrum

The ability of the labrum to resist anterior translation of the humeral head on the glenoid is linearly related to the height of this restraint. If a soft-tissue Bankart tear is present, it must be repaired in a way that restores the height of the glenoid-labral wall. Repairing the labrum up onto the glenoid rim rather than to the side of the glenoid neck effectively restores this restraint. One cadaveric biomechanical study of a surgically created Bankart lesion suggested that three points of fixation were more effective against resisting translations than were two points of fixation. If a significant bony Bankart lesion is present, it must be repaired to restore the height of the glenoid rim and labrum. In another cadaveric study of anteroinferior glenoid rim fractures more than 20% of the glenoid height (average, 6.8 mm wide), significant reduction in dislocation force and a marked decrease in passive external rotation were found when the capsule was repaired directly to the fracture site. No difference in instability was found in the provocative position, underscoring that a competent, tight anteroinferior capsule on maximum stretch will maintain the glenoid head in its proper location. The instability was found in abduction and internal rotation, a midrange position where labral height is more important to resisting dislocation. Any bony Bankart lesion that compromises the height of the anteroinferior glenoid rim and leaves a "trough" for the head to escape should be repaired at surgery. If the patient has an atrophic or flat labrum, measures to augment the rim at surgery may be used. Some authors report using barrel stitches to thicken the capsule and labrum anteroinferiorly. In extreme and revision cases, bone blocks and allografts have been reported.

The amount of capsular imbrication at surgery must be tailored to the specific clinical setting. Primary repairs for first-time anterior dislocations in young, active patients require little capsular imbrication. These repairs usually can be accomplished either arthroscopically or by open procedures with good success. One exception is the humeral avulsion of the glenohumeral ligament (HAGL) lesion, which generally necessitates an open approach with a lateral capsulotomy for repair. One study found that patients with a HAGL lesion tended to be older than those with instability from other causes, that the injury resulted from violent trauma in 94% of patients, and that 17% had concomitant damage to the rotator cuff.

Open Versus Arthroscopic Repair

Recurrent anterior instability has been addressed by both open and arthroscopic methods. Higher recurrence rates have been reported for arthroscopic repairs, possibly because it is more difficult to address capsular laxity as effectively arthroscopically and because arthroscopic techniques generate less anterior scarring. Long-standing anterior instability with years of recurrent dislocations will have, in addition to the labral pathology, a component of capsular laxity that should be addressed at surgery to minimize recurrence.

When treating MDI, an inferior shift should be included in any surgical reconstruction. Arthroscopic reconstructions for MDI using a variety of techniques have been described. Most recent reports indicate considerably higher recurrence rates for arthroscopic repairs of MDI than for open capsular shifts, particularly considering the marked success seen in Pollock and associates' recent study. For patients undergoing revision surgery for MDI, if significant scarring prevents an adequate shift, both anterior and posterior approaches may be required to address instability in all directions. An open technique using a T-shaped capsulotomy with a vertical capsular incision on the humeral side allows for the most dramatic reduction of capsular volume in severe cases and can be used with a spectrum of instabilities, from recurrent traumatic lesions to severe MDI.

Technique-Specific Complications

Many of the complications seen with surgery for instability are technique-specific. Arthroscopic staple capsulorrhaphy, which has been largely abandoned, showed recurrence rates of 11% to 33% at an average follow-up of 2 to 4 years. Migration of hardware with pain, as well as articular and capsular damage, was commonly seen. Arthroscopic transglenoid suture capsulorrhaphy is technically demanding and has shown failure rates considerably higher than those reported by the initial investigators. Reported complications unique to this technique include permanent damage to the suprascapular nerve from the pin placed to pass the sutures or from the sutures tied over the infraspinatous fascia. Irritation over the posterior soft tissues, often requiring removal of the stitches, also has been reported. Rarer complications such as posterior glenoid neck fracture, synovial cyst formation requiring removal, and pneumothorax also have been reported. The failure rate associated with Suretac (Smith & Nephew; Memphis, TN) capsulorrhaphy is 0 to 37%. Loosening, migration, loose-body production with dissociation of the head of the tack from the shaft, synovitis, and foreign-body granuloma formation have all been reported. Suture anchors have been reported to cause articular damage and painful crepitus if seated improperly or left proud or if late migration from the anchor bed occurs.

Thermal capsulorrhaphy, which has been described as an arthroscopic treatment of capsular redundancy, has been associated with stiffness, adhesive capsulitis, axillary nerve injury, and recurrence. No long-term outcome studies of this procedure are available. If too much energy is delivered to the inferior capsule, the axillary nerve can sustain thermal injury. Nerve deficits are usually transitory, though the deficit can be permanent. One investigator has recommended using less energy in the thin axillary pouch and avoiding "shrinking" the capsule from the 5 o'clock to 7 o'clock position. Too much energy delivered to the capsule can irrevocably damage the capsule, creating absent capsule syndrome. Excessive heat (ie, that which causes more than 35% shrinkage) permanently destroys the capsule, leading to recurrent instability and disastrous consequences for revision. The other problem with shrinkage techniques is that the biologic response varies and requires close monitoring postoperatively to make sure the patient does not get too stiff or move too soon and loosen the capsule. Risk factors for poor outcome after thermal capsulorrhaphy in one reported series included MDI, participation in contact sports, revision surgery, and multiple preoperative dislocations.

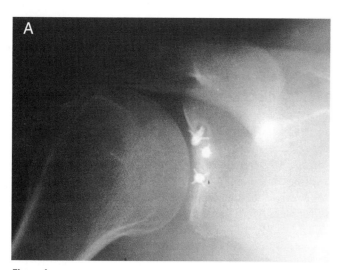

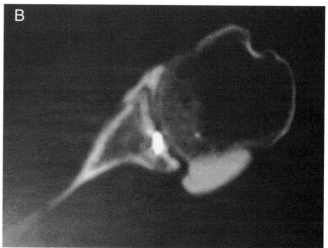

Figure 1 A shoulder 1 year after three anchors were placed posteriorly for an open posterior capsular shift. Painful glenohumeral crepitus began insidiously 3 months prior to imaging. Radiographs, CT, and MRI showed the center anchor seated in bone. **A,** Radiograph shows lucency around the top and bottom anchors, indicating loosening. **B,** MR arthrogram shows superior anchor in the joint. Anchor was put in too shallowly posteriorly, causing the tip to lie in the articular cartilage. The anchors were removed arthroscopically.

Implant Complications

Capsular and labral repairs to bone have been accomplished through bone tunnels or with some form of fixation, including staples, screws, tacks, and suture anchors. Whatever technique is used, the principles remain the same: restoring the labrum height and tailoring the capsular imbrication (with or without a shift) as appropriate. In one study, screws were loose in 50% of patients in whom a previous Bristow procedure was revised. Tacks are reportedly easy to use and reduce soft tissue to bone over a surface area. Polyglyconate tacks have been associated with loose body production, pain, restricted motion, synovitis, recurrent instability, and foreign body granuloma formation. Failure of such an implant can mimic a postoperative infection. Polylactic acid implants reportedly have a longer in vivo strength retention profile. Granuloma formation and implant failure with loose body production has not been as much of a problem with polylactic acid implants, though each implant will generate its own track record. In testing, most suture anchors fail through the suture. Improper placement of the fixation device can lead to prominent intra-articular hardware, painful crepitus, and glenohumeral articular cartilage destruction. Metal and plastic implants can migrate into the joint and cause late proud hardware symptoms with new-onset painful crepitus and articular cartilage destruction. Radiographs and CT scans (Fig. 1) can evaluate the position of metal implants. Permanent plastic implants may not be seen on these studies, and arthroscopy may be needed to evaluate late, new-onset, painful glenohumeral crepitus. Prominent painful intra-articular hardware often can be removed arthroscopically.

Rehabilitation Errors

Soft-tissue repairs heal to other soft tissue and to bone over time. Aggressive, early motion may destroy or stretch the repair. Waiting too long to start motion may doom a patient to debilitating stiffness. For arthroscopic and open anterior reconstructions in unidirectional, traumatic instability, rehabilitation goals are graduated after surgery (Table 1). The goals of this graduated program are to avoid stiffness while protecting the capsular reconstruction and subscapularis repair. For open capsular shifts for MDI, stiffness is less of a problem and recurrent instability can occur if rehabilitation pushes active motion too soon. Most authors agree that for true atraumatic MDI, the shoulder should be braced after surgery in a position that takes tension off of the capsular repair for 6 to 8 weeks—some external rotation for posterior repairs and some internal rotation for anterior repairs. Arthroscopic repairs must be followed closely postoperatively, particularly if radiofrequency capsulorrhaphy is performed. The biologic response to this technique is highly variable, and active motion may have to be either accelerated or stopped, depending on how stiff the patient is at each postoperative visit.

Recurrence

Reinjury

Reinjury in athletes who participate in contact sports has been described well in the literature. Open repairs are preferred in athletes who participate in sports without a premium on overhead motion, as they appear to withstand the rigors of contact sports more reliably than do arthroscopic repairs. Patients with underlying collagen disorders (eg, Ehlers-Danlos syndrome) have a ten-

TABLE 1 | Postoperative Physical Therapy Program After Instability Surgery			
After Surgery	**Forward Flexion**	**External Rotation**	**Activity**
Immediate	0°	0°	Keep swathed and in sling at all times. Extend elbow with palm on stomach; work wrist and fingers. (No resistive exercise or active or resisted internal rotation.)
1 week	0°	0°	Remove dressing and begin to shower. Change clean, dry cloth or gauze pad under armpit daily to avoid fungus infection.
2 weeks	120°	20°	Remove from sling for active ROM to limits. Wear sling in public and sling and swath while asleep.*
4 weeks	140°	40°	Remove from sling for active ROM to limits.*
6 weeks	160°	60°	Remove from sling for active ROM to limits. Start light resistive exercise <u>except</u> in internal rotation.
3 months	95% of the unaffected side		Can begin throwing, plyometrics. Light resistive internal rotation; can increase resistance in all other directions.
4 months	97% of the unaffected side		Full resistance in all directions.
6 months	98% of the unaffected side		Full contact sports.

*Discard sling if the shoulder is stiffer than parameters; keep in sling and use slow therapy if the shoulder is easily beyond parameters; ROM = range of motion

dency to stretch out their capsule again after repair, and recurrent instability can develop. Recurrence rates increase with length of follow-up in all types of instability and reconstructions.

Failure

Reported recurrence rates after reconstruction vary depending on the definition of recurrence (subluxation, dislocation, or positive apprehension sign), the length of follow-up, and the procedure performed. The older, nonanatomic repairs typically result in limited motion. This helps to prevent recurrent instability but can also cause painful stiffness, fixed painful subluxations (Fig. 2), and, eventually, glenohumeral arthritis. The average rate of recurrent dislocation after open reconstructions of various types and different durations of follow-up is about 3%. The rate increases with length of follow-up. With MDI, dislocations often do not occur preoperatively, so recurrence must be defined as symptomatic recurrent subluxations. Anteroinferior instability is effectively treated with open capsular shift procedures. One series included 42 shoulders with MDI reconstructed with the T-plasty modification of the Bankart technique. Patient satisfaction was 95%, though symptomatic recurrent instability occurred in 4 of the 42 shoulders. In another series, athletes had a 2.9% redislocation rate at 4-year

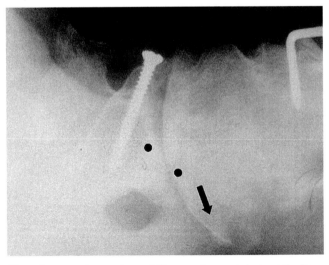

Figure 2 Tight anterior capsular repair. The arrow shows posterior translation. The center of the humeral head has translated behind the center of the glenoid. The black dots represent the centers of the humeral head and glenoid and highlight the posterior translation.

follow-up; another 11% experienced painful clicking or snapping without clear subluxation. An 11% recurrence of MDI after repair was reported in a series of 43 patients with a minimum 2-year follow-up. Recurrence rates following open repair of posterior and posteroinferior instability have been reported as 50% or greater.

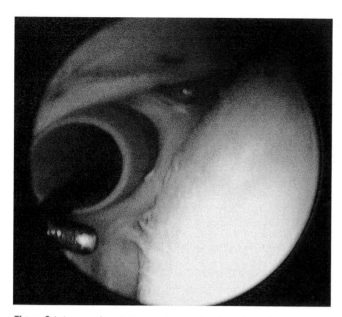

Figure 3 Arthroscopy for selective anterior capsular release to regain motion revealed evidence of degenerative chondrosis of the posterior humeral head from fixed posterior subluxation. Releases and manipulation allowed 70° of external rotation with the arm at the patient's side, which was symmetric with the contralateral side.

A recent series reviewed open posteroinferior capsular shifts in patients with recurrent posterior instability and MDI with a predominant posterior component. At 5-year follow-up, 23 of 24 patients who underwent an open posteroinferior capsular shift as the initial repair had successful results. In a separate report, 52 patients with MDI underwent an open inferior capsular shift as their first procedure on the side of predominant instability. At an average follow-up of 5 years, 96% of the shoulders remained stable. Results were good or excellent in 94%. Eighty-six percent of the athletes returned to sports, but only 69% reached their premorbid level of performance. All of the 15 posterior shifts remained stable.

Comorbidities Leading to Perceived Failure

A patient who experiences persistent postoperative shoulder pain may regard the surgery as a failure, even if the pain is not caused by the instability. Comorbidities such as cervical spondylosis and acromioclavicular arthritis should be identified and discussed with patients preoperatively so that they can formulate realistic expectations about outcomes of surgery. Acromioclavicular arthritis, impingement syndrome, and rotator cuff pathology can be addressed at surgery. Early glenohumeral arthritis and partial tears of the cuff, which can be débrided, should be noted as well and discussed with the patient as potential causes of continued postoperative pain.

Other Postoperative Complications

Stiffness

Excessive tightness after instability surgery can cause persistent pain and disability. The most common complaints noted in one study of long-term follow-up after Bankart repair were decreased range of motion (particularly in external rotation with the arm at the side) and intermittent pain. Tensioning the capsular flaps during T-capsulorrhaphy in some external rotation and abduction or adduction for the inferior and superior flaps, respectively, can help the surgeon avoid overtightening the capsule. After capsule closure, the surgeon should ensure that at least 20° to 30° of external rotation is maintained. The subscapularis splitting approach was designed to minimize motion loss; this approach may be indicated in athletes for whom shoulder motion is critical, as in throwers. Arthroscopic techniques are reported to result in less loss of motion on average. This may be because arthroscopic procedures result in less capsular imbrication and extracapsular scarring than do open techniques. Less scarring also has been implicated as a cause of higher rates of recurrence with arthroscopic techniques.

Another cause of permanent stiffness may be inadequate rehabilitation after reconstruction. The best way to avoid this is with a closely monitored, physician-directed, graduated therapy program following the initial procedure. If the shoulder is tight and motion is not restored after a concerted effort at aggressive stretching, then selective releases may be required to restore motion and relieve pain. This should be done no earlier than 6 months after the index procedure and only if no progress is being made in intensive physical therapy. Examination under anesthesia can determine the areas where the capsule is overly tight. If the patient lacks significant external rotation with the arm in adduction, then the rotator interval and anterosuperior capsule are implicated. If extracapsular scarring is not excessive, selective capsular releases can be performed arthroscopically to regain motion without making the shoulder unstable (Fig. 3). For stiffness with significant extracapsular scarring, open releases may be required. If the subscapularis insertion is not detached, aggressive postoperative stretching can be pursued. Releases for stiffness after instability reconstructions usually do not result in recurrent instability, though this remains a concern.

Arthritis

Degenerative glenohumeral arthritis can occur after stabilization surgery for instability (Fig. 4). This may result from postoperative, iatrogenic subluxations from overtightening, from persistent MDI, from inadequate or inappropriate surgery, from nonanatomic repairs, or as a complication of hardware. The cause of degenerative

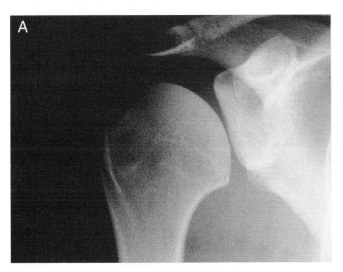

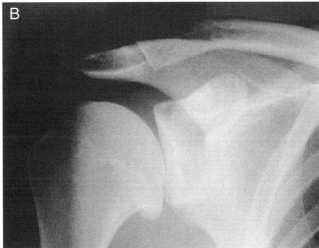

Figure 4 Arthrosis following inferior capsular shift for MDI. **A,** Postoperative radiograph. **B,** Early degenerative changes are apparent 12 years later.

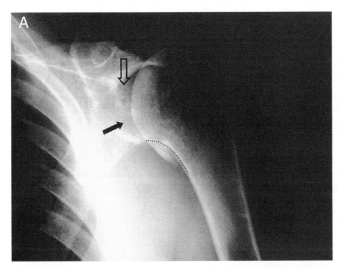

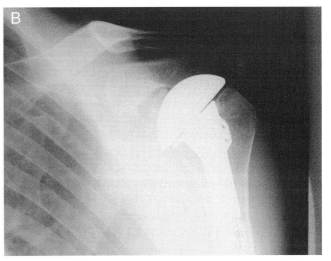

Figure 5 Radiographs of the shoulder of a 35-year-old man with painful glenohumeral arthritis and stiffness after multiple instability reconstructions in his late teens and early twenties. **A,** Dotted line outlines native cortex and shows size of inferior osteophyte. Arrows indicate nonmetallic anchor hole from prior repair for instability. **B,** AP radiograph of hemiarthroplasty with biologic resurfacing of glenoid with reflected capsule.

glenohumeral arthritis is often multifactorial. In a study of 66 shoulders an average of 22 years after undergoing the Putti-Platt procedure, arthrosis was evident radiographically in 61% of patients. In one series, symptomatic arthrosis progressed to the point where prosthetic replacement was needed an average of 16 years after the initial stabilization procedure (Figs. 5 and 6). In another report, the average age of similar patients was 38 years. Soft-tissue contractures on the side of the surgery with fixed humeral subluxation and rim erosion opposite the repair are common findings in this population.

Nerve Injuries

Nerve injuries can occur around the shoulder with both arthroscopic and open shoulder surgery. The axillary nerve courses from anterior to posterior, off the posterior cord of the brachial plexus, 3 to 5 mm medial to the musculotendinous junction of the inferolateral border of the subscapularis, and lies in contact with the inferior glenohumeral joint capsule until it exits the quadrangular space. The axillary nerve then reflects anteriorly, running on the deep surface of the deltoid from posterior to anterior. This nerve is at risk during inferior capsular dissection, during suture placement through the inferior capsule, and with retraction on the subscapularis medially and the deltoid laterally. In cadaveric sectioning studies, the inferior part of a deltoid split approach averages 9 mm above the anterior branch of the nerve for a standard anterolateral approach and 6.5 mm for a more anterior approach. The standard posterior arthroscopy portal averages 18 mm above the main trunk of the

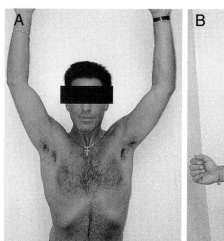 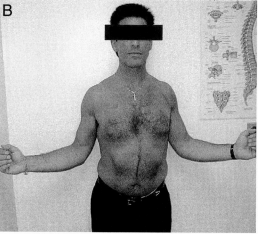 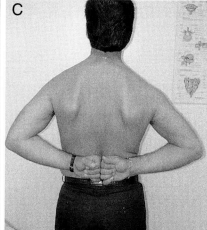

Figure 6 Same patient as in Figure 5, 1 year after left humeral head replacement with fascial arthroplasty. The patient plays golf and lifts light weights. **A,** Maximum forward flexion compared with the normal side. **B,** Maximum external rotation. **C,** Maximum internal rotation.

nerve. Arthroscopically placed sutures are most safely placed 1 cm from the glenoid margin, averaging 7 mm from the axillary nerve. The musculocutaneous nerve enters the medial coracobrachialis 3.1 to 8.2 cm from the coracoid, with branches entering as close as 1.7 cm. Caution during muscle retraction is warranted. The suprascapular nerve lies within 2 cm of the glenoid rim and is as close as 1 cm at the posterior middle glenoid. This should be kept in mind during posterior open approaches.

To avoid injury to the suprascapular or axillary nerves, care should be taken to avoid excessive medial or inferior placement or direction of the trochar through the posterior portal during arthroscopy. The anterior portal must be lateral to the coracoid and not directed too inferior or medial to avoid musculocutaneous nerve damage. The lateral portal can jeopardize the axillary nerve if it is placed too inferiorly, and advancing instruments too medially over the glenoid can result in suprascapular nerve damage.

The incidence of nerve deficits after open anterior instability repairs was 8.2% (23 of 232 shoulders) in one series. One third were sensory, and two thirds were sensorimotor. Eighteen of 23 completely resolved. Three patients had a persistent sensory deficit, and one had a persistent motor deficit (biceps weakness). Traction injury was implicated most often, and no lesions were explored. In a large series of arthroscopy patients, 7% (21 of 304) had sensory deficits 2 weeks postoperatively, most involving sensory branches of the reflected axillary nerve, implicating the lateral portal. More than half of these recovered completely. Structural nerve injuries such as laceration or incorporation in a suture line are rare after instability repairs. Unless this type of injury is suspected, nerve deficits should be followed; electrical studies are ordered only if no improvement is seen 6 weeks postoperatively.

Infection

Deep and overall infection rates of 0.3% to 1.4% have been reported after open stabilization procedures in two series reviewing more than 1,500 shoulders. As with all postoperative infections, a high index of suspicion, early recognition, appropriate cultures, early irrigation and débridement (repeated as necessary), and antibiotics based on results of cultures and sensitivities are the hallmarks of successful treatment. Implants may need to be removed, and suture anchors or tacks may be difficult to extract without open exposure and additional damage to bone. Significant postoperative hematomas may need to be débrided to avoid persistent drainage and infection.

Results of Revision Surgery

Results of revisions for failed instability reconstruction depend on several factors: the reason for failure, the residual pathology, the clinical setting, and the surgical approach used previously and for revision. Fifty patients were reviewed at an average of 4.7 years after revision stabilization surgery for recurrent anteroinferior instability following prior reconstruction. The results of open revisions for failed arthroscopic stabilizations were excellent. One of seven patients had a Bankart lesion, but all had unaddressed capsular laxity. Scarring was minimal in this population. Excellent results were obtained with revision surgery for all previously reconstructed patients who had recurrent instability after a significant traumatic event. Only 67% of patients with atraumatic onset of recurrent instability after their prior procedures had satisfactory outcomes with open revision. Forty-four percent of patients who had undergone more than one prior procedure had recurrence after revision surgery, as opposed to only 17% in patients who had had only one previous surgery. More scarring was present in patients with more than one prior procedure. Seven of the 11 patients with failed results after attempted revision surgery were voluntary dislocators. Revisions for failed MDI stabilizations have less success than revisions for failed reconstructions for anterior instability. In one series, only 39% of patients who underwent revision surgery for failed MDI reconstructions had good or excellent results, as opposed to 78% for failed anterior reconstructions. Autografts or allografts including possible bone blocks may be needed to reconstruct bony and capsular deficiencies in shoulders that have undergone multiple failed reconstructions.

Annotated Bibliography

General

Flatow EL, Warner JJP: Instability of the shoulder: Complex problems and failed repairs: Part 1. Relevant biomechanics, multidirectional instability and severe loss on glenoid and humeral bone. *J Bone Joint Surg Am* 1998;80:122-140.

Review of recent literature concerning relevant biomechanics, multidirectional instability, and severe bone loss on both sides of the joint.

Flatow EL, Miniaci A, Evans PJ, Simonian PT, Warren RF: Instability of the shoulder: Complex problems and failed repairs: Part 2. Failed repairs. *J Bone Joint Surg Am* 1998;80:284-298.

A review of recent literature concerning open shoulder instability and surgical complications is presented. Specific pitfalls, their avoidance, causes of failure, and surgical solutions at revision as well as results of revision surgery are discussed.

Mair SD, Hawkins RJ: Open shoulder instability surgery: Complications. *Clin Sports Med* 1999;18:719-736.

Complications reported after open shoulder instability operations were reviewed. Complications were characterized by improper diagnosis, recurrence, loss of function, degenerative changes, and neurovascular and "other" complications. Discussion includes how to avoid various complications by making the right diagnosis and applying the appropriate technique.

Shaffer BS, Tibone JE: Arthroscopic shoulder instability surgery: Complications. *Clin Sports Med* 1999;18:737-767.

An excellent review of recent literature concerning arthroscopic instability surgery complications is presented. Documented complications are discussed, their causes are delineated, and strategies are presented to avoid them.

Considerations in Choice of Treatment

Cole BJ, L'Insalata J, Irrgang J, Warner JJ: Comparison of arthroscopic and open anterior shoulder stabilization: A two to six-year follow-up study. *J Bone Joint Surg Am* 2000;82:1108-1114.

Twenty-two patients with inferior translation ≥ 2 cm; capsular rupture; thinned, patulous capsule; or no discrete ligaments visualized at arthroscopy were selected for open capsular repair. Thirty-seven patients with ≤ 1 cm inferior translation, translation over the anterior glenoid rim, a Bankart lesion, and discrete glenohumeral ligaments were selected for arthroscopic repair. Twenty-four percent of the arthroscopic and 18% of the open procedures were unsatisfactory at mean follow-up of 54 months. Shoulders with episodes of recurrent instability or a positive apprehension sign on follow-up were deemed failures. Not all patients with a positive apprehension sign felt unstable. All cases of recurrent instability after arthroscopic repair (16%) were the result of contact sports or a fall within 2 years after the repair. Nine percent of the patients treated with open repair had recurrent instability.

Fuchs B, Jost B, Gerber C: Posterior-inferior capsular shift for the treatment of recurrent, voluntary posterior subluxation of the shoulder. *J Bone Joint Surg Am* 2000; 82:16-25.

Twenty-four patients (26 shoulders) were operated on for posterior instability and assessed on average 7.6 years after open posterior-inferior capsular shift. All patients could exhibit their instability voluntarily and had involuntary instability. None of the patients had psychiatric disorders. Patients rated their shoulders as 16 excellent, 8 good, and 2 fair. The relative Constant score was 91%. Of the cases of recurrence that occurred in six shoulders (23%), three were associated with previous posterior surgery and three with a new traumatic event. Open posterior reconstruction for voluntary instability in patients without psychiatric disorders produced reasonable results.

Kirkley A, Griffin S, Richards C, Miniaci A, Mohtadi N: Prospective randomized clinical trial comparing the effectiveness of immediate arthroscopic stabilization versus immobilization and rehabilitation in first traumatic anterior dislocations of the shoulder. *Arthroscopy* 1999;15:507-514.

Forty patients younger than age 30 years at the time of the first traumatic anterior dislocation were randomized to two groups: those who underwent 3 weeks of immobilization followed by rehabilitation, and those who underwent immediate arthroscopic stabilization followed by identical immobilization and rehabilitation protocols. There was a statistically significant rate of redislocation at 2 years (47% for the first group and 15.9% for the second group). At 33 months, no difference in motion was recorded. Improvement in disease-specific quality of life was afforded by early arthroscopic stabilization for first-time traumatic anterior dislocations.

Pollock RG, Owens JM, Flatow EL, Bigliani LU: Operative results of the inferior capsular shift procedure for multidirectional instability of the shoulder. *J Bone Joint Surg Am* 2000;82:919-928.

The inferior capsular shift procedure for MDI was used on the predominant side of the instability as the index procedure on 52 shoulders (34 anterior and 18 posterior approaches); follow-up averaged 61 months. Ninety-four percent of the patients had good or excellent results, with 96% of the patients still stable at follow-up. Two of the 34 anteroinferior shifts and none of the 15 posteroinferior shifts began to subluxate again postoperatively. Eighty-six percent of the athletes returned to sports, but only 69% returned to their premorbid level of competition.

Roberts SN, Taylor DE, Brown JN, Hayes MG, Saies A: Open and arthroscopic techniques for the treatment of traumatic anterior shoulder instability in Australian Rules football players. *J Shoulder Elbow Surg* 1999;8: 403-409.

This study reported a 70% recurrence of instability on return to Australian Rules Football after arthroscopic suture anchor repair, 38% recurrence (three fourths of which occurred after minimal trauma after repair with polyglyconate tacks and 30% recurrence (50% by violent trauma) after open reconstruction. This underscores that for athletes who participate in contact sports, open repairs may significantly reduce recurrence over arthroscopic techniques.

Savoie FH, Field LD: Thermal versus suture treatment of symptomatic capsular laxity. *Clin Sports Med* 2000; 19:63-75.

Thirty patients were treated for MDI with thermal capsulorrhaphy and rotator interval plication and followed for 2 years. Two had symptomatic recurrence. Results were similar for arthroscopic reconstruction using sutures.

Technical Pitfalls

Anderson K, Warren RF, Altchek DW, Craig EV, O'Brien SJ: Risk factors for early failure after thermal capsulorrhaphy. *Am J Sports Med* 2002;30:103-107.

In this series, 106 patients underwent thermal capsulorrhaphy at a mean follow-up of more than 6 years, and 15 patients experienced recurrent instability. Previous operations and multiple dislocations were risk factors for poor outcome. Although not statistically significant, patients with injuries from contact sports and MDI tended to do less well with thermal techniques, and the authors recommended caution using thermal capsulorrhaphy in these patients.

Black KP, Schneider DJ, Yu JR, Jacobs CR: Biomechanics of the Bankart Repair: The relationship between glenohumeral translation and labral fixation site. *Am J Sports Med* 1999;27:339-344.

The authors studied glenohumeral translations in nine cadaveric shoulders following repair of a surgically created Bankart lesion. They determined that failure to carefully repair the labrum to the inferior glenoid rim during a Bankart reconstruction might contribute to recurrent instability.

Bokor DJ, Conboy VB, Olson C: Anterior instability of the glenohumeral joint with humeral avulsion of the glenohumeral ligament: A review of 41 cases. *J Bone Joint Surg Br* 1999;81:93-96.

The authors retrospectively reviewed 547 shoulders in 529 patients who underwent surgery for instability. Lateral avulsion of the capsule was considered to be the cause of instability in 41 of the patients. These patients were older on average than patients who had instability from other causes.

Burkart A, Imhoff AB, Roscher E: Foreign-body reaction to the bioabsorbable Suretac device. *Arthroscopy* 2000;16:91-95.

The authors determined that arthroscopic shoulder stabilization with the Suretac device (Acufex Microsurgical; Mansfield, MA) offered some technical advantages when compared with other approaches; however, the device's biodegradability may make it prone to early failure in patients with SLAP lesions.

Higgins LD, Warner JJ: Arthroscopic Bankart repair: Operative technique and surgical pitfalls. *Clin Sports Med* 2000;19:49-62.

Step-by-step review and description of technical pitfalls to avoid during arthroscopic Bankart repair. Radiofrequency thermal capsulorrhaphy was not addressed.

Itoi E, Lee SB, Berglund LJ, Berge LL, An KN: The effect of a glenoid defect on anteroinferior stability of the shoulder after Bankart repair: A cadaveric study. *J Bone Joint Surg Am* 2000;82:35-46.

This cadaveric biomechanical study evaluated the effects of reconstructing a bony Bankart lesion with repair of the capsule back to the fractured edge of the glenoid without fixing the bony fragment. Treating bony Bankart fractures wider than one fifth the height of the glenoid face in this manner resulted in significant decrease in force of translation to dislocation and loss of external rotation of 25°.

Silver MD, Daigneault JP: Symptomatic interarticular migration of glenoid suture anchors. *Arthroscopy* 2000; 16:102-105.

Case report of intra-articular suture anchor used for Bankart repair that migrated into the joint several weeks after index procedure. New onset painful glenohumeral crepitus developed as a result. Destruction of anterior humeral articular cartilage was seen during arthroscopy to remove the anchor.

Recurrence

Brems JJ: Arthritis of dislocation. *Orthop Clin North Am* 1998;29:453-466.

Excellent review of arthritis of instability and risk factors of arthrosis after capsulorrhaphy.

Boardman ND, Cofield RH: Neurologic complications of shoulder surgery. *Clin Orthop* 1999;368:44-53.

Thorough review of current literature regarding nerve complications with different shoulder surgeries is presented. Relevant anatomy of axillary, suprascapular, and musculocutaneous nerves is covered, as well as incidence of nerve injury.

Ho E, Cofield RH, Balm MR, Hattrup SJ, Rowland CM: Neurologic complications of surgery for anterior shoulder instability. *J Shoulder Elbow Surg* 1999;8:266-270.

The authors studied 282 patients who underwent anterior reconstruction for recurrent glenohumeral instability. Neurologic deficit occurred in 23 patients (8.2%) following surgery. The authors determined that neurologic injuries presumably were a result of traction and prognosis was generally good. The injury did not interfere with outcome of the surgery.

van der Zwaag HM, Brand R, Obermann WR, Rozing PM: Glenohumeral osteoarthrosis after Putti-Platt repair. *J Shoulder Elbow Surg* 1999;8:252-258.

The authors studied 66 of 139 shoulders (46%) at a mean follow-up of 22 years after Putti-Platt repair for recurrent anterior dislocation of the glenohumeral joint. They determined that the rate of glenohumeral arthrosis increased following a Putti-Platt procedure and correlates with length of time since surgery.

Results of Revision Surgery

Levine WN, Arroyo JS, Pollock RG, Flatow EL, Bigliani LU: Open revision stabilization surgery for recurrent anterior glenohumeral instability. *Am J Sports Med* 2000;28:156-160.

Fifty patients treated with revision anterior stabilization procedures for recurrence after prior reconstruction were reviewed. Thirty-nine had good or excellent results. Eleven were unsatisfactory, seven of which had voluntary dislocations. Risk factors for poor outcome at revision include atraumatic recurrence, voluntary dislocations, and multiple prior stabilization attempts.

Classic Bibliography

Young DC, Rockwood CA Jr: Complications of a failed Bristow procedure and their management. *J Bone Joint Surg Am* 1991;73:969-981.

Section 3

Rotator Cuff Impingement

Section Editors:
Christian Gerber, MD
Gilles Walch, MD

Chapter 13

Rotator Cuff Disorders: Anatomy, Function, Pathogenesis, and Natural History

Christopher M. Jobe, MD

Introduction

Over the past 5 years, three ideas that are critical to improved understanding of the rotator cuff have continued to evolve. First, rotator cuff disease is a true syndrome, a collection of signs and symptoms (and altered anatomy) that arises from more than one cause. Second, rotator cuff disease relates not only to the coracoacromial arch but also to other structures and events, such as dislocation. Current knowledge has gone beyond regarding subacromial impingement as the sole cause of rotator cuff disease to a more complicated understanding. And last, the complexity of shoulder function has become increasingly apparent.

These developments are reviewed as they relate to anatomy, function, pathogenesis, and natural history, along with a review of implications for future research and, to that end, some less recent anatomic material that has not been fully correlated with function and pathogenesis.

Anatomy

Gross Anatomy

The most recent studies on the anatomy of the rotator cuff are driven by several clinical considerations. Sur-geons currently need to know the nature of the anatomy they are trying to reconstruct, the manner in which cuff damage occurs and the predicted outcomes of that damage, and, as surgical techniques advance, the variety of muscle-tendon units available for tendon transfer.

The structure of the muscles of the rotator cuff varies from a parallel arrangement of the fibers to a pennate arrangement. A pennate arrangement limits muscle excursion to generate greater force. In the supraspinatus muscle, the fibers are more parallel in the posterior area and more pennate or conical in the anterior area. Therefore, the anterior supraspinatus is a more powerful force generator than is the posterior supraspinatus. A similar comparison can be made between the upper and lower subscapularis. The upper subscapularis is multipennate, whereas the lower subscapularis is more parallel. The upper subscapularis is therefore a more powerful force generator, whereas the lower subscapularis has a much longer excursion, which allows abduction and external rotation.

Categorizing the muscles of the cuff in terms of relative strength and muscle excursion can be useful in understanding function and the requirements for muscle transfer (Table 1), although these values are complicated by relationships within the individual muscles. For comparison, Table 2 lists parameters for other shoulder mus-

TABLE 1	Rotator Cuff Muscles: Excursion and Relative Strength		
Muscle Unit	**Structure**	**Excursion (cm)**	**Relative Strength**
Supraspinatus	Pennate	6.7	0.8
Infraspinatus	Pennate	8.6	1.4
Subscapularis	Multipennate	7.3	2.6
Teres minor	Longitudinal	8.8	0.8

Adapted with permission from Herzberg G, Urien JP, Dimnet J: Potential excursion and relative tension of the muscles in the shoulder girdle: Relevance to tendon transfers. J Shoulder Elbow Surg 1999;8:430-437.

TABLE 2 | Parameters for Other Shoulder Muscles

Muscle	Structure	Excursion (cm)	Relative Tension	Cuff Transfer Described
Upper trapezoid (clavicular)	Longitudinal	13.8	2.6	–
Upper trapezoid (acromial)	Longitudinal	10.1	3.5	Supraspinatus
Middle trapezius	Longitudinal	10.4	2.9	–
Lower trapezius	Longitudinal	14.8	2.7	–
Levator scapulae	Longitudinal	15.3	1.7	–
Rhomboidei	Longitudinal	12.5	4.0	–
Upper serratus	Longitudinal	11.1	3.9	–
Lower serratus	Longitudinal	17.6	5.6	–
Pectoralis minor	Longitudinal	13.2	2.1	Subscapularis
Latissimus dorsi	Longitudinal	33.9	5.9	Infraspinatus and subscapularis
Pectoralis major (clavicular)	Longitudinal	14.5	2.3	Subscapularis (entire pectoralis)
Pectoralis major (sternal)	Longitudinal	18.8	5.4	Subscapularis
Teres major	Longitudinal	14.9	4.3	Infraspinatus
Anterior deltoid	Longitudinal	11.5	3.4	Supraspinatus
Middle deltoid (anterior)	Multipennate	9.2	3.0	–
Middle deltoid (posterior)	Multipennate	9.0	10.8	–
Posterior deltoid	Longitudinal	13.9	3.7	–

Adapted with permission from Herzberg G, Urien JP, Dimnet J: Potential excursion and relative tension of the muscles in the shoulder girdle: Relevance to tendon transfers. J Shoulder Elbow Surg 1999;8:430-437.

cles. Additional information needed for tendon transfer includes the line of pull and the phase or timing of contraction of the muscle. Complications relating to size, such as the difficulty in passing the thick teres major under the acromion, are not addressed by the data included in these tables.

The tendons of the rotator cuff fuse near their bony insertions into one continuous cuff of tendon, except in the lower cuff, where the muscle fibers themselves insert onto the bone in what is called an indirect insertion. In addition to the tendon insertion, the cuff is reinforced by the coracohumeral ligament, with two important extensions: a contribution to the restraint of the biceps at the upper groove (Fig. 1), and the rotator cuff cable (Fig. 2), or fasciculus obliquus. The coracohumeral ligament has its origin at the upper inside of the curve of the coracoid, where it is V-shaped; it overlies the interval between the upper subscapularis tendon and the anterior supraspinatus tendon. In addition to inserting onto the humerus, the ligament reinforces the rotator cuff tendons, particularly the supraspinatus and infraspinatus. The fibers of this ligament run on both the superficial, or bursa, side and the interior, or capsular, side of the tendons, perpendicular to the forces generated by the

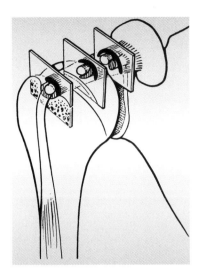

Figure 1 The interrelationship of the coracohumeral ligament with the biceps and the superior glenohumeral ligament. In addition to forming the roof or bursal side of the rotator interval, the coracohumeral ligament combines with the superior glenohumeral ligament to form a sling that contains the biceps tendon. *(Reproduced with permission from Habermeyer P, Walch G: The biceps tendon and rotator cuff disease, in Burkhead WZ (ed): Rotator Cuff Disorders. Philadelphia, PA, Williams & Wilkins, 1996, pp 142-159.)*

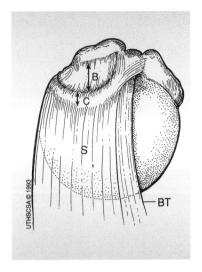

Figure 2 The rotator cuff seen from above. The rotator cuff cable, C, is shown at its attachment to the two tuberosities and running posteriorly to a more posterior tuberosity attachment. The supraspinatus tendon is thus interrelated with (from front to back) the upper fibers of subscapularis, the biceps sling and the infraspinatus.
B = medial-lateral diameter of rotator crescent; S = supraspinatus; BT = biceps tendon. *(Copyright © 1993 Unitversity of Texas Health Science Center San Antonio.)*

muscles. This inner contribution of the rotator cuff, which is visible on arthroscopy and is readily seen on histology, is the rotator cuff cable. The function of this structure is obvious when the supraspinatus is torn; in the normal shoulder, its function may be to distribute the force generated by the different regions of the supraspinatus.

In the areas of the tuberosities, the tendon fibers attach directly to the bone. In the inferior, or neck area, of the humerus, the insertion tends to be muscular, or indirect. In addition, the tendon fibers run obliquely into adjacent tendons, thereby creating a true cuff of tendons.

The relationship at the bicipital groove (Fig. 3) is particularly important: upper fibers of the subscapularis, along with fibers of the superior glenohumeral ligament, insert onto the upper portion of the lesser tuberosity and continue laterally into the depth of the bicipital groove, forming the true floor of the upper groove. Conversely, the fibers of the anterior supraspinatus tendon, along with the coracohumeral ligament, continue inferiorly over the groove, forming the roof of the bicipital groove. Some of the fibers of these tendons run in the opposite direction, thereby forming a ring around the biceps tendon.

The rotator cuff tendons are adjacent to two ball-and-socket articulations. The inner, or glenohumeral, joint involves two round articulating structures: the convex humeral head and the concave glenoid-labrum combination. When the cartilage is taken into account, the shapes of these two surfaces conform very closely. The other ball-and-socket joint, the scapulohumeral articulation, is less obvious from skeletal anatomy or on radiographs, but it is more obvious from cross-sectional anatomy and on MRI scans (Fig. 4). The inner round surface consists of rotator cuff tendons and tuberosity, and the socket is made up of acromion, coracoid, and coracoacromial ligament. The glenohumeral and the scapulohumeral articulations have the same center of rotation. There are forces across the scapulohumeral

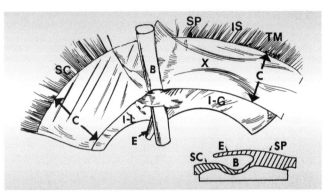

Figure 3 The undersurface of a rotator cuff dissection, illustrating the sling of tissue around the biceps (B). This sling of tissue is cut sharply off the floor of the bicipital groove and represents mainly the fibers of the superior glenohumeral ligament. E represents the roof of the bicipital groove, formed by the coracohumeral ligament. X is the other continuation of the coracohumeral ligament of the rotator cuff cable. SC = subscapularis; SP = supraspinatus; IS = infraspinatus; TM = teres major; C = capsule; I-L = insertion of lesser tuberosity; I-G = insertion on greater tuberosity. *(Reproduced with permission from Harryman DT, Clark JM Jr: Anatomy of the rotator cuff, in Burkhead WZ (ed): Rotator Cuff Disorders. Philadelphia, PA, Williams & Wilkins, 1996, pp 23-35.)*

articulation even with normal function, and there are normal distributions of the forces or stresses.

Researchers continue to study the effect of shoulder position on relationships between structures. Of particular interest are the relationships occurring in the end-range positions: abduction and external rotation; full flexion and internal rotation (Neer position); and forward flexion and internal rotation with horizontal adduction. Each of these positions involves the close approach and contact of a rotator cuff tendon and its tuberosity to the glenoid and labrum. In the first two positions, the greater tuberosity and the supraspinatus tendon approach the glenoid and upper labrum, as has been shown by earlier studies. Recent studies have shown that in flexion-adduction and internal rotation, the subscapularis tendon and the lesser tuberosity approach and contact the anterior superior labrum (Fig. 5).

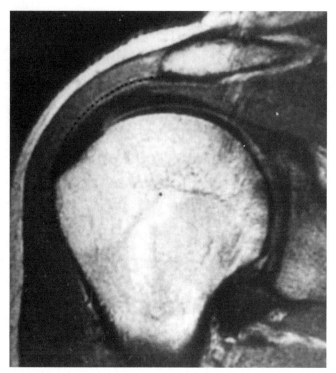

Figure 4 A coronal MRI scan showing the two round articulations of the shoulder. The inner surface is formed by the articular surface of the humeral head. Note that the greater tuberosity and supraspinatus tendon form another perfectly round surface. *(Reproduced with permission from Gagey O, Hue E: Mechanics of the deltoid muscle: A new approach. Clin Orthop 2000;375:250-257.)*

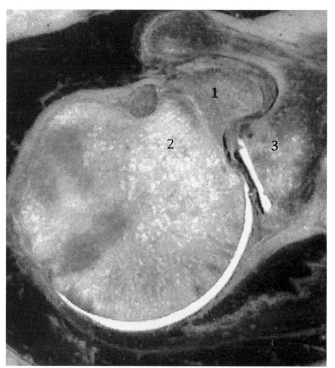

Figure 5 An anatomic cross-section showing anterior internal impingement in flexion-adduction and internal rotation of the shoulder. Note the greater tuberosity and attached supraspinatus (1), the lesser tuberosity and attached subscapularis (2), and the anterior superior glenoid and labrum (3). The biceps is seen between the two tuberosities. Note the contact between the labrum and the subscapularis and biceps pulley.

Histologic Anatomy

The histology of the rotator cuff tendon has been studied previously, but it bears discussion here because some of this information has not been correlated fully with biomechanics or pathology. The tendons of the upper cuff (supraspinatus and infraspinatus) are joined together in a true cufflike fashion as they approach the humerus (Table 3). The fibers within the tendons, particularly the third layer, are not parallel to the axis of the pull of the muscle. Although this arrangement is beneficial in surgery because it allows a more secure suture, the biomechanical implications have not been explored fully. Assuming that collagen fibers are laid down in response to tension, fiber orientation may produce a sort of biologic snapshot of lines of stress. The oblique orientation of some of the fibers indicates that some lines of stress are not generated solely by the muscle bearing the same name as the tendon (Fig. 6).

In the subscapularis tendon, the collagen fibers are parallel and tightly packed without the layering seen in the supraspinatus and infraspinatus. The fibers splay a little at the insertion. The outer fibers may continue over the bicipital groove, especially at the upper end of the groove. If the anchor of the roof of the groove to the lesser tuberosity comes loose, the tendon of the long head of the biceps can dislocate medially while seeming to leave an outer layer of the subscapularis intact. In fact, the situation may appear surgically normal from the bursal surface.

Biomechanical Function

Current understanding of rotator cuff biomechanics suggests that the name "rotator cuff" may be a misnomer because joint compression may be its most important function, rather than rotation. The cuff enables shoulder function by (1) compressing the joint to improve stability, (2) resisting sliding or translation (either anterior-posterior or inferior-superior), and (3) providing some rotation about any or all of the three major axes (AP, medial-lateral, or humeral shaft). Joint stability is almost entirely a cuff function in midrange positions because all passive restraints are lax in these positions.

Essential to an understanding of these functions is the concept that the humeral head maintains a relatively constant position in relation to the glenoid during shoulder rotation. The rotator cuff muscles are closer than any other muscles to the axes of rotation and therefore have shorter lever arms to affect rotation. Compression is affected less by lever arm length than by alignment of the muscle rector. Recent work has shown the compression effect to be relatively independent of shoulder

TABLE 3 | Layers of the Rotator Cuff: Layers of Supraspinatus and Infraspinatus

Layer	Contents of the Layer	Orientation of Fibers
1	Superficial contribution from the coracohumeral ligament; arterioles	Oblique to long axis
2	Large-diameter fibers	Parallel
3	Smaller fibers Not uniform in orientation; interdigitating	45° oblique
4	Loose connective tissue; contains the deep coracohumeral ligament contribution (rotator cuff cable)	Oblique to perpendicular
5	Capsule	Random

Adapted with permission from Harryman DT, Clark JM Jr: Anatomy of the rotator cuff, in Burkhead WZ (ed): Rotator Cuff Disorders. Philadelphia, PA, Williams & Wilkins, 1996, pp 23-35.

position. The effect of the cuff on sliding motion or translation of the head varies greatly with position: the infraspinatus is a very effective head depressor with the arm at 90° of abduction and neutral rotation, but it is a head elevator at the same amount of abduction but with external rotation. The subscapularis, on the other hand, is a more effective head depressor in external rotation. The subscapularis produces almost no AP translation in abduction and external rotation. This may contribute to understanding why the subscapularis fires so strongly at the initiation of the acceleration phase of throwing in the higher level overhead athlete.

There has been a renewed interest in the contribution of the subscapularis to rotation about the axis of the shaft. Several powerful muscles contribute to internal rotation, but tears of the subscapularis can be revealed by testing function at the extreme of internal rotation (the belly press and lift-off tests), indicating the importance of the subscapularis at this end range of motion. Further evidence of this unique function of the subscapularis is the fact that no other muscle can be substituted for the subscapularis without sacrificing these last few degrees of internal rotation; however, much of the patient's function may otherwise improve. The patient with a subscapular tear keenly feels the loss of joint compression and stabilization provided by that muscle.

The infraspinatus and teres minor are the only two muscles that produce external rotation, and large tears in this region of the cuff have profound effects on motion and strength, which can be observed on physical examination. Some patients with cuff tears will have fairly normal-appearing kinematics when the arm is in elevation or abduction, but with larger tears, there will be a loss of strength.

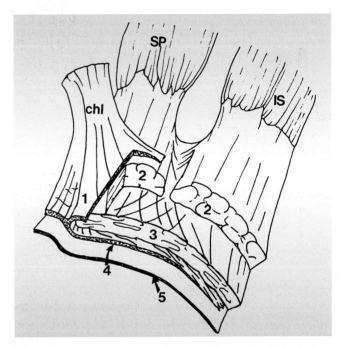

Figure 6 Diagram showing the layers of the supraspinatus (SP) and infraspinatus (IS) along with the contribution of the coracohumeral ligament (chl). The transverse contribution of the chl (layers 1 and 4) and the oblique intertwining of the fibers of layer 3 illustrate the complex relationship of these structures. Layer 5 is the joint capsule of the glenohumeral joint *(Reproduced with permission from Harryman DT, Clark JM Jr: Anatomy of the rotator cuff, in Burkhead WZ (ed): Rotator Cuff Disorders. Philadelphia, PA, Williams & Wilkins, 1996, pp 23-35.)*

Abduction, although powered by the deltoid, requires a relatively constant fulcrum. This is provided by joint compression. It is further assisted by head depression, as described earlier. In normal shoulders, fatigue of the rotator cuff muscles allows increased translation of the humeral head, especially superiorly. The portion of the cuff above the centroid may contribute to abduction,

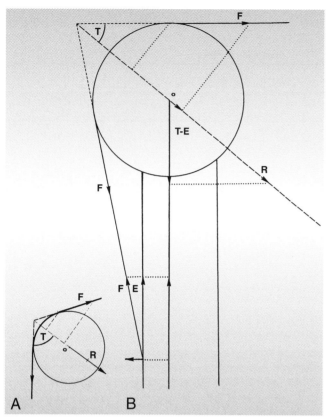

Figure 7 The mechanical model of the pulley effect of the deltoid. **A,** Diagram showing the pulley effect on a round object in general. **B,** Diagram in which the model is applied specifically to the shoulder, in which F is the force of the indicated section of deltoid, T is one half the angle formed by the two deltoid tangents to the round cuff-tuberosity combination. E is the angle of approach of the deltoid to the shaft, and R is resulting force. *(Reproduced with permission from Gagey O, Hue E: Mechanics of the deltoid muscle: A new approach. Clin Orthop 2000;375: 250-257.)*

with the largest contribution coming from the sub-scapularis (52% of the rotator cuff contribution).

Contributions From Other Muscles

Other muscles assist the muscles of the rotator cuff, either by providing some of the same function or by providing a more optimal mechanical environment. The assistance of the deltoid in head depression is an example of the first type of contribution (Fig. 7). With the arm in adduction at the initiation of elevation, the pull of the deltoid muscle is nearly parallel to the glenoid surface, producing a well-documented upward shear component. A recent study has pointed out that a pulley-like arrangement is created by the more powerful anterior lateral portion of the deltoid being draped over the prominence of the greater tuberosity. This creates a force that opposes the upward pull of the deltoid and adds to joint compression and therefore stability. The existence of this force contributes to an understanding of (1) why deltoid rehabilitation is the cornerstone of nonsurgical and postoperative care; (2) why deltoid dysfunction mitigates against a successful outcome

in repair and tendon transfer, and (3) how some patients with massive tears are able to elevate the arm.

The second type of contribution from other muscles, that of creating a better environment for cuff function, is exemplified by the scapular stabilizers. Recent studies have continued to focus on the muscles controlling the scapula, particularly their function during athletic activities. Upward rotation of the scapula in the coronal plane is essential for prevention of subacromial disease. The most obvious example of failure of this mechanism is limb-girdle dystrophy. Shoulder pain associated with this disorder is treated not with acromioplasty but with scapulothoracic fusion, fixing the scapula in a position of some upward rotation in both the coronal and sagittal planes. This position increases the mechanical efficiency of the abductor muscles by allowing them to operate at the peak of the length-tension curve, where maximum force is produced. It places the glenoid under the humerus, so that gravity contributes to joint compression. In the athlete, similar mechanical considerations make mobility and stability of the scapula essential.

Function Remote to the Shoulder

Earlier studies of total body kinematics of athletes, especially those participating in throwing and racquet sports, have revealed that the shoulder is a transfer point at which energy developed elsewhere in the body is transmitted to the upper limb and back. Kinetic energy is initiated by a controlled forward fall of the entire body. The energy thus developed is directed by appropriate athletic technique into smaller and smaller segments of the body. In this fashion a given amount of energy will produce high velocities in the upper limb ($KE = \frac{1}{2}mV^2$). The reversal of this process during the follow-through stage dissipates the energy throughout the entire body, especially through the large muscles of the lower limbs and pelvic girdle. Weakness, stiffness, or lack of coordination in the trunk or lower limbs might result in improper transfer of energy to the upper limb during acceleration or delayed dissipation during follow-through, thereby producing injury in the shoulder.

Mechanics of the (Outer) Scapulohumeral Articulation

Stereophotogrammetry has shown that some compression of the cuff by the overlying coracoacromial arch is normal. Control of upward movement of the humeral head should be considered a normal function of the rotator cuff. Upward movement of the head and cuff also generates tension within the coracoacromial ligament. This ligament has been noted to regenerate even after removal, indicating that an ongoing force pattern directs the alignment of the newly formed collagen.

Pathogenesis

Aging and physical loading both have been suggested as causes for rotator cuff disease and its associated findings. According to the first school of thought, aging leads to degenerative cuff damage, particularly at the insertion of the cuff (enthesopathy) as demonstrated by fiber thickening and granulation tissue. The damaged cuff then malfunctions, leading to disorders in the subacromial area. According to the second theory, damage to the cuff secondary to loading is the primary event, leading then to cuff malfunction and further damage.

Current evidence supports the second theory: that physical forces are the primary cause of rotator cuff disorders. Intact cuffs show very few time-related changes in the area of the insertion. The tendon becomes somewhat thinner, but the vessel pattern does not change, and when degenerative changes do occur they are localized to the inner region of the tendon insertion rather than the outer region. This localized distribution is indicative of physical causes, as opposed to a uniform distribution, which might point to aging. Degenerative changes also arise more commonly in the supraspinatus than in the other tendons. Aging may play a role to the extent that the older person who sustains microscopic damage arising from loading usually recovers more slowly than does a younger patient. In addition, stiffness in the shoulder and in remote areas of the kinetic chain may affect dynamic events in the shoulder.

Given that the primary cause of rotator cuff damage is loading, the next question is whether the type of loading involved is a normal tension load that occurs in too great a quantity or accumulates because of increased frequency or an abnormal type of load such as shear or compression. Currently, the most common cause of tendon failure is thought to be abnormal loading. Failure caused by tension alone is unusual but does occur. Tension failure most often occurs in patients younger than age 40 years.

Identifying the source of the abnormal loading is critical for determining treatment. Does the damaging event occur from a static or structural cause, such as an unyielding hooked acromion affecting a normally functioning shoulder? Or is it a dynamic event, in which the humeral head and rotator cuff are caused to move against an unyielding structure? Acromioplasty has become one of the most frequently performed operations in North America; therefore, accurate diagnosis would benefit a large number of patients.

Current evidence indicates that there are both static and dynamic causes of rotator cuff disease. Impingement syndrome, therefore, is exactly what its name suggests—a syndrome, ie, a collection of symptoms, signs, and pathologies arising from different primary causes. The clinician's skills are needed to determine the primary cause.

Static Causes

Static causes of rotator cuff damage involve abnormalities of the coracoacromial arch, which lead to areas of higher than normal compression of the rotator cuff. Such abnormalities have been referred to as subacromial roughness or discontinuity of the arch. The primary example of this is the type III acromion, in which the curvature of the undersurface is not smooth. This lack of roundness can lead to higher compression in some of the regions where the rotator cuff articulates with the arch. A similar abnormality of acromial morphology occurs in the coronal plane: a higher incidence of rotator cuff disease has been found in people with a laterally downward sloping acromion.

Another abnormality is os acromiale, or an unfused acromial apophysis. This condition can cause subacromial roughness in two ways: by allowing the shape of the anterior acromion to change, and by allowing growth of osteophytes along the edges of the nonunion.

Secondary changes have also been cited as causes of static impingement. Ossification of the acromion at the origin of the coracohumeral ligament alters the shape of the affected side of the scapulohumeral articulation. Hypertrophy of the coracoacromial ligament may change the nature of the articulation in a fashion not visible on radiographs. As a result of these secondary changes, a problem previously caused by dynamic factors may have a static component. This interrelationship muddies an already confusing picture: structures that predispose to cuff injury do not always result in injury (eg, not all type III acromia produce cuff disease), and not all structural changes are primary (eg, ossification of the coracoacromial ligament may occur secondary to a dynamic impingement).

Dynamic Causes

In shoulders with rotator cuff damage of dynamic origin (Table 4), the coracoacromial arch and other subacromial structures may be, initially at least, normal. Abnormal motion of the head and cuff relative to the scapula is the primary cause of this cuff damage, although continued abnormal motion may lead to permanent structural changes that will then need to be addressed in treatment, along with the dynamic problem. The abnormal rotator cuff contact is of two types. External impingement exists when the bursal side of the cuff contacts the coracoacromial arch. Internal impingement exists when the inner fibers of the cuff contact the upper labrum and its adjacent structures.

External impingement has been studied the longest, and a number of causes have been documented. Muscle weakness, which has been shown to allow the humeral head to rise higher toward the acromion, is considered

TABLE 4 | Dynamic Causes of Rotator Cuff Injury

External Impingement	Internal Impingement
Cuff weakness	Cuff weakness (subscapularis)
Tight posterior capsule	Type II superior labrum anterior-posterior
Shoulder instability	Scapular dysfunction
Use of wheelchairs and crutches	Stiffness
Scapular dysfunction	Weakness
Limb girdle dystrophy	Poor scapulohumeral rhythm
Serratus palsy	Trunk or lower limb weakness
Poor conditioning	Poor athletic technique
Trunk and lower limb weakness	
Poor athletic technique	

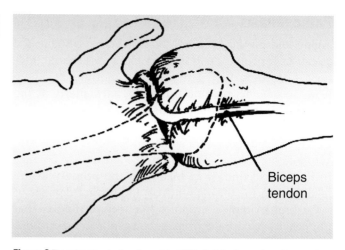

Figure 8 The relocation test performed in 120° of abduction and maximum external rotation. In this position, the lesser tuberosity can move farther posteriorly, creating an abrupt change in the path of the biceps.

the most common cause, especially in athletes. A second cause is a tight posterior capsule, which pushes the head in an anterior-superior direction when the shoulder is brought into flexion. Conversely, looseness of the superior shoulder, as in an anterior type II superior labrum anterior-posterior lesion, can allow motion toward the coracoacromial arch. Weakness in the muscles controlling the scapula can mimic these causes and aggravate the problem. Trunk or lower limb weakness or improper kinetics can also mimic scapular muscle dysfunction. In addition, an upward force on the humerus caused by the chronic use of crutches or a wheelchair as is seen in paraplegia creates a condition called the weight-bearing acromion. As might be predicted, this last cause is more resistant to treatment than the other dynamic causes because the precipitating cause cannot be eliminated.

Internal impingement has been seen in two areas: posterior and anterior. Posterior internal impingement occurs in the end-range positions between abduction and external rotation and full elevation in external and internal rotation (Neer position). The position of extreme abduction and external rotation of the shoulder is seen in athletes who participate in racquet or throwing sports. Anterior internal impingement occurs in the position of forward flexion, internal rotation, and adduction.

In posterior impingement, the greater tuberosity and its attached cuff tendons make contact with the superior labrum and attached biceps anchor. This does not require overstretch of the anterior capsule, but the same mechanism may lead to overstretch of the anterior capsule. An interesting finding is that in 120° of shoulder

abduction and external rotation the biceps tendon is sharply angled posteriorly, which may play a role in labral damage (Fig. 8). Internal impingement places several structures at risk, and damage to more than one of the following structures is not unusual: the supraspinatus, the upper labrum, the greater tuberosity, the bone or cartilage of the glenoid, or the anterior capsule (Fig. 9).

Anterior internal impingement likewise places more than one structure at risk. Damage can occur to the inner fibers of the subscapularis, the upper anterior labrum, the biceps tendon, or combinations thereof (Fig. 5).

Natural History

The natural history of rotator cuff disorders comprises three factors: structure, symptoms, and mechanics (Fig. 10). There are several reasons all three factors must be considered.

First, many patients with structural damage are asymptomatic. In one study, partial or complete rotator cuff tears were found in 23% of asymptomatic volunteers in a 50- to 59-year-old cohort and in 51% of those older than age 80 years. Admittedly, MRI data tend to overestimate the incidence, but clearly a tear may not produce symptoms, just as the symptomatic patient may not have a tear. In addition, the presence of a tear in a patient with pain does not indicate necessarily that the tear is the cause of the pain.

Second, mechanics and symptomatology do not correlate well. Increased glenohumeral translation is found in shoulders with cuff tears irrespective of the presence or absence of pain.

Finally, the effect of treatment may differ among the three factors. Repair of a large tear may greatly relieve pain and partially improve function, yet be considered a

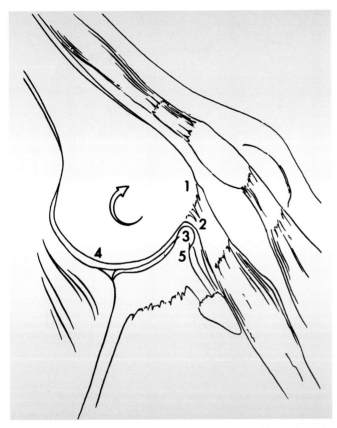

Figure 9 An anatomic cross section in the impingement sign position (flexion and internal rotation). Note that the tuberosity (1) is beyond the acromion and that the supraspinatus (2) and labrum (3) are making contact. Later secondary changes can occur in the anterior capsule (4) (stretch and instability) and the glenoid (5) (sclerosis or fracture). *(Reproduced with permission from Jobe CM: Posterior superior glenoid impingement: Expanded spectrum. Arthroscopy 1995;11:530-536.)*

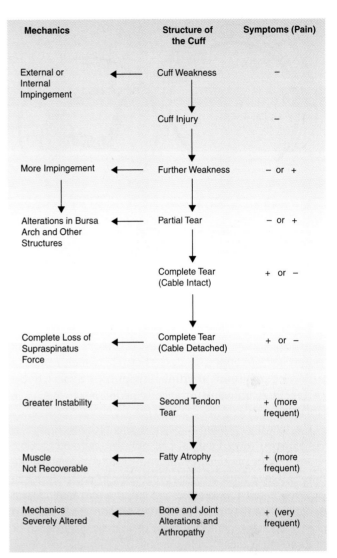

Mechanics	Structure of the Cuff	Symptoms (Pain)
External or Internal Impingement	Cuff Weakness	−
	Cuff Injury	−
More Impingement	Further Weakness	− or +
Alterations in Bursa Arch and Other Structures	Partial Tear	− or +
	Complete Tear (Cable Intact)	+ or −
Complete Loss of Supraspinatus Force	Complete Tear (Cable Detached)	+ or −
Greater Instability	Second Tendon Tear	+ (more frequent)
Muscle Not Recoverable	Fatty Atrophy	+ (more frequent)
Mechanics Severely Altered	Bone and Joint Alterations and Arthropathy	+ (very frequent)

Figure 10 Natural history of rotator cuff disorders.

failure in terms of structural improvement as shown on MRI.

Despite the lack of correlation between structure, symptoms, and mechanics, a general natural history of rotator cuff damage is believed to occur and is described here. Structural changes are the focus of the discussion, with function and symptoms mentioned where relevant. In addition to the structural changes in the cuff, simultaneous or secondary changes in adjacent structures must be considered. After initial injury to the cuff from a mechanical source and the resulting continued dysfunction, permanent changes may also occur in the bursa, acromion, coracoacromial ligament, labrum, tuberosity, or glenoid. These secondary changes can in turn influence the mechanics of the shoulder. Pain is usually indicative of inflammation; even with subacromial alteration, the patient may be pain free.

Changes in the bursa and coracoacromial arch may necessitate surgery even though the cuff is intact and the muscles and range of motion have responded to rehabilitation. Similarly, a concomitant superior labrum anterior-posterior lesion may require attention.

Most frequently the early changes in the tendon are small or microscopic and involve changes in the collagen fibers, usually on the articular side of the cuff. These changes may progress to become an incomplete tear. If small, these tears may have no effect on mechanics, but if they are painful, cuff weakness and dysfunction may result.

If damage continues, a single tendon tear may occur, usually in the supraspinatus. Transverse fibers, especially the rotator cuff cable, may hold the supraspinatus in extension, causing much of its force to be transmitted to the humerus. On the other hand, detachment of one end of the rotator cuff cable may cause a separate mechanical problem in the subacromial space. When one end of the cable detaches, a portion of the transverse tear retracts, creating a triangular defect. With time, there is muscle shortening and contracture of adjacent soft tissues such as the capsule under the retracted tendon corner or the coracohumeral ligament.

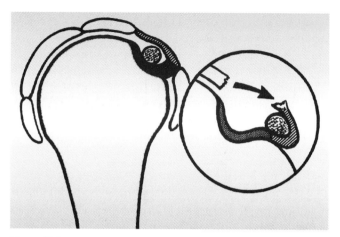

Figure 11 Damage to one part of the biceps sling, in this case the lateral attachment of the coracohumeral ligament, allows the long head of the biceps to subluxate medially. *(Reproduced with permission from Habermeyer P, Walch G: The biceps tendon and rotator cuff disease, in Burkhead WZ (ed): Rotator Cuff Disorders. Philadelphia, PA, Williams & Wilkins, 1996, pp 142-159.)*

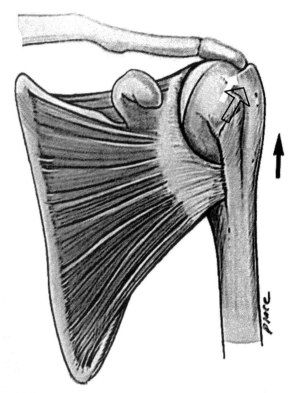

Figure 12 Altered mechanics caused by a rotator cuff tear. The large tear has removed any cuff contribution to abduction. The humeral head has moved superiorly (black arrow), altering the length-tension curve of the deltoid. Finally, the acromion has "captured" the tuberosity. For movement to occur, the center of rotation would have to shift (white arrow) to the acromion, severely shortening the lever arm of the deltoid. *(Adapted with permission from Burkhart: A unified biomechanicale rationale for the treatment of rotator cuff tears: Debridement versus repair, in Burkhead WZ (ed): Rotator Cuff Disorders. Philadelphia, PA, Williams & Wilkins, 1996, pp 293-312.)*

Disruption of the attachment of the coracohumeral ligament to the humerus may result in subluxation of the biceps tendon disease (Fig. 11), which can lead to biceps irritation, attrition, atrophy, or hypertrophy. In fact it is unusual for biceps problems to occur in isolation.

The tear may remain static, or it may progress in one or both of two ways. First, lack of pull-through and chronic shortening of the muscle will lead to fatty atrophy of the muscle. Once fatty atrophy progresses to a certain level, function is not recoverable. Second, the tear may extend to an adjacent tendon. Such two-tendon tears will not always be accompanied by pain or a gross disturbance of motion, but a measurable amount of weakness will most certainly be found in testing individual muscles. At this point, or even earlier, the mechanical alterations in the shoulder are so large that the original mechanical problems seem irrelevant, but they still need to be kept in mind.

The condition may progress further, to the point that the relationship of the humeral head to the glenoid changes. The humeral head rises and also may be unstable in either the anterior or posterior direction, depending on which second tendon is torn. With sufficient upward progression of the humeral head, the greater tuberosity may articulate against the lateral edge of the acromion (Fig. 12) and cause the center of rotation to move from the center of the humeral head to the point of contact. This shortens the lever arm of the deltoid, rendering it essentially ineffective and making abduction impossible. This occurs in addition to whatever changes in motion are brought about by pain.

Arthrosis may eventually result if the humeral head erodes into the upper glenoid and the undersurface of the acromion. As upward and medial migration of the head progresses, the lower glenoid may articulate against the humeral shaft. The progression of the disease is not relentless, and it is somewhat difficult to predict in which patients it will progress. This natural history should not be cited, however, as an argument for early surgical intervention.

Natural History in the Competitive Overhead Athlete

Although symptoms of early rotator cuff disease usually do not correlate closely with structural damage in the general population, the disease has been found to follow a fairly predictable course in competitive overhead athletes. This predictability is attributed to the highly demanding nature of these athletes' activities and the regularity with which they are performed.

Internal impingement of the cuff and greater tuberosity against the posterior superior labrum and glenoid is the mechanism of injury. Causes can include a weak subscapularis, insufficient scapular mobility and stability, or improper technique, including anything from shoulder placement to foot placement and muscle weakness anywhere along the kinetic chain.

Early symptoms include stiffness and a feeling of slowness during warm-up. Early in the course of the disease, when there is no pain, the shoulder will respond to rest, rehabilitation, and correction of technique. If the disease is allowed to progress, however, the cuff will become painful at the initiation of the acceleration phase of the overhead activity. The shoulder will also demonstrate a positive relocation test (ie, reduction of pain when the humeral head is relocated to make optimal contact with the glenoid). At this stage the same program of rest, rehabilitation, and correction of technique will still be effective in most shoulders.

If the disease progresses further, one or more of the following lesions requiring surgery may occur: anterior instability, a superior labrum anterior-posterior lesion, or a stress fracture of the glenoid. These lesions may be suspected if a shoulder fails to respond to an appropriate rehabilitation and technique correction program. The close association of symptoms with tissue injury in this group of patients is evidence that demand plays a role in the natural history of symptoms. Perhaps shoulders of nonathletes with rotator cuff damage would also follow the natural history described here if they were subjected to persistent high-demand activity.

Natural History With Intervention Through Rehabilitation or Surgery

Prognosis seems to depend on restorability of mechanics and how the prognosis is measured, for example, athletic performance versus pain relief versus structural integrity. If the cuff is intact, restoring the normal mechanics should eliminate symptoms and prevent progression, at least in the short term. With incomplete or smaller and more recent tears, repair is easier and fatty atrophy will not have occurred. With larger, more chronic tears the rate of recurrence or failure to heal is higher and restoring strength and kinematics much less likely. These tears, however, may have a good prognosis for pain relief.

For cuffs that require surgical repair, a good result at 1 year tends to be present at 10 years. However, at least one study has found a paradoxically poor prognosis in massive tears in which the duration between onset of symptoms and the date of surgery is short. This paradox may be explained in that the duration prior to surgery occurs in response to the increased severity of the original symptoms and pathomechanics. Thus, the poor prognosis may be the result of surgeon behavior rather than the true chronicity of the tear.

Permanently lost muscles can be substituted by tendon transfer, such as substituting the latissimus dorsi for the infraspinatus. This strategy seems to provide good pain relief and some improvement in motion and head location, but offers little chance of restoring full function. Long-term results of tendon transfers are not yet available. Some studies cite better results when transfer is done as part of the primary repair attempt, but at least one recent study shows satisfactory results in failed primary repairs.

In hemiarthroplasty for cuff tear arthropathy, results seem to reflect the preoperative status of the patient. Pain relief is frequently achieved, but postoperative motion does not improve much.

Summary

The health of the rotator cuff and its two adjacent articulations, the glenohumeral joint and the scapulohumeral articulation, is highly dependent on proper mechanics. Conversely, these mechanics are highly dependent on the rotator cuff. Investigations into rotator cuff disease must consider the initiating pathodynamics, the status of the cuff, and secondary changes in adjacent structures.

Annotated Bibliography

Anatomy

Banas MP; Miller RJ; Totterman S: Relationship between the lateral acromion angle and rotator cuff disease. *J Shoulder Elbow Surg* 1995;6:454-461.

This article describes an additional variation in acromial morphology, a lateral downward sloping in the coronal plane, that may make a "static" contribution to rotator cuff disease.

Gagey O, Hue E: Mechanics of the deltoid muscle: A new approach. *Clin Orthop* 2000;375:250-257.

This study demonstrates the effects of a downward force on the proximal humerus at the initiation of elevation. This mechanism may help to explain good motion in shoulders with large or massive cuff tears.

Harryman DT, Clark JM Jr: Anatomy of the rotator cuff, in Burkhead WZ (ed): *Rotator Cuff Disorders.* Philadelphia, PA, Williams & Wilkins, 1996, pp 23-35.

This study provides a complete and detailed description of the anatomy of the rotator cuff tendons with microscopic delineation of the fiber orientation. If, as we assume, fiber orientation is an indication of tensile forces, results of this study will provide guidance not only for the surgeon, but for future biomechanical studies of the shoulder.

Herzberg G, Urien JP, Dimnet J: Potential excursion and relative tension of the muscles in the shoulder girdle: Relevance to tendon transfers. *J Shoulder Elbow Surg* 1999;8:430-437.

Because the stability and function of the shoulder are dynamic, muscle transfers are being used with increasing frequency to compensate for muscle deficits. This article discusses the muscles available for such transfers.

Biomechanical Function

Soslowsky LJ, Carpenter JE, Buccieri JS, Flatow EL: Biomechanics of the rotator cuff. *Orthop Clin North Am* 1997;28:17-30.

This article reviews the biomechanics of the rotator cuff.

Yamaguchi K, Sher JS, Andersen WK, et al: Glenohumeral motion in patients with rotator cuff tears: A comparison of asymptomatic and symptomatic shoulders. *J Shoulder Elbow Surg* 2000;9:6-11.

This study demonstrates abnormal migration of the head in rotator cuff tears. The migration is unrelated to symptoms, however.

Pathogenesis

Ishii H, Brunet JA, Welsh RP, Uhthoff HK: "Bursal reactions" in rotator cuff tearing, the impingement syndrome, and calcifying tendonitis. *J Shoulder Elbow Surg* 1997;6:131-136.

This study found that histologically, what appears to the surgeon to be inflammation is often a healing response. The authors recommend that resectioning of bursal tissue be limited to the amount needed to restore motion.

Sano H, Ishii H, Trudeo G, Uhthoff HK: Histologic evidence of degeneration at the insertion of three rotator cuff tendons: A comparative study with human cadaveric shoulders. *J Shoulder Elbow Surg* 1999;8:574-579.

This study examined the anatomic distribution of tendon degeneration, finding degeneration more prominent on the inner half of the tendons, and with a higher incidence in the supraspinatus. These findings suggest that degeneration is more related to local factors such as mechanics rather than to general factors such as age and general health.

Natural History

Gerber C, Sebesta A: Impingement of the deep surface of the subscapularis tendon and the reflection pulley on the anterosuperior glenoid rim: A preliminary report. *J Shoulder Elbow Surg* 2000;9:483-490.

This article is the first clinical report of anterior internal impingement.

Hyvonen P, Lohi S, Jalovaara P: Open acromioplasty does not prevent the progression of an impingement syndrome to a tear: Nine-year follow-up of 96 cases. *J Bone Joint Surg Br* 1998;80:813-816.

This study followed 96 shoulders with previous acromioplasties and found that some with initial successful outcomes proceeded on to rotator cuff tears. This suggests that cuff pathology may arise from a cause other than acromial morphology.

Jost B, Pfirrmann CW, Gerber C, Switzerland Z: Clinical outcome after structural failure of rotator cuff repairs. *J Bone Joint Surg Am* 2000;82:304-314.

This article demonstrates that the structural success of a rotator cuff is a somewhat better predictor of mechanical success (muscle function) than it is of symptomatic success. Patients reported decreased pain and improved function following surgery, even if the rotator cuff reruptured. Strength may also increase if retear is smaller than the original tear.

Payne LZ, Deng XH, Craig EV, Torzilli PA, Warren RF: The combined dynamic and static contributions to subacromial impingement: A biomechanical analysis. *Am J Sports Med* 1997;25:801-808.

This cadaveric study measured the combined effect of muscle forces and acromial structure on subacromial impingement. It demonstrates how a group of patients with similar symptoms can be divided into subgroups according to whether the impingement has a static or dynamic etiology.

Soslowsky LJ, Thomopoulos S, Tun S, et al: Overuse activity injures the supraspinatus tendon in an animal model: A histologic and biomechanical study. *J Shoulder Elbow Surg* 2000;9:79-84.

The authors of this article developed an animal model to allow the study of the effect of overuse activity on rotator cuff disease.

Thomazeau H, Boukobza E, Morcet N, Chaperon J, Langlais F: Prediction of rotator cuff repair results by magnetic resonance imaging. *Clin Orthop* 1997;344:275-283.

Function of the muscles is essential to shoulder function. In this study, fatty degeneration of the muscle belly of the supraspinatus correlated with mechanical results or muscle strength, but not with pain or range of motion.

Wang JC, Shapiro MS: Changes in acromial morphology with age. *J Shoulder Elbow Surg* 1997;6:55-59.

This study shows that structural changes predisposing to impingement may increase with age; ie, static causes of impingement may arise later in life.

Chapter 14

Natural History and Nonsurgical Treatment of Rotator Cuff Disorders

Cyrus J. Lashgari, MD

Ken Yamaguchi, MD

Introduction

Rotator cuff disease ranks among the most prevalent of musculoskeletal disorders. Previous studies on the epidemiology of rotator cuff disease have found a high incidence of cuff tears among individuals older than age 55 years. Based on the latest census information, approximately 17 million individuals in the United States may be at risk for disabilities secondary to rotator cuff tears. Rotator cuff disease may also become increasingly important as the population ages.

This chapter reviews the latest information obtained from studies on the natural history of rotator cuff tears, which can help clinicians decide whether nonsurgical or surgical treatment is indicated. However, despite the clinical importance of rotator cuff tears, surprisingly little information is available regarding their natural history, perhaps because so many patients undergo surgery following the development of symptoms. Indications for nonsurgical treatment are presented based on current understanding of the natural history of rotator cuff disease, and guidelines for nonsurgical treatment are reviewed.

Prevalence

Cadaveric studies have shown that the prevalence of full-thickness rotator cuff tears ranges from 7% to 40%. Because these were cadaveric studies, correlation of tear prevalence with symptoms or demographic factors was not possible. Recent studies using both MRI and ultrasound have shown that a high percentage of tears in the elderly population may be asymptomatic. In one study, the overall prevalence of rotator cuff tears was 34% in a group of 96 asymptomatic patients examined using MRI, but in those patients older than age 60 years, the prevalence increased to 54%. A later study that used ultrasound to examine 411 asymptomatic volunteers revealed similar results. Looking only at full-thickness rotator cuff tears, the authors of this study found an age-related increase from 13% in patients between age 50 and 59

years to a remarkable 51% in patients older than age 80 years. As did the patients in the earlier study, these patients were functioning normally and without pain despite the presence of a full-thickness rotator cuff tear.

Clearly, the presence of a tear diagnosed by an imaging study alone does not warrant surgical intervention. It remains unclear why asymptomatic tears become symptomatic in certain individuals. Recently, a longitudinal analysis of asymptomatic tears was performed as a model to evaluate the natural history of rotator cuff tears. The authors studied asymptomatic tears discovered during routine bilateral ultrasound examinations on patients who had contralateral symptomatic rotator cuff tears. Results of a concurrent study at the same institution, in which ultrasound evaluation was compared to surgical findings in 100 consecutive patients, demonstrated that ultrasound was a highly accurate tool with which to conduct a longitudinal analysis of asymptomatic tears.

During a 5-year review of patients undergoing bilateral ultrasounds, the authors followed 45 patients. All patients completed a comprehensive questionnaire that included an American Shoulder and Elbow Surgeons shoulder score, an analog pain scale, an evaluation of activities of daily living, and outcome questions. Twenty-three patients underwent repeat ultrasounds and a standardized physical examination. Of the 45 patients, 23 (51%) became symptomatic (Fig. 1), with 15 reporting moderate to severe pain and 16 reporting night pain. Overall, the shoulder scores decreased from 89.9 to 64.4. There was no correlation with activity level, increased use, age, hand dominance, or sex. Of the 23 patients who returned for repeat ultrasounds, 9 were asymptomatic and 14 were symptomatic. Only two of the nine asymptomatic patients showed tear progression, compared with 7 of the 14 symptomatic patients.

It should be noted that the patients in this study already had a symptomatic rotator cuff tear on one side and so may represent a population with intrinsic cuff

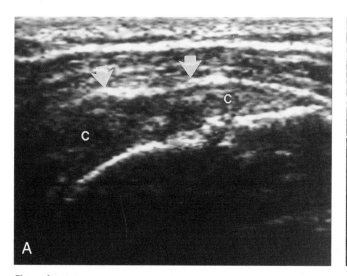 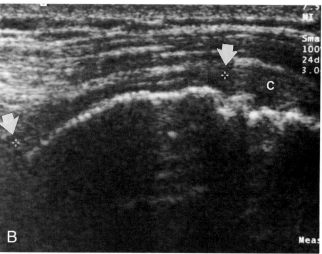

Figure 1 A, A representative ultrasound from a patient with symptomatic progression of a previously asymptomatic rotator cuff tear. A coronal ultrasound performed in 1991 showed a 1.3-cm supraspinatus tear. The arrows indicate the approximate length of the tear. **B,** A repeat ultrasound performed in 1997 showed progression of the tear to 2.4 cm. In this study, seven of 14 patients with newly symptomatic rotator cuff tears showed tear progression over time, in comparison with only two of nine patients who remained asymptomatic. *(Reproduced with permission from Yamaguchi K, Tetro AM, Blam O, Evanoff BA, Teefey SA, Middleton WD: Natural history of asymptomatic rotator cuff tears: A longitudinal analysis of asymptomatic tears detected sonographically.* J Shoulder Elbow Surg *2001;10:199-203.)*

weakness. Therefore, the results may overestimate the rate of symptom and tear progression in patients with bilateral asymptomatic tears. Despite these limitations, this study is relevant to a significant portion of the population because bilateral tears are common in the older population. It appears that a high percentage of patients with asymptomatic tears are at risk for symptom development as well as tear size progression over time.

Relationship Between Cuff Disease and Glenohumeral Kinematics

Many authors have studied the relationship between glenohumeral kinematics and rotator cuff tears in an effort to understand why symptoms develop. An early study looked at the kinematic patterns of 12 shoulders with massive, irreparable cuff tears, dividing the patients into three groups. One group had normal shoulder kinematics and a stable glenohumeral fulcrum despite the presence of the tear. These patients had normal shoulder motion and good strength because only the supraspinatus and a small portion of the infraspinatus were involved. This may have allowed for the preservation of essential force couples in the transverse and coronal planes. The other two groups, who showed superior and/or anterior subluxation with shoulder motion, had tears extending farther into the posterior or anterior cuff, which may have affected the force couples around the shoulder. The author observed that normal function is possible in the presence of a massive tear if the force couple involving the posterior cuff is intact. He compared the forces in these shoulders to those in a suspen-

sion bridge, concluding that tear extension is unlikely in these circumstances.

In a later study, glenohumeral motion was examined in normal subjects and in patients with both asymptomatic and symptomatic rotator cuff tears. Both groups with full-thickness tears showed progressive superior migration of the humerus on the glenoid with increasing arm elevation from 30° to 150°. This motion was significantly different from that in the group of normal volunteers who showed ball-in-socket kinematics after 30° of elevation. This study showed that painless, normal shoulder motion was possible despite abnormal glenohumeral kinematics. The authors concluded that symptoms are likely the result of multiple factors and that abnormal glenohumeral kinematics do not need to be treated in the asymptomatic patient.

Healing Patterns

Data from the previously mentioned study on the natural history of asymptomatic tears also confirmed the widely held belief that rotator cuff tears do not heal spontaneously. No decrease in tear size was observed in any of the 23 repeat ultrasound examinations. Healing of rotator cuff defects has been investigated in numerous recent studies using both humans and animals. In one study, a controlled defect was created in the supraspinatus tendons of 36 rats. After 3, 6, or 12 weeks, the supraspinatus tendon was examined both histologically and biomechanically. There were persistent defects in 78% of the specimens, and the tissue properties remained an order of magnitude lower than those of control tendons. Over the 12 weeks the authors noted highly cellular, vascularized tissue with disordered collagen attempting to heal the defect, but this tissue was of a very poor quality. They concluded that an active but ineffective healing process occurs in response to the defect.

In an earlier study, surgical specimens of torn rotator cuffs were examined to identify the pathology and pathogenesis of this process. The distal stump showed hypervascular areas, but the proximal stumps were avascular and contained abundant chondrocytes. There was no active repair response in the proximal stump or in the area between the stumps. These studies support the belief that torn rotator cuffs do not heal spontaneously.

Chronic changes that occur within nonhealing rotator cuff tendons and the risk of tear extension are important aspects of the natural history of rotator cuff disorders. A longitudinal study using ultrasound found tear extension in 39% of patients. This is especially important given the evidence that full-thickness rotator cuff tears do not heal spontaneously. It has long been noted that rotator cuff tears retract and form adhesions, complicating surgical repair. The tendon deteriorates over time, often leaving only tissue-paper–quality tendon for repair. Fatty degeneration and muscle atrophy occur and probably are permanent changes in long-standing cuff tears (Fig. 2). These chronic changes produce a weak shoulder with altered glenohumeral kinematics. Finally, degenerative joint changes also occur in long-standing tears, with a small percentage progressing to rotator cuff tear arthropathy.

Indications for Nonsurgical Care

In deciding between nonsurgical and surgical management, the risks and benefits of each approach should be understood. The benefits of nonsurgical care include avoiding surgery and its inherent complications. Although these are considerable benefits, the treating physician should note that there are important potential risks as well, including recurrent symptoms, tear extension, and chronic changes as discussed earlier. The risk of recurrence is unknown, but it can be estimated based on results of the study on asymptomatic patients followed by ultrasound that showed a 51% chance of becoming symptomatic. The benefits of surgical treatment include long-term pain relief and the possible cessation of chronic changes. The risks of surgery are well known and include infection, nerve injury, and most importantly, deltoid injury.

Information obtained from natural history studies can be used to identify the potential risks and benefits of nonsurgical treatment for full-thickness rotator cuff tears. Patients with rotator cuff tears generally can be divided into three categories based on the risk for

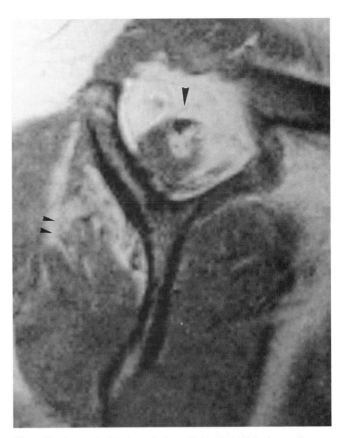

Figure 2 MRI scan showing supraspinatus and intraspinatus fatty degeneration and atrophy that can occur with long-standing rotator cuff tears. This fatty degeneration and atrophy has been correlated with a deterioration in functional outcome following repair. *(Reproduced with permission from Jost B, Pfirrmann CW, Gerber C, Switzerland Z: Clinical outcome after structural failure of rotator cuff repairs.* J Bone Joint Surg Am *2000;82:304-314.)*

development of irreversible changes to the rotator cuff with prolonged nonsurgical therapy. Consideration of these risks will dictate the timing of surgical repair to help prevent these changes, which include muscle atrophy, muscle fatty degeneration, changes in tendon morphology, and degenerative joint changes. In addition, with prolonged nonsurgical treatment, further adverse chronic changes can occur, including enlargement of the tear with time and the formation of adhesions in a retracted position, both of which can make surgical repair at a later date more difficult and extensive. Given these considerations, patients with rotator cuff tears can be grouped as follows: those not at risk for irreversible changes in the near future (group I); those at risk for irreversible changes to the rotator cuff with prolonged nonsurgical treatment (group II); and those in whom irreversible changes have already occurred (group III).

Group I patients have intact rotator cuffs with tendinitis or have only partial-thickness tears. Although there is a small risk that irreversible changes will develop when these patients are treated nonsurgically, they do run the risk of altered joint kinematics, prolonged pain, and muscle weakness. Because these symptoms are readily reversible with surgery, a relatively long course of nonsurgical treatment can be prescribed with minimal risk to the patient. Moreover, the advisability of prescribing a longer course of nonsurgical care in this group is further substantiated by the high success rate seen with nonsurgical treatment measures. In a recent retrospective study of 616 patients, the results of nonsurgical treatment for subacromial impingement syndrome were assessed. Overall, 67% of patients had a satisfactory result, and of these only 18% experienced a recurrence over time.

Group II includes patients with small- to medium-sized tears, a patient age of younger than 60 years, acute tears of any size, and/or tears and a recent loss of function. This group is at risk for tear extension, recurrent symptoms if they do respond to initial nonsurgical management, and, most importantly, irreversible changes in the cuff and glenohumeral joint. Because of the significant risk associated with nonsurgical treatment, early surgical repair may be preferable for these patients.

Group III consists of patients with large, chronic tears and those who are older than age 70 years. These patients already have had irreversible changes in their cuff or glenohumeral joint. Therefore, there is very little risk in attempting nonsurgical therapy except for prolonged pain. The fact that these patients have abnormal glenohumeral kinematics does not preclude them from having both pain-free and near-normal function. Therefore, these patients should undergo a trial of nonsurgical management.

General Strategies of Nonsurgical Management

Historically, nonsurgical management has proved quite successful for rotator cuff tendinitis. Studies over the last 10 years show a success rate between 70% and 80% with nonsurgical management. Options include steroid injections, nonsteroidal medication, modalities such as ultrasound, activity modification, and rehabilitation exercises that emphasize both stretching and strengthening of the rotator cuff and periscapular musculature. Unfortunately, very few controlled trials have conclusively demonstrated that any of these options are of benefit in the treatment of rotator cuff tears. The rehabilitation exercises described in this chapter are not a detailed description of rehabilitation protocols, but rather a review of recent articles.

Corticosteroid Injection

The potential deleterious effects of steroid injections are well known, including tendon atrophy and decreased quality of the tissue available for repair. For these rea-

sons, no more than three injections are recommended, spaced at least 3 months apart. Steroid injections remain quite popular despite the significant risks. They are most useful for patients experiencing night pain and to help enhance rehabilitation by decreasing pain. These injections are best indicated for patients in groups I or III.

A recent prospective, randomized, controlled, double-blind clinical study evaluated the efficacy of steroid injections in patients with subacromial impingement syndrome. Forty patients were involved, with one group receiving just 6 mL of lidocaine alone and the other receiving a combination of 4 mL of lidocaine and 80 mg (2 mL) of triamcinolone acetonide. The group receiving combination therapy reported significantly more pain relief (84%) than did the group receiving lidocaine alone (36%). In addition, the group receiving combination therapy experienced a significant increase in active forward elevation and external rotation and significantly fewer patients with a positive Neer impingement sign. Although this study did not include patients with rotator cuff tears and it included only short-term follow-up (33 weeks), it did provide evidence that steroids decrease pain and improve motion—two very important aspects of a successful nonsurgical management strategy. A review of 13 controlled studies published between 1955 and 1993 assessed the efficacy of steroid injections for treatment of rotator cuff tendinitis. Most of the studies were found to be poor in quality, leaving most questions about the proper use of steroids unanswered. Taken together, however, the studies point to the effectiveness of local steroid injections over placebo and nonsteroidal anti-inflammatory drugs (NSAIDs) in treating tendinitis. In particular, steroid injections were most useful for pain control.

To evaluate the adverse effects of steroid injections on the rotator cuff, a recent study was conducted on 30 rats, which were injected either three or five times with either triamcinolone at an equivalent human dosage or with saline solution. The supraspinatus and infraspinatus tendons were evaluated both macroscopically and microscopically in a blinded fashion. The tendons of two of seven rats that received five steroid injections showed clear structural changes, and microscopic changes were seen in four of the seven. Inflammatory cells were found between collagen bundles, and the bundles exhibited signs of necrosis and fragmentation. None of these changes was found in the rats injected with saline solution or in the rats injected with triamcinolone three times. In addition, the rats treated with steroids lost weight compared with the rats injected with saline solution. The authors believed this weight loss was the result of systemic effects of injected steroids. This study supports the cautious, limited use of steroid injections for patients with rotator cuff tears.

Nonsteroidal Anti-inflammatory Drugs

NSAIDs, which have both anti-inflammatory and analgesic properties, are an integral part of most nonsurgical treatment protocols for rotator cuff tears. Despite the widespread use of NSAIDs, no good controlled trials have been conducted to examine their efficacy in the treatment of rotator cuff disorders. A recently performed meta-analysis reviewed all controlled trials studying NSAIDs and steroid injections for the treatment of shoulder pain associated with several different shoulder problems, including frozen shoulder, rotator cuff tendinitis, and osteoarthritis. The studies were poor in quality, with varied selection criteria and outcome measures. The only tentative conclusions were that both NSAIDs and steroid injections are superior to placebo in increasing abduction in patients with rotator cuff tendinitis. However, steroid injections did not confer any further benefit for those patients taking NSAIDs. Even without good controlled trials, use of NSAIDs remains widespread for patients with rotator cuff tears.

Ultrasound, Phonophoresis, and Iontophoresis

Ultrasound

Ultrasound has been used in the treatment of various musculoskeletal injuries for many years. The high-frequency vibrations (1 to 3 mHz) pass into the body, creating both thermal and nonthermal effects. The heat increases blood flow locally and may decrease pain and muscular spasm. The nonthermal effects of ultrasound are less well defined. It is believed that the cellular permeability and metabolism of the local tissue are altered, creating a more favorable environment for healing.

Past studies have shown the effectiveness of ultrasound for some orthopaedic complaints, but case-controlled studies have shown no benefits of ultrasound over exercise for the treatment of rotator cuff tears. Although there is no recent literature on this subject, a double-blind study from the 1980s investigated the effectiveness of ultrasound for the treatment of subacromial bursitis. The authors wanted to evaluate the effectiveness of ultrasound compared to range-of-motion exercises with or without NSAIDs in decreasing pain and increasing range of motion. Twenty patients were randomized to receive true or sham ultrasound three times a week for 4 weeks. The physician, physical therapist, and patients were all blinded during the study. The range of motion, level of pain, and ability to perform five functional tasks were compared, and no significant differences were found. Despite these results, the use of ultrasound continues to be widespread.

Phonophoresis

Phonophoresis is a technique by which ultrasound is used to deliver medication transdermally. Multiple types of medication have been used, including corticosteroids, local anesthetics, and NSAIDs. Both the thermal and nonthermal properties of ultrasound have been credited for delivering these drugs into the subcutaneous tissues. The thermal effects include a local increase in blood flow and dilation of sweat glands and hair follicles. The increased cellular permeability, a nonthermal effect, may also cause subcutaneous penetration. This subcutaneous penetration decreases systemic side effects of the drugs, and the first-pass effect by the liver is avoided. Although several studies of the efficacy of phonophoresis have shown promising results, these studies have methodologic shortcomings that cast doubt on their conclusions.

Authors of a recent article reviewed 49 patients with a variety of orthopaedic conditions. Patients were matched according to their condition and then randomly assigned to either ultrasound alone or ultrasound with a corticosteroid (fluocinonide). The patients and examining physicians were blinded to eliminate experimental bias. The patients were asked to mark their pain level on a visual analog scale before and after 3 weeks of treatment. Patients also were evaluated using a pressure algometer designed to test the ability of the area of maximal tenderness to withstand pressure. No significant difference was found between the two groups for any measured category, with both showing significant pain relief. The authors concluded that phonophoresis with fluocinonide was of no additional benefit in reducing pain and pressure sensitivity.

Iontophoresis

Iontophoresis is a process by which electric current is used to deliver medication, most commonly steroids, locally into the skin. As with phonophoresis, the systemic side effects of the drug are avoided, although there is a risk of chemical burns. No recent literature supports the use of iontophoresis, and the data currently available do not conclusively prove its effectiveness. Because of this paucity of supportive information, iontophoresis is used infrequently by physical therapists. Its use is limited to situations when other nonsurgical treatments have failed.

Rehabilitation Exercises

Exercise is the most important aspect of nonsurgical therapy for rotator cuff disorders. Initially, the patient should rest, avoiding provocative activities. When the acute inflammation and pain decrease, stretching and strengthening exercises can begin. The goal of stretching exercises is to restore a full range of motion through long, slow stretches with minimal pain. Initially, internal rotation and extension should be avoided. Once range of motion has improved and pain has decreased, strengthening of the rotator cuff and surrounding musculature can begin. There are two philosophies regarding strengthening of the rotator cuff. One supports improving kinematics by maximizing the force couples of the remaining cuff tissue. The other believes that restoration of the force couples is not necessary and that maximizing the deltoid strength will decrease pain and improve function. Regardless of theory, multiple studies have shown a 50% to 80% success rate following surgical intervention for full-thickness tears.

Opinions differ as to the need for supervision by a physical therapist during rehabilitation. A recent study looked at self-training versus physical therapist-supervised rehabilitation. Forty-three patients who underwent arthroscopic subacromial decompression and were found to have intact cuffs were randomized to either self-training or training with a physical therapist. The patients were evaluated by an independent observer after 3, 6, and 12 months. There was no statistical difference in return to work or improvement in functional outcomes. These data lend support to physicians who have developed specific rehabilitation protocols for their patients with impingement or rotator cuff tears. Physician-supervised rehabilitation also improves doctor-patient communication and may improve compliance. Physical therapists probably benefit patients who need more encouragement and guidance during the early phases of rehabilitation.

In recent studies, investigators have tried to elucidate the principal actions of the rotator cuff and parascapular muscles. This information could influence rehabilitation protocols, maximizing a patient's functional return. Muscle moment arms of the deltoid, rotator cuff, and scapulohumeral muscle groups during four specified glenohumeral motions were studied using cadaveric specimens. The anterior deltoid, middle deltoid, and supraspinatus were the largest elevators, whereas the scapulohumeral muscles (teres major, latissimus dorsi, and pectoralis major) were the main depressors. The infraspinatus initially was an elevator, but it became a depressor at 50° of elevation. The subscapularis worked in an opposite fashion, initially as a depressor and later as an elevator. The main difference between these and earlier reports was in the relative roles of the deltoid and supraspinatus in elevation. As the arm is elevated, the supraspinatus moment arm becomes quite small compared with that of the deltoid, emphasizing the importance of the anterior and middle deltoid. In a second study, 14 shoulder muscles were evaluated using electromyographic data from five subjects. The data confirmed the concept of the rotator cuff as a humeral head stabilizer of the glenohumeral joint. Clearly, strengthening of both the deltoid and the remaining rotator cuff musculature in patients with tears is important for rehabilitation.

A recent article in which normal shoulders in 12 male volunteers were studied using the radiographic techniques of Poppen and Walker showed that endurance is also important for these muscles. True AP radiographs of the glenohumeral joint in 0°, 45°, 90°, and 135° of scapular abduction were taken before and after muscle fatigue of the deltoid and rotator cuff. The patients used a dumbbell until there was a confirmed decrease in strength of at least 30%. The radiographs were viewed in a random, blinded fashion. Before muscle fatigue, the radiographs showed no change in position of the humeral head relative to the glenoid at any degree of abduction. After muscle fatigue, humeral head excursion averaged 2.5 mm, and the superior migration was statistically significant at 45°, 90°, and 135° of abduction. Results of this study suggest that muscle fatigue of the rotator cuff disrupts its function as a dynamic stabilizer. Superior migration of the humeral head may lead to mechanical impingement of the rotator cuff with the coracoacromial arch. Rotator cuff endurance as well as strengthening exercises could improve dynamic stabilization, possibly preventing symptomatic impingement and propagation of a rotator cuff tear. Another recent study, however, shows normal, painless function in patients with rotator cuff tears. These patients were found to have the same abnormal superior head migration as patients with symptomatic rotator cuff tears. Although the importance of normal glenohumeral kinematics remains uncertain, strengthening of the rotator cuff should remain a cornerstone of rehabilitation.

Summary

Continued research needs to be devoted to understanding the natural history of rotator cuff tears. Recent studies have shown progression of tears, symptomatic flare-ups, and irreversible changes in rotator cuffs managed nonsurgically. These data allow the grouping of patients with rotator cuff tears into three categories based on risk-benefit ratios. Nonsurgical care should be maximized for patients with impingement symptoms only, with partial-thickness tears, with chronic massive tears, and for elderly patients. Nonsurgical management starts with restoring motion once pain is controlled, followed by strengthening of both the rotator cuff and surrounding musculature. The proper selection of candidates should lead to the high success rate quoted by multiple authors. Surgical management should be considered when prolonged nonsurgical treatment fails. In contrast, early surgery should be considered for tears that are acute, small or medium, associated with shoulder loss of function, or occur in a younger patient. Prolonged nonsurgical care in these patients risks tear propagation and irreversible changes to the cuff, which may complicate rotator cuff repair.

Annotated Bibliography

Prevalence

Tempelhof S, Rupp S, Seil R: Age-related prevalence of rotator cuff tears in asymptomatic shoulders. *J Shoulder Elbow Surg* 1999;8:296-299.

The authors studied 411 asymptomatic patients using ultrasound. An age-related increase in full-thickness rotator cuff tears was found. Overall, tears were found in 23% of patients: 51% of patients older than age 80 years, and 13% of patients between age 50 and 59 years. The reasons that tears become symptomatic during this normal aging process are uncertain.

Relationship Between Cuff Disease and Glenohumeral Kinematics

Arwert HJ, de Groot J, Van Woensel WW, Rozing PM: Electromyography of shoulder muscles in relation to force direction. *J Shoulder Elbow Surg* 1997;6:360-370.

Electromyogram studies of 14 muscles around the shoulder were performed on five normal subjects. The arm was held in three positions and the principal action of the individual muscles was determined for each position. The rotator cuff muscles were found to stabilize the glenohumeral joint.

Chen SK, Simonian PT, Wickiewicz TL, Otis JC, Warren RF: Radiographic evaluation of glenohumeral kinematics: A muscle fatigue model. *J Shoulder Elbow Surg* 1999;8:49-52.

This study reviewed the impact of muscle fatigue on glenohumeral kinematics. Twelve normal volunteers had a series of radiographs taken of their shoulder at different levels of abduction before and after deltoid and rotator cuff exercises. The fatigue caused superior migration of the humeral head in all abducted positions.

Kuechle DK, Newman SR, Itoi E, Morrey BF, An KN: Shoulder muscle moment arms during horizontal flexion and elevation. *J Shoulder Elbow Surg* 1997;6:429-439.

Evaluation of the moment arms of 10 shoulder muscles during different shoulder motions confirmed some previous information on the function of these muscles. The roles of the supraspinatus, infraspinatus, and subscapularis, however, were questioned.

Yamaguchi K, Sher JS, Andersen WK, et al: Glenohumeral motion in patients with rotator cuff tears: A comparison of asymptomatic and symptomatic shoulders. *J Shoulder Elbow Surg* 2000;9:6-11.

This article compares glenohumeral kinematics in patients without rotator cuff tears, with asymptomatic rotator cuff tears, and with symptomatic rotator cuff tears. The two rotator cuff tear groups, unlike the normal group, showed superior translation of the humeral head. This study demonstrated that painless, normal shoulder motion is possible despite abnormal glenohumeral kinematics.

Healing Patterns

Carpenter JE, Thomopoulos S, Flanagan CL, DeBano CM, Soslowsky LJ: Rotator cuff defect healing: A biomechanical and histologic analysis in an animal model. *J Shoulder Elbow Surg* 1998;7:599-605.

The authors investigated the healing of rotator cuff defects in rats histologically and biomechanically; 78% of the specimens had persistent defects after 12 weeks. Biomechanical properties improved over the 12 weeks, indicating some healing, but the tissue quality remained poor compared to normal tendon. The healing response in the rotator cuff is inadequate.

Indications for Nonsurgical Care

Morrison DS, Frogameni AD, Woodworth P: Non-operative treatment of subacromial impingement syndrome. *J Bone Joint Surg Am* 1997;79:732-737.

In this retrospective review of 616 patients with subacromial impingement syndrome, all patients underwent supervised physical therapy and were taking NSAIDs. Of the patients, 67% had a satisfactory outcome; however, 18% of these patients experienced a recurrence of their symptoms. Of patients with symptoms of less than 4 weeks' duration, 78% had a satisfactory result, versus 67% who had symptoms for more than 6 months. Patients with type I acromions had better results than those with type II or III (91% versus 68% and 64%, respectively).

Yamaguchi K, Tetro AM, Blam O, Evanoff BA, Teffey SA, Middleton WD: Natural history of asymptomatic rotator cuff tears: A longitudinal analysis of asymptomatic tears detected sonographically. *J Shoulder Elbow Surg* 2001;10:199-203.

In this study, the natural history of asymptomatic rotator cuff tears was reviewed over a 5-year period. Ultrasound was used to initially document bilateral rotator cuff tears in 58 patients with unilateral shoulder pain. Forty-five patients responded to a comprehensive questionnaire at a mean of 2.8 years later; of these, 23 also had a physical examination and repeat ultrasound. Of the 45 patients, 23 previously asymptomatic patients (51%) had become symptomatic. Of the 23 patients who returned for ultrasound, nine were asymptomatic and 14 were symptomatic. Nine of the 23 patients (39%) had tear progression.

General Strategies of Nonsurgical Management

Anderson NH, Sojbjerg JO, Johannsen HV, Sneppen O: Self-training versus physiotherapist-supervised rehabilitation of the shoulder in patients treated with arthroscopic subacromial decompression: A clinical randomized study. *J Shoulder Elbow Surg* 1999;8:99-101.

This clinical prospective study reviewed the rehabilitation of 43 consecutive patients who had undergone arthroscopic subacromial decompression for impingement. No difference was found between patients who underwent supervised rehabilitation and those who self-trained.

Blair B, Rokito AS, Cuomo F, Jarolem K, Zuckerman JD: Efficacy of injections of corticosteroids for subacromial impingement syndrome. *J Bone Joint Surg Am* 1996;78:1685-1689.

This prospective, randomized, double-blind study looked at the short-term efficacy of subacromial injections. Forty patients were randomized to receive lidocaine or lidocaine with triamcinolone. At 33 weeks, 84% of the steroid group experienced decreased pain, compared with 36% of the lidocaine group.

Klaiman MD, Shrader JA, Danoff JV, Hicks JE, Pesce WJ, Ferland J: Phonophoresis versus ultrasound in the treatment of common musculoskeletal conditions. *Med Sci Sports Exerc* 1998;30:1349-1355.

Forty-nine patients with varying orthopaedic conditions were randomly assigned in a double-blind fashion to receive either phonophoresis or ultrasound alone. Although both groups experienced decreased pain, there was no significant difference between the two groups. A control group was lacking.

Tillander B, Franzen LE, Karlsson MH, Norlin R: Effect of steroid injections on the rotator cuff: An experimental study in rats. *J Shoulder Elbow Surg* 1999;8:271-274.

Thirty rats were injected three to five times with a steroid or normal saline solution. Histologic evaluation showed focal inflammation, necrosis, and fragmentation of collagen bundles in the rats that received five injections of steroids. There were no pathologic findings in the control groups or in the rats that received three steroid injections. Prudent use of steroids is recommended.

Classic Bibliography

Bassett RW, Cofield RH: Acute tears of the rotator cuff: The timing of surgical repair. *Clin Orthop* 1983;175:18-24.

Bokor DJ, Hawkins RJ, Huckell GH, Angelo RL, Schickendantz MS: Results of nonoperative management of full-thickness tears of the rotator cuff. *Clin Orthop* 1993;294:103-110.

Burkhart SS: Fluoroscopic comparison of kinematic patterns in massive rotator cuff tears: A suspension bridge model. *Clin Orthop* 1992;284:144-152.

Downing DS, Weinstein A: Ultrasound therapy of subacromial bursitis: A double blind trial. *Phys Ther* 1986;66:194-199.

Itoi E, Tabata S: Conservative treatment of rotator cuff tears. *Clin Orthop* 1992;275:165-173.

Neer CS: Impingement lesions. *Clin Orthop* 1983;173:70-77.

Sher JS, Uribe JW, Posada A, Murphy BJ, Zlatkin, MB: Abnormal findings on magnetic resonance images of asymptomatic shoulders. *J Bone Joint Surg Am* 1995;77:10-15.

Chapter 15

Surgical Treatment of Partial-Thickness Tears

Roger C. Dunteman, MD

Hiroaki Fukuda, MD

Stephen J. Snyder, MD

Introduction

Even though incomplete and intratendinous tears of the rotator cuff were first described by Codman in 1934, a unified approach to the management of rotator cuff pathology was lacking. Neer's description of the impingement lesion in 1972 greatly enhanced understanding of the pathophysiology as well as the treatment of lesions involving the rotator cuff. However, the most significant advancement in the diagnosis and treatment of partial-thickness rotator cuff tears (PTRCTs) did not occur until the advent of shoulder arthroscopy. PTRCTs are now a well-established clinical entity, yet there is no consensus in regards to surgical management. Recommended treatment varies widely from simple débridement of the torn tendon to subacromial decompression to excision of the degenerative tendon and repair. Surgery may be performed using an open, arthroscopically assisted (mini-open), or entirely arthroscopic procedure. The advantages and disadvantages of open and arthroscopic procedures may lie in the balance between precision and morbidity.

Several factors influence the decision to perform surgery, including the patient's preference, age, demands, response to nonsurgical treatment, the type and extent of tearing, the underlying pathology, and the surgeon's skill and experience. Therefore, a proper understanding of the diverse causes of PTRCTs is essential for a successful outcome.

Pathophysiology

PTRCTs typically involve the supraspinatus tendon, although the other components of the rotator cuff can be involved. These tears are located on the articular surface, the bursal surface, or within the tendon (intratendinous) (Fig. 1). Intratendinous tears are defined as having no communication with the articular or bursal surface. Clinical studies have shown there is an increased propensity for articular surface tears, with a reported incidence of two to three times that of bursal surface tears. Selective vascular injection studies have demonstrated a uniform area of hypovascularity or critical zone at the articular surface close to the insertion of the supraspinatus tendon. Results of histologic and biomechanical studies in 60 cadaveric supraspinatus tendons also have shown that the articular surface has thinner collagen bundles in a less orderly array than the large, parallel bundles along the bursal surface. Consequently, the ultimate stress to failure is half that of the bursal surface. The poor vascularity and decreased biomechanical properties of the articular surface are most likely significant factors in the pathogenesis of articular-sided tears.

Increasing evidence suggests that PTRCTs progress. Serial arthrography has been used to illustrate the progression of a partial-thickness tear to a complete tear in 11 of 40 patients (28%) and enlargement of the PTRCT in 21 of 40 patients (53%). Only four patients (10%) in this study demonstrated complete healing of a partial tear. Rehabilitation or arthroscopic treatment (subacromial decompression) has not been shown to delay or prevent the progression of a partial-thickness tear to a complete tear. Furthermore, débridement of a PTRCT does not appear to invoke an active healing response, and histologic sections of PTRCTs show no signs indicative of ongoing repair.

Some agreement exists as to use of the depth of the tendon tearing in selecting treatment method. Most clinicians agree that tears involving more than 50% of the tendon thickness (average cuff thickness, 9 to 12 mm) should influence the surgeon to perform open repair. There seems to be no consensus of opinion for treatment based on the tear surface area. In addition, the timing of surgical intervention after nonsurgical treatment has not been well defined, ranging from a few months to 1.5 years.

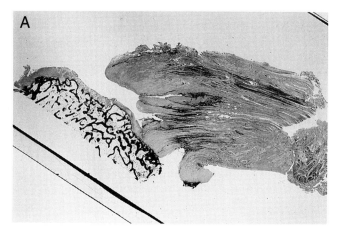

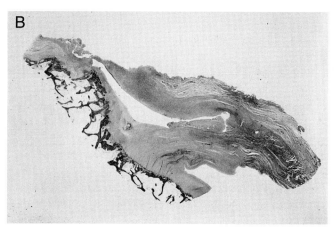

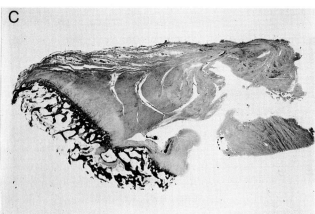

Figure 1 A, Photomicrograph of a bursal-sided partial-thickness rotator cuff tear involving more than one-half thickness of the supraspinatus tendon in a 57-year-old man (Stain, Azan, original magnification, x 1). (*Reproduced with permission from Fukuda H, Kazutoshi H, Yamanaka K: Pathology and pathogenesis of bursal-side rotator cuff tears viewed from en bloc histologic sections. Clin Orthop 1990;254: 75-80.*) **B,** Photomicrograph of an intratendinous tear in the midlayer of the supraspinatus tendon in a 42-year-old man, the distal end of which is close to the bursal floor (Stain, Azan, original magnification, x 1). **C,** Photomicrograph of a joint-sided or articular surface tear in a 41-year-old man that communicates with an intratendinous tear oriented parallel to the tendon fibers. The distal end of the intratendinous tear is in continuity with a local disruption of the enthesis by granulation tissue. The torn portion of the tendon demonstrates marked degeneration. The insertion area facing the bursa is edematous (Stain, Azan, original magnification, x 1). (*Reproduced with permission from Fukuda H, Hamada K, Nakajima T, Tomonaga A: Pathology and pathogenesis of the intratendinous tearing of the rotator cuff viewed from en bloc histologic sections. Clin Orthop 1994;304:60-67.*)

Clinical Findings

It is sometimes difficult to differentiate between a full-thickness tear, a partial-thickness tear, or tendinosis. Partial-thickness tears often are found in patients younger than age 45 years, with pain as the predominant complaint. These tears are common in athletes who participate in repetitive overhead sports such as tennis, baseball, volleyball, or swimming, with pain persisting for several hours after cessation of the activity. Particular attention should be directed to any symptoms of glenohumeral instability in the throwing athlete. The athlete initially will report stiffness and difficulty warming up for the throwing activity. Later stages of instability can cause posterior shoulder pain while throwing during the late cocking phase.

Physical examination usually reveals a painful arc of motion from 60° to 120° of flexion. Pain with occasional weakness during resisted isometric contraction of the involved muscle is common. For example, resisted elevation with the arm held in 90° of abduction, 30° of forward flexion, and full internal rotation (Jobe sign) tests the supraspinatus tendon. Resisted external rotation with the arm at the patient's side in neutral rotation with the elbow flexed 90° tests the infraspinatus tendon.

More recently, attempts have been made to differentiate partial-thickness tears from full-thickness tears through various lag signs. The external rotation lag sign for partial ruptures of the supraspinatus tendon is universally negative, whereas a positive sign is observed in nearly all complete tears. The Neer (pain with passive forward elevation) and Hawkins (pain with passive internal rotation with the arm at 90° of forward flexion) impingement signs are usually positive. A thorough instability examination must be performed in the throwing athlete to assess for the possibility of posterior internal rotator cuff impingement caused by anterior shoulder instability. Decreased internal rotation secondary to contracture of the posterior capsule is another common finding.

Imaging

Plain radiographs of the shoulder usually yield nonspecific findings in relation to rotator cuff pathology but are helpful in diagnosing other types of shoulder pathology (glenohumeral arthritis, acromioclavicular arthritis, and calcific tendinitis). The supraspinatus outlet view will delineate the bony architecture of the coracoacromial arch and identify any bony abnormalities, such as a hooked acromion, anterior acromial spur, or inferior acromioclavicular osteophyte. Evaluation of the rotator cuff requires an imaging modality that can identify the different stages of tendon disease from frank tear to partial tear to subtle signs of tendinosis. Traditionally, conventional arthrography, bursography, and ultrasound have been used with varying degrees of success in detecting a complete rotator cuff tear; however, the accurate diagnosis of a partial-thickness tear has been disappointing.

Currently, conventional MRI is the modality of choice for evaluating rotator cuff pathology, but it also has been an unreliable tool in the detection of partial-thickness tears. Because of the difficulties in detecting subtle injuries to the rotator cuff, a combination of MRI with intra-articular contrast (gadolinium) was developed to better delineate abnormalities of the rotator cuff. Using arthroscopy as the standard, magnetic resonance arthrography has been shown to be the most accurate, sensitive, and specific modality in the diagnosis of PTRCTs when compared with standard MRI (Fig 2). It is a useful adjunct when conventional MRI is inconclusive.

Classification

Although Neer's classic work described three stages of impingement lesions, PTRCTs were not accurately depicted in Neer's staging system. Therefore, a classification system based on the integrity of the rotator cuff was proposed: grade 1, bursitis and/or tendinitis (pretear); grade 2, partial-thickness tears; grade 3, full-thickness tears. Partial-thickness tears were further classified based on the depth and size of the lesion: grade 1 tears measure less than 25% of the tendon thickness or less than 3 mm; grade 2 tears measure less than 50% of the tendon thickness or 3 to 6 mm; and grade 3 tears measure greater than 50% of the thickness of the tendon or greater than 6 mm. A third system classifies PTRCTs based on the location and size of the tear. The location of the tear was designated as A indicating the articular surface and B indicating the bursal surface of the rotator cuff. The size and severity of the tear was graded from 0 to 4 (Table 1). For example, a 1.5-cm area of articular surface disruption with a normal bursal surface would be designated A2B0.

Open Surgical Techniques

With the patient in the beach chair position, an antero-superior approach is used because of its excellent exposure of the subacromial bursa and the supraspinatus tendon and its environs, with minimum deltoid detachment (2.0 cm). The tendon repair is preceded by anterior acromioplasty for those older than age 40 years. For patients younger than age 40 years, a coracoacro-

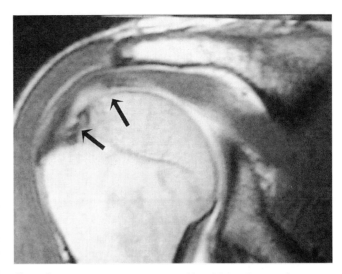

Figure 2 A magnetic resonance arthrogram with gadolinium demonstrating a partial articular supraspinatus tendon avulsion (PASTA) lesion.

mial ligament section would be preferable unless there is an obvious skeletal abnormality.

Bursal-sided tears are identified, but synovial proliferation may mask the small cuff defect. To detect both intratendinous and articular surface (joint-sided) tears, the critical portion of the supraspinatus tendon and the adjacent area should be carefully palpated for a thinned area. Puckering may be seen when elevating the arm or milking the tendon digitally or with a probe.

The color test, an intraoperative cuff-staining test, can be used to more accurately diagnose and localize articular surface tears and the intratendinous extensions during open surgery. Indigo carmine or methylene blue (3 mL mixed with 17 mL of normal saline solution) is injected into the glenohumeral joint. The shoulder is then put through a range of motion. Torn cuff tissue is preferentially stained by the dye. The sheath of the long head of the biceps brachii and the rotator interval normally are stained, and they should be used for surgical orientation. The color test proved positive when more than 50% of the tendon thickness was involved and was reported to detect articular surface tears in 65% of patients.

Incising the tendon along its fibers for direct visualization of the insubstance or undersurface of the tendon is also a helpful diagnostic maneuver. During diagnostic arthroscopy performed before open surgery, an articular surface tear can be tagged with suture passed through a spinal needle to assist in locating the tear from the bursal side. The torn portion of the tendon is then excised in an elliptical or isosceles fashion until the healthier tissue is met and oversewn side-to-side or to a trough in the anatomic neck or the greater tuberosity.

Besides pure intratendinous tears, intratendinous laminations are associated with approximately 50% of bur-

TABLE 1 | Classification of Partial-Thickness Rotator Cuff Tears

Grade	Description
0	A normal rotator cuff
1	An area on the surface of the rotator cuff where the synovium is inflamed and there is mild superficial fraying of the tendon; < 1 cm in size
2	A moderate-sized lesion with actual fiber disruption; < 2 cm in size
3	A moderate-to-severe lesion with fiber disruption and fragmentation; < 3 cm in size
4	A severe lesion with complex disruption, flap formation, and retraction of the partial-thickness flaps; > 3 cm in size

(Reproduced with permission from Snyder SJ: Arthroscopic evaluation and treatment of the rotator cuff, in Pennington J, McCurdy P (eds): Shoulder Arthroscopy. New York, NY, McGraw-Hill, 1994, pp 148-149.)

sal-sided and articular surface tears. Such laminations also are found frequently in full-thickness tears, and if they are completely excised, the subsequent cuff closure may become difficult. In this situation, some authors recommend suturing (in-and-out suture) of the superficial and deep cuff layers after thorough débridement of the inner surfaces (Fig. 3). The color test or use of topical dye facilitates débridement to distinguish degenerated tissue (stained) from normal tissue (less stained). This suture technique is based on an in situ hybridization study, which demonstrated abundant signal-positive cells containing procollagen α1 type I messenger RNA in intratendinous laminations of torn supraspinatus tendons obtained at surgery. Although the short-term results with this technique are promising, intratendinous tears and any types of cuff tears associated with sizable intratendinous extensions remain an unsolved therapeutic problem.

Postoperative rehabilitation is the same as after the repair for full-thickness cuff tears and should be surgeon-oriented and individualized because only the surgeon can judge the quality of both the tendon and the repair. The goal is to restore a full range of shoulder motion by early passive motion and to gain strength later. Approximately 5 to 6 weeks are necessary for the strong reattachment of the deltoid before active elevation of the arm is allowed. Six to 12 months are needed for the return of full use of the arm after successful repair of the cuff tear.

These combined open procedures for PTRCTs, with acromioplasty and tenorrhaphy after excision of the diseased portion, can provide several advantages: (1) a good tendon repair and anchoring can be accomplished; (2) decompression is reinforced by tenorrhaphy; (3) hidden lesions can be identified by inspection, palpation, mobilization, color test, and tendon exploration; (4) tissue repair is enhanced by excision; (5) progression of the tear can be prevented by a good repair; (6) con-

comitant intratendinous lamination can be treated; and (7) tendon surgery can be performed with the same exposure with minimal risk.

Recently, articular surface tears in young throwers and other overhead athletes that developed secondary to internal impingement were described. The pathomechanism is considered repetitive contact between the undersurface of the supraspinatus tendon and the posterosuperior glenoid through subtle instability during the late cocking phase of the throwing motion. The choice of treatment for this pathology is still controversial.

Mini-open Technique

A combined arthroscopic and open surgical approach has been developed to decrease the morbidity to the anterior deltoid. After arthroscopic subacromial decompression, a mini-open technique is performed using the short deltoid-splitting approach. Care should be taken to avoid avulsion of the deltoid from the anterior acromion by overzealous retraction. If needed, more exposure can be obtained by detaching the anterior deltoid an additional 2.0 cm.

Results

Pertinent literature has been scarce, often with small clinical series, short follow-up time, and differing treatment regimens, making comparison difficult. However, in the surgical treatment of PTRCTs, including arthroscopic acromioplasty and débridement, overall satisfactory (excellent or good) results ranged from 50% to 94%, with an unweighted mean of 81% and a median of 84%. Of note, the three studies with the highest percentages of satisfactory results were those in which a standard open acromioplasty was performed, often in association with tendon repair. Late outcome after open acromioplasty for stage 2 impingement recently was reported, with a mean follow-up of 9.5 years. The primary result was good, but after an average of 5 years, 12% of the shoulders deteriorated with development of a rotator cuff tear. The authors concluded that the abnormal supraspinatus tendon may tear even after the subacromial impingement is removed.

Results of another study with an arthrographic follow-up of 40 articular surface tears for approximately 2 years indicated that 10% of the tears decreased in size and 10% disappeared, but the remaining 80% of tears had enlarged or progressed to full-thickness tears. At present, if surgery is indicated for the PTRCT, the standard open anterior acromioplasty and tendon repair after excision of the diseased portion appear to be the most reliable in yielding satisfactory results.

Arthroscopy

Before the advent of arthroscopy, the treatment of PTRCTs was difficult. The diagnosis and treatment of bursal-sided tears was possible with an open procedure; however, the diagnosis and treatment of articular lesions was often problematic. As MRI and arthroscopy improved, so did the diagnosis and subsequent treatment of PTRCTs.

Because partial-thickness tears often are secondary to other conditions affecting the shoulder, an accurate diagnosis is essential. Treatment must be directed at the primary problem, such as impingement or instability. Following treatment of the primary diagnosis, the partial-thickness tear can be addressed. Arthroscopy provides visualization of both the articular and bursal surfaces as well as the ability to treat either lesion. Débridement of partial tendon tears, subacromial decompression, and rotator cuff repair can be done comfortably using arthroscopic techniques.

Arthroscopic Assessment

A thorough diagnostic examination of the glenohumeral joint is conducted to visualize the articular surface of the rotator cuff and to identify any intra-articular pathology. If a partial articular surface tear is found, a suture marker is placed through the area of the tear by using an 18-gauge spinal needle and No. 1 absorbable suture. A diagnostic bursoscopy is performed, and the suture marker is identified on the bursal surface. The extent and depth of partial tearing can be assessed further following débridement of the frayed and fragmented tissue. If there is no arthroscopic evidence of bursal or articular involvement and a preoperative MRI demonstrates intratendinous tearing, palpation of the rotator cuff with a probe can help localize the lesion. Only after completing a thorough assessment of the articular and bursal surfaces, as well as the subacromial space from both the anterior and posterior portals, can a treatment decision be made.

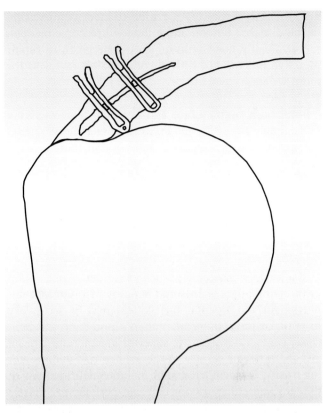

Figure 3 Depiction of the in-and-out suture by which the superficial and deep cuff layers are approximated after débridement of the inner surfaces of an intratendinous lamination.

Surgical Recommendations

Several factors must be considered when determining whether a partial tear can be treated with decompression alone or with decompression and repair, including the depth and the location of the tear, the patient's activity level, and the bony architecture of the coracoacromial arch.

The location of the partial tear dictates whether a subacromial decompression (acromioplasty) should be performed. Because bursal-sided tears almost always are associated with outlet impingement, they usually require an acromioplasty whether the tear is débrided or repaired. In situations with a flat acromion, limited bursectomy and release of the coracoacromial ligament should suffice. Articular-sided or intratendinous tears usually do not require a decompression unless there is evidence of subacromial impingement (fraying of the coracoacromial ligament, bursitis) or bony pathology (hooked acromion, anterior acromial spur, inferior acromioclavicular osteophyte).

Following decompression, the depth of the partial tear is the primary factor influencing management. Most authors agree that a tear that involves more than 50% of the thickness of the tendon should be repaired regardless of the location (bursal, articular, or intratendinous). These partial tears can be treated with excision of the diseased tendon and either arthroscopic or open repair. Finally, consideration should be given to repair in active individuals, with decompression reserved for more sedentary patients.

The ideal patient for repair is an active individual with normal bony architecture and a partial tear involving more than 50% of the tendon thickness. However, inactive patients with significant bony outlet impingement and a partial tear involving less than 50% of the tendon are good candidates for decompression and débridement. Because most patients do not fall into either of these two groups, management is best dictated by surgical experience.

A subset of articular surface tears in which the supraspinatus tendon impinges on the posterosuperior aspect of the glenoid causing an articular surface tear is found in throwing athletes. In some patients with internal impingement, the articular surface tear may be secondary to anterior instability rather than physiologic and anatomic contact between the superior glenoid and labrum and the articular surface of the rotator cuff and greater tuberosity. Surgical treatment includes débridement of the tear and either rotator cuff and periscapular muscle strengthening or anterior capsular reconstruction.

Partial Articular Supraspinatus Tendon Avulsion Lesion

A subset of partial-thickness tears is particularly amenable to arthroscopic repair. These tears are classified as either A3 or A4 according to the classification based on location and size of tear, and often represent a partial articular supraspinatus tendon avulsion (PASTA) lesion (Fig. 2). When there is at least 25% good-quality bursal tendon remaining, a transtendon arthroscopic repair is performed. The purpose of this approach is to allow preservation of any remaining good-quality tendon on the bursal surface as well as to reestablish the rotator cuff footprint at its original humeral insertion site at the articular edge.

Results

Débridement With or Without Acromioplasty
The earliest results of arthroscopic débridement of a PTRCT without subacromial decompression yielded controversial results. Satisfactory outcomes varied widely from 50% to 85%. As the ability to perform arthroscopic subacromial decompression increased, much more consistent results were obtained, and satisfactory results ranged between 75% and 86%. However, isolated articular surface tears were found to have more unsatisfactory results. This distinction between bursal and articular surface tears led to selective subacromial decompression. All bursal surface tears are treated with subacromial decompression, whereas isolated articular surface tears usually do not require decompression and can be treated with débridement alone unless there is evidence of subacromial impingement. Despite these reasonably good clinical results, débridement and/or subacromial decompression has not been shown to alter the natural history or progression of partial-thickness tears to complete tears.

Repair
The extent of partial tear involvement and the remaining tendon thickness dictate treatment and whether a repair should be performed. Repair, either arthroscopic or open, is warranted when more than 50% of the tendon thickness is involved or when there is severe degeneration. A comparison study of 65 patients with significant partial-thickness tears who were treated with either acromioplasty and débridement or acromioplasty and mini-open repair was undertaken to determine significant differences with respect to outcome. Patients with extensive tears involving more than 50% of the tendon thickness were treated with repair. The arthroscopic débridement and acromioplasty group had less postoperative pain and a faster recovery; however, improved long-term results and fewer reoperations were found in the mini-open repair group. Similar findings have been reported with open acromioplasty and open repair. Consequently, strong consideration should be given to repairing significant partial-thickness tears.

Summary

PTRCTs are commonly encountered during routine shoulder arthroscopy. Visualization of both the articular and bursal surfaces is mandatory to determine the level of rotator cuff disease and formulate a treatment strategy. Because these tears often are a secondary finding, recognition of the primary pathology is critical. Treatment of the primary problem usually remedies the partial tear. However, when there is significant partial-thickness tearing, an arthroscopic or open repair of the diseased tendon will give the most consistent results.

Annotated Bibliography

Open Surgical Techniques

Breazeale NM, Craig EV: Partial-thickness rotator cuff tears: Pathogenesis and treatment. *Orthop Clin North Am* 1997;28:145-155.

This review article addresses important aspects of the pathogenesis, imaging, and treatment of the PTRCT. A review of the relevant literature is included.

Fukuda H, Hamada K, Nakajima T, Yamada N, Tomonaga A, Goto M: Partial-thickness tears of the rotator cuff: A clinicopathological review based on 66 surgically verified cases. *Int Orthop* 1996;20:257-265.

This review article discusses 66 surgically verified PTRCTs. Satisfactory results (94%) were obtained after a combined procedure of open anterior acromioplasty and subsequent tenorrhaphy after excision of the torn portion of the tendon.

Hamada K, Fukuda H, Yamada N, Gotoh M, Yamakawa H: Management of intratendinous extension based on basic research, in Skirving AP (ed): *Shoulder Surgery: The Asian Perspective.* Perth, Australia, The Asian Shoulder Association, 1997, vol 2, pp 202-204.

Based on the presence of signal-positive cells for procollagen $\alpha 1$ type I messenger RNA in torn supraspinatus tendons, eight extensive intratendinous tears were sutured, approximating the superficial and deep layers (in-and-out suture) after débridement in between, to obtain a promising result.

Hamada K, Tomonaga A, Gotoh M, Yamakawa H, Fukuda H: Intrinsic healing capacity and tearing process of torn supraspinatus tendons: In situ hybridization study of $\alpha 1(I)$ procollagen mRNA. *J Orthop Res* 1997; 15:24-32.

In this study, in situ hybridization was used to identify cells containing $\alpha 1$ (I) procollagen messenger RNA in order to determine the healing potential and healing process of torn supraspinatus tendons. It was determined that torn supraspinatus tendons may have an intrinsic ability for healing during the intermediate/late phases of healing.

Hyvönen P, Lohi S, Jalovaara P: Open acromioplasty does not prevent the progression of an impingement syndrome to a tear: Nine-year follow-up of 96 cases. *J Bone Joint Surg Br* 1998;80:813-816.

The late outcome after open acromioplasty for stage 2 impingement was reported with a mean follow-up of 9.5 years. The abnormal supraspinatus tendon may tear even after subacromial impingement is removed.

Jobe CM: Superior glenoid impingement. *Orthop Clin North Am* 1997;28:137-143.

This article discusses superior glenoid impingement and the structures it places at risk for injury.

Arthroscopy

Fukuda H: Partial-thickness rotator cuff tears: A modern view on Codman's classic. *J Shoulder Elbow Surg* 2000;9:163-168.

This review article compares Codman's observations on PTRCTs in 1934 with a current view based on 66 surgically verified cases. It is stressed that PTRCTs deserve more attention because they are common and can be disabling.

Hertel R, Ballmer FT, Lambert SM, Gerber C: Lag signs in the diagnosis of rotator cuff rupture. *J Shoulder Elbow Surg* 1996;5:307-313.

In this prospective study, the value of lag signs was assessed in the evaluation of rotator cuff rupture in 100 consecutive painful shoulders with stage 1 to 3 impingement.

McConville OR, Iannotti JP: Partial-thickness tears of the rotator cuff: Evaluation and management. *J Am Acad Orthop Surg* 1999;7:32-43.

This is a review of the pathogenesis, diagnosis, treatment, and treatment results of PTRCTs.

Paley KJ, Jobe FW, Pink MM, Kvitne RS, ElAttrache NS: Arthroscopic findings in the overhand throwing athlete: Evidence for posterior internal impingement of the rotator cuff. *Arthroscopy* 2000;16:35-40.

Arthroscopic examination in 41 professional overhand throwing athletes demonstrated undersurface rotator cuff fraying in 93% and posterosuperior labral fraying in 88%. These findings support the concept of impingement of the posterior cuff undersurface with the posterosuperior glenoid rim.

Weber SC: Arthroscopic debridement and acromioplasty versus mini-open repair in the treatment of significant partial-thickness rotator cuff tears. *Arthroscopy* 1999;15:126-131.

A comparison between patients with significant PTRCTs treated with an acromioplasty and débridement were compared to patients treated with a mini-open repair. Functional results were significantly improved in the repair group. Healing of the partial tear never was observed.

Wright SA, Cofield RH: Management of partial-thickness rotator cuff tears. *J Shoulder Elbow Surg* 1996;5: 458-466.

Thirty-nine patients treated with acromioplasty, débridement, and open tendon suturing were followed for an average of 55 months. Twenty-three patients (59%) obtained an excellent result, 10 (26%) had a satisfactory result, and six (15%) had an unsatisfactory result.

Classic Bibliography

Altcheck DW, Warren RF, Wickiewicz TL, Skyhar MJ, Ortiz G, Schwartz E: Arthroscopic acromioplasty: Technique and results. *J Bone Joint Surg Am* 1990;72: 1198-1207.

Andrews JR, Broussard TS, Carson WG: Arthroscopy of the shoulder in the management of partial tears of the rotator cuff: A preliminary report. *Arthroscopy* 1985;1:117-122.

Codman EA (ed): *The Shoulder: Rupture of the Supraspinatus Tendon and Other Lesions in or About The Subacromial Burse.* Boston, MA, Thomas Todd, 1934.

Ellman H: Diagnosis and treatment of incomplete rotator cuff tears. *Clin Orthop* 1990;254:64-74.

Esch JC, Ozerkis LR, Helgager JA, Kane N, Lilliott N: Arthroscopic subacromial decompression: Results according to the degree of rotator cuff tear. *Arthroscopy* 1988; 4:241-249.

Fukuda H, Hamada K, Nakajima T, Tomonaga A: Pathology and pathogenesis of the intratendinous tearing of the rotator cuff viewed from en bloc histologic sections. *Clin Orthop* 1994;304:60-67.

Fukuda H, Hamada K, Yamanaka K: Pathology and pathogenesis of bursal-side rotator cuff tears viewed from en bloc histologic sections. *Clin Orthop* 1990; 254:75-80.

Fukuda H, Mikasa M, Ogawa K, Yamanaka K, Hamada K: "The color test": An intraoperative staining test for joint-side rotator cuff tearing and its extension. *J Shoulder Elbow Surg* 1992;1:86-90.

Gartsman GM: Arthroscopic acromioplasty for lesions of the rotator cuff. *J Bone Joint Surg Am* 1990;72: 169-180.

Gartsman GM, Milne JC: Articular surface partial-thickness rotator cuff tears. *J Shoulder Elbow Surg* 1995; 4:409-415.

Hodler J, Kursunoglu-Brahme S, Snyder SJ, et al: Rotator cuff disease: Assessment with MR arthrography versus standard MR imaging in 36 patients with arthroscopic confirmation. *Radiology* 1992;182:431-436.

Itoi E, Tabata S: Incomplete rotator cuff tears: Results of operative treatment. *Clin Orthop* 1992;284:128-135.

Lohr JF, Uhthoff HK: The microvascular pattern of the supraspinatus tendon. *Clin Orthop* 1990;254:35-38.

Nakajima T, Rokuuma N, Hamada K, Tomatsu T, Fukuda H: Histologic and biomechanical characteristics of the supraspinatus tendon: reference to rotator cuff tearing. *J Shoulder Elbow Surg* 1994;3:79-87.

Neer CS II: Anterior acromioplasty for the chronic impingement syndrome in the shoulder: A preliminary report. *J Bone Joint Surg Am* 1972;54:41-50.

Ogilvie-Harris DJ, Wiley AM: Arthroscopic surgery of the shoulder: A general appraisal. *J Bone Joint Surg Br* 1986;68:201-207.

Roye RP, Grana WA, Yates CK: Arthroscopic subacromial decompression: Two- to seven-year follow-up. *Arthroscopy* 1995;11:301-306.

Snyder SJ, Pachelli AF, Del Pizzo W, Friedman MJ, Ferkel RD, Pattee G: Partial thickness rotator cuff tears: Results of arthroscopic treatment. *Arthroscopy* 1991; 7:1-7.

Tabata S, Sano H, Itoi E: Treatment of partial-thickness tears of the rotator cuff, in Wu JJ, Fukuda H, Shih L-Y, Chan KM, Soong TH (eds): *Shoulder Surgery: The Asian Perspective.* Taipei, Taiwan, Orthopaedics Department Veterans General Hospital, 1995, pp 193-195.

Walch G, Boileau P, Noel E, Donell ST: Impingement of the deep surface of the supraspinatus tendon on the posterosuperior glenoid rim: An arthroscopic study. *J Shoulder Elbow Surg* 1992;1:238-245.

Yamanaka K, Matsumoto T: The joint side tear of the rotator cuff: A follow-up study by arthrography. *Clin Orthop* 1994;304:68-73.

Chapter 16

Surgical Treatment of Full-Thickness Tears

Robert H. Cofield, MD

Gary M. Gartsman, MD

Introduction

The supraspinatus tendon is found in the rotator cuff and is the tendon most commonly torn in humans. Repair of rotator cuff tears is one of the most frequently performed musculoskeletal surgical procedures. The rate at which open surgery of these tears is performed varies considerably in different geographic locations and appears to be unrelated to the size of the physician workforce. In addition, the role of arthroscopy in the management of rotator cuff lesions is evolving. In the last decade, shoulder arthroscopy has advanced from its use as a diagnostic tool to an effective treatment option for stage 2 impingement and acromioclavicular joint arthritis. Arthroscopic decompression also has been described in the management of more severe rotator cuff lesions such as partial-thickness tears. Recently, repair of full-thickness rotator cuff tears using arthroscopic techniques has been described. The advantages of arthroscopic repair include smaller skin incisions, glenohumeral joint inspection, treatment of intra-articular lesions, no deltoid detachment, less soft-tissue dissection, less pain, and more rapid rehabilitation.

Open Surgery

Indications

Recent reports on indications for surgery have focused on selected subgroups or factors associated with rotator cuff tears. In people younger than age 40 years who have rotator cuff tears, an acute injury often is involved. The results of surgical repair can be quite good, but the procedure is not as dramatically effective as it is in older patients. Surgical repair of rotator cuff tears in the elderly can be very effective, even in patients with larger tears.

Rotator cuff tears can occur in association with primary anterior shoulder dislocation. The frequency of these tears increases dramatically with age and is more pronounced in women. The tearing in and of itself can engender shoulder instability.

Injuries associated with the typical supraspinatus tendon tear can include traumatic tears of the rotator interval (either in association with other tears or alone) or subtle subscapularis tears. Subscapularis tears often are associated with abnormalities of the long head of the biceps, including instability of this tendon with medial displacement into the joint.

Some attention, particularly in Europe, has been directed to CT and MRI of the rotator cuff muscles, assessing for fatty infiltration, atrophy, and cross-sectional area (MRI). Extreme atrophy (or fatty infiltration) may discourage surgical repair of the corresponding tendon.

The surgeon must look for associated infraclavicular brachial plexus injuries or cervical radiculopathies that may coexist with rotator cuff tears. Treatment of the nerve injury also may be necessary to avoid an unexpectedly poor result.

Surgical Exposure

The anterosuperior exposure continues to be favored for open surgery. Some surgeons prefer deltoid splitting distal to the acromioclavicular joint; others prefer to perform the split at the anterolateral corner of the shoulder between the anterior and middle segments of the deltoid muscle (Fig. 1). If the deltoid muscle is detached from its origin, a common component of exposure, the detachment is along the anterior aspect of the acromion and typically extends for a distance of approximately 2 cm. In selected cases of subscapularis tearing, the preferable approach would be through the deltopectoral interval to facilitate safe dissection beneath the conjoined tendon group. The skin incision in this situation should be positioned so that it can be extended superiorly to incorporate a deltoid split if surgery on the superior aspect of the shoulder is contemplated.

Acromion

Further study of the mechanical environment of the subacromial space has reaffirmed that with impingement,

A

B

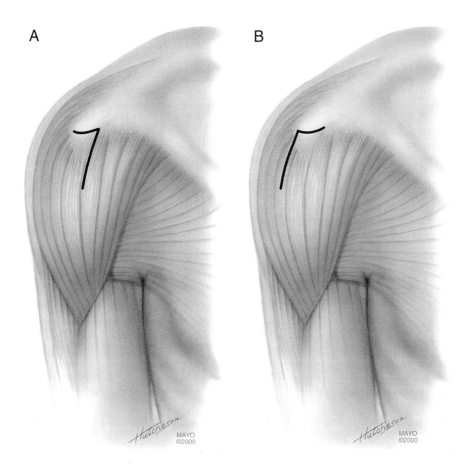

Figure 1 A, Traditional method of exposure through the deltoid muscle for rotator cuff repair. The deltoid muscle and fascia are carefully incised for 2 cm on the anterior aspect of the acromion and split distally from the acromioclavicular joint for 4 cm. **B,** More recently, some surgeons have preferred a similar detachment of fascial tissue from the anterior aspect of the acromion but with a split of the deltoid for 4 cm along the anterolateral corner of the acromion between the anterior and middle portions of the deltoid muscle. *(Reproduced with permission from the Mayo Foundation, Rochester, Minnesota.)*

high stresses are created in and around the critical zone. These stresses may occur on the bursal surface, the articular surface, or within the tendon itself. Acromia are classified into three types: type I (flat), type II (curved), and type III (hooked). During further study of this classification, some investigators have found it difficult to consistently categorize each acromion, either on repeated evaluations by the same observer or among different observers. This finding indicates that less diagnostic relevance should be placed on the assessment of acromial morphology and more on the clinical picture and the state of the rotator cuff tendons. MRI offers little additional information about the basic acromial shape. However, it can define certain additional structural arrangements, such as an acromial angle, which measures the amount of curvature, or a lateral acromial angle, which evaluates the tipping of the acromion relative to the face of the glenoid. Both of these angles have an association with rotator cuff disease.

Shaving the undersurface of the anteroinferior acromion, as suggested by Neer, continues to be standard. This procedure renders a slightly curved or hooked undersurface of the acromion flat in reference to the slope of the posteroinferior aspect of the acromion (Fig. 2). A few surgeons have suggested an additional vertical osteotomy to remove the part of the acromion

that protrudes anterior to the clavicle, while others have suggested avoiding acromioplasty if the tear is large to massive and anterosuperior subluxation would be likely in the postoperative period.

Os acromiale may occur more frequently than has been suspected. It is most readily diagnosed on an axillary radiograph. When an os acromiale occurs at the preacromion site, this small fragment can be excised at the time of rotator cuff surgery. When it occurs at the mesoacromion or meta-acromion site, internal fixation with cannulated screws, tension band wiring, and autogenous bone grafting generally are recommended to ensure a superior result. With these techniques the fusion rate is quite high. Some patients have experienced continually painful and weak shoulders following excision of larger fragments.

When an anteroinferior acromioplasty is performed, the coracoacromial ligament is released, and often a segment of the ligament is resected. Little additional support has appeared in the literature for repair of the ligament following acromioplasty.

Distal Clavicle

No difference in acromioclavicular joint position has been identified in patients with or without rotator cuff tears, and there is no difference in the presence or absence of joint space narrowing. However, patients with rotator cuff tears have larger and more osteophytic reaction about the joint. Some surgeons never excise the distal clavicle when performing rotator cuff repair but bevel the undersurface of the joint to open the supraspinatus outlet; others always excise the distal clavicle. However, most surgeons seem to be selective, excising the distal clavicle when some component of the preoperative pain is localized to the acromioclavicular joint, there is tenderness over the joint, and there are radiographic changes of degenerative arthritis. In addition, some surgeons require that shoulder pain be relieved with an injection before the distal clavicle is excised in conjunction with rotator cuff repair.

When distal clavicle excision is performed in symptomatic individuals with demonstrated structural changes, the exposure is as shown in Figure 3. The incision of the deltoid origin from the anterior aspect of the acromion is extended medially over the anterosuperior aspect of the acromioclavicular joint to the superior aspect of the distal clavicle between the trapezius and deltoid muscles. The deltoid muscle is elevated from the anterior aspect of the distal clavicle. The trapezius fascia and muscle are left in continuity. The distal 1.0 to 1.2 cm of the clavicle is resected, leaving not only the trapezius fascia and muscle intact but also the ligamentous tissue across the posterior aspect of the resected area, connecting the posterior aspect of the acromioclavicular joint and the remaining distal clavicle. Larger amounts of resection have been associated with poorer outcomes. The incised deltoid muscle is then advanced into the resected area, suturing it to the trapezius.

Subacromial/Subdeltoid Bursa

Localized bursal reaction is associated with rotator cuff tears. The tissue changes include formation of perivascular new collagen and predominantly type III collagen. The abnormal bursa should be excised to facilitate appropriate observation of the tendon tear and to eliminate the subacromial impingement that has occurred from the hypertrophy of this tissue. Additional bursal excision seems unnecessary and undesirable.

Long Head of the Biceps Tendon

Additional mechanical study of this tendon has shown that there is increased translation of the humeral head in abduction after loss of the long head of the biceps tendon. This study also has shown that the long head of the biceps tendon is an active depressor of the humeral head in shoulders with lesions of the rotator cuff. Therefore, tenodesis of the long head of the biceps tendon is performed only if the tendon is unstable (ie, dislocated medially) or if a substantial portion of the tendon has undergone attritional changes. Involvement of at least 50% of the tendon width has been suggested as an indi-

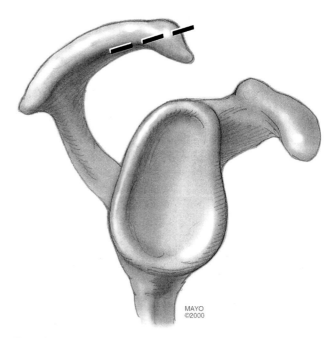

Figure 2 A lateral view of the anteroinferior acromioplasty with the osteotomy beginning about two thirds of the way from the inferior to the superior aspect of the anterior acromion and extending posteroinferiorly to the mid segment of the acromion. This creates a flat undersurface of the acromion, eliminating the anteroinferior curvature or hook formation. *(Reproduced with permission from the Mayo Foundation, Rochester, Minnesota.)*

cation for tenodesis of the long head of the biceps tendon in conjunction with rotator cuff repair.

Tendon Repair

Tendon mobilization may include capsulotomy proximal to the tear outside the labrum-biceps anchor complex. This procedure is performed in addition to freeing the tendon from scarred bursa and contracture around the base of the coracoid.

Recently, less attention has been directed toward augmenting tendon healing than toward assessing the mechanical strength of tendon fixation, with attention to the tendon, suture, and bone links of the repair. The most typical suture suggested has been of the horizontal mattress type. Authors of one study suggested that simple sutures may be better in certain circumstances, and authors of another study indicated quite clearly that a more complex suture-grasping technique would improve the strength of the interface between the rotator cuff tendon and the suture. The Mason-Allen configuration of suturing has been suggested. Although longer-lasting resorbable suture material has been advocated by some surgeons, most seem to favor nonabsorbable suture material. Larger suture sizes also are favored, ranging from 0 to No. 3. The technique of forming a deep trough in the humeral head is being replaced in favor of forming a shallow trough (5 mm or less) or no trough at all. The usual area of tendon insertion of fibrous tissue and fibrocartilage is cleared, exposing a mixture of cortical and firm subcortical cancellous bone

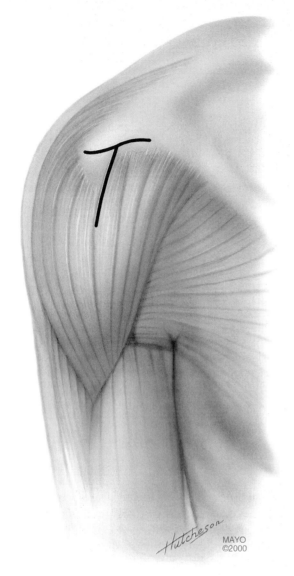

Figure 3 Exposure for distal clavicle resection in conjunction with rotator cuff repair. *(Reproduced with permission from the Mayo Foundation, Rochester, Minnesota.)*

(Fig. 4). For transosseous sutures, fixation strength will be increased with suturing sites approximately 1 cm distal to the tip of the greater tuberosity and creation of a slightly wider bony bridge (approximately 1 cm) between suture exit sites. Metallic or other suture anchors can be equivalent in fixation strength to conventional transosseous attachments, and in certain circumstances, such as in mechanical testing with cyclic loading, the anchors may be somewhat better. Strength of fixation can vary significantly among anchoring devices. Whatever bony fixation method is selected, the surgeon should be aware that early active mobilization and use of the limb must be avoided because the strength of any type of fixation is much less than that required for arm use.

In positioning the rotator cuff tendon for repair, the tension of the repair should, in general, be similar to the tension in adjacent, untorn, rotator cuff tissue. Passive tension by lateral traction may be increased with certain repair techniques, and this increase may result in incomplete restoration of muscle contractile properties. It is possible to advance the attachment medially somewhat without impairing the moment arm of the supraspinatus tendon. Satisfactory results have been achieved with tendon advancement of 3 mm and 10 mm; with 17 mm of medial advancement of the tendon, a significant reduction in the supraspinatus moment arm occurs.

Subscapularis transfer as an adjunct to rotator cuff repair may be useful in special circumstances; however, this procedure should be used cautiously in patients with full preoperative elevation because of the risk of adversely affecting postoperative elevation should the transfer not heal well. Similarly, patients with ample active range of motion before surgery may lose active motion after surgery if there is excessive mobilization of the adjacent muscle-tendon units, including detaching and repositioning of the remaining insertion of the infraspinatus tendon.

Postoperative Support and Rehabilitation

In the postoperative period, the limb cannot go unprotected because of the vast difference between the security of the tendon repair and the forces about the shoulder required for typical daily activities. A shoulder immobilizer or sling is suggested following most repairs, with the use of a splint in perhaps 25% or fewer of patients. A splint typically is believed to be most useful when the quality of the tendon tissues is compromised by degenerative changes or when the repair is mainly posterosuperior and stretching it by internal rotation is not desirable.

Early passive range of motion within safe limits determined at surgery seems to be the standard, with therapy beginning within the first days after surgery. An active motion program should not be initiated for 5 to 8 weeks. Training someone to assist the patient with a home program of passive motion exercises has been found to be as safe and effective as using a physical therapist-supervised program. The least amount of muscle activity as measured using electromyography occurs with Codman exercises, assisted passive motion exercises, and a continuous passive motion machine. More activity occurs with wand-assisted motion exercises, and even more activity occurs in the muscles about the shoulder with pulley exercises. Patient outcomes after use of the usual physical therapy programs do not differ from outcomes after the use of a continuous passive motion machine for 4 weeks. Pain and disability, range of motion, and later isometric strength are the same with both treatments. The cost is somewhat increased with use of a passive motion machine. Typically, strengthening exercises are delayed for 8 to 12 weeks following surgery.

Results and Factors Affecting Outcome

Results of clinical series indicate that results are excellent or good in more than 85% of patients and less than 95% of patients. Preoperative tear size is the dominant feature in determining the eventual outcome. In general, shoulders that have undergone rotator cuff repair have good results but they do exhibit a slight decrease in strength and range of motion. Again, recovery of strength is related to tear size, with average return of strength varying between 85% and 90% of the opposite normal shoulder for flexion, abduction, and external rotation. The return of strength is less consistent with larger tear sizes.

Postoperative MRI can be used to predict results. In one study, approximately 50% of the tendons were continuous and thick, 25% were continuous and thin, and somewhat less than 25% of the tendons exhibited some retearing. Often, the tearing was smaller than that seen on the original MRI or at surgery. Even with retearing, most patients will have a satisfactory outcome with a reduction in pain and improvement in active movement and strength.

Patient series that included only massive rotator cuff tears again illustrate the generally satisfactory nature of this procedure. Patients had a reduction in pain, an average improvement in active movement, and improvement in strength over a period of time of more than 1 year.

Patients with isolated subscapularis tears also can have good results; however, results are better with a shorter delay between injury and surgical treatment. In some series, patients with workers' compensation benefits have worse results, whereas in others, workers' compensation has no effect on patient outcome.

Questionnaires assessing general health status indicate reliable and significant improvement following rotator cuff repair. Patients surveyed by telephone respond somewhat more favorably than those surveyed by mail. Patients lost to follow-up may not be doing as well as those who have responded to the typical follow-up mechanisms.

Complications and Reoperations

Failure of tendon healing is the substantial postoperative problem; other complications, including stiffness, are much more rare. Arthrocutaneous fistulas can develop after rotator cuff repair; development often is associated with some degree of deltoid avulsion. Early débridement and deltoid reattachment are suggested.

Infection occurs in less than 1% of patients. This infection can be related to *Staphylococcus aureus* but most often is associated with less virulent organisms, such as

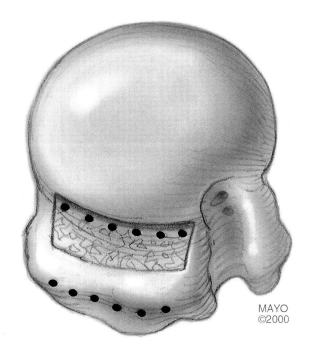

Figure 4 Preparation of the humeral bed for rotator cuff tendon attachment. An area approximately 1 cm wide from lateral to medial is exposed on the humeral head near the usual tendon insertion site. The area is cleaned of soft tissue, and the cortical bone is partially removed to expose a mixture of cortical and firm subcortical cancellous bone. Formation of a bony trough is not necessary. Transosseous sutures are placed 8 to 10 mm lateral and distal to the exposed attachment area, and connecting holes are prepared along the medial aspect of the bed for tendon attachment. *(Reproduced with permission from the Mayo Foundation, Rochester, Minnesota.)*

Propionibacterium, coagulase negative *Staphylococcus*, or *Peptostreptococcus*. In addition to antibiotics, treatment includes débridement, deltoid repair, rotator cuff repair as possible, and physiotherapy. In spite of the infection, the outcome will be good or excellent in 33% of affected patients, fair in 33%, and poor in 33%.

The incidence of iatrogenic suprascapular nerve injury is low but does occur on occasion. Clinically significant postoperative deltoid detachment is uncommon; it usually can be avoided by careful reattachment of the deltoid through bone, avoidance of lateral acromioplasty, avoidance of detachment of the middle deltoid, and detachment of the anterior deltoid over an area less than 2 cm in length (Fig. 5).

Should symptoms persist following surgical repair and rehabilitation, MRI is valuable for diagnosis but may be compromised by the presence of confusing scar tissue or metal artifacts.

Arthroscopy

Preoperative Evaluation

A complete patient history and physical examination of the upper extremity and cervical spine is vital. Elements in the patient's history are reviewed for indications as to the

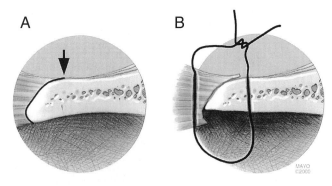

Figure 5 During detachment of the deltoid from the anterior acromion, careful attention is paid to removing all the fascia with the thin slip of deltoid muscle that is released. This is then reattached to bone through the anterior aspect of the acromion. **A,** The arrow indicates the initiation point for incision of the deltoid from the bone. The incision continues anteriorly along the acromion. **B,** The position of suture placement is shown. The suture is placed in the acromion using a trochar needle. It is then placed through the deltoid, incorporating the deep and superficial fascial layers. *(Reproduced with permission from the Mayo Foundation, Rochester, Minnesota.)*

etiology of the cuff tear. Most lesions are secondary to the impingement process but partial- and full-thickness rotator cuff tears also can be found in patients with glenohumeral instability or an episode of macrotrauma. The patient's desired activity level should also be noted.

AP, axillary, and scapular outlet radiographic views are obtained and examined for the presence of anterior acromial sclerosis, anterior acromial osteophytes, and acromial shape. MRI studies provide additional data on the location and extent of the tendon lesion. Gadolinium contrast is a helpful addition to MRI in the younger athletic individual in whom the possibility of labral or ligamentous damage exists.

Indications

The indications for arthroscopic rotator cuff repair are identical to those for an open repair and should not in any way be altered or broadened in the mistaken belief that arthroscopic repair is a lesser procedure. Although the skin incisions may be smaller and the deltoid is left attached, all elements of an open repair are performed arthroscopically. Patients who are unable to tolerate either the surgery or postoperative rehabilitation of an open procedure are not candidates for an arthroscopic rotator cuff repair. Surgery is performed for persistent pain interfering with activities of daily living, work, or sports that is unresponsive to a 6- to 12-month period of nonsurgical care.

Surgical Technique

Glenohumeral Joint

Although traditional open surgical methods have a documented history of success in the management of rotator cuff tears, not all patients respond successfully. It is possible that untreated intra-articular glenohumeral joint lesions may account for some of the poor results after open rotator cuff repair.

A clear advantage of arthroscopy is that the glenohumeral joint is well visualized and intra-articular lesions that were not seen with an open repair technique can now be diagnosed and treated. These intra-articular findings include partial rotator cuff tears, labrum tears, ligament damage, and cartilage lesions.

Glenohumeral joint abnormalities are common in patients with complete rotator cuff tears, but most of the abnormalities are minor. Lesions are considered significant if they (1) require surgical treatment, (2) change the postoperative rehabilitation, or (3) alter the expected goals of the procedure. Significant lesions are found in only 12.5% of patients (25 of 200).

Treatment of the intra-articular lesion can improve the final outcome. Patients with full-thickness rotator cuff tears undergoing arthroscopic repair were analyzed using the University of California at Los Angeles (UCLA) scale, which measures shoulder outcomes. Mean preoperative scores were 23.7 for the normal group (without intra-articular lesions) and 10.9 for the group with a major glenohumeral lesion. Postoperative UCLA scores were 31.2 for the normal group and 29.9 for the group with a major glenohumeral lesion, differences that are not statistically significant ($P = 0.23$). The comparison indicates that identification and treatment of intra-articular lesions resulted in these patients achieving results comparable to those of patients without intra-articular lesions.

Subacromial Space

Tear Classification The arthroscope is inserted into the subacromial space immediately beneath the acromion and then rotated so that it is pointed directly down at the rotator cuff tear. With small to medium tears, the size geometry of the tear is easily perceived. The length of the tear from anterior to posterior and the amount of medial retraction are noted. Straight medial retraction or retraction in an elliptical shape are the most common findings. As tear size increases, the surgeon's ability to perceive tear geometry becomes more difficult. Reverse L-shaped tears with a longitudinal component along the rotator interval will allow the tear to rotate posteriorly. L-shaped tears have a longitudinal limb posteriorly, often at the junction of the supraspinatus and infraspinatus in addition to the lateral detachment at the greater tuberosity. V-shaped tears with their apex pointed medially have the longitudinal component in addition to a lateral detachment. Only when tear geometry is perceived can the surgeon perform an effective repair.

One technique to help the surgeon determine tear geometry is to pull on the tear edge with a grasper in an attempt to determine its anatomic location. The surgeon should pull on the tendon edge while varying elevation and rotation until a best fit is obtained. A mechanical arm holder is then secured to maintain the arm position.

Acromioplasty If the tear is reparable, the surgeon should then evaluate the acromion. The purpose of acromioplasty is to create adequate space for the rotator cuff tendons. In classic rotator cuff tears, the anterolateral acromion is part of the impingement process, and the surgeon need not be concerned as to whether the acromial spur caused or was a result of the cuff tear. If the spur compromises the space for the cuff or if there is clear evidence of impingement (coracoacromial ligament or acromial undersurface fraying), the surgeon may perform an acromioplasty. As the thickness and shape of the acromion varies, the amount of bone removed during acromioplasty also varies. If the acromion is flat and there is adequate space for the cuff, then acromioplasty is not performed.

Acromioclavicular Joint Inferior AC joint osteophytes are removed if necessary, as determined by preoperative radiograph or inspection at the time of surgery. The AC joint is removed only for preoperative symptoms of pain localized to it and for AC joint tenderness on physical examination.

Repair Site Preparation Most surgeons do not advocate creation of a bone trough. Simple decortication with a power burr is all that is necessary. The area of bone preparation corresponds to the anterior to posterior margins of the tear. It extends from a point immediately lateral to the articular surface of the humeral head to the greater tuberosity.

Anchor Placement The number of anchors depends on the length of the rotator cuff tear and whether the anchor is loaded with one or two sutures. Tears involving two or more tendons generally require three to four anchors. Some surgeons place the anchors just lateral to the articular margin of the humeral head and place the anchor directly through the tendon. Others place the anchors lateral to the greater tuberosity for the following reasons: (1) The anchor is placed in bone with an intact cortical surface instead of in the prepared bed of the repair site. (2) Lateral placement allows the anchors to be positioned so that the line of tendon pull is 90° to the direction of the anchor, which minimizes anchor pullout. (3) The tendon is repaired anatomically. As the anchors are moved medially onto the superior surface of the tuberosity, the tendon-healing site also is moved medially.

The anchors are placed proportionally along the length of the greater tuberosity corresponding to the length of the torn tendon, beginning anteriorly approximately 1 cm posterior to the bicipital groove and pro-

ceeding posteriorly. The anchors are placed through the lateral cannula and their sutures withdrawn out the anterior cannula with a crochet hook. The arm is gradually internally rotated to allow anchor insertion posteriorly. All anchors are placed in the bone before any tendon suturing starts.

Suture Placement Once the suture anchors have been placed, the braided sutures must be passed through the torn tendon. The soft-tissue grasper is passed through the lateral cannula, and the precise location for the tendon repair, as well as the location and spacing of each suture, is estimated. The sutures should be evenly spaced from the anterior tendon edge to its posterior margin. The sutures are placed approximately 5 mm from the tendon edge.

If the tear is transverse, all sutures may be placed the same distance from the tendon edge and the full length of the tear repaired anatomically to its insertion site on the greater tuberosity. As the tear becomes more elliptical, some adjustments are needed. The central portion of the tear is retracted more than the anterior and posterior margins, and attempts to repair the central portion anatomically may result in failure because the central portion of the tendon may be permanently shortened. In this situation, the surgeon may elect to repair the anterior and posterior margins anatomically and repair the central portion more medially.

Other Lesions

Teres minor lesions are well visualized and are repaired with the technique described above, but the anchors usually must be inserted through a separate posterolateral incision. Subscapularis tears that are limited to the superior 25% may be repaired arthroscopically after the arm is elevated and externally rotated. Full-thickness subscapularis tears are repaired through a separate anterior open deltopectoral approach. Biceps subluxation or dislocation occurs medially through a tear of the superior subscapularis and is stabilized by arthroscopic subscapularis repair. Partial biceps tendon tears greater than 50% are tenodesed arthroscopically.

Postoperative Management

A sling maintains the arm in 15° of abduction, and an ice pack wrap decreases swelling and pain in the shoulder. Passive motions in elevation and external rotation are started the afternoon of surgery and continue at home for 6 weeks. At 6 weeks, patients begin active range-of-motion exercises and continue until week 12, when strengthening is begun. Muscles strengthened with rubber tubing include the deltoid, infraspinatus, supraspinatus, scapular rotators, and biceps. Patients continue range-of-motion and strengthening exercises for 1 year.

Results

The results of arthroscopic repair of full-thickness rotator cuff tears are satisfactory and equal the results reported from open repair. According to one study, at final evaluation, 90% of patients rated their satisfaction with the shoulder as good to excellent. Postoperative pain relief was self-assessed as good to excellent in 78% of patients. Shoulder function was improved in all 10 areas of the American Shoulder and Elbow Surgeons' activities of daily living functional evaluation, and 90% assessed shoulder function as good to excellent. Patients were particularly pleased with the improved ability to sleep comfortably. Active range of motion was improved in all measured planes with a preoperative mean constant motion score of 27.2 (out of a possible 40) and a postoperative score of 37.9. Strength improved from 7.5 lb preoperatively to 14.0 lb postoperatively. Patient self-assessed levels of general health were improved in all scales and summary measures of the SF-36 Health Survey with the exception of General Health and the Mental Component Summary.

Annotated Bibliography

Open Surgery

Gartsman GM, Taverna E: The incidence of glenohumeral joint abnormalities associated with full-thickness, reparable rotator cuff tears. *Arthroscopy* 1997;13:450-455.

This article describes the type and incidence of glenohumeral joint lesions found in patients with full-thickness rotator cuff tears.

Gerber C, Hersche O, Farron A: Isolated rupture of the subscapularis tendon. *J Bone Joint Surg Am* 1996;98:1015-1023.

In this study of 16 consecutive mostly middle-aged male patients with an isolated rupture of the subscapularis tendon, surgical repair afforded good results. Results were better when there was only a short delay between injury and surgery.

Hersche O, Gerber C: Passive tension in the supraspinatus musculotendinous unit after long-standing rupture of its tendon: A preliminary report. *J Shoulder Elbow Surg* 1998;7:393-396.

The authors remind surgeons to attempt to restore near-normal length at the time of surgical repair of supraspinatus musculotendinous unit so that active force generation by this muscle is minimally compromised.

Iannotti JP, Bernot MP, Kuhlman JR, Kelley MJ, Williams GR: Postoperative assessment of shoulder function: A prospective study of full-thickness rotator cuff tears. *J Shoulder Elbow Surg* 1996;5:449-457.

This contemporary analysis of surgical results clearly demonstrates the value of rotator cuff repair to patients. The size of the rotator cuff tear is the dominant determinant of outcome.

Jost B, Pfirrmann CW, Gerber C: Clinical outcome after structural failure of rotator cuff repairs. *J Bone Joint Surg Am* 2000;82:304-314.

Even after structural failure of the rotator cuff repair, pain can be reduced, and active elevation and strength can be improved. Often, the remaining tear is smaller than the initial one.

Kronberg M, Wahlstrom P, Brostrom LA: Shoulder function after surgical repair of rotator cuff tears. *J Shoulder Elbow Surg* 1997;6:125-130.

Authors of this contemporary assessment of the outcome of rotator cuff repair conclude that there is substantial improvement after surgery, but a slight decrease in range of motion and muscle strength will remain.

Luo ZP, Hsu HC, Grabowski JJ, Morrey BF, An KN: Mechanical environment associated with rotator cuff tears. *J Shoulder Elbow Surg* 1998;7:616-620.

The authors present a two-dimensional finite element model demonstrating that subacromial impingement causes high stresses in the usual critical zone on the bursal side, the articular side, and within the rotator cuff tendon.

Mansat P, Cofield RH, Kersten TE, Rowland CM: Complications of rotator cuff repair. *Orthop Clin North Am* 1997;28:205-213.

This article is the first comprehensive review on this subject. Failure of tendon healing dominates; all other complications are infrequent.

Rokito AS, Cuomo F, Gallagher MA, Zuckerman JD: Long-term functional outcome of repair of large and massive chronic tears of the rotator cuff. *J Bone Joint Surg Am* 1999;81:991-997.

The authors document effective surgical outcome following repair of massive tears, with patient satisfaction and increase in strength and range of motion, improvement in function, and reduction in pain. Strength is slow to return but can, on average, approach 80% of normal.

Sher JS, Iannotti JP, Warner JJ, Groff Y, Williams GR: Surgical treatment of postoperative deltoid origin disruption. *Clin Orthop* 1997;343:93-98.

This uncommon but significant problem is outlined. Poorer outcomes are associated with prior lateral acromionectomy, involvement of the middle deltoid, a massive rotator cuff tear, and a residual deltoid defect larger than 2 cm.

Thomazeau H, Boukobza E, Morcet N, Chaperon J, Langlais F: Prediction of rotator cuff repair results by magnetic resonance imaging. *Clin Orthop* 1997;344: 275-283.

In this study, preoperative MRI findings correlate strongly with clinical outcome. Healing of the tendon repair is very important.

Worland RL, Arredondo J, Angles F, Lopez-Jimenez F: Repair of massive rotator cuff tears in patients older than 70 years. *J Shoulder Elbow Surg* 1999;8:26-30.

This is one of several recent articles that indicate that age and tear size are not an absolute contraindication to surgical repair. Good results can be achieved in many patients with surgical repair of the rotator cuff tendons.

Arthroscopy

Burkhart SS, Johnson TC, Wirth MA, Athanasiou KA: Cyclic loading of transosseous rotator cuff repairs: Tension overload as a possible cause of failure. *Arthroscopy* 1997;13:172-176.

This is one of a series of articles describing the most recent concepts of rotator cuff tendon tear and repair.

Craft DV, Moseley JB, Cawley PW, Noble PC: Fixation strength of rotator cuff repairs with suture anchors and transosseous suture technique. *J Shoulder Elbow Surg* 1996;5:32-40.

This study compared fixation strength with a variety of mechanical anchors and the traditional bone tunnel technique. Suture anchor design has improved to the point where fixation is equivalent to the more traditional bone tunnel technique.

Gartsman GM: Arthroscopic assessment of rotator cuff tear reparability. *Arthroscopy* 1996;12:546-549.

This article describes the accuracy of arthroscopic assessment of rotator cuff tear size when compared to open techniques.

Gartsman GM, Brinker MR, Khan M: Early effectiveness of arthroscopic repair for full-thickness tears of the rotator cuff: An outcome analysis. *J Bone Joint Surg Am* 1998;80:33-40.

This article describes the effectiveness of arthroscopic rotator cuff repair as measured by the SF-36.

Gartsman GM, Hammerman SM: Arthroscopic biceps tenodesis: Operative technique. *Arthroscopy* 2000;16: 550-552.

This is a description of technique for arthroscopic biceps tenodesis.

Gartsman GM, Hammerman SM: Arthroscopic rotator cuff repair, in Warren RF (ed): *Techniques in Shoulder and Elbow Surgery*. Philadelphia, PA, Lippincott Williams & Wilkins, 2000, pp 2-8.

This is the most current and complete description of the surgical technique for arthroscopic repair.

Gartsman GM, Khan M, Hammerman SM: Arthroscopic repair of full-thickness tears of the rotator cuff. *J Bone Joint Surg Am* 1998;80:832-840.

This article describes patient population and results of rotator cuff repair with arthroscopic technique.

Classic Bibliography

Gerber C, Schneeberger AG, Beck M, Schlegel U: Mechanical strength of repairs of the rotator cuff. *J Bone Joint Surg Br* 1994;76:371-380.

Neer CS II: Anterior acromioplasty for the chronic impingement syndrome in the shoulder: A preliminary report. *J Bone Joint Surg Am* 1972;54:41-50.

Chapter 17

Complications of Rotator Cuff Surgery

Brian S. Cohen, MD

Armodios M. Hatzidakis, MD

Anthony A. Romeo, MD

Introduction

Continued shoulder pain and debility are disappointing, yet not uncommon, complications of rotator cuff (RC) surgery. Persistent pain and decreased function are general conditions that can be attributed to discrete and identifiable factors, such as an incorrect or incomplete diagnosis, surgical technical errors, or inappropriate rehabilitation, that can be traced to the surgeon. The causes of complications such as postoperative infection and reflex sympathetic dystrophy cannot be completely controlled by the surgeon. The focus of this chapter is to identify the complications that can occur following RC surgery and their causes and discuss how these complications can be minimized by good surgical decision making, technique, and patient counseling before and after surgery.

Incorrect or Incomplete Diagnosis

Continued pain and debility can occur even after the most technically satisfying, tension-free RC repair, especially if concomitant conditions are not identified. The surgeon must make a complete and correct diagnosis to maximize the chances of postoperative success. Conditions associated or confused with RC disease include cervical spine disease, suprascapular neuropathy, axillary neuropathy, thoracic outlet syndrome, acromioclavicular (AC) joint pathology, biceps tendinopathy, glenohumeral instability, glenohumeral arthritis, labral tears, and adhesive capsulitis. Any of these conditions may actually be the prime cause of the patient's shoulder pain or a secondary cause that can result in persistent pain even after successful RC repair. A complete history and physical examination must be performed to identify signs and symptoms of these associated conditions as well as those of RC tear. When the examination is supplemented by plain radiographs and specialized imaging, such as MRI, associated conditions can be addressed before or during surgery to prevent persistent postoperative pain and debility.

Neurologic Diagnoses

Pain referred to the shoulder is sometimes related to a pathologic condition of the cervical spine such as cervical disk disease, facet disease, or arthritis. A complete examination of the neck must be performed before any shoulder surgery is performed. Range of motion of the neck, Spurling's maneuver, and a complete neurologic history and examination of the involved upper extremity must be performed in every patient with shoulder pain. If cervical pathology seems to be the prime cause of an individual's shoulder pain, the patient should be referred to an appropriate specialist for evaluation and treatment. If cervical spine disease is an important secondary cause of the patient's pain, the surgeon must communicate with the specialist to formulate an effective surgical plan.

Shoulder pain secondary to suprascapular nerve entrapment usually has a different history than that of an RC tear. Suprascapular neuropathy is more common in younger patients who participate in sports that require raising the arms overhead and who have had limited trauma to their shoulder. These patients are unlikely to have a large RC tear. If suprascapular neuropathy is suspected, an MRI study should be obtained to evaluate the possibility that a ganglion cyst is compressing the nerve. If the diagnosis remains elusive and MRI demonstrates an intact cuff, an electromyography examination should be performed. Because suprascapular neuropathy is treated differently than an RC tear, it is important to make the correct diagnosis to avoid performing ineffective surgery (see chapter 53).

Isolated injury to the axillary nerve may be caused by shoulder trauma, such as a proximal humerus fracture or shoulder dislocation, or it may be the result of overzealous retraction and/or splitting of the deltoid during RC repair. Patients may have early shoulder pain and weakness followed by deltoid atrophy. For proper patient care, the surgeon must be aware of this potential clinical entity and its confusion with RC injury, particularly in patients older than age 40 years with a dislocated shoulder who may have both an axillary nerve injury and RC injury. Following a dislocation, older patients have a higher risk for an associated RC injury than do younger patients. During the physical examination, the surgeon must confirm that all heads of the deltoid contract voluntarily. Earlier studies have shown that the sensory examination is notoriously unreliable in patients with axillary nerve injury. Neurologic diagnostic tests such as EMG and nerve conduction studies should be ordered for patients with clinical findings that are suspicious of axillary nerve injury, especially patients in whom RC repairs have failed following deltoid-splitting incisions. MRI of the shoulder can help distinguish these injuries as well, demonstrating deltoid edema and/or atrophy in patients with an axillary nerve injury and a retracted cuff tendon in patients with an RC tear.

Thoracic outlet syndrome is a condition that also can cause shoulder pain. Usually, thoracic outlet syndrome results from vascular or neural compression, which causes distal symptoms of paresthesias, pain, and blanching (see chapter 38).

Acromioclavicular Joint Pathology

One of the most common challenges in the diagnosis of RC problems is the extent to which the AC joint affects the patient's shoulder pain. Clinically significant AC pathology is seen in association with RC disease in approximately 10% to 15% of patients undergoing RC repair. Part of the challenge of making a correct diagnosis is the lack of correlation between radiographic findings and symptoms that are specific to the AC joint. The AC joint normally begins to degenerate in the third decade of life; however, degenerative radiographic findings do not become apparent until the fourth and fifth decade. The most important information regarding the AC joint is obtained from a careful preoperative clinical examination. Pain that occurs with palpation over the AC joint, worsens with cross-body (horizontal) adduction, and is alleviated with an injection of local anesthetic into the AC joint are confirmation that the AC joint is an important part of the patient's problem. Prominent undersurface AC spurring may also result in RC abrasion, and retearing may occur if the spurs are left behind. Failure to address symptomatic AC joint pathology with a distal clavicle resection will result in persistent postoperative pain and impairment.

Long Head of the Biceps Tendon

The functional role of the biceps tendon in the shoulder is controversial, but there is no doubt that the long head of the biceps (LHB) tendon can be a significant source of pain and dysfunction. Persistent pain and patient dissatisfaction following RC surgery is often secondary

to persistent LHB tendon pathology. Positive clinical findings include reproducible pain with palpation of the LHB tendon, radiation of pain down the anterior aspect of the arm following the path of the biceps muscle (but not proceeding beyond the elbow), and a positive Speed, Yergason, or active compression test. Positive signs of LHB tendon pathology should warn the surgeon that the substance and stability of the biceps tendon must be carefully and completely examined intraoperatively.

Labral and Intra-articular Pathology

Intra-articular pathology that can result in an incorrect diagnosis includes subtle forms of instability and labral pathology. Injuries such as partial cuff tears secondary to internal impingement in overhead athletes are particularly challenging to integrate into the presentation of cuff conditions. A careful history and physical examination, supported by advanced imaging studies, assists in clarification of the diagnosis. Following cuff débridement and acromioplasty, higher failure rates occur in patients younger than age 40 years with RC symptoms than in patients age 50 to 60 years who present with a classic impingement syndrome. Labral tears that cause instability and superior labral anterior-posterior tears can also result in shoulder symptoms that can be confused with an RC tear. A careful history and examination will aid the clinician in making the correct diagnosis. Instability and superior labral anterior-posterior lesion testing and imaging should be performed. Arthroscopy of the glenohumeral joint is particularly helpful in diagnosing and instituting proper treatment of labral tears. Failure to appreciate labral tears is a potential complication of conventional open RC repair, because the glenohumeral joint is not well visualized unless there is a large tear.

Glenohumeral Arthritis and Stiffness

RC tears also can be associated with glenohumeral degenerative joint disease in patients with shoulder pain. Range of motion often is restricted in all planes, particularly rotation. Close attention should be paid to good quality AP and axillary radiographs for narrowing of the joint space and glenohumeral spurs because these findings are sometimes subtle. In patients with otherwise subtle glenohumeral narrowing, a true AP radiograph with the arm actively abducted to 30° to 45° can sometimes markedly narrow the joint, secondary to compression by the RC. Treatment of the RC without addressing glenohumeral arthritis may result in improved function, but pain relief is unpredictable. The decision to replace the surfaces of the joint should be based on the degree of humeral head and glenoid surface degeneration.

Preoperative stiffness is common in patients with RC tears. A complete history and physical examination of the patient with a stiff and painful shoulder is essential to determine the cause and location of pathology. Loss of external rotation with the arm at the side indicates contracture involving the anterosuperior aspect of the shoulder (or glenohumeral arthritis), while limitation of external rotation and abduction usually results from contracture of the anteroinferior capsule. Loss of internal rotation indicates posterior capsular tightness. Although some degree of stiffness is common, a global restriction of motion (without glenohumeral arthritis) indicates a more extensive process, namely adhesive capsulitis (frozen shoulder). Most patients with adhesive capsulitis are between age 40 and 60 years. The hallmark of adhesive capsulitis is loss of passive external rotation with no prior significant trauma to the shoulder. RC disease alone is highly unlikely to restrict passive external rotation. The diagnosis of adhesive capsulitis must be made before surgery. A shoulder that is stiff before RC surgery is likely to remain stiff after repair. The pain the patient hopes to resolve may be unchanged or worse after surgery. The stiffness usually does not respond to nonsurgical treatment and interferes with the normal recovery after RC repair. Adequate treatment of severe stiffness and adhesive capsulitis includes frequent daily stretching so that most of the stiffness is eliminated before RC repair. If the stiffness cannot be resolved before surgery, a capsular release can be performed before surgery or included with the RC repair. The benefits of a staged or all-in-one procedure have not been documented in the literature. In these difficult situations, the patient should be warned of a much higher likelihood of postoperative stiffness that may require another procedure.

Postoperative stiffness also can be a difficult problem. Puckering of the skin in the subacromial region combined with a loss of motion usually are complications of surgery, secondary to adhesions in the subacromial space, injury to the axillary nerve, or partial detachment of the deltoid. Repeat rotator cuff surgery in patients with postoperative stiffness is fraught with difficulty and uncertain results. However, if revision of an RC repair is chosen, an adequate subacromial and glenohumeral adhesion and contracture release must be performed to mobilize the repair tissue and allow supple motion after surgery.

Secondary Gain

One final consideration in the preoperative evaluation is the environment in which the patient believes his or her problem began. RC problems that occur at work or as part of a compensable (legal) injury have a less favorable prognosis than do noncompensable injuries. The duration of symptoms and persistent impairment remain greater for these patients, even after repair. The

surgeon should realize that these factors impart a negative influence on any treatment rendered. Furthermore, these factors should be considered when suggesting prognosis. For example, a 50-year-old man who engages in heavy, strenuous labor in whom a large full-thickness RC tear develops is unlikely to return to his preinjury level of work responsibilities despite appropriate treatment of the RC tear.

Preoperative Counseling and Patient Expectations

Patients who have recovered from RC repair tend to be satisfied with the outcome of surgery, and they sometimes believe that their shoulders have regained normal function with no pain. Nonetheless, it is important to emphasize that the patient may experience some subjective functional deficit or imperfect pain relief. Functional improvement following RC surgery usually is less predictable than pain relief. A successful outcome is more common in younger patients with an acute injury, especially a one-tendon minimally retracted tear; older patients with a more chronic history have a less predictable functional result. In general, RC repair for the patient with long-standing pathology and significant pain can result in predictable pain relief, but functional recovery may be less than anticipated. To prepare the patient psychologically and with realistic expectations, it should be emphasized during preoperative discussions that the goal of surgery on a viable repairable cuff is to eliminate most of the patient's pain and restore as much function as possible.

Complications Related to Surgical Technique

Repair Failure (Rerupture)

The integrity of the cuff attachment to bone offers the best chance of restoring normal shoulder mechanics and maintaining long-term shoulder comfort and function. Patients with intact cuff repairs at follow-up have better strength and overall function than those patients in whom the repair did not remain intact, regardless of their comfort level and satisfaction. Recently, the continuity of the restored tendon has been evaluated by postoperative ultrasound. The literature suggests that repair failure is related to the preoperative size of the cuff tear and degeneration of the muscles. The number of tendons involved, the amount of retraction, and the extent of fatty degeneration can be quantified on an arthrogram, CT, or MRI. Large cuff injuries involving two or more RC tendons have a later risk of repair failure of more than 40%. More than two thirds of RC repairs on tendons retracted to the level of the glenoid will fail to heal to the humerus. A lower but significant incidence of rerupture of between 10% and 20% occurs in patients with smaller, single tendon tears. Factors such as retraction and fatty degeneration may play a large role in the failure to heal, even with tears considered small based on the area of the tendon involved. The risk of repair failure appears to be unrelated to the surgical approach or method of suture-tendon fixation.

Surgical management of a torn RC can be accomplished with one of three surgical techniques: conventional open repair, arthroscopic-assisted mini-open repair, and all-arthroscopic repair. Each approach has its own advantages and associated complications. The approach chosen should be based on the surgeon's ability to perform the most reliable repair.

Repairing the Rotator Cuff With Undue Tension
The goal of RC surgery is to balance the forces of the soft tissue around the glenohumeral joint by repairing the RC to the humerus. To minimize tension on the repair, RC tears should be repaired according to patterns of RC retraction, using principles of margin convergence. Simple traction of the retracted edge of the tendon to the tuberosity can result in an overtensioned repair. Most overtensioned repairs will eventually fail. An abduction orthosis that reduces initial tension on the repair is unlikely to promote healing of an overtensioned tendon. An overtensioned cuff repair that remains intact will result in stiffness and pain. A partial repair and débridement is more likely to prevent stiffness and complete repair failure than an overtensioned "watertight" repair.

Complications of Open and Mini-Open Rotator Cuff Surgery

Deltoid Detachment
Although deltoid detachment has been described as occurring with an overaggressive arthroscopic acromioplasty, this complication traditionally has been associated with open RC repair. The conventional open approach is characterized by exposure of the cuff tear through a deltoid split between the anterior and middle thirds of the muscle. Surgical exposure can be improved by elevating the tendinous origin of the deltoid sharply from the anterior acromion. Deltoid detachment is the most devastating complication following any approach for RC surgery, and revision surgery for this complication has a high failure rate. Deltoid repair to the acromion must be secure, either to good quality tendinous tissue or by using transosseous sutures through the acromion. The periosteum surrounding the acromion should be included in the deltoid origin detachment. Overly aggressive and unnecces-

sary bone resection should be avoided. A good guide to an appropriate bone resection is to make the anterior extent of the acromion resection level with the anterior clavicle in the sagittal plane. Early recognition of deltoid detachment postoperatively is necessary for a successful outcome. Treatment consists of prompt deltoid repair for acute avulsions and a very conservative postoperative rehabilitation protocol that includes the use of an abduction brace for 6 weeks, passive motion only for the first 6 weeks, and no strengthening exercises until 3 months after the repair. Chronic deltoid detachments with an atrophic anterior deltoid have a greater than 50% risk of a poor surgical outcome following treatment. Deltoidplasty (rotation of the middle deltoid anteriorly) may help to reduce pain, but the final result is inferior to an acute deltoid repair.

Nerve Injury
The mini-open approach allows access to the RC through a lateral deltoid muscle-splitting incision. During this technique, the deltoid is not removed from the acromion, thus avoiding the potential problem of deltoid detachment. The most serious potential complication of this surgical approach is injury of the axillary nerve. The course of the axillary nerve has been well described. The anterior terminal branch runs from posterior to anterior along the undersurface of the deltoid muscle approximately 5 cm inferior to the lateral and anterior edge of the acromion, innervating the anterior two thirds of the deltoid muscle. The nerve is at risk for injury if the deltoid split is extended too far distally. Many authors suggest a maximum distance or "safe zone" of 3.5 to 5 cm from the acromial edge. Another method of determining the level of the axillary nerve is to identify the reflection of the subacromial bursa underneath the deltoid. The deltoid split can be extended to within 1 cm of the bursal reflection because the axillary nerve is distal to the reflection. However, this anatomic relationship should not be relied upon during revision surgery because the soft-tissue planes are usually altered by scars and adhesions. In addition, the nerve can be injured proximally during the mobilization and repair of a torn subscapularis.

Intraoperatively, the risk of axillary nerve injury can be avoided by placing a stay suture at the apex of the deltoid split, preventing extension of the split from excessive deltoid retraction. Postoperatively, recognition of the injury is important. Patients will present initially with weakness during shoulder abduction and forward elevation, sometimes with an associated loss of skin sensation over the lateral upper arm. A long-standing nerve injury will be accompanied by atrophy of the deltoid anterior to the surgical incision. EMG can confirm the diagnosis and establish the severity of the injury. An axillary neurapraxia can be managed nonsurgically with range-of-motion exercises to prevent shoulder stiffness. Transection of the nerve is a devastating complication. Although exploration and repair of a transected axillary nerve can be performed, the best treatment is to protect the nerve during surgery.

Loss of the anterior deltoid can be treated with rotation of the deltoid anteriorly, similar to the treatment of deltoid detachment. Although in theory this rotational deltoidplasty may be beneficial in patients with axillary nerve injury from a deltoid split, the results in this patient group are unknown.

Complications of All-Arthroscopic Repair

A potential advantage of arthroscopic cuff repairs is decreased postoperative pain and a possible decrease in the risk of postoperative stiffness. Arthroscopic repair of the RC requires fixation of the tendon with techniques that are different from those of classic open repairs. Therefore, the strength and integrity of arthroscopic repairs compared with open repairs is a concern. However, recent postoperative imaging studies have demonstrated that the integrity of the arthroscopic repair is similar to that of the open technique at similar follow-up periods.

Complications of arthroscopic cuff repairs can be avoided, beginning with patient positioning. Attention to proper padding helps prevent pressure neurapraxia. Because excessive traction on the extremity may be responsible for transient paresthesias, with an incidence as high as 30% in some early series, surgeons who use the lateral decubitus position must avoid excessive traction. Current methods should result in a less than 5% incidence of transient paresthesias. Proper portal placement is crucial to avoid neurovascular injuries. The axillary and suprascapular nerves are at risk for injury with improper posterior or posterior-inferior portal placement. The axillary nerve and musculocutaneous nerves are at risk with malpositioned lateral and anterior portals, respectively.

During an arthroscopic RC repair, fluid extravasation into the surrounding soft tissues occurs. However, the typical swollen or distended appearance of the shoulder has not been associated with a persistent pathologic increase in the intramuscular pressure of the deltoid muscle. Intramuscular pressure returns to normal levels very quickly, within 30 minutes following the procedure. Compartment syndromes of the deltoid have not been reported. Because of the potential risk, pump pressures greater than 50 mm Hg are not recommended and arthroscopic procedures should last less than 2 hours.

Complications specific to newer methods of tendon fixation include loss of fixation of bone anchors or bioabsorbable tacks. With bone anchors, especially bioabsorbable anchors, the surgeon should assess the fixation strength during surgery. If the anchor easily backs out, either a larger or different type of anchor is required. In general, a well-seated metal bone anchor does not displace even with a recurrent tendon tear; it is the suture, knot, or tissue that fails.

Successful results using bioabsorbable tacks have been reported using clinically based outcomes focusing on pain relief and motion, but objective evidence of strength recovery and tendon repair integrity has not been reported. Tacks that absorb over 1 to 2 years may be associated with a sudden onset of pain and crepitation 3 to 6 months after the repair, caused by displacement of the head from the shaft of the tack. The displaced tack head can create mechanical symptoms in the subacromial space. This phenomenon may be secondary to variable rates of hydrolysis in the tissue next to the tack (tendon versus bone), mechanical failure resulting from excessive strain on the tack from the force of the RC, or failure because of improper insertion that is not recognized at the time of the procedure. The best treatment is a thorough arthroscopic débridement and, if necessary, a revision of the RC repair.

Postoperative Stiffness Following Rotator Cuff Repair

Significant range-of-motion restriction can occur postoperatively in shoulders that had relatively normal motion preoperatively. Complex regional pain syndrome, or reflex sympathetic dystrophy, can also ensue after RC repair. These conditions are particularly difficult to treat effectively. The glenohumeral capsule can contract and become scarred, and adhesions can occur at the humeroscapular motion interface. The humeroscapular motion interface is the "articulation" of the RC, humeral head, and biceps tendon on the articular side and the coracoacromial arch, deltoid, and coracoid muscles on the bursal side. Up to 4 cm of gliding motion has been measured across this articulation in normal shoulders. Loss of motion across this interface can be a source of significant shoulder pain following surgery or trauma to the shoulder and may mimic an impingement syndrome or cuff injury. Adhesions in this interface have been described as causing a "captured shoulder." Although not clearly reported in the literature, postoperative loss of motion secondary to humeroscapular adhesions or capsular contractions may be as high as 5% to 10%. Postoperative stiffness following an RC repair may or may not be associated with repair failure. Paradoxically, the cuff repair usually remains intact.

Treatment of a stiff shoulder following RC repair is distinctly different than that for a stiff shoulder caused by idiopathic adhesive capsulitis. Patients with adhesive capsulitis, especially those with insulin-dependent diabetes, may be successfully treated with aggressive physical therapy and an occasional closed manipulation or arthroscopic release. Physical therapy and manipulations sometimes are not effective in the postoperative stiff shoulder and may be harmful to the repaired tendons. Manipulation may effectively release part of the glenohumeral capsule contracture, but it has minimal effect on the adhesions in the subacromial region. Therefore, the recommended treatment is an arthroscopic evaluation, release of the glenohumeral capsule, and débridement of subacromial adhesions. The advantage of arthroscopic treatment is the ability to selectively free the humeroscapular articulation and release the glenohumeral capsule without injuring the RC tendons. Patients with reflex sympathetic dystrophy should be treated with adequate pain medication, physical therapy with special attention to desensitization, and, in selected patients, sympathetic blocks.

Complications Related to Associated Procedures Performed During Cuff Surgery

Acromioplasty

Over the last 30 years, many reports have supported acromioplasty as an important procedure associated with improved patient comfort and healing following RC repair. However, recent reports have questioned the value of acromioplasty as a routine part of RC repair. Performing a subacromial decompression in conjunction with RC repair creates a bleeding bony surface that is in close proximity to the RC, potentially increasing the risk of adhesions forming in the humeroscapular interface. Other complications of surgery on the acromion include either an inadequate or excessive resection of bone or a dome acromioplasty, which occurs in approximately 3% to 11% of RC repairs. An inadequate decompression may result in persistent symptoms of subacromial abrasion of the RC. Patients who demonstrate impingement-type symptoms and have evidence of simple inadequate decompression on a supraspinatus outlet radiographic view should be treated initially with close observation, physical therapy, and anti-inflammatory medication. Subacromial steroid injections should be avoided during the first 3 months after surgery so that the repaired RC can heal. A revision acromioplasty is indicated for persistent impingement findings.

Risks of excessive removal of parts of the acromion include the potential for an acromial fracture, deltoid detachment, or loss of the integrity of the coracoacromial arch with superior humeral migration (with massive RC tears). All of these complications are devastating. Revision surgery is unlikely to provide pain relief and functional results similar to a properly performed index procedure.

Deltoid detachment requires aggressive treatment. Patients who have a violation of the coracoacromial arch but an intact RC may be asymptomatic secondary to the stabilizing effect of the cuff on the humeral head. However, patients with RC insufficiency and loss of the continuity of the coracoacromial arch are subject to anterosuperior instability of the humeral head. At this time, there is no consistently successful treatment of anterosuperior instability, only unpredictable salvage procedures. Release of the coracoacromial ligament and acromioplasty are not advisable for massive, potentially irreparable tears. If the ligament is released in a patient with an inadequately repaired RC, the surgeon should repair the ligament back to the acromion, although the effectiveness of this approach has not been fully confirmed.

A common technical error during an acromioplasty is an inadequate resection of the medial and lateral edges of the acromion, as well as of the anterior prominence. This pattern is referred to as a dome acromioplasty. Patients with a dome acromioplasty have symptoms of continued subacromial irritation with potential irritation of the repaired tendon and a significant risk of acromial fracture. Awareness of a dome acromioplasty is important to avoid acromial fracture during revision surgery. The revision should include removal of the bone at the edges of the acromion, but not in the central portion. When performing a revision arthroscopic acromioplasty, viewing the acromion from the lateral portal provides the best visual assessment of the acromion profile. Alternatively, the revision surgery can be performed via an open approach with meticulous deltoid repair at closure. An open approach is recommended when deltoid detachment is suspected. The acromial thickness should be evaluated using a preoperative supraspinatus outlet radiograph to plan the amount of bone that needs to be resected.

Distal Clavicle Resection and Coplaning

Complications following a distal clavicle resection include either an inadequate resection of bone with persistent pain and crepitation or an overly aggressive resection of bone with instability of the lateral clavicle. Persistent pain at the AC joint following RC surgery requires further evaluation, especially if it persists beyond 6 months. Radiologic examination of the AC joint with a Zanca view (an AP radiograph of the AC joint with the beam aimed 15° cephalad and using 50% of the normal power for a shoulder radiograph) and an axillary lateral view may demonstrate incomplete decompression of the AC joint. Excess bone or heterotopic bone that develops after the resection is most commonly located in the posterosuperior portion of the joint and is best seen on the axillary lateral view. If the radiograph suggests heterotopic ossification, revision surgery through an open approach is advisable to decrease the risk of recurrent ectopic bone formation.

Excessive resection of the lateral clavicle can lead to instability. Because the attachment of the superior and posterior ligaments of the AC joint can be as close as 7 mm from the joint, resection of more than 7 mm with detachment of the ligaments and capsule can result in anteroposterior instability or horizontal instability of the AC joint. Resection of more than 2 cm of the lateral clavicle can disrupt the coracoclavicular ligaments, resulting in horizontal instability of the AC joint. Therefore, for an arthroscopic distal clavicle resection, the goal should be a resection of up to 7 mm of bone from the clavicle, with an additional 1 to 3 mm from the medial acromion to create a space of approximately 1 cm. For open distal clavicle resection, up to 1.5 cm of lateral clavicle can be safely removed, followed by a meticulous closure of the AC capsule and deltotrapezial fascia. Surgical stabilization via reconstruction of the coracoclavicular ligaments may be required if symptoms persist.

Arthroscopic acromioplasty is sometimes combined with resection of part of the lateral inferior clavicle that protrudes into the subacromial space. Coplaning of the undersurface of the AC joint is controversial. Some authors believe that coplaning increases the risk of AC joint pain; others believe that it leads to decreased pain secondary to decompression of the RC (see chapters 49 and 50). Aggressive coplaning violates the AC joint, potentially resulting in AC arthrosis and continued pain after successful RC repair.

Long Head of the Biceps Tenotomy

At the time of surgery, the intra-articular portion of the biceps can best be evaluated with an arthroscopic examination. Extra-articular evaluation has been described only with open surgery until recently, but it can also be evaluated at the time of subacromial arthroscopy by opening the tendon sheath distal to the attachments of the coracohumeral and superior glenohumeral ligaments. Fraying or disruption of more than 50% is an indication for biceps tenotomy. In some patients with a positive clinical examination for biceps symptoms, pathology involving less than 50% of the tendon width also may be an indication for biceps tenotomy or tenodesis. Instability of the biceps, most commonly seen in conjunction with a subscapularis tear, is a clear indication for biceps tenotomy or tenodesis. If these problems are not addressed at the time of RC repair, pain is likely to continue even after successful RC healing.

The main complication related to tenotomy is an associated deformity of the biceps muscle, commonly referred to as a Popeye deformity. This is caused by distal retraction of the LHB, resulting in a "balled-up" appearance of the distal biceps muscle. Although this deformity usually does not result in functional problems, many patients prefer that their arm have a relatively normal appearance. This is possible with tenodesis of the LHB tendon. Tenodesis methods have varied from traditional open approaches to newer arthroscopic techniques. The results are the same as long as the tendon heals to the surgical repair site. Disruption of the tenodesis can occur, but revision tenodesis usually is not needed. When an initial tenodesis fails, patients usually are disappointed in the appearance of the deformity but pleasantly surprised by the lack of pain.

Infection

The risk of infection following RC repair is low (approximately 1.5%). Infections may present early or late, and their location may be superficial or deep. Superficial wound infections are characterized by pain, erythema, and increased warmth, with or without drainage. Deeper infections may have the same presentation with more significant pain and swelling as well as an inability to move the shoulder. However, some deep infections involving the subacromial space present with few superficial findings and minimal systemic symptoms. Persistent stiffness and pain after surgery, failure to progress with physical therapy, and subtle systemic symptoms such as low-grade fevers or night sweats should alert the surgeon to the possible presence of infection. MRI may demonstrate fluid in the subacromial space and the glenohumeral joint but cannot confirm the diagnosis. Aspiration and subsequent positive cultures can confirm the diagnosis, but frequently the decision to proceed with urgent surgical treatment is based on a high index of suspicion. Treatment of superficial wound or skin infections may be treated with local wound care in addition to intravenous antibiotics that cover *Staphylococcus* and *Streptococcus* organisms. *Propionibacterium acnes* is a normal skin bacterium that is a relatively common pathogen in shoulder infections. Because this bacterium grows slowly, cultures in patients with suspected infection and negative cultures after 3 to 4 days should be observed for 3 to 4 weeks.

Deep infections require aggressive treatment. Laboratory findings such as an elevated erythrocyte sedimentation rate, C-reactive protein, and white blood cell count can be helpful in establishing the diagnosis. Diagnosis may be confirmed with glenohumeral aspiration, but if deep infection is of concern, arthroscopic or open irrigation and débridement is warranted. Intraoperative Gram stain and culture should be obtained prior to the administration of antibiotics. An incision, irrigation, and débridement of the subacromial space, biceps tendon sheath, and glenohumeral joint should be performed. Deep infections require the removal of all foreign material, including non-absorbable sutures and metallic suture anchors, which may require the takedown of a repaired tendon. Closed suction drains are used following surgery and generally removed 24 to 72 hours following the procedure. Intravenous antibiotics should start after cultures are obtained and can be adjusted appropriately according to Gram stain and culture results. Eradication of the infection supersedes the primary goal of RC repair. Once the infection is completely resolved, revision surgery is based on the patient's continued symptoms and functional deficits.

Infection after arthroscopic repairs has been reported in approximately 1% to 2% of patients. The risk may be higher (up to 5%) with a mini-open approach after arthroscopic acromioplasty and other arthroscopically performed procedures such as distal clavicle resection. Recommendations to prevent infection include the routine use of preoperative antibiotics and performing a separate skin preparation and draping after arthroscopic acromioplasty, before starting the RC repair approach.

Anesthesia-Related Complications

Three types of anesthesia are used most commonly during RC surgery: general anesthesia, interscalene regional anesthesia, or a combination of both. The patient and anesthesiologist should choose the type of anesthesia to be used, based on associated risks and benefits. The surgeon should understand the different anesthesia approaches available so that the patient can be counseled appropriately during preoperative education.

Major complications occur less than 1% of the time that general anesthesia is used. Patients with significant comorbid medical conditions, especially pulmonary problems, are at a greater risk for significant complications with general anesthesia than with regional anesthesia. The more common complications of general anesthesia in patients following elective shoulder surgery include nausea, inability to void, and significant pain following surgery that requires intravenous or intramuscular medication. The most common complication of an interscalene block is inadequate anesthesia (in up to 10% of patients). Other events associated with an interscalene block include Horner's syndrome or a recurrent laryngeal nerve block. Both of these are temporary complications and of no long-term consequence to the patient. A more serious, but less common, event related to interscalene block is an intravascular injection of the anesthetic medication, which can cause a seizure or delirium. Finally, some patients will complain of radicular pain distributed into their thumb and index finger, most likely as a result of the inadvertent needle injury to fibers of C6. For most patients, this pain is temporary and should resolve in 6 to 12 weeks.

Recently, in the United States, the trend for RC surgery has been to perform the procedure as an ambulatory or outpatient surgery. Sometimes a patient who undergoes outpatient surgery requires admission to the hospital, most commonly for pain control. Analysis of both general anesthesia and interscalene block has shown that, in a medical center staffed by anesthesiologists who are well trained in regional anesthesia, far fewer side effects and hospital admissions occur with regional anesthesia than with general anesthesia. However, the anesthetic approach used remains the choice of the anesthesia team and surgeon.

Summary

RC surgery is a successful and reproducible procedure when performed in a patient with clinically significant RC pathology. Pain relief is more predictable than functional recovery in most patients, and patients should be apprised as such before surgery so that they have realistic expectations. The final result depends on a complete history and physical examination with a comprehensive diagnosis that considers all important etiologies of shoulder pain.

The most common complication following an RC repair is failure of the surgical repair. Although studies have shown that the integrity of the repair is related to functionality of the shoulder, many patients with a failed repair are satisfied following surgery because of significant pain relief. Integrity of the repair does not appear to be related to the chosen technique, but each procedure has its own associated complications. The most devastating complications include deltoid detachment, acromion fracture, and axillary nerve injury. All of these complications can be prevented by meticulous surgical technique. Even though the risk of infection is low, the surgeon must be vigilant to the often subtle signs because early treatment may prevent chronic pain and permanent dysfunction. The ultimate result or maximum medical improvement following RC repair surgery may not be achieved for at least 1 year. Therefore, the patient and surgeon should pursue an enduring, long-term rehabilitative approach following RC surgery, unless a clearly defined complication is recognized.

Annotated Bibliography

Introduction

Matsen FA III, Arntz CT, Lippitt SB: Rotator cuff, in Rockwood CA Jr, Matsen FA III, Wirth MA, Harryman DT II (eds): *The Shoulder*, ed 2. Philadelphia, PA, WB Saunders, 1998, vol 2, pp 755-839.

This is an excellent review of RC disorders, including complications.

Incorrect or Incomplete Diagnosis

Karas EH, Iannotti JP: Failed repair of the rotator cuff: Evaluation and treatment of complications. *Instr Course Lect* 1998;47:87-95.

Overall satisfaction after primary repair of the RC was reported to be as high as 91% in a series of 340 shoulders. This success was made possible by improved surgical techniques over the last several decades. However, RC repairs can fail because of an incomplete or incorrect diagnosis, postoperative complications, surgical technique errors, and rehabilitation errors or poor performance. The authors discuss these factors and future treatment options.

Complications Related to Surgical Technique

Berjano P, Gonzalez BG, Olmedo JF, Perez-Espana LA, Munilla MG: Complications in arthroscopic shoulder surgery. *Arthroscopy* 1998;14:785-788.

In this retrospective evaluation of 179 consecutive arthroscopic (n = 141) and combined open and arthroscopic (n = 38) procedures, the overall complication rate was 9.49% (5.26% for combined procedures and 10.63% for arthroscopic procedures).

Boardman ND III, Cofield RH: Neurologic complications of shoulder surgery. *Clin Orthop* 1999;368:44-53.

The authors discuss the nerves that are most at risk for injury during shoulder surgery. The suprascapular nerve may be as close as 1 cm to the glenoid rim, the axillary nerve may be 3 mm from the inferior shoulder capsule and the musculocutaneous nerve may be as close as 3.1 cm from the coracoid. Three-dimensional knowledge of the anatomy of nerves is essential to prevent injuries during arthroscopic surgery.

Burkhart SS, Athanasiou KA, Wirth MA: Margin convergence: A method of reducing strain in massive rotator cuff tears. *Arthroscopy* 1996;12:335-338.

Increased security of fixation in RC repair is usually achieved by increasing the strength of fixation. The principle of margin convergence can be applied to RC repair as a means to enhance security of fixation by decreasing the mechanical strain at the margins of the tear.

Burkhart SS, Johnson TC, Wirth MA, Athanasiou KA: Cyclic loading of transosseous rotator cuff repairs: Tension overload as a possible cause of failure. *Arthroscopy* 1997;13:172-176.

RC tears were created and repaired in 16 cadaver shoulders and cyclically loaded. The central suture always failed first and by the largest magnitude, suggesting that cuff tears that are repaired under tension will undergo gradual failure with physiologic cyclic loading.

Jost B, Pfirrmann CW, Gerber C, Switzerland Z: Clinical outcome after structural failure of rotator cuff repairs. *J Bone Joint Surg Am* 2000;82:304-314.

Twenty of 65 consecutive RC repairs exhibited structural failure on postoperative MRI at a mean 38-month follow-up. Reruptures usually involved the originally torn tendon but were smaller than the original tear in 16 of the 20 patients. Fatty degeneration of the RC muscles tended to progress in these patients, but age-adjusted Constant scores still improved from 49% to 83% (P = 0.0001). The clinical outcome was significantly correlated with the size of the new tear, stage of postoperative fatty RC muscle degeneration, postoperative acromiohumeral distance, and degree of postoperative degenerative joint disease (P < 0.05).

Sher JS, Iannotti JP, Warner JJ, Groff Y, Williams GR: Surgical treatment of postoperative deltoid origin disruption. *Clin Orthop* 1997;343:93-98.

Results were 4% excellent, 29% good, and 67% unsatisfactory in 24 patients who underwent direct repair or rotational deltoidplasty reconstruction of a detached muscle origin after shoulder surgery. A poor outcome was associated with a prior lateral acrominectomy, involvement of the middle deltoid, a massive RC tear with weakness in external rotation, and a residual defect of greater than 2 cm.

Postoperative Stiffness Following Rotator Cuff Repair

Warner JJ, Greis PE: The treatment of stiffness of the shoulder after repair of the rotator cuff. *Instr Course Lect* 1998;47:67-75.

The authors review the variables involved in the loss of motion that may occur following rotator cuff repair as well as describe an approach to evaluate and treat stiffness in the shoulder.

Complications Related to Associated Procedures Performed During Cuff Surgery

Blazar PE, Iannotti JP, Williams GR: Anteroposterior instability of the distal clavicle after distal clavicle resection. *Clin Orthop* 1998;348:114-120.

Seventeen isolated distal clavicle resections were reviewed to assess translation of the AC articulation in the anteroposterior plane and its relationship to patient outcome. The total translation averaged 8.7 mm and was significantly greater than that of the contralateral shoulder. Patients' postoperative visual analog pain scales correlated with the magnitude of translation.

Anesthesia-Related Complications

D'Alessio JG, Rosenblum M, Shea KP, Freitas DG: A retrospective comparison of interscalene block and general anesthesia for ambulatory surgery shoulder arthroscopy. *Reg Anesth* 1995;20:62-68.

In this study of 263 patients, which was designed to determine whether interscalene block is a reliable approach to anesthesia in ambulatory surgery when compared with general anesthesia, 160 patients had a general anesthetic and 103 had interscalene block. Regional anesthesia required significantly less total nonsurgical intraoperative time use and also decreased the time spent in the postanesthesia care unit. It also resulted in fewer unplanned hospital admissions.

Ready BL: Anesthesia for shoulder procedures, in Rockwood CA Jr, Matsen FA III, Wirth MA, Harryman DT II (eds): *The Shoulder*, ed 2. Philadelphia, PA, WB Saunders, 1998, pp 277-289.

The authors review anesthesia techniques that are helpful for shoulder procedures and their attendant complications.

Classic Bibliography

Blom S, Dahlback LO: Nerve injuries in dislocations of the shoulder joint and fractures of the neck of the humerus: A clinical and electromyographical study. *Acta Chir Scand* 1970;136:461-466.

Brown AR, Weiss R, Greenberg C, Flatow EL, Bigliani LU: Interscalene block for shoulder arthroscopy: Comparison with general anesthesia. *Arthroscopy* 1993;9:295-300.

Gazielly DF, Gleyze P, Montagnon C: Functional and anatomical results after rotator cuff repair. *Clin Orthop* 1994;304:43-53.

Goutallier D, Postel JM, Bernageau J, Lavau L, Voisin MC: Fatty muscle degeneration in cuff ruptures: Pre- and postoperative evaluation by CT scan. *Clin Orthop* 1994;304:78-83.

Harryman DT II, Mack LA, Wang KY, Jackins SE, Richardson ML, Matsen FA III: Repairs of the rotator cuff: Correlation of functional results with integrity of the cuff. *J Bone Joint Surg Am* 1991;73:982-989.

Hawkins RJ, Misamore GW, Hobeika PE: Surgery for full-thickness rotator-cuff tears. *J Bone Joint Surg Am* 1985;67:1349-1355.

Lee YF, Cohn L, Tooke SM: Intramuscular deltoid pressure during shoulder arthroscopy. *Arthroscopy* 1989;5:209-212.

Liu SH, Baker CL: Arthroscopically assisted rotator cuff repair: Correlation of functional results with integrity of the cuff. *Arthroscopy* 1994;10:54-60.

Pasila M, Jaroma H, Kiviluoto O, Sundholm A: Early complications of primary shoulder dislocations. *Acta Orthop Scand* 1978;49:260-263.

Paulos LE, Franklin JL: Arthroscopic shoulder decompression development and application: A five year experience. *Am J Sports Med* 1990;18:235-244.

Yamanaka K, Matsumoto T: The joint side tear of the rotator cuff: A followup study by arthrography. *Clin Orthop* 1994;304:68-73.

Chapter 18

Massive Rotator Cuff Tears

Christian Gerber, MD

Gilles Walch, MD

Introduction

The rotator cuff undergoes progressive degenerative changes; therefore, the risk of tendon tears increases with advancing age, as does the size of the tear. Many authors consider a tear massive if its maximum diameter is greater than 5 cm. This definition is not always adequate, however, because patients vary widely in height and size, tears may be measured before or after resection of non-viable tendon tissue, and tears appear larger if the humerus is pushed cranially and smaller if the humerus is pulled distally. It therefore has been suggested that the amount of tendinous disinsertion at the tuberosities should be measured and a tear defined as massive if disinsertion of at least two complete tendons is present.

The superior border of the subscapularis and the anterior border of the supraspinatus are easily defined. The posterior border of the supraspinatus and thereby the superior border of the infraspinatus are found by virtual prolongation of the scapular spine to the greater tuberosity with the arm held in neutral rotation. In open surgery, this is accomplished by placing the two branches of a pair of forceps on either side of the scapular spine and observing where the forceps meet the greater tuberosity. Arthroscopically, the posterior rotator interval is identified by identifying the scapular spine. The muscle fibers coming from the infraspinatus fossa to the insertion on the greater tuberosity identify the superior-most portion of the infraspinatus. The teres minor is more difficult to identify but is usually defined by a small tuberosity that is distal and medial to the infraspinatus insertion and usually must be palpated.

Critical Associated Findings

Massive tears, especially if the infraspinatus is affected, lead to static superior subluxation of the humeral head so that the acromiohumeral distance as measured on an AP radiograph with the arm in neutral rotation becomes smaller than 7 mm. If such static superior subluxation has occurred, direct repair of a tear is very likely to fail, and other options, such as tendon transfers, should be considered. If proximal migration increases, so-called subacromial arthritis may develop. This should be clearly distinguished from rotator cuff tear arthropathy, which consists of (massive) rotator cuff tearing, static superior subluxation, and arthropathy (eg, destruction of the humeral head and eccentric erosion of the glenoid).

Massive tendon tears are associated with profound changes of the respective muscles. Fatty degeneration of the musculature has been described and classified on the basis of CT scans (Table 1), and a recent study has shown that, with some reservations, this staging system can be adapted to MRI of the shoulder. Massive tears also are associated with marked atrophy of the respective muscles. The structural changes in the rotator cuff muscles also are associated with profound changes in their stress-strain behavior, which compromise the stability and healing of tendon-to-bone repairs.

Atrophy may reverse somewhat after successful tendon repair, but fatty degeneration does not. Moreover, fatty degeneration appears to be the single factor most prognostic for reparability and recovery of strength after rotator cuff repair.

The tendon of the long head of the biceps may be normal, or it may be pathologic, subluxated, dislocated, or torn. Anterior dislocation of the biceps tendon into the joint is proof of a subscapularis tear and transforms the long biceps from a potential head depressor to a raiser. Biceps tenotomy with or without tenodesis, which is recommended in Europe as treatment for painful, massive rotator cuff tears in the elderly, is definitely indicated under these circumstances. Repair or preservation of a degenerated biceps tendon is rarely indicated.

Epidemiology

Massive rotator cuff tears are exceedingly rare in the asymptomatic working population and, unlike small

TABLE 1	Classification of Fatty Degeneration of Muscle
Stage	**Appearance of Muscle**
0	No fatty streaks
1	Occasional fatty streaks
2	Substantial fatty infiltration but less fat than muscle
3	Equal amounts of fat and muscle
4	Predominance of fat over muscle

tears, are not a normal variant in persons younger than age 70 years. In persons older than age 70 years, large and even massive tears also may be found in asymptomatic shoulders. Natural history studies have shown that the spontaneous outcome of a massive rotator cuff tear in a young individual who requires use of the arm with the elbow away from the side is not satisfactory. However, the spontaneous outcome may be satisfactory for the elderly patient who has pain but very few functional demands on the arm.

Disability

Patients with massive rotator cuff tears may or may not experience pain. Anterosuperior tears are usually more painful than posterosuperior tears. Pathologic changes in the long biceps tendon have been associated with pain. Massive rotator cuff tears always cause loss of strength when the arm is elevated or abducted but usually do not cause disability when the elbow is at the side. The type of treatment to be undertaken depends on the disability of the individual patient. A patient with low functional demands and a tear of the nondominant arm may require a different type of treatment than a patient with high functional demands and an identical structural lesion of the dominant arm.

Treatment

If a massive rotator cuff tear is diagnosed, a rapid decision about treatment is necessary only if a traumatic event has occurred. Asymptomatic partial- or full-thickness rotator cuff tears may be enlarged by trauma, transforming a well-functioning shoulder into a completely dysfunctional arm. In such a situation, a conventional, true (central beam parallel to the joint line) AP radiograph of the shoulder taken with the arm in neutral rotation is mandatory. An acromiohumeral distance of less than 7 mm indicates that a massive rotator cuff

tear must have been present before the current injury, which severely compromises the possibility of successful repair. An acromiohumeral distance greater than 7 mm in the presence of a proven rotator cuff tear indicates that the traumatic event has caused or enlarged a mechanically compensated rupture of the rotator cuff, which can probably be repaired.

Low Functional Demands

In addition to the extent of the lesion, which is best determined by the degree of fatty degeneration of the musculature, treatment decisions should be based primarily on the functional demands of the patient. A patient's functional demands are low if he or she uses the arm almost exclusively with the elbow at the side and can compensate for the dysfunction with the opposite arm. If a pseudoparalysis with tolerable pain has gradually developed in a patient with low functional demands and a massive rotator cuff tear, and the patient has pronounced muscular wasting and an acromiohumeral distance of less than 7 mm, skillful neglect with occasional intermittent physical therapy may be the most advisable form of treatment.

A new constrained prosthesis, which has not yet been approved in the United States, has been used with short-term and midterm success in Europe for elderly patients with a complete pseudoparalysis. Results with this prosthesis should be observed closely because it has a spectacular potential for short-term to midterm results in well-selected patients.

A patient with low functional demands who has a massive cuff tear with significant pain usually does not require immediate surgical intervention because there is no proof that early surgical intervention provides superior pain management. Nonsurgical treatment, which may include subacromial (intra-articular) injection of steroids, should be the first approach. If this fails, arthroscopic evaluation should be considered. If the long head of the biceps is still present, a biceps tenotomy with débridement of inflamed parabursal tissues is indicated. Most authors perform an acromioplasty, but there is no proof that this improves the prognosis. Débridement will not restore anterior elevation of a pseudoparalytic shoulder, and biceps tenotomy without a large anterior acromioplasty, which can be effective in treatment of pain, has not been observed to cause pseudoparalysis.

High Functional Demands

Laborers and individuals who require the use of the affected arm above shoulder level are considered to have high functional demands on the shoulder. If a young patient with a previously asymptomatic, strong shoulder sustains trauma with an associated rotator cuff tear, surgical repair is advocated as soon as the shoulder has free passive mobility. Techniques of direct repair recently have been studied in vitro and in vivo. The use of No. 3 polyester suture, a modified Mason-Allen tendon-grasping technique, and augmentation of a weak cortical bone by means of a plate over which sutures are tied have yielded holding characteristics that are superior to more conventional techniques. Also, one study has shown that if such repair techniques are used, reruptures are very likely to be smaller than the original tear, and the patient has less pain and improved strength, even in the event of a rerupture. An attempt at repair therefore seems unquestionably justified.

If a young patient with high functional demands and a massive rotator cuff tear has a gradually developed pseudoparalysis with tolerable pain, a careful analysis of the extent of the structural damage is mandatory. Repair is indicated if the acromiohumeral distance is 7 mm or more and if on CT or MRI the musculature still seems adequate (< stage 3). In the more likely situation of significant fatty degeneration and atrophy, partial repairs with additional tendon transfers may be necessary. The results to be expected will, however, not be as good as with successful direct repairs.

If the acromiohumeral distance is less than 7 mm, direct repair is ineffective. Under these conditions equatorial (partial) repair plus latissimus dorsi transfer for restoration of external rotation or pectoralis major transfer for anterosuperior coverage may be considered. However, there is little hope that significant overhead strength will be restored.

In the situation with chronic pseudoparalysis, absence of pain, an acromiohumeral distance of less than 7 mm, and severe atrophy of at least two complete muscles, the chances of functional restoration using any reconstructive procedures are minimal. Fortunately, this situation is exceedingly rare in young manual laborers. Although use of shoulder fusion is extremely rare, it should be considered for the exceptional young patient with very high functional demands and complete destruction of the cuff.

Hemiarthroplasty probably has a role only in very large tears that are associated with significant glenohumeral arthritis. The hemiarthroplasty should not be expected to lead to substantial functional improvement, but it may relieve the pain caused by osteoarthritis. Overall, the results of hemiarthroplasty in the presence of massive tears are fair.

Postoperative Rehabilitation

There is relatively little disagreement regarding the techniques of massive rotator cuff tear repair, but there is major disagreement regarding aftercare. Functional

rehabilitation after biceps tenotomy and débridement is undebated. If a massive tear has been repaired, however, the need for an abduction splint is controversial; there are no results from randomized trials. In humans, it has been shown that abduction of only 30° substantially reduces tension on a supraspinatus repair. In vivo studies in sheep have shown that almost any repair technique will fail unless the repair is protected from weight bearing. Thus, protection of a repair with an abduction splint for approximately 6 weeks seems much better supported by evidence than keeping the arm at the side.

Failed Repair of Massive Rotator Cuff Defects

The treatment of massive rotator cuff defects is complex, but the further management of patients in whom attempts at repair of those defects failed is even more complex. The cause of failure must be established first. Causes include inappropriate patient selection (failure to deselect patients with preoperative static superior subluxation, dynamic anterosuperior subluxation, or preoperative severe fatty degeneration of the rotator cuff muscles), inadequate repair, insufficient or excessive rehabilitation, or postoperative complications (infection, stiffness, deltoid disinsertion, or ossification). As one study demonstrated, rerupture may occur after repair of large and massive cuff tears even if patient selection, repair, and rehabilitation are adequate. However, the results may be acceptable because of the high patient satisfaction rate. Nevertheless, a failed massive rotator cuff defect usually is responsible for severe disability, pain, weakness, inability to perform activities of daily living, and partial or complete paralysis on anterior elevation and external rotation.

Despite recognition of the causes of the failure, reoperation does not necessarily guarantee success. One study reported 48% unsatisfactory results, another 58% poor results, and in another, 67% of patients reported unsatisfactory pain relief. The authors of the latter study warned patients not to expect improved function. Damage to the deltoid may be extremely serious. The authors of one series reported only 50% satisfactory results of reoperation when deltoid damage was present. A recent study involving 24 patients demonstrated that the surgical treatment of postoperative disruption of the deltoid origin led to unsatisfactory results in 67% of patients.

Once it has been established that a repeat surgical attempt is necessary, the decision process is similar to that for primary massive rotator cuff defects. Options include débridement and decompression, local tissue repair, free grafts, distant muscle transfers, arthroplasty, or arthrodesis. Unfortunately, not much evidence exists in the literature to guide the decision-making process.

A recent study involved 17 patients in whom surgical treatment of a massive rotator cuff tear was unsuccessful; thes patients were managed with transfer of a latissimus dorsi muscle as a salvage operation. Fourteen of the 17 patients were satisfied following surgical treatment because they reported significant pain relief and significant improvement in function. Fifteen patients stated that they would have the surgical procedure again. Seven of eight patients with a detached or nonfunctional anterior portion of the deltoid had substantial improvement.

Annotated Bibliography

Critical Associated Findings

Fuchs B, Weishaput D, Zanetti M, Hodler J, Gerber C: Fatty degeneration of the muscles of the rotator cuff: Assessment by computed tomography versus magnetic resonance imaging. *J Shoulder Elbow Surg* 1999;8: 599-605.

The classification of Goutallier can partly be adapted to MRI, which tends to overestimate fatty degeneration.

Gaenslen ES, Satterlee CC, Hinson GW: Magnetic resonance imaging for evolution of failed repairs of the rotator cuff. *J Bone Joint Surg Am* 1996;78:1391-1396.

Thirty reoperated shoulders in 29 patients were preoperatively imaged by MRI. Positive and negative predictive values were between 80% and 90% for complete and partial tears and between 80% and 100% for intact cuffs.

Neviaser RJ: Evaluation and management of failed rotator cuff repairs. *Orthop Clin North Am* 1997;28: 215-224.

This study maintains that the decision to perform revision rotator cuff reconstruction should be based on the clinical problem, not the mere presence of a cuff defect. A functional deltoid is critical to the success of such surgery. Reconstructive procedures on the cuff include direct repair, interpositional grafting, and tendon transfers associated with an appropriate decompression. Decompression without repair carries a significant risk of creating a severe functional loss and a poor outcome.

Epidemiology

Milgrom C, Schaffler M, Gilbert S, van Holsbeeck M: Rotator-cuff changes in asymptomatic adults: The effect of age, hand dominance and gender. *J Bone Joint Surg Br* 1995;77:296-298.

Although small tears are frequent findings in persons older than age 40 to 50 years, massive tears are not observed in asymptomatic individuals of working age.

Walch GBA, Calderone S, Robinson AHN: The 'dropping' and 'hornblower's' signs in evaluation of rotator-cuff tears. *J Bone Joint Surg Br* 1998;80:624-628.

This article shows that dysfunction of the shoulder is better correlated with degree of fatty degeneration than with tendon tear size.

Treatment

Aoki M, Okamura K, Fukushima S, Takahashi T, Ogino T: Transfer of latissimus dorsi for irreparable rotator-cuff tears. *J Bone Joint Surg Br* 1996;78:761-766.

Twelve irreparable tears were treated with latissimus dorsi transfer. Results were good to excellent only if the subscapularis was intact.

Cordasco FA, Bigliani LU: The treatment of failed rotator cuff repairs. *Instr Course Lect* 1998;47:77-86.

Conservative treatment should be considered in selected patients with failed rotator cuff repairs. Deltoid detachment, altered acromion, and poor quality of cuff are poor prognostic factors.

Field LD, Dines DM, Zabinski SJ, Warren RF: Hemiarthoplasty of the shoulder for rotator cuff arthropathy. *J Shoulder Elbow Surg* 1997;6:18-23.

Of 16 hemiarthroplasties for rotator cuff arthropathy, 10 did well. Previous acromioplasty seemed to compromise the result.

Gartsman GM: Massive, irreparable tears of the rotator cuff: Results of operative debridement and subacromial decompression. *J Bone Joint Surg Am* 1997;79: 715-721.

Following débridement and subacromial decompression, pain and range of motion were improved, but the Constant score increased only from 39% to 66%. The results in these 33 patients were much less favorable than repair of comparable tears by the author.

Gartsman GM, Khan M, Hammerman SM: Arthroscopic repair of full-thickness tears of the rotator cuff. *J Bone Joint Surg Am* 1998;80:832-840.

This series demonstrates that even very large and massive tears can successfully be treated arthroscopically.

Gerber C, Fuchs B, Hodler J: The results of repair of massive tears of the rotator cuff. *J Bone Joint Surg Am* 2000;82:505-515.

Twenty-nine massive tears treated with a laboratory-tested repair yielded good to excellent results despite a significant failure rate. Muscle atrophy recovered in the supraspinatus; fatty degeneration never recovered.

Gerber C, Hersche O: Tendon transfers for the treatment of irreparable rotator cuff defects. *Orthop Clin North Am* 1997;28:195-203.

This is an overview of the current possibilities of tendon transfer surgery for rotator cuff disease.

Gerber C, Schneeberger AG, Perren SM, Nyffeler RW: Experimental rotator cuff repair. A preliminary study. *J Bone Joint Surg Am* 1999;81:1281-1290.

The authors of this complex study in sheep documented that rotator cuff repairs must be protected from weight bearing and that repair with a Mason-Allen tendon-grasping technique and cortical bone augmentation improves healing rate in the experimental animal.

Rokito AS, Cuomo F, Gallagher MA, Zuckerman JD: Long-term functional outcome of repair of large and massive chronic tears of the rotator cuff. *J Bone Joint Surg Am* 1999;81:991-997.

The authors reported 30 consecutive cases with good results; however, strength never returned to normal.

Sher JS, Iannotti JP, Warner JJ, et al: Surgical treatment of postoperative deltoid origin disruption. *Clin Orthop* 1997;343:93-98.

Twenty-four patients underwent direct repair or rotational deltoidplasty reconstruction of a detached muscle origin after shoulder surgery. Overall, one excellent (4%), seven good (29%), and 16 unsatisfactory (67%) results were obtained.

Walch G, Madonia G, Pozzi I, Riand N, Levigne C: Arthroscopic tenotomy of the long head of the biceps in rotator cuff ruptures, in Gazielly DF, Gleyze P, Thomas T (eds): *The Cuff*. Paris, France, Elsevier, 1997, pp 350-355.

The author reported 87 cases, with 85% satisfactory results. Elevation is compromised if the subscapularis is torn. Pain relief is reliable and is not improved by additional acromiplasty.

Williams GR, Rockwood CA: Hemiarthroplasty in rotator cuff deficient shoulders. *J Shoulder Elbow Surg* 1996;5:362-367.

In 21 shoulders with irreparable rotator cuff tears and arthritis, active elevation was improved by 50°. Only 12 patients became pain free.

Postoperative Rehabilitation

Erggelet C, Eggensperleger G, Steinwachs M, et al: Postoperative ossification of the shoulder: Incidence and clinical impact. *Arch Orthop Trauma Surg* 1999; 119:168-170

Heterotopic ossification was found in 28 of 106 rotator cuff repairs. Clinical outcome was not significantly influenced.

Failed Repair of Massive Rotator Cuff Defects

Jost B, Pfirrmann CW, Gerber C, Switzerland Z: Clinical outcome after structural failure of rotator cuff repairs. *J Bone Joint Surg Am* 2000;82:304-314.

MRI detected 20 structural failures of rotator cuff repair. The subjective shoulder value averaged 75% of the value for a normal shoulder. Eleven patients were very satisfied with the result, six were satisfied, two were disappointed, and one was dissatisfied. An attempt at rotator cuff repair significantly decreases pain and improves function and strength even if MRI documents that the repair has failed. The potential for rerupture should not be considered a formal contraindication to an attempt at repair if optimal functional recovery is the goal of treatment.

Karas EH, Iannotti JP: Failed repair of the rotator cuff. *J Bone Joint Surg Am* 1997;79:784-793.

This is an overview of causes and potential treatment options for a failed rotator cuff repair.

Karas SE, Giaghello TL: Subscapularis transfer for reconstruction of massive tears of the rotator cuff. *J Bone Joint Surg Am* 1996;78:239-245.

Following subscapularis transportation for repair of massive tears, 17 of 20 patients were satisfied with the results, but two lost active elevation.

Miniacci A, Macleod M: Transfer of the latissimus dorsi muscle after failed repair of a massive tear of the rotator cuff: A two to five year review. *J Bone Joint Surg Am* 1999;81:1120-1127.

In this study, 17 failures of massive tear repair were managed with a transfer of a latissimus dorsi muscle; 14 had significant pain relief and significant improvement of function. Seven of eight patients with a detached or nonfunctional anterior portion of the deltoid had substantial improvement.

Resch H, Povacz P, Ritter E, Matschi W: Transfer of the pectoralis major muscle for the treatment of irreparable rupture of the subscapularis tendon. *J Bone Joint Surg Am* 2000;82:372-382.

Subcoracoid transposition of the subscapularis yielded good results for isolated or combined subscapularis tears.

Settecerri JJ, Pitner MA, Rock AG, et al: Infection after rotator cuff repair. *J Shoulder Elbow Surg* 1999;8:1-5.

In 16 patients treated for infection following rotator cuff repair, treatment required intravenous antibiotics and multiple procedures. A satisfactory result was obtained in 16 patients.

Classic Bibliography

Bigliani LU, Cordasco FA, McLlveen SJ, et al: Operative treatment of failed repairs of the rotator cuff. *J Bone Joint Surg Am* 1992;74:1505-1515.

Bigliani LU, McIlveen SJ, Cordasco F, Musso E: Operative repair of massive rotator cuff tears: Long term results. *J Shoulder Elbow Surg* 1992;1:120-130.

De Orio JK, Cofield RH: Results of a second attempt at surgical repair of a failed initial rotator-cuff repair. *J Bone Joint Surg Am* 1994;66:563-567.

Gerber C, Schneeberger AG, Beck M, Schlegel U: Mechanical strength of repairs of the rotator cuff. *J Bone Joint Surg Br* 1994;76:371-380.

Goutallier D, Postel JM, Bernageau J, Lavau L, Voisin MC: Fatty muscle degeneration in cuff ruptures. *Clin Orthop* 1994;304:78-83.

Montgomery TJ, Yerger B, Savoie FH: Management of rotator cuff tears: Comparison of arthroscopic debridement and surgical repair. *J Shoulder Elbow Surg* 1994; 3:71-78.

Neviaser RJ, Neviaser TJ: Re-operation for failed rotator cuff repair: Analysis of fifty cases. *J Shoulder Elbow Surg* 1992;1:283-286.

Rockwood CAJ, Williams GR, Burkhead WZ: Débridement of degenerative, irreparable lesions of the rotator cuff. *J Bone Joint Surg Am* 1995;77:857-866.

Satterlee CC, Neer CS: Re-operation for failed rotator cuff repairs. *J Should Elbow Surg Suppl* 1993;2:510.

Walch G, Maréchal E, Maupas J, Liotard JP: Traitement des ruptures de la coiffe des rotateurs: Facteurs de pronostic. *Rev Chir Orthop Reparatrice Appar Mot* 1992;78:379-388.

Chapter 19

Cuff Tear Arthropathy

Evan L. Flatow, MD

David L. Glaser, MD

Armodios M. Hatzidakis, MD

Suzanne L. Miller, MD

Tom R. Norris, MD

Matthew L. Ramsey, MD

Gerald R. Williams, Jr, MD

Introduction

Symptomatic arthritis of the glenohumeral joint in the setting of rotator cuff deficiency poses a complex problem for the orthopaedic surgeon. Numerous authors have described this condition, beginning with the pathoanatomic description by Adams and Smith in the late 19th century. Derived from clinical observations, several theories have evolved to describe this relationship, including localized rheumatoid arthritis (RA), rapidly destructive arthritis of the shoulder, hemorrhagic shoulder of the elderly, Milwaukee shoulder syndrome/crystal-associated arthritis, and cuff tear arthropathy.

The term cuff tear arthropathy (CTA) was first used in 1983 to describe glenohumeral arthritis in the setting of a massive rotator cuff tear with characteristic superior migration of the proximal humerus. These patients had no evidence of concurrent pathology such as RA, osteoarthritis (OA), or crystal-induced arthropathy. Its pathogenesis remains poorly understood, and its management remains controversial.

Glenohumeral arthritis associated with rotator cuff pathology is now recognized as a common end point for several different pathologic processes. Although arthropathy develops in only a small percentage of patients with rotator cuff tears, the patients who are affected have massive rotator cuff tears, bone loss, and poor joint mechanics that make CTA a severe functional problem that is difficult to treat effectively by conventional surgical methods.

Etiology

Despite a considerable amount of discussion and scientific investigation, the pathogenesis of CTA remains unknown. In part, this is because different names have been given to what is probably a similar condition. In 1983, Neer and associates described the clinical and pathologic findings of 26 patients with massive rotator cuff tears and glenohumeral joint loss. Characteristics of this patient population included a higher prevalence of pathology in the dominant shoulder (although common bilaterally), an average age of 69 years, and a 3:1 female-to-male ratio. According to one theory, mechanical and nutritional factors were believed to be critical to the development of CTA. Because CTA was not thought to be associated with degenerative arthritis in other joints, a massive rotator cuff tear was suggested as the initial event in the pathogenesis. Force couple balance between the rotator cuff and the deltoid and compressive effects generated by the rotator cuff are lost as a rotator cuff tear enlarges, and superior and anterosuperior migration develops with consequent loss of concentric glenohumeral articulation. Inactivity, disuse, and leaking of the synovial fluid were nutritional factors that contributed to the complete syndrome of CTA (Fig. 1). Leaking of the synovial fluid away from the joint surfaces makes nutrients less available for diffusion into the articular cartilage. Furthermore, the decrease in motion associated with CTA causes chronic disuse osteopenia, which results in structural alterations in the articular cartilage as well as biochemical changes in the water and glycosaminoglycan content.

The rheumatology literature has emphasized biochemical factors as an etiology of the development of CTA in reports describing the so-called Milwaukee shoulder. The clinical similarities between CTA as described by Neer and associates and crystal-associated arthropathy seen with the Milwaukee shoulder syndrome suggest that calcium phosphate crystals may have a role in the pathogenesis of CTA. The exact origin of the crystals is unknown, and it is not clear whether the crystals are the cause or effect of arthritis. Nonetheless, some investigations have found that these crystals (hydroxyapatite, octacalcium phosphate, or tricalcium phosphate) form in diseased synovium and articular cartilage and are released into the synovial fluid. Subsequent phagocytosis of these crystals by phagocytic synovial cells is believed to induce a secretory response that releases

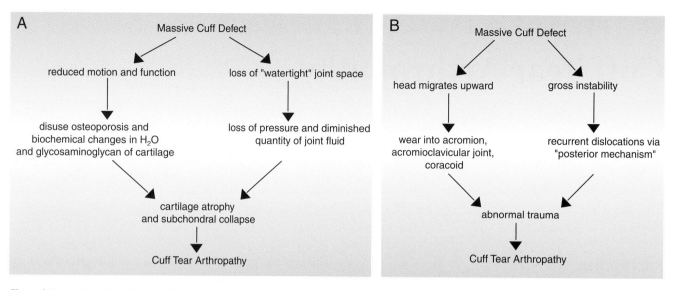

Figure 1 Neer and associates' theory on the pathogenesis of rotator cuff arthropathy. In the setting of a massive rotator cuff tear, both nutritional (**A**) and mechanical (**B**) factors contribute to the development of rotator cuff arthropathy. *(Reproduced with permission from Neer CS II, Craig EV, Fukuda H: Cuff-tear arthropathy. J Bone Joint Surg Am 1983;65:1232-1244.)*

matrix-degrading proteins (metalloproteinases, such as collagenase and stromelysin) that destroy the rotator cuff tendon and the articular cartilage. As the tissue is damaged, additional crystals are released, resulting in a vicious circle.

In addition to Milwaukee shoulder, other crystal-associated arthropathies share a similar clinical picture with CTA as described by Neer and associates. Large quantities of basic calcium phosphate crystals have been found in patients with CTA without the characteristic inflammatory response seen in Milwaukee shoulder. Basic calcium phosphate crystals have also been found in association with other processes and conditions, such as OA and aging. This information suggests that crystal deposition may not play a role in the development of this disease process but may only represent a common end point in several types of destructive arthropathy.

Clinical Evaluation

Patients most commonly have long-standing and progressively increasing pain that is worse at night, usually without a history of a significant traumatic event. The pain intensifies with use and activity. Patients also report loss of motion and recurrent swelling. Prior treatment often will have included periods of immobilization, physical therapy, and attempts at rotator cuff repair. Although many patients report having received one or multiple corticosteroid injections, there is no proven correlation between these injections and progression of the disease.

Clinical inspection of the shoulder often reveals atrophy of the supraspinatus and infraspinatus fossae with swelling or a fluid sign. The fluid sign is a swollen fluid-

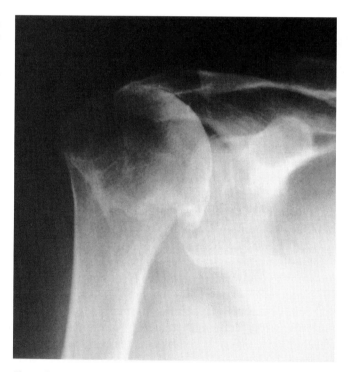

Figure 2 A typical radiograph demonstrating the upward migration of the humeral head with "snowcap" subarticular sclerosis and an area of collapse of the proximal aspect of the humeral articular surface without the large osteophytes typically seen in OA.

filled appearance to the superficial shoulder that arises from profuse leakage of glenohumeral joint fluid into the subacromial bursa. Aspiration of the joint often reveals a bloody effusion resulting from chronic impingement. In some patients, large ecchymosis may develop, prompting a fruitless hematologic work-up for a clotting disorder. Further examination reveals crepitus, loss of both passive

TABLE 1 | Differential Diagnosis of Cuff Tear Arthropathy

Diagnosis	Humeral Head	Rotator Cuff	Long Head of Biceps	Evidence of Subacromial Impingement	Other
Cuff tear arthropathy	Atrophic cartilage and osteoporosis, with areas of collapse and eburnation	Massive tear	Ruptured or dislocated	Yes	No trauma; negative laboratory findings
OA	Sclerotic, enlarged with osteophytes	Intact	Intact	No	
RA	Marginal or pannus erosion	Intact in 70%	Rupture in 15%	Occasionally (due to weak cuff muscle)	Multiple joints involved; distinctive laboratory findings
Infection	Chondrolysis and osteolysis	Intact	Intact	No	Hot, swollen joint; purulence; positive culture or tuberculosis tests
Old trauma (old dislocation)	May have fractures	Tuberosity fragments if torn	Usually intact	No	History of trauma
Metabolic disease (gout, ochronosis, pseudogout)	Crystals or discoloration, radiographs like OA	Intact	Intact	No	Systemic findings
Osteonecrosis (steroid, sickling, alcoholism)	Subchondral collapse, thick cartilage flap	Intact	Intact	No	Glenoid spared; predisposing factor
Neuroarthropathy (syringomyelia, lues)	Disorganization of joint, subsynovial fragments	Intact	Intact	No	Neural signs

(Reproduced with permission from Neer CS II, Craig EV, Fukuda H: Cuff-tear arthropathy. J Bone Joint Surg Am 1983;65:1232-1244.)

and active motion, rotator cuff weakness, and, often, rupture of the tendon of the long head of the biceps. Attempts at forward elevation or abduction usually show the characteristic superior "hiking" of the shoulder consistent with a massive rotator cuff tear. Glenohumeral movement elicits pain. Anterosuperior instability also may be present, which is even more painful, disabling, and difficult to treat than "standard" CTA.

Radiographic findings include loss of glenohumeral joint space with an area of subarticular sclerosis and collapse of the proximal aspect of the humeral articular surface, without the large osteophytes typically seen in OA (Fig. 2). Proximal migration of the humeral head erodes the undersurface of the acromion, progressing to the acromioclavicular joint and distal clavicle. Superior and medial erosion results in an acetabularization of the glenoid/acromion and rounding off of the greater tuberosity (femoralization of the humeral head) with subarticular sclerosis (snowcap sign) and cystic changes.

Neer and associates considered an area of collapse near the proximal aspect of the humeral surface to be a requirement for diagnosis. With further collapse, the joint medializes, sometimes eroding into the coracoid. Anterior subluxation or dislocations also may be demonstrated, especially if the coracoacromial arch has been violated.

Management of a cuff-deficient arthritic shoulder is dependent on the underlying etiology. It is important to rule out other causes that could present a similar clinical picture, such as RA, infection, old trauma, osteonecrosis, metabolic bone disease, or neuroarthropathy (Table 1). Three distinct conditions exist in which patients present with a rotator cuff tear or insufficiency and glenohumeral arthritis. These are RA, primary OA independent of the rotator cuff tear, and CTA. Patients with RA may have systemic symptoms, involvement of other joints, and characteristic laboratory findings. In addition, patients with RA have poor quality soft tissues with a destructive pannus. Patients with RA have concentric glenoid wear with severely osteopenic bone. Characteristics of OA include subchondral sclerosis, humeral head osteophytes, glenoid osteophytes, and posterior glenoid erosion. Infection and metabolic disease also are important to consider in the differential diagnosis, and, if suspected, they can be ruled out by joint aspiration and evaluation of fluid. The criteria necessary for the diagnosis of CTA are a massive chronic tear of the rotator cuff accompanied by glenohumeral cartilage destruction, osteoporosis of the subchondral bone of the humeral head, and humeral head collapse. It is important to distinguish between CTA and a massive chronic rotator cuff tear without arthropathy, so that prosthetic replacement is not performed needlessly.

Treatment

Nonsurgical Management

When faced with glenohumeral arthritis and a rotator cuff tear, many orthopaedic surgeons feel compelled to immediately recommend surgical intervention. However, it is important to keep in mind that radiographic findings do not always correlate with pain and function and that surgery does not always produce a satisfactory outcome. A course of rest and anti-inflammatory medication followed by physical therapy to maintain motion should be considered in patients who have mild to moderate symptoms. The goal of treatment is relatively pain-free performance of the activities of daily living.

Surgical Management

The primary goal of treatment is the resolution of the patient's pain. Pain usually is well controlled with surgery, but improvement in other parameters, such as range of motion and strength, is less predictable. It is very important for the patient to understand the guarded prognosis. Unrelenting pain, despite extensive nonsurgical management, is the primary indication for surgery. The rotator cuff-deficient shoulder provides a challenge in arthroplasty for numerous reasons. First, the rotator cuff may be irreparable or nonfunctional even if repaired secondary to irreversible muscle atrophy. Second, severe bone loss may make prosthetic reconstruction difficult. Third, the coracoacromial arch is a very important stabilizer, yet painful contact with tuberosity excrescences may be present. Options for surgical treatment have included arthroscopic lavage and débridement, arthrodesis, constrained arthroplasty, unconstrained total shoulder arthroplasty, humeral head replacement (hemiarthroplasty), and semiconstrained total shoulder arthroplasty. Most orthopaedic surgeons consider hemiarthroplasty the treatment of choice in

the United States at this time, with the reverse ball-in-socket prosthesis becoming a superior standard of care in Europe.

Arthroscopic Lavage and Débridement

Arthroscopic joint irrigation may offer short-term reduction of pain, especially in the setting of crystal-associated CTA. However, with severe cuff and glenohumeral disease, long-term results are not predictable. It is crucial that an acromioplasty and release or resection of the coracoacromial ligament is not performed. Compromise of the coracoacromial arch may result in anterosuperior instability, a functionally devastating complication. Several authors have attributed a poor outcome following hemiarthroplasty to either a prior acromioplasty or a deltoid injury during a prior surgery.

Glenohumeral Arthrodesis

Arthrodesis generally is indicated only for patients with a deficient anterior deltoid that is caused by either previous surgery or trauma. Shoulder fusion is a poor choice for most patients with CTA. Many patients have bilateral cuff disease, which makes an arthrodesis difficult to tolerate. Also, because these patients tend to be older, there is a greater risk for surgical complications. Bone quality makes hardware purchase less secure and healing of the fusion less predictable. Older patients do not often tolerate the fused shoulder well even if it heals successfully. Stress is shifted to the scapulothoracic articulation, causing many patients to have unacceptable periscapular pain and trapezial spasm following arthrodesis.

Resection Arthroplasty

Although potentially pain relieving, resection arthroplasty is not recommended as an initial procedure because it usually produces a flail shoulder and increased dysfunction. The procedure is not always complication free because medial and superior migration of the proximal humerus can occur. The option should be reserved for those patients who have had multiple failed attempts at surgical treatment or intractable infections following surgery.

Constrained Total Shoulder Arthroplasty

In the early 1970s, constrained total shoulder arthroplasty seemed to offer promise as a solution for patients with CTA because a stable fulcrum for deltoid function was created, obviating the need for the rotator cuff. However, as happens with other constrained systems, high component-bone interface stresses lead to early loosening, implant dissociation, and fracture. In one

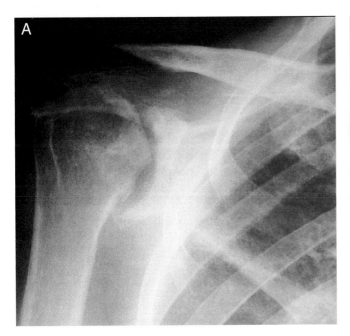 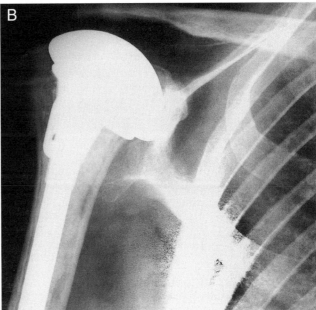

Figure 3 A, Preoperative radiograph showing findings of upward migration of the humeral head and erosion of the acromion. **B,** Postoperative radiograph of the shoulder treated with a humeral hemiarthroplasty.

series, more than 60% of constrained total shoulders had to be revised at short-term follow-up. Because of these problems, constrained total shoulder arthroplasty has been largely abandoned.

Unconstrained Total Shoulder Arthroplasty

Unconstrained total shoulder replacement lowers the shear stresses on the glenoid prosthesis at the expense of mechanical stability, making the presence of an intact cuff a requirement for long-term survival. Early studies, specifically on CTA, have demonstrated an overall reduction of pain with limited improvement of motion with short-term follow-up. However, eccentric forces across the glenohumeral joint in the cuff-deficient shoulder result in superior migration of the humeral head and rim loading of the superior glenoid. One group of authors named this the "rocking-horse effect," referring to these eccentric forces. They linked this theory to clinical results, noting radiographic signs of loosening of the glenoid component in 7 of 14 patients with a cuff-deficient shoulder at 2 years. None of the other 16 patients with an intact cuff demonstrated loosening. The authors theorized that the high-riding humeral component caused excessive compressive stresses on the superior rim of the glenoid, leading to superior tilt and rim wear. In a shoulder with a cuff defect, total shoulder arthroplasty is indicated only when the cuff is either reconstructable or strong enough to stabilize the humeral head concentrically to the glenoid by compression. This is almost never possible or advisable in a patient with CTA.

Hemiarthroplasty

Since the early 1990s, hemiarthroplasty has emerged as the most popular treatment of CTA (Fig. 3). In the past, the use of oversized heads intended to fit the radius of curvature of the coracoacromial arch was advocated. Theoretically, the oversized head fits over the tuberosities and allows for full tensioning of the deltoid with articulation with the coracoacromial arch and superior glenoid in full abduction and forward flexion. Recently, the consensus has been to not "overstuff the joint" to avoid pain from soft-tissue tension, potential antero-superior instability, and posterior capsular tightness associated with large humeral heads. Major contraindications to hemiarthroplasty are infection, loss of the coracoacromial arch, and a deficient deltoid.

One study examined the role of glenoid resurfacing in 30 shoulders with rotator cuff deficiency and glenohumeral arthritis that underwent prosthetic replacement. Thirteen shoulders had a diagnosis of CTA. Nine shoulders underwent humeral head replacement, and four had an unconstrained total shoulder arthroplasty. Satisfactory results were obtained in 11 of 13 patients with CTA. No significant difference was found between groups in terms of patient satisfaction or pain relief. Shoulders treated with hemiarthroplasty did gain significantly more active elevation (52° versus 2°) and had decreased anesthesia time and blood loss. The authors believed function was better when the humeral head replacement respected the "new fulcrum" under the coracoacromial arch.

Another series included 16 patients treated with hemi-

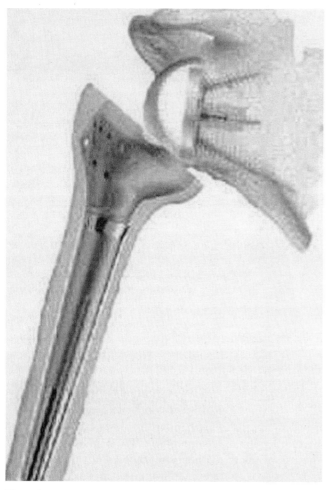

Figure 4 A reverse ball-and-socket semiconstrained total shoulder replacement. A polyethylene insert attached to the humeral component articulates with the metal glenoid component, which is fixed to the native glenoid with screws.

arthroplasty for CTA using Neer and associates' limited goal criteria. Of 12 patients with good deltoid function, 10 were rated successful. Four of the six patients with unsuccessful results had previous surgery, including acromioplasty. Two patients were left deltoid-deficient from their previous surgery. From this study, it is important to note that disruption of the coracoacromial arch at any time in the patient's life may jeopardize hemiarthroplasty in the future. Marginally successful attempts have been made to repair the coracoacromial arch using fascia lata grafts, iliac crest bone struts, and augmentation of the superior aspect of the glenoid rim using bone from the humeral head.

A recent study reviewed 15 patients who underwent shoulder hemiarthroplasty for CTA with mean follow-up at slightly more than 2 years. Special attention was directed at not using excessively large humeral heads. Overall patient satisfaction was 87%. University of California at Los Angeles scores and active range of motion in forward elevation and external rotation increased sig-

nificantly. The authors concluded that hemiarthroplasty, without using excessively large humeral heads, can result in a satisfactory outcome.

The two most important technical considerations are maintaining the integrity of both the coracoacromial arch and the deltoid muscle. The coracoacromial arch is the last restraint to anterosuperior migration of the humeral head and provides a fulcrum for potential glenohumeral motion. Violation of the coracoacromial arch during surgery on the rotator cuff-deficient shoulder can result in painful and debilitating anterosuperior instability postoperatively. Damage to the axillary nerve or avulsion of the deltoid origin can be equally devastating.

Selection of an appropriately sized humeral head that carefully balances the remaining rotator cuff tendons has been shown to offer a good alternative to tenuous tendon repairs and extensive tendon transfers. Whether or not to repair the rotator cuff and to what extent a surgeon should attempt to mobilize and repair the cuff are questions that must be answered for each patient. By definition, CTA includes a massive rotator cuff tear that in most cases is irreparable. Attempting extensive mobilization and trying to obtain a watertight repair with flimsy degenerative cuff tissue is not advisable. There often is fatty degeneration of the cuff musculature that would obviate any worthwhile function of a "complete" repair or transfer, if even possible. A judicious, low-tension, anteroposterior force couple balancing repair is probably more worthwhile. Even with these principles applied, however, functional gains tend to be limited.

Semiconstrained Total Shoulder Arthroplasty

Hooded glenoid components were developed in an effort to overcome the drawbacks of the constrained prosthesis. Long-term data on the function of the components are sparse. Neer attempted to use hooded glenoid components 200% and 600% larger than the standard glenoid components. The 600% larger component was placed in 2 of 12 patients and was subsequently abandoned because of inability to repair the rotator cuff. The 200% larger component also was found to interfere with cuff repair and showed a significant amount of radiolucent lines in the remaining 10 patients. These components are associated with glenoid loosening and decreased postoperative range of motion, which has caused their use to fall out of favor.

In the late 1980s, an inverted, reversed ball-and-socket shoulder prosthesis (Delta, DePuy, France) with a humeral cup articulating on a spherical glenoid component was introduced (Fig. 4). The prosthesis is semiconstrained because the articulating parts are congruent but not "locked together." This prosthesis moves the center of rotation medially, providing a center of rotation closer to the glenoid bone, theoretically decreasing the shear stresses on the glenoid component, which is fixed with screws. The center of rotation also is moved distally, increasing the length of the deltoid lever arm. This design theoretically improves function and stability while decreasing the forces responsible for loosening. Results in Europe have been promising, with good 5- to 7-year results. Preliminary reports show better pain relief and functional results than conventional hemiarthroplasty for CTA. The reverse ball-and-socket prosthesis also may be helpful in patients with anterosuperior instability. However, use of this prosthesis in the United States has not yet been approved by the US Food and Drug Administration (FDA). Long-term follow-up studies are needed to clarify its role for this very challenging patient group.

Summary

Cuff tear arthropathy remains a difficult problem to treat. Over the years, the term CTA has been used loosely to describe different pathologic processes resulting in glenohumeral arthritis and rotator cuff tears; at the same time, different names have been used to describe CTA. Determining the underlying etiology of glenohumeral arthritis in the rotator cuff-deficient shoulder will allow for improved understanding of the disease process, better surgical planning, and more accurate outcome expectations. Helping the patient understand the complexity of the disease while setting realistic goals during management is beneficial to the patient and surgeon. Fully constrained and unconstrained total shoulder arthroplasty are doomed to failure in these patients. The current treatment of choice is humeral head replacement with preservation of the coracoacromial arch, with the goal of pain relief rather than range of motion and return of strength. Hemiarthroplasty should not be performed in patients with an incompetent coracoacromial arch because debilitating anterosuperior instability is likely to develop. In the future, semiconstrained arthroplasty with an improved reverse ball-and-socket design may be a better surgical option than hemiarthroplasty for patients with CTA, pending long-term results of study in Europe and FDA approval in the United States.

Annotated Bibliography

Etiology

Hsu HC, Luo ZP, Cofield RH, An KN: Influence of rotator cuff tearing on glenohumeral stability. *J Shoulder Elbow Surg* 1997;6:413-422.

This study further supports Neer's mechanical hypothesis. Why so few rotator cuff tears progress to CTA remains unexplained. The authors used cadaveric shoulder specimens to demonstrate the effects that different sized rotator cuff tears in different locations had on glenohumeral stability.

Jensen KL, Williams GR Jr, Russell IJ, Rockwood CA Jr: Rotator cuff tear arthropathy. *J Bone Joint Surg Am* 1999;81:1312-1324.

This is the most recent and comprehensive review of rotator cuff tear arthropathy. The article includes historic review, etiology, diagnosis, and treatment of the disease.

Treatment

Cantrell JS, Itamura JM, Burkhead WZ Jr: Rotator cuff tear arthropathy, in Warner JJP, Iannotti JP, Gerber C (eds): *Complex and Revision Problems in Shoulder Surgery.* Philadelphia, PA, Lippincott-Raven, 1997, pp 303-318.

In this excellent, well-illustrated overview of the topic, the senior author outlines his preferred method of treatment (hemiarthroplasty), which is based on a case series of 18 patients managed with four different techniques: bipolar replacement, hemiarthroplasty with a large head, hemiarthroplasty with a small head, and total shoulder arthroplasty. The status of the subscapularis in guiding surgical management is discussed.

Collins DN, Harryman DT II: Arthroplasty for arthritis and rotator cuff deficiency. *Orthop Clin North Am* 1997; 28:225-239.

This is a good summary of the major issues in treating CTA. The authors prefer proximal humeral replacement arthroplasty, and special techniques of this procedure are presented.

De Buttet M, Bouchon Y, Capon D, Delfosse J: Abstract: Grammont shoulder arthroplasty for osteoarthritis with massive rotator cuff tears: Report of 71 cases. *J Shoulder Elbow Surg* 1997;6:197.

This abstract reports the use of the reversed shoulder prosthesis developed by P. Grammont to treat 71 cases of OA with massive rotator cuff tear. Follow-up was only about 2 years, with 49 patients with good to excellent results. There were no cases of radiolucent lines or implant loosening. There were three revisions secondary to technical problems. The authors acknowledge the importance of longer follow-up.

DiGiovanni J, Marra G, Park JY, Bigliani LU: Hemiarthroplasty for glenohumeral arthritis with massive rotator cuff tears. *Orthop Clin North Am* 1998;29:477-489.

This article is an in-depth review of the pathophysiology and treatment options for glenohumeral arthritis with massive rotator cuff tears. The surgical technique for hemiarthroplasty is described.

Field LD, Dines DM, Zabinski SJ, Warren RF: Hemiarthroplasty of the shoulder for rotator cuff arthropathy. *J Shoulder Elbow Surg* 1997;6:18-23.

Sixteen patients underwent hemiarthroplasty for rotator cuff arthropathy with a modular head large enough to articulate with the coracoacromial arch but not so large as to prevent approximately 50% of humeral head translation on the glenoid. Average follow-up was 33 months. Results in 10 patients were rated as successful and as unsuccessful in 6. Failures were attributed to prior acromioplasty. Ten of the 12 patients with good deltoid function and an adequate coracoacromial arch had results rated as successful.

Gartsman GM: Arthroscopic treatment of rotator cuff disease. *J Shoulder Elbow Surg* 1995;4:228-241.

This is an excellent summary of the arthroscopic treatment of rotator cuff disease including CTA.

Vrettos BC, Wallace WA, Neumann L: Abstract: Bipolar hemiarthroplasty of the shoulder for the elderly patient with rotator cuff arthropathy *J Bone Joint Surg Br* 1998;80(suppl 1):106.

This abstract reports poor results in six of seven patients treated with a bipolar device. A full description of this study has not been published.

Williams GR Jr, Rockwood CA Jr: Hemiarthroplasty in rotator cuff-deficient shoulders. *J Shoulder Elbow Surg* 1996;5:362-367.

Hemiarthroplasty results for 21 shoulders with CTA are provided. Follow-up was an average of 4 years. The authors recommend preservation of the coracoacromial ligament, débridement of the rotator cuff without repair, and balance of the remaining cuff tendons by altering the size of the humeral head.

Worland RL, Arredondo J: Bipolar shoulder arthroplasty for painful conditions of the shoulder. *J Arthroplasty* 1998;13:631-637.

The authors present a large study of 182 bipolar replacements, with 27 specifically implanted in patients with CTA. Follow-up was 2.9 years (range, 2 to 6 years), with an overall success rate of 72%. The patients with CTA generally did worse than those with other diagnoses.

Worland RL, Jessup DE, Arredondo J, Warburton KJ: Bipolar shoulder arthroplasty for rotator cuff arthropathy. *J Shoulder Elbow Surg* 1997;6:512-515.

The authors report on a series of 33 patients with CTA, with 22 of them having an average follow-up of 28 months (range, 24 to 48 months). All patients had preserved passive motion and good deltoid function. The authors report uniformly improved function and reduced pain in all patients.

Zuckerman JD, Scott AJ, Gallagher MA: Hemiarthroplasty for cuff tear arthropathy. *J Shoulder Elbow Surg* 2000;9:169-172.

This most recent series in the literature reviews the results of 15 hemiarthroplasties performed for CTA. At an average of 28.2 months, 87% of patients expressed overall satisfaction with their surgery. Increases were seen in range of motion and ability to perform activities of daily living.

Classic Bibliography

Amstutz HC, Thomas BJ, Kabo JM, Jinnah RH, Dorey FJ: The Dana total shoulder arthroplasty. *J Bone Joint Surg Am* 1988;70:1174-1182.

Arntz CT, Jackins S, Matsen FA III: Prosthetic replacement of the shoulder for the treatment of defects in the rotator cuff and the surface of the glenohumeral joint. *J Bone Joint Surg Am* 1993;75:485-491.

Barrett WP, Franklin JL, Jackins SE, Wyss CR, Matsen FA III: Total shoulder arthroplasty. *J Bone Joint Surg Am* 1987;69:865-872.

Barrett WP, Thornhill TS, Thomas WH, Gebhart EM, Sledge CB: Nonconstrained total shoulder arthroplasty in patients with polyarticular rheumatoid arthritis. *J Arthroplasty* 1989;4:91-96.

Caporali R, Rossi S, Montecucco C: Letter: Tidal irrigation in Milwaukee shoulder syndrome. *J Rheumatol* 1994;21:1781-1782.

Cofield RH: Total shoulder arthroplasty with the Neer prosthesis. *J Bone Joint Surg Am* 1984;66:899-906.

Coughlin MJ, Morris JM, West WF: The semiconstrained total shoulder arthroplasty. *J Bone Joint Surg Am* 1979; 61:574-581.

Franklin JL, Barrett WP, Jackins SE, Matsen FA III: Glenoid loosening in total shoulder arthroplasty: Association with rotator cuff deficiency. *J Arthroplasty* 1988; 3:39-46.

Grammont PM, Baulot E: Delta shoulder prosthesis for rotator cuff rupture. *Orthopedics* 1993;16:65-68.

Gristina AG, Romano RL, Kammire GC, Webb LX: Total shoulder replacement. *Orthop Clin North Am* 1987;18:445-453.

Hawkins RJ, Bell RH, Jallay B: Total shoulder arthroplasty. *Clin Orthop* 1989;242:188-194.

Laurence M: Replacement arthroplasty of the rotator cuff deficient shoulder. *J Bone Joint Surg Br* 1991;73: 916-919.

Lettin AW, Copeland SA, Scales JT: The Stanmore total shoulder replacement. *J Bone Joint Surg Br* 1982;64: 47-51.

Matsen FA III, Arntz CT, Harryman DT II: Rotator cuff tear arthropathy, in Bigliani LU (ed): *Complications of Shoulder Surgery*. Baltimore, MD, Williams & Wilkins, 1993, pp 44-58.

McCarty DJ, Halverson PB, Carrera GF, Brewer BJ, Kozin F: "Milwaukee shoulder": Association of microspheroids containing hydroxyapatite crystals, active collagenase, and neutral protease with rotator cuff defects. I: Clinical aspects. *Arthritis Rheum* 1981;24:464-473.

McElwain JP, English E: The early results of porous-coated total shoulder arthroplasty. *Clin Orthop* 1987; 218:217-224.

Neer CS II, Craig EV, Fukuda H: Cuff-tear arthropathy. *J Bone Joint Surg Am* 1983;65:1232-1244.

Neer CS II, Watson KC, Stanton FJ: Recent experience in total shoulder replacement. *J Bone Joint Surg Am* 1982;64:319-337.

Pollock RG, Deliz ED, McIlveen SJ, Flatow EL, Bigliani LU: Prosthetic replacement in rotator cuff-deficient shoulders. *J Shoulder Elbow Surg* 1992;1:173-186.

Post M, Haskell SS, Jablon M: Total shoulder replacement with a constrained prosthesis. *J Bone Joint Surg Am* 1980;62:327-335.

Post M, Jablon M: Constrained total shoulder arthroplasty: Long-term follow-up observations. *Clin Orthop* 1983;173:109-116.

Post M, Jablon M, Miller H, Singh M: Constrained total shoulder joint replacement: A critical review. *Clin Orthop* 1979;144:135-150.

Section 4

Trauma/Fracture

Section Editor:
Andrew Green, MD

Chapter 20

Proximal Humeral Fractures

Andrew Green, MD

Introduction

Proximal humeral fractures are common injuries and occur at about 70% the incidence of hip fractures. Most proximal humeral fractures are minimally displaced and can be treated successfully without surgery. Less commonly, surgical treatment is indicated for displaced fractures. Although nonsurgical treatment is usually straightforward, surgical treatment can be difficult. A variety of factors including associated soft-tissue injuries (neurovascular and rotator cuff), preexisting shoulder abnormalities, and patient factors impact the outcome. With the aging of the US population and the associated increased prevalence of osteoporosis, the incidence of proximal humeral fractures will increase. These epidemiologic factors will further challenge clinicians to produce satisfactory outcomes. New developments in surgical implants and techniques have facilitated surgical treatment. Important advances in the outcome evaluation of shoulder disorders are helping orthopaedic surgeons to recognize the impact of proximal humeral fractures on patients and to direct treatment selection.

Anatomy

The relevant anatomy has been discussed adequately in many other publications. The proximal humerus comprises four segments, including the greater and lesser tuberosities, the articular segment, and the humeral shaft. The tuberosities attach to the articular segment at the anatomic neck and are the sites of attachment for the glenohumeral capsule and ligaments and the rotator cuff tendons. The greater tuberosity has three facets for the insertions of the supraspinatus, infraspinatus, and teres minor tendons; the subscapularis tendon inserts on the lesser tuberosity. The insertions of the rotator cuff tendons are broad and extend up to 2 cm beyond the edge of the articular surface. The intertubercular groove lies between the tuberosities and forms the conduit for the tendon of the long head of the biceps as it passes from its intra-articular position in the glenohumeral joint into the arm. In addition, the deltoid, pectoralis major, latissimus dorsi, and teres major insert on the humerus distal to the surgical neck. The soft-tissue attachments contribute to the displacement of the fracture fragments.

The vascular anatomy of the proximal humerus has an important role in the pathophysiology of proximal humeral fractures. The anterior humeral circumflex artery continues under the biceps tendon and gives rise to the ascending branch, which supplies most of the articular segment. The posterior humeral circumflex artery gives rise to vessels that enter the posterior medial aspect of the humeral head and supply a smaller part of the articular segment. Injury of the arterial supply to the articular segment, especially the ascending branch of the anterior humeral circumflex artery, can result in osteonecrosis.

Classification of Fractures

Codman recognized that most proximal humeral fractures occur along the physeal scars of the proximal humerus. Based on this early observation, Neer developed the four-part classification system that remains the most recognized and used standard for assessing proximal humeral fractures. He described six different variations of displaced proximal humeral fractures and defined displacement as 45° of angulation or 1 cm of displacement of a part. More recent literature suggests that even greater tuberosity displacements of 5 mm or less can have a clinically significant impact. A recent study of the normal anatomy of the proximal humerus demonstrated that the greater tuberosity is on average 8 ± 3.2 mm below the top of the articular segment. Thus, even small amounts of greater tuberosity displacement can be problematic.

More recently, the AO/ASIF/OTA Comprehensive Long Bone Classification system has been adopted. This is a more detailed classification system in which proximal humeral fractures are classified into three main

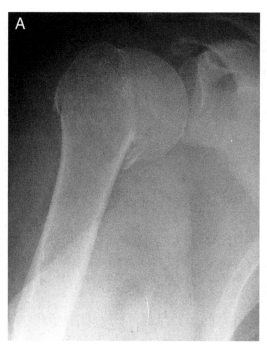
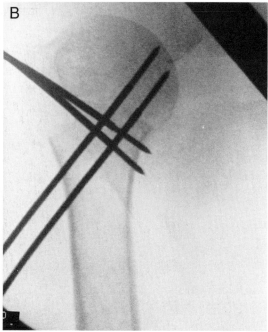

Figure 1 A, Displaced (angulated) two-part surgical neck fracture. **B,** After treatment with closed reduction and percutaneous pinning.

groups and three additional subgroups. It is less commonly referenced than the Neer system. In contrast to Neer's classification, the Comprehensive Long Bone Classification system clearly identifies the valgus impacted anatomic neck fracture as distinct from other four-part fractures. Valgus impacted fractures, unlike true four-part fractures, can have partial preservation of the vascularity to the articular segment through the intact medial capsule.

Unfortunately, all fracture classification systems have limited interobserver reliability. Two recent studies demonstrated this for proximal humeral fractures. Another study found that the addition of CT scans did not improve the interobserver reliability of proximal humeral fracture classification with the Neer and Comprehensive Long Bone Classification systems. Nevertheless, these classification systems are clinically useful because they help clinicians to triage different injuries to appropriate treatment in order to achieve an optimal outcome.

Associated Injuries

Peripheral nerve injuries are the most common injuries associated with proximal humeral fractures. They occur in as many as one third of patients and are more common with increasing age. In one reported study, the incidence of nerve injury with proximal humeral fracture-dislocation was greater than 50% after age 50 years. The axillary nerve is the most commonly injured peripheral nerve. This injury most likely is related to the anatomy of the nerve, which branches from the posterior cord as it passes deep to the conjoined tendon, under the sub-

scapularis muscle, and through the quadrilateral space before wrapping around the proximal humerus. In addition, axillary nerve injury often occurs in combination with other peripheral nerve injuries. Some of these combined injuries are infraclavicular brachial plexus injuries. Unfortunately, recovery of associated nerve injuries is often incomplete.

Vascular injuries are a rare complication of proximal humeral fractures and fracture-dislocations. They usually involve the axillary artery, its branches, or the axillary vein. Vascular injuries most commonly occur in older patients who have fragile atherosclerotic vessels. An associated vascular injury must be treated as an emergency, and timely evaluation with arteriography is imperative. Because of the extensive collateral blood supply around the shoulder, a distal pulse can sometimes be palpated in the presence of a significant proximal vascular injury.

Evaluation

A standardized approach to the evaluation of the injured shoulder is followed. This approach includes a detailed history that defines any comorbid conditions, preexisting shoulder problems, and the mechanism of injury. The social history is particularly important in elderly patients. Observation of the patient should include assessment of his or her ambulatory and general physical condition. A careful and detailed physical examination can help the clinician determine whether there is associated neurologic injury. Although it can be difficult to precisely evaluate shoulder girdle muscle strength in the acute injury setting, voluntary isometric muscle con-

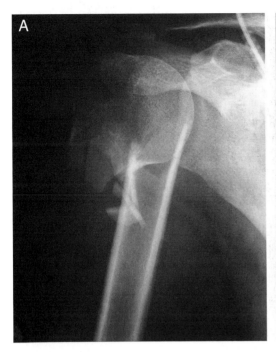
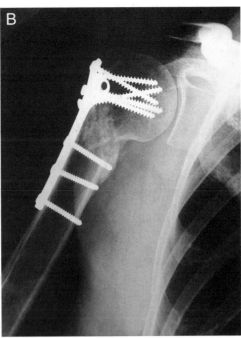

Figure 2 A, Plain radiograph of a 48-year-old woman demonstrates a displaced two-part surgical neck fracture. **B,** Nearly anatomic position was achieved with ORIF with a modified AO small fragment cloverleaf plate (Synthes, Paoli, PA).

traction usually can be elicited to obtain a complete motor examination. Sensory examination, particularly of the axillary nerve, can be misleading because it is possible to have intact sensation and abnormal motor function. Electrodiagnostic studies should be obtained if a neurologic deficit does not resolve after 3 weeks.

Radiographic evaluation of the injured shoulder should always include the shoulder trauma series with a true AP, scapular Y view, and axillary lateral view. Additional AP views in internal and external rotation can provide more details about a fracture of the greater tuberosity as well as help to identify an occult surgical neck fracture.

In some cases, CT imaging is required to further define the extent of tuberosity displacement or articular segment fracture. In occasional cases, standard axial imaging does not clearly demonstrate the amount of fracture displacement in the vertical axis of the body. Coronal and three-dimensional reconstruction CT occasionally is used to define the displacement of a proximal humeral fracture. Advanced imaging should be considered when there is a question of the amount of displacement and the choice of treatment is in question.

MRI rarely is indicated for routine evaluation of a proximal humeral fracture. However, if plain radiographs fail to demonstrate a fracture and the clinical course is not progressing satisfactorily, MRI is an appropriate study and can demonstrate occult nondisplaced fractures, rotator cuff tearing, occult articular injury, or osteonecrosis.

Nonsurgical Treatment

Nondisplaced fractures are treated nonsurgically. When the fracture is impacted or stable, early range-of-motion exercises can be initiated. If the fracture is unstable, a period of immobilization is required. Most nondisplaced fractures are stable enough to begin motion exercises within 2 to 4 weeks after the injury.

Some fracture-dislocations can be reduced closed. The most common fracture-dislocation is an anterior greater tuberosity fracture-dislocation. Most of these injuries reduce anatomically with closed reduction. However, great care should be taken whenever a fracture-dislocation is reduced closed. If any difficulty is encountered or if there is concern about causing iatrogenic displacement, then a reduction under general anesthesia or interscalene nerve block should be considered.

The amount of acceptable fracture displacement depends on several factors. The anatomic pattern and the patient's premorbid functional status are important considerations. Despite Neer's criteria for displacement, most authors agree that the shoulder has very little tolerance for greater tuberosity displacement. In fact, most suggest that displacement of greater than 5 mm can result in substantial dysfunction either from impingement or rotator cuff tear. More recently, it was suggested that fractures with 3 mm of displacement should be reduced in athletes and laborers who are involved in overhead activity. Lesser tuberosity fractures are rare. Medial displacement of the lesser tuberosity can cause internal rotation weakness, block internal rotation, or result in subcoracoid impingement. Surgical neck angulation, which is usually directed apex anterolateral, limits shoulder elevation and can lead to subacromial impingement. In some cases, because of comorbid factors, nonsurgical treatment is the most appropriate treatment despite substantial displacement.

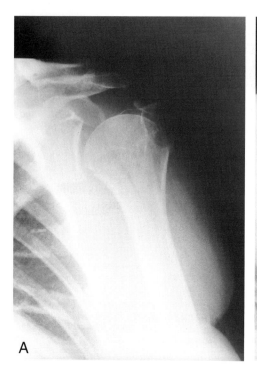

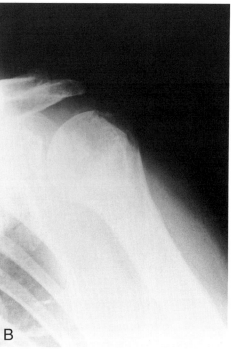

Figure 3 True AP radiographs of a valgus impacted proximal humeral fracture. **A,** The injury film demonstrates the valgus position of the articular segment, which is impacted between the tuberosities. **B,** The postoperative film demonstrates anatomic repositioning of the articular segment after open reduction and minimal internal fixation with heavy sutures.

Surgical Treatment

Some fractures can be adequately treated with closed reduction and percutaneous pinning, for which many of the same principles as those of open reduction and internal fixation (ORIF) apply. The best results of closed reduction and percutaneous pinning have been reported for two-part surgical neck fractures (Fig. 1), but some authors have reported using the technique for three- and four-part fractures. More unstable and comminuted fractures and more severe osteopenia can compromise the results of this technique. Early motion should be avoided because the fixation is not as secure as with ORIF.

The indications for ORIF of displaced proximal humeral fractures are not clear-cut. Although Neer defined displacement, the effect of displacement on the outcome of treatment is difficult to determine. The outcome of surgical treatment depends on many factors in addition to the quality of the reduction of the fracture.

Surgical treatment of proximal humeral fractures can be difficult. The complex anatomy of the shoulder girdle, difficulty achieving and maintaining anatomic reduction and stable fixation, and variations in the patient's ability to participate with a prolonged and rigorous rehabilitation program are all factors that impact on the eventual outcome. Few orthopaedists have extensive clinical experience with the surgical treatment of proximal humeral fractures.

The surgical approach depends on the specific fracture. Most fractures, including surgical neck, three-part, and four-part fractures, are approached through a deltopectoral approach. A superior deltoid splitting approach (similar to open rotator cuff repair) can be used for ORIF of greater tuberosity fractures and some valgus impacted fractures.

Many different internal fixation techniques have been described, including interosseous sutures or wires, pins, screws, plates and screws, and intramedullary rods. No single technique can be used in every patient with a specific fracture pattern. Comminution and osteopenia affect the stability or rigidity achieved by any fixation technique. Good bone is the exception, and techniques that achieve both interfragmentary and axial stability without excessive soft-tissue dissection are most likely to be successful.

Screw fixation is often unsuccessful because there is poor purchase in the humeral head. The best screw fixation can be achieved in the central aspect of the articular segment, where the cancellous bone is the thickest. Screw fixation of the greater tuberosity can fail because although the screw may have purchase in the humeral head articular segment, the fragile tuberosity may displace around the screw. Plate and screw fixation is best reserved for younger patients with good bone quality (Fig. 2). When heavy suture fixation is used, the sutures can be placed through the bone or around the tuberosity fragments at the rotator cuff insertion. The latter is usually a stronger technique.

Metaphyseal comminution is particularly problematic. When there is medial comminution at the surgical neck or proximal shaft area, maintaining humeral length and the position of the articular segment is especially difficult. Varus malunion is a common sequela of comminution at the medial aspect of the surgical neck. Intramedullary fixation and fixed-angle plate and screw

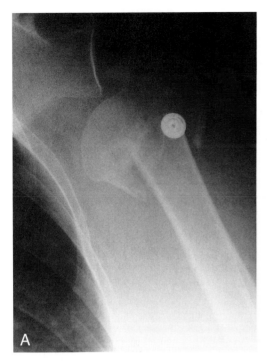

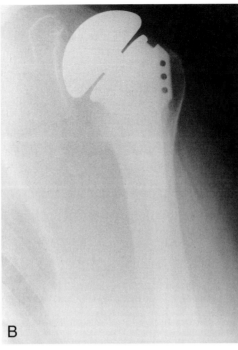

Figure 4 A, True AP radiograph of a head-splitting three-part proximal humeral fracture in a 70-year-old woman. **B,** Postoperative radiograph after successful treatment with a humeral head replacement.

devices can improve axial stability; conventional plate and screw fixation is prone to failure in this situation. In all instances, extraneous dissection should be avoided to preserve the vascularity to the articular segment.

The strength and stability achieved by a variety of fixation techniques were evaluated in several recent biomechanical studies. In one study, multiple-pin fixation was compared with locked antegrade intramedullary rodding for three-part greater tuberosity fractures, and the latter construct was found to be superior. In another study, the addition of intramedullary rodding to a tension band construct significantly improved the fixation strength. Results of yet another study confirmed the common belief that the quality of the bone of the proximal humerus has a significant effect on the strength of specific fracture fixation constructs.

Articular segment fractures are problematic because of the risk of arthritis caused by articular incongruity as well as humeral head collapse secondary to osteonecrosis. Some simple articular fractures can be reduced and fixed internally. The articular reduction can be palpated through the rotator cuff interval and visualized with fluoroscopic imaging. Articular comminution is difficult to reduce without direct fracture exposure. Most fractures with significant articular comminution are treated with prosthetic replacement.

Valgus impacted four-part fractures treated with ORIF have a lower risk of osteonecrosis than do true four-part fractures (Fig. 3). Open reduction of true four-part fractures is controversial because there is a high risk of osteonecrosis. Achieving an anatomic reduction is critical when performing ORIF. When there is osteo-

necrosis in the presence of an anatomic reduction, the clinical outcome is better. Late reconstruction after failed closed or open treatment is difficult. In one study of fracture management, late shoulder arthroplasty had worse results than did primary humeral head replacement. In another study, the results of late reconstruction were correlated with the authors' ability to correct problems encountered at surgery, such as malunion, nonunion, stiffness, and arthritis.

Humeral head replacement is recommended for most four-part fractures and fracture-dislocations. In addition, some authors advocate humeral head replacement for some three-part fractures, especially comminuted fractures in the elderly (Fig. 4). Recent advances in implant design have included modular humeral components. Modularity has several advantages, including facilitating reconstruction of the variable anatomy of the proximal humerus and revision from humeral head replacement to total shoulder replacement. Posterior fracture-dislocations with impaction of greater than 40% of the articular segment can be treated with humeral head replacement. Recent reports have described osteochondral reconstruction of large anterior and posterior humeral head impaction defects.

Complications

In addition to associated injuries, complications or poor results are not uncommon after proximal humeral fractures. Poor results after nonsurgical treatment are most commonly related to shoulder stiffness and limited motion or to the consequences of displacement of the

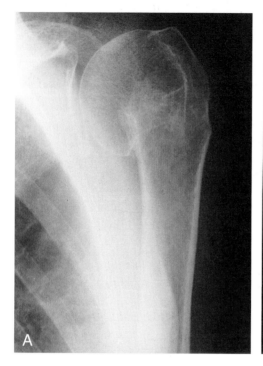

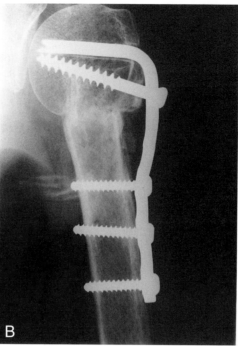

Figure 5 Plain radiographs of a patient who presented with pain and limited shoulder motion after sustaining a surgical neck fracture. **A,** Plain radiograph demonstrates a varus malunion. **B,** The malunion was successfully treated with an osteotomy and internal fixation with an angled blade plate.

greater tuberosity. Even small amounts of superior displacement of the greater tuberosity can cause subacromial impingement. In fact, subacromial scarring without displacement can be sufficient to cause impingement. Surgical neck angulation and malunion are relatively common. The typical angulation is apex anterolateral, and there is usually an associated loss of shoulder elevation and abduction (Fig. 5). In addition, capsular contracture can occur and limit motion. Shoulder stiffness is best avoided by initiating passive motion exercises early in the rehabilitation process.

Although osteonecrosis is more common after four-part fractures, it also can occur after surgical treatment of less complex fractures. In contrast, osteonecrosis is rare after nondisplaced fractures or nonsurgical treatment of two- or three-part fractures. Posttraumatic arthritis usually occurs after articular segment fractures or malunions.

Outcomes

There has been a recent interest in the evaluation of the outcome of various shoulder disorders. Most studies have focused on the treatment of atraumatic disorders. No outcome measure is specifically designed to evaluate the outcome of shoulder fractures.

Results of a recent study demonstrated that the outcome of nonsurgical treatment of nondisplaced proximal humeral fractures often is limited. The outcome of nonsurgical treatment of nondisplaced and minimally displaced proximal humeral fractures was fair or poor in 23% of patients. Consequently, it is not surprising

that the results of surgical treatment of proximal humeral fractures are frequently less than optimal.

Reports of several recent studies indicated variable outcomes of surgical treatment of more severe proximal humeral fractures. It is difficult to determine why authors of some studies report better outcomes than others, although varying patient populations, surgeon skill, and observer bias undoubtedly have an effect. Authors of studies in which modern outcome assessments are used tend to report poorer outcomes for ORIF of more complex fractures, especially four-part fractures.

Summary

Although proximal humeral fractures are common, there is much to be learned to improve the outcome of treatment. Improvements in understanding of the pathophysiology of proximal humeral fractures, in surgical techniques, and in assessment of outcomes provide the opportunity to achieve this goal.

Annotated Bibliography

Beredjiklian PK, Iannotti JP, Norris TR, Williams GR: Operative treatment of malunion of a fracture of the proximal aspect of the humerus. *J Bone Joint Surg Am* 1998;80:1484-1497.

The authors performed a retrospective study of surgical treatment of malunion of the proximal humerus. The outcome was evaluated with a categorical rating. Many patients with satisfactory results had substantial functional limitations. The authors were able to correlate the results with their ability to correct the pathologic anatomy.

Bosch U, Skutek M, Fremerey RW, Tscherne H: Outcome after primary and secondary hemiarthroplasty in elderly patients with fractures of the proximal humerus. *J Shoulder Elbow Surg* 1998;7:479-484.

In a series of 39 patients with three- and four-part fractures of the proximal humerus that were treated with humeral head replacement, the authors found that the results of early surgery were better than the results of late reconstruction. They did not perform total shoulder arthroplasty in any of the late reconstructions.

Bernstein J, Adler LM, Blank JE, Dalsey RM, Williams GR, Iannotti JP: Evaluation of the Neer system of classification of proximal humeral fractures with computerized tomographic scans and plain radiographs. *J Bone Joint Surg Am* 1996;78:1371-1375.

The study evaluated the intraobserver reliability and interobserver reproducibility of the Neer classification system on the basis of review of plain radiographs and CT scans of 20 fractures. The addition of CT scans was associated with a slight increase in the intraobserver reliability but no increase in the interobserver reproducibility. The interobserver reproducibility of the responses of the senior shoulder surgeons regarding diagnosis and treatment did not change when CT images were used in addition to plain radiographs.

Chen CY, Chao EK, Tu YK, Ueng SW, Shih CH: Closed management and percutaneous fixation of unstable proximal humerus fractures. *J Trauma* 1998;45:1039-1045.

Treatment of 19 patients with two- and three-part proximal humeral fractures yielded satisfactory results.

Gerber C, Hersche O, Berberat C: The clinical relevance of posttraumatic avascular necrosis of the humeral head. *J Shoulder Elbow Surg* 1998;7:586-590

Twenty-five patients with posttraumatic osteonecrosis of the humeral head were reviewed. The overall shoulder function according to the Constant score was 51% of an age- and sex-matched normal control group. The clinical outcome was related to the anatomic alignment of the healed proximal humerus. The authors noted that a proximal humeral fracture that is at risk for osteonecrosis has to be reduced anatomically. If anatomic reduction cannot be obtained, other treatment such as humeral head replacement should be considered.

Herscovici D Jr, Saunders DT, Johnson MP, Sanders R, DiPasquale T: Percutaneous fixation of proximal humeral fractures. *Clin Orthop* 2000;375:97-104.

The authors evaluated the results of percutaneous fixation of displaced proximal humeral fractures. Despite high union rates, they observed varus malunion and loss of pin fixation as complications of this technique. They recommended using multiple, heavier, terminally threaded pins with wide spacing in the articular segment.

Instrum K, Fennell C, Shrive N, Damson E, Sonnabend D, Hollinshead R: Semitubular blade plate fixation in proximal humeral fractures: A biomechanical study in a cadaveric model. *J Shoulder Elbow Surg* 1998;7:462-466.

The authors compared the strength of fixation of a surgical neck osteotomy of the proximal humerus fixed with either an AO T-plate or a blade plate constructed from a semitubular plate. The blade plate construct was significantly better ($P < 0.05$) when the specimens were subjected to submaximal cyclic loading.

Kannus P, Palvanen M, Niemi S, Parkkari J, Jarvinen M, Vuori I: Increasing number and incidence of osteoporotic fractures of the proximal humerus in elderly people. *BMJ* 1996;313:1051-1052.

This epidemiologic study of all patients with proximal humeral fractures admitted to Finnish hospitals during six different 2- and 3-year periods between 1970 and 1993 demonstrated a steady increase in the age-specific incidences of fractures of the proximal humerus for males and females of all ages. Based on population trends, the authors predicted that the number of proximal humeral fractures would increase exponentially for the next 20 to 30 years.

Ko JY, Yamamoto R: Surgical treatment of complex fracture of the proximal humerus. *Clin Orthop* 1996; 327:225-237.

This is a retrospective review of the results of open reduction and minimal internal fixation with or without external fixation for 16 three- and four-part fractures and fracture-dislocations of the proximal humerus. There were 12 three-part greater tuberosity fractures (six with dislocation), and four four-part fractures (three with dislocation). At a mean follow-up of 3.8 years, 14 of the 16 patients had a satisfactory (eight) or excellent (six) result based on the Neer criteria. The type of fracture did not correlate with the results.

Koval KJ, Blair B, Takei R, Kummer FJ, Zuckerman JD: Surgical neck fractures of the proximal humerus: A laboratory evaluation of ten fixation techniques. *J Trauma* 1996;40:778-783.

The authors studied the stability and ultimate strength of 10 different fixation techniques for surgical neck fractures of the proximal humerus. They used fresh frozen (nonosteopenic) and embalmed (osteopenic) specimens. In the fresh frozen group, T-plate and screws was the strongest technique. Ender rods with tension band fixation was the next strongest. In the embalmed group, four Schanz pins (one pin through the greater tuberosity) provided the strongest fixation, followed by the T-plate and screws. Tension band fixation was the weakest in both groups.

Koval KJ, Gallagher MA, Marsicano JG, Cuomo F, McShinawy A, Zuckerman JD: Functional outcome after minimally displaced fractures of the proximal part of the humerus. *J Bone Joint Surg Am* 1997;79:203-207.

In a retrospective study of 104 patients, the authors found that the outcome of nonsurgical treatment of non- and minimally displaced proximal humeral fractures was fair or poor in 23% of cases. They found that earlier initiation of motion exercises improved the outcome.

Movin T, Sjödén GO, Ahrengart L: Poor function after shoulder replacement in fracture patients: A retrospective evaluation of 29 patients followed for 2-12 years. *Acta Orthop Scand* 1998;69:392-396.

The authors evaluated 29 proximal humeral fractures treated with humeral head replacement. There were 18 acute and 11 late replacements. Overall, the results were worse than in most other reports. The mean Constant score was 38. The timing of surgery did not affect the outcomes. The use of a modular implant did not affect the outcome.

Orthopaedic Trauma Association Committee for Coding and Classification: Fracture and Dislocation Compendium. *J Orthop Trauma* 1996;10(suppl 1):1-155.

This publication describes a fracture classification system that was proposed by the Committee for Coding and Classification of the Orthopaedic Trauma Association. It is based on the early work of Maurice Muller and associates at the AO/ASIF Documentation Center in Bern, Switzerland.

Resch H, Povacz P, Fröhlich R, Wambacher M: Percutaneous fixation of three- and four-part fractures of the proximal humerus. *J Bone Joint Surg Br* 1997;79:295-300.

Twenty-seven patients, 9 with three-part and 18 with four-part proximal humeral fractures that were treated with percutaneous pinning, were reviewed at mean 2-year follow-up. The mean patient age was 54 years (25 to 68 years). All of the three-part fractures had good to very good functional results. The mean Constant score for the four-part fractures was 87% that of the age and gender match control. Overall patient satisfaction was universal.

Wheeler DL, Colville MR: Biomechanical comparison of intramedullary and percutaneous pin fixation for proximal humeral fracture fixation. *J Orthop Trauma* 1997;11:363-367.

The authors compared the biomechanics of fixation of three-part proximal humeral fractures with that of either percutaneous pinning or locked intramedullary rodding. They tested the fixation stiffness and durability under cyclic rotational loading and torsional loading to failure. The specific intramedullary device that they tested provided superior resistance to cyclic loading.

Williams GR Jr, Copley LA, Iannotti JP, Lisser SP: The influence of intramedullary fixation on figure-of-eight wiring for surgical neck fractures of the proximal humerus: A biomechanical comparison. *J Shoulder Elbow Surg* 1997;6:423-428.

The authors evaluated the effect of the addition of intramedullary fixation to figure-of-8 wire for internal fixation of a surgical neck osteotomy of the proximal humerus. The addition of two Ender rods increased the resistance of maximal torsional load by 1.5 times. In addition, they did not find a significant correlation between the mean maximal load to failure and the bone mineral density of the specimens.

Wretenberg P, Ekelund A: Acute hemiarthroplasty after proximal humerus fracture in old patients: A retrospective evaluation of 18 patients followed for 2-7 years. *Acta Orthop Scand* 1997;68:121-123.

The mean patient age in this study, 82 years, was older than that in most other reported studies. Eleven of the patients were pain free. Range of motion and function were limited.

Zyto K, Ahrengart L, Sperber A, Tornkvist H: Treatment of displaced proximal humeral fractures in elderly patients. *J Bone Joint Surg Br* 1997;79:412-417.

This randomized prospective study of elderly patients compared the outcome of closed treatment and ORIF with minimal fixation. There were mostly three-part fractures. There was no significant difference in the outcome of treatment.

Zyto K, Wallace WA, Frostick SP, Preston BJ: Outcome after hemiarthroplasty for three-and four-part fractures of the proximal humerus. *J Shoulder Elbow Surg* 1998;7:85-89.

This study was a retrospective review of the outcome of hemiarthroplasty for three- and four-part proximal humeral fractures. There were 27 patients, 17 with three-part and 10 with four-part fractures. The authors were disappointed with the results because the patients had limited motion, as well as a high incidence of pain and disability.

Zyto K: Non-operative treatment of comminuted fractures of the proximal humerus in elderly patients. *Injury* 1998;29:349-352.

The authors identified 58 patients who had three- or four-part proximal humeral fractures. At greater than 10-year follow-up, 38 patients were deceased and five were lost to follow-up. Long-term follow-up of the remaining 15 patients (17 shoulders), whose fractures were treated nonsurgically, demonstrated minimal pain, limited function, and high degree of patient satisfaction. The mean Constant score was 59 for the patients with three-part fractures and 47 for patients with four-part fractures.

Classic Bibliography

Codman EA: *The Shoulder.* Boston, MA, T Todd, 1934.

Connor PM, Boatright JR, D'Alessandro DF: Posterior fracture-dislocation of the shoulder: Treatment with acute osteochondral grafting. *J Shoulder Elbow Surg* 1997;6:480-485.

Esser RD: Open reduction and internal fixation of three- and four-part fractures of the proximal humerus. *Clin Orthop* 1994;299:244-251.

Neer CS II: Displaced proximal humeral fractures: I. Classification and evaluation. *J Bone Joint Surg Am* 1970;52:1077-1089.

Neer CS II: Displaced proximal humeral fractures: II. Treatment of three-part and four-part displacement. *J Bone Joint Surg Am* 1970;52:1090-1103.

Norris TR, Green A, McGuigan FX: Late prosthetic shoulder arthroplasty for displaced proximal humerus fractures. *J Shoulder Elbow Surg* 1995;4:271-280

Schai P, Imhoff A, Preiss S: Comminuted humeral head fractures: A multicenter analysis. *J Shoulder Elbow Surg* 1995;4:319-330.

Chapter 21

Clavicular Fractures and Sternoclavicular Dislocations

Andrew Green, MD

Sean Griggs, MD

William C. Doukas, MD, LTC

Carl J. Basamania, MD

Introduction

Clavicular fractures, one of the most common types of fracture, are easily recognized because of the prominent subcutaneous position of the clavicle. In most cases, nonsurgical treatment results in healing and a satisfactory outcome. However, healing does not always occur with nonsurgical treatment nor does the outcome always meet patient expectations. Nonunion, although relatively uncommon, can be quite disabling. Malunion also can be problematic and can present unique challenges to the treating physician. Sternoclavicular dislocations are rare and often are not identified on initial presentation. Anterior dislocations are more common than posterior dislocations and treatment is different for each condition. Most clavicular injuries are treated nonsurgically; therefore, experience with their surgical management is limited.

Anatomy

The clavicle is the first bone to ossify. This occurs during the fifth week of gestation. It is also the only long bone to ossify by intramembranous ossification. Ossification occurs centrally until about age 5 years, when the medial and lateral epiphyseal growth plates develop. Subsequent longitudinal growth occurs primarily by enchondral ossification at the medial end. The sternal epiphysis does not fuse until sometime between the ages of 20 and 25 years. Consequently, sternoclavicular injuries in adolescence are usually physeal fractures.

The clavicle is the only bone linking the shoulder girdle to the axial skeleton. The sternoclavicular joint is a synovial articulation supported by very strong ligaments, including the intra-articular disk ligament, the costoclavicular (rhomboid) ligament, the interclavicular ligament, and the capsular ligament (Fig. 1). This unique diarthrodial joint permits 3° of freedom of movement and thus functions with ball-and-socket mechanics. Laterally, the entire upper extremity is suspended from the clavicle by the coracoclavicular and acromioclavicular ligaments.

The shape of the clavicle has important anatomic and functional implications. From the superior view it forms an S-shape, with the convexity of the curves directed posteromedially and anterolaterally. The middle third is essentially tubular, with transition zones through the apices of the curves both medially and laterally. Medially, the bone flares with metaphyseal expansion in all planes, whereas laterally, the bone becomes wider in the AP plane and flatter in its superior-inferior dimensions. Because of this S-shape, forces transmitted through the clavicle from the lateral aspect of the shoulder generate shear forces across the middle third, where most clavicle fractures occur. The middle third is thickest and strongest to help protect the underlying neurovascular structures, and injury to these vital structures is relatively uncommon. The medial cord of the brachial plexus, which ultimately gives rise to the ulnar nerve, is located beneath the clavicle and above the first rib, where it is vulnerable to direct injury from middle-third fractures. Likewise, ulnar nerve symptoms are most common when there is compressive neuropathy associated with malunion or hypertrophic callus formation following middle-third fractures. Vascular injuries most commonly affect the subclavian artery and warrant immediate vascular consultation.

The blood supply to the clavicle has important implications for fracture healing. Early reports described a single main nutrient artery. Injection studies indicate that three arteries, the suprascapular, thoracoacromial, and internal thoracic (mammary), are the source of the blood supply to the clavicle. No nutrient artery was identified; however, the main blood supply was found to be primarily periosteal. Therefore, extensive soft-tissue stripping, either at the time of injury or during treatment, may jeopardize or delay healing.

Despite being relatively constrained, the clavicle rotates through a substantial arc of motion in all planes. Approximately 50° of rotation occurs through the long axis of the clavicle, primarily laterally through the acro-

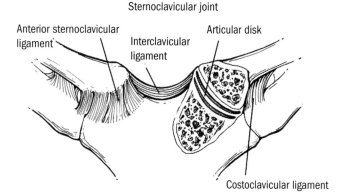

Figure 1 Anatomy of the sternoclavicular joint. *(Reproduced with permission from Tibone J, et al: The shoulder: Functional anatomy, biomechanics and kinesiology, in DeLee JC, Drez D (eds): Orthopaedic Sports Medicine: Principles and Practice. Philadelphia, PA, WB Saunders, 1994.)*

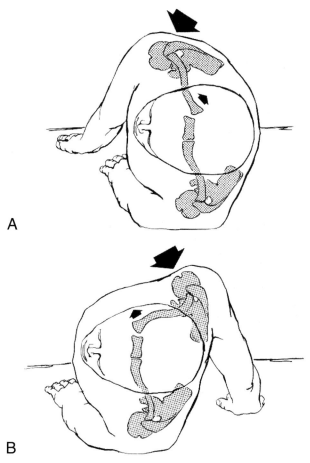

A

B

Figure 2 Mechanism of sternoclavicular joint injuries. **A,** A posterolateral compressive force is applied to the shoulder, and the medial end of the clavicle is displaced posteriorly. **B,** A lateral compressive force is applied to the anterior shoulder resulting in an anterior sternoclavicular dislocation. *(Reproduced with permission from Rockwood CA, Green DP (eds): Fractures, ed 2. Philadelphia, PA, JB Lippincott, 1984.)*

mioclavicular joint. This motion is amplified by the lateral curvature of the clavicle and has been likened to the action of a crankshaft. This mechanism accounts for nearly half the arc of motion for scapulothoracic elevation. Scapulothoracic abduction and elevation both are affected by the relationship of the clavicle to the thorax; therefore, fixation of the clavicle at the sternoclavicular or acromioclavicular joint will significantly decrease overall shoulder motion.

Etiology and Epidemiology

Epidemiologic studies indicate that clavicular fractures are more common in males. Most clavicular fractures occur as a result of a fall onto the lateral aspect of the affected shoulder or, less commonly, as a result of a direct blow to the clavicle. Fractures can occur anywhere along the clavicle. Indirect mechanisms, such as falling onto an outstretched hand, are less common and more typically result in middle-third fractures. Stress fractures are uncommon and can occur in athletes involved in repetitive overhead activities or upper extremity weight training, or after radiation.

Motor vehicle accidents and sports activities are the most common causes of traumatic sternoclavicular dislocations, which can be the result of either direct or indirect forces. Direct forces almost always lead to posterior dislocations, whereas indirect forces, depending on the position of the shoulder and the direction of the force, may lead to either anterior or posterior dislocations (Fig. 2). Indirect forces are the most common mechanism of injury to the sternoclavicular joint.

Atraumatic sternoclavicular instability is uncommon. It often is associated with generalized hyperlaxity and may be a voluntary condition.

Classification

Clavicular fractures are classified according to their anatomic location. Traditionally, this involves division of the clavicle into thirds along its long axis; each third can be further subdivided into specific fracture patterns.

Distal-third fractures are subclassified into four types. Type I fractures occur lateral to the costoclavicular ligaments but do not extend into the acromioclavicular joint. Type II fractures are further subdivided based on the fracture pattern relative to the coracoclavicular ligaments. Type IIA fractures occur just medial to the coracoclavicular ligaments, which remain intact. In type IIB fractures, the conoid ligament is disrupted, and the trapezoid ligament remains attached to the lateral fragment. Type III fractures involve intra-articular extension into the acromioclavicular joint without ligamentous disruption. Type IV fractures occur in skeletally immature patients and involve disruption of the periosteal sleeve surrounding the distal metaphyseal clavicle, which is then displaced superiorly. These epiphyseal injuries mimic acromioclavicular separations and have been called pseudodislocations. The costoclavicular ligaments are attached to the periosteal sleeve; therefore, this fracture pattern tends to remodel over time because it generally occurs in patients younger than age 16 years.

Fractures of the medial third of the clavicle are rare. They are classified into five types: type I, minimally displaced; type II, displaced; type III, intra-articular; type IV, physeal separation; and type V, comminuted.

Clinical Evaluation

Physical Examination

Because of their subcutaneous location, clavicular fractures are easily recognized by inspection and direct palpation. Crepitus is often apparent at the fracture site, along with swelling and ecchymosis. The extent of deformity is related to the location of the fracture and the amount of displacement. Fractures of the middle third tend to occur just lateral to the clavicular head of the sternocleidomastoid muscle, where there are no ligamentous or muscular attachments and the clavicle is thinnest. The apex of the deformity is typically superior, with the medial fragment elevated by the upward pull of the clavicular head of the sternocleidomastoid muscle and the lateral fragment pulled downward and inward by the weight of the arm (through the costoclavicular ligaments) and the pull of the clavicular head of the pectoralis major muscle.

A small percentage of clavicular fractures occur in association with more severe injuries, including scapular fractures, scapulothoracic dissociation, rib fractures, pneumothorax, and neurovascular compromise. These associated injuries indicate more severe trauma and require appropriate clinical and radiologic evaluation. A chest radiograph should be obtained in this setting, as well as an arteriogram if vascular injury is suspected.

Sternoclavicular injuries are associated with characteristic asymmetry of the involved joint and the uninvolved side. Local tenderness is especially exacerbated by lateral compression of the shoulder girdle. With an anterior dislocation, the medial aspect of the clavicle is prominent and may be fixed or mobile. With posterior dislocations, a depression is present, although it may not always be readily apparent. Although anterior dislocations are often accompanied by relatively benign symptoms, posterior injuries can result in significant comorbidities, including vascular or airway compromise and mediastinal injury, that may necessitate more urgent evaluation. In either case, imaging studies often are required to confirm the diagnosis.

Radiologic Evaluation

Most clavicular fractures can be confirmed with a standard AP radiograph of the shoulder. For middle-third fractures, this radiograph should include views of the sternoclavicular and acromioclavicular joints as well as the superior lung field. Additional orthogonal views can help determine the amount of displacement and shortening: a 45° cephalic tilt view to evaluate superior-inferior displacement, and a 45° caudal tilt to better evaluate displacement in the AP plane. The apical oblique view (20° cephalic tilt perpendicular to the plane of the scapula) can help delineate more subtle fracture patterns.

Distal-third fractures are best evaluated with a 15° cephalic tilt AP view with reduced voltage that is centered on the acromioclavicular joint (Zanca view). This radiograph profiles the clavicle away from the scapula and enhances visualization of the acromioclavicular joint for better evaluation of intra-articular fracture extension. An axillary lateral view can demonstrate AP displacement. CT or MRI generally is not required, although a CT scan may help to delineate intra-articular involvement.

Medial-third fractures are easiest to see on a standard AP projection, but often a "serendipity view" (40° cephalic tilt AP centered on the manubrium) should be included, especially if there is suspected involvement of the sternoclavicular joint. Because medial injuries are difficult to evaluate on standard radiographs, a CT scan usually is required. CT scans are also useful to evaluate the underlying soft-tissue structures.

Treatment and Results

During the past 5 years, numerous studies of the treatment of acute fractures and nonunions of the clavicle have been published. Most middle-third clavicle fractures are successfully treated nonsurgically. Nondisplaced fractures almost always unite and have few sequelae. Closed methods to obtain and maintain reduction of displaced middle-third fractures are poorly tolerated by most patients; because their efficacy is questionable, these techniques have been abandoned. Recommended options for treatment include a sling (with or without a swathe), a figure-of-8 harness, or a combination of both. There is little clinical data to support one form of treatment over another. Union rates are high with either method, and functional results generally have been reported as good. A recent study reported that nonsurgical treatment of ipsilateral clavicular and scapular fractures resulted in excellent results in most cases.

Recent studies of nonsurgical treatment of clavicle shaft fractures demonstrate that the amount of displacement and shortening correlates with the rate of healing

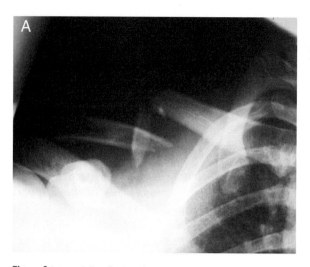 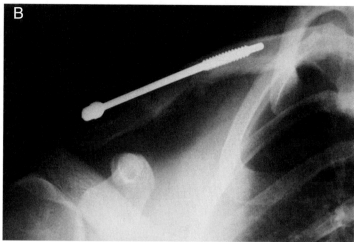

Figure 3 Intramedullary fixation of an acute, middle-third clavicular fracture. **A,** Comminuted, displaced middle-third clavicle fracture. **B,** ORIF was done with an intramedullary screw.

and symptomatic problems. Despite these findings, other studies still recommend nonsurgical treatment in almost all cases of middle-third clavicle fractures.

Indications for primary surgical treatment of acute middle-third fractures include open fractures, concomitant displaced scapular neck fractures that disrupt the superior shoulder suspensory complex, the presence of neurovascular or skin compromise, and patients with multiple trauma who need assistance with early mobilization. More recently, fractures with marked displacement and/or soft-tissue interposition have been considered for primary surgical treatment. Surgical treatment also can be considered for some high-demand patients, such as heavy laborers or athletes, and for patients who object to a marked deformity, but careful patient selection and extensive preoperative counseling are required because of the potential pitfalls of surgical treatment in these patients.

In some studies of open reduction and internal fixation (ORIF) with plate and screws, the overall satisfaction rates approach 95% despite a high incidence of supraclavicular nerve injury and subsequent removal of symptomatic hardware. No deficits were found in strength and range of motion. In other studies, the complication rates were high and could be attributed to patient compliance issues.

Any open approach to the midclavicle places the supraclavicular nerves at risk. These nerves should be identified during the procedure and protected to avoid dysesthesia or painful neuromas. Incisions can be minimized to match what is required for the implant and should be made along Langer's lines to avoid unsightly scarring.

Although most middle-third clavicle fractures heal uneventfully, some of these fractures become problematic if healing is delayed or occurs with significant defor-

mity. Historical arguments against surgical treatment of displaced clavicle shaft fractures included the high risk of complications (extensive scarring, neurovascular damage, and implant failure and/or migration) and high rates of postoperative nonunion. Much of this concern has been relieved by the development of stronger implants and improved surgical technique. Current options include contoured rigid plate fixation with either a 3.5-mm reconstruction plate or a 3.5-mm (limited contact) dynamic compression plate using AO/ASIF techniques and intramedullary fixation (Fig. 3).

Treatment of distal-third fractures depends on the type of fracture. Type I fractures are inherently stable and heal uneventfully. A simple sling is used until acute symptoms subside and a range-of-motion program can be instituted. Type II fractures are more challenging to treat because of the increased risk of healing problems. Although nonsurgical treatment can be effective, results of nonsurgical treatment were poor in some recent studies, and in other studies results of surgical treatment were excellent. Coracoclavicular fixation is advocated in the latter studies and can be done by several techniques, including screw fixation or the use of Dacron tape or resorbable suture (Fig. 4). Type III fractures without coracoclavicular instability are treated nonsurgically.

Anterior sternoclavicular dislocations are usually unstable, and maintenance of closed reduction is difficult. In the acute setting, the dislocation can be reduced with the patient under intravenous sedation in the emergency department. A bolster is placed between the scapulae, with traction applied while the arm is abducted and slightly extended. Although reduction may occur, dislocation usually recurs immediately on removing these forces. This result has led many authors to recommend the use of a sling in this setting until symptoms resolve. If

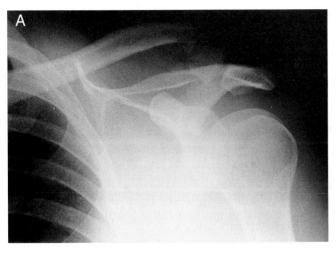
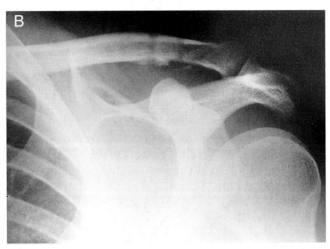

Figure 4 ORIF of a displaced distal-third clavicular fracture with coracoclavicular suture fixation. **A,** AP internal rotation view of the shoulder shows displaced fracture of the distal third of the clavicle. **B,** ORIF was performed with heavy suture coracoclavicular fixation.

reduction can be maintained with the shoulders retracted, the use of a figure-of-8 harness or cast may be effective. Open management of anterior sternoclavicular dislocations is rarely indicated, and the use of pin fixation has been condemned because of pin migration and catastrophic complications, including death. Chronic anterior dislocations are best left untreated because reconstructive procedures have less predictable results.

Posterior sternoclavicular dislocations that are seen in the acute setting accompanied by signs or symptoms related to retrosternal compromise warrant urgent evaluation. Closed reduction should be attempted in the operating room after appropriate coordination with a thoracic surgeon. Closed reduction maneuvers are similar to those done for anterior dislocations but may require placement of a sterile towel clip around the clavicle to assist with reduction. If closed reduction is unsuccessful or unstable, open treatment is indicated. The reduction is often stable in the acute setting, and thus stability can be maintained with suture repair of the anterior capsule. Postoperatively, a sling can be worn for approximately 8 weeks to allow soft-tissue healing.

Symptoms dictate treatment of chronic sternoclavicular dislocations. Chronic anterior dislocations seldom require anything more than supportive care. Chronic posterior dislocations, on the other hand, require the same thorough evaluation as that mandated in the acute setting. If surgical treatment is warranted, partial resection of the medial clavicle with soft-tissue reconstruction is the procedure of choice.

Sternoclavicular injuries in adolescents are usually physeal injuries that, like injuries to the lateral clavicle, have tremendous potential for remodeling. Signs and symptoms are similar to those for adults and vary with the direction of displacement. Anterior displaced injuries are treated with support and observation; with posterior injuries in adolescents, the same treatment protocols are followed as are used for adults, with overall results reported as good.

Complications

Nonunion

Lack of progression to union over a 3-month period constitutes delayed union. Failure to heal within 6 months constitutes nonunion. In most studies of middle-third clavicle fractures, the reported incidence of nonunion is 1% to 4%. In other recent studies, however, reported rates have been closer to 15% to 20%. Factors influencing nonunion include severity of displacement and comminution, fracture location, and effectiveness of immobilization.

Nonunion can be present without pain or functional deficit and remain asymptomatic indefinitely. More commonly, persistent pain at the fracture site causes the patient to seek further treatment. ORIF of the nonunion can be performed with intramedullary fixation or plate and screws. Atrophic nonunion requires bone grafting, whereas hypertrophic nonunion can be treated with ORIF with a compression plate. Atrophic nonunion and shortening may require intercalary structural bone graft. Success rates between 85% and 95% have been reported in several studies. Intramedullary fixation minimizes soft-tissue dissection, allows fragments to compress, and has the added advantage of ease of hardware removal. Partial or total clavulectomy remains an option as a salvage procedure in the face of failed surgical treatment or chronic infection.

Malunion

There are no specific criteria to define a clinically significant malunion. Both objectively and subjectively, this type of malunion is difficult to assess and delineate; therefore, rates most likely are underreported and misleading. Malunion generally involves shortening with angular deformities with or without brachial plexopathy. Associated weakness and decreased function may be present. Clavicular shortening, leading to anteromedialization of the shoulder girdle, may contribute to the dysfunction. Some studies suggest that shortening in excess of 15 mm leads to weakness and an overall decline in function. However, other studies refute these findings. Some patients complain of pain associated with significant shortening; additionally, some patients report dissatisfaction with the cosmetic appearance.

For middle-third fractures, excessive callus formation can cause a compression brachial plexopathy or thoracic outlet syndrome, most commonly affecting the medial cord of the brachial plexus and resulting in ulnar nerve symptoms. Treatment involves osteotomy of the malunion with bone grafting and internal fixation. Length can be difficult to reestablish in the chronic setting secondary to long-standing soft-tissue contractures. These sequelae may be preventable with early surgical treatment of acute displaced middle-third fractures.

Neurovascular Injuries

Although the neurovascular bundle is located close to the clavicle, acute neurovascular injuries are quite rare; however, fatalities secondary to laceration of the subclavian artery after middle-third clavicle fractures have been reported. Posterior sternoclavicular dislocations pose the greatest risk to these structures in the acute setting. Malunion of middle-third fractures, on the other hand, is more commonly associated with neurovascular compromise in the chronic setting.

Posttraumatic Arthritis

Intra-articular fractures of the medial or lateral clavicle may predispose to the development of posttraumatic arthritis. Some authors also have suggested that acromioclavicular arthritis also is a sequela of middle-third fractures. Although it is not uncommon for radiographic changes to be present in older individuals, these changes are often clinically silent and unrelated to previous clavicle fracture. Acromioclavicular arthritis is easily treated with a limited resection of the distal clavicle that preserves the costoclavicular ligaments. Involvement of the sternoclavicular joint may require a balanced reconstructive resectional arthroplasty so that problems of joint instability may be avoided.

Annotated Bibliography

Ballmer FT, Lambert SM, Hertel R: Decortication and plate osteosynthesis for nonunion of the clavicle. *J Shoulder Elbow Surg* 1998;7:581-585.

This is a retrospective review of the treatment of 37 clavicular nonunions with decortication and plate fixation. Eighty-six percent involved the midshaft of the clavicle. Nine patients had tricortical intercalary bone graft to regain length. The union rate was 95%. At an average follow-up of 8.6 years 86% had pain-free range of motion.

Bosch U, Skutek M, Peters G, et al: Extension osteotomy of malunited clavicular fractures. *J Shoulder Elbow Surg* 1998;7:402-405.

The authors reported on four cases of clavicular malunion that presented with shoulder pain and glenohumeral dysfunction, but no neurovascular dysfunction. They obtained good results with an extension osteotomy, plate fixation, and interposition iliac crest bone graft.

Bostman O, Manninen M, Pihlajamaki H: Complications of plate fixation in fresh displaced midclavicular fractures. *J Trauma* 1997;43:778-783.

The results of ORIF of 103 acute midshaft clavicular fractures were reviewed. The cases represented 9.5% of all midshaft clavicular fractures seen. The complication rate was 23%, with a 7.8% infection rate. Fracture comminution and a state of alcohol intoxication on admission were associated with an increased risk of complications. The authors warn against surgical treatment for noncompliant patients.

Bradbury N, Hutchinson J, Hahn D, et al: Clavicle nonunion. 31/32 healed after plate fixation and bone grafting. *Acta Orthop Scand* 1996;67:367-370.

The authors compared the use of 3.5-mm direct compression plates with 3.5-mm reconstruction plates in a matched series. There was no difference in the outcomes. The reconstruction plates were thought to be easier to contour to the clavicle.

Edwards SG, Whittle AP, Wood GW II: Nonoperative treatment of ipsilateral fractures of the scapula and clavicle. *J Bone Joint Surg Am* 2000;82:774-780.

Twenty patients with an ipsilateral fracture of the scapula and clavicle were treated nonsurgically. One patient developed nonunion of the clavicle. The results were excellent in almost all cases. The authors concluded that nonsurgical treatment of these injuries can give predictable results equal to or better than those reported for patients undergoing surgical treatment.

Edelson JG: Clavicular fractures and ipsilateral acromioclavicular arthrosis. *J Shoulder Elbow Surg* 1996;5: 181-185.

More than 300 specimens were examined and there was no association between clavicular fracture and acromioclavicular arthritis. In addition, 20 patients were examined at an average of 26 years after a clavicular fracture, and no association was found.

Goldberg JA, Bruce WJ, Sonnabend DH, et al: Type 2 fractures of the distal clavicle: A new surgical technique. *J Shoulder Elbow Surg* 1997;6:380-382.

The authors treated type II distal-third clavicular fractures with coracoclavicular suture fixation in addition to interosseous suture fixation of the clavicle. All of the fractures healed, eight of the nine patients were pain free, and no complications were reported.

Hessmann M, Kirchner R, Baumgaertel F: Treatment of unstable distal clavicular fractures with and without lesions of the acromioclavicular joint. *Injury* 1996;27: 47-52.

The authors reviewed 39 cases of unstable distal-third clavicular fractures. They found that the results of nonsurgical treatment were worse than the results of surgical treatment.

Hill JM, McGuire MH, Crosby LA: Closed treatment of displaced middle-third fractures of the clavicle gives poor results. *J Bone Joint Surg Br* 1997;79:537-539.

The authors reviewed the results of nonsurgical treatment of 52 of 66 completely displaced midshaft clavicular fractures in adults. Fifteen percent developed nonunion and 31% had unsatisfactory results. Twenty-five percent had mild to moderate residual pain, 29% had some evidence of brachial plexus irritation, and 54% had cosmetic complaints. Shortening of greater than 20 mm had a significant association with nonunion and unsatisfactory result. ORIF was recommended for severely displaced midshaft clavicular fractures.

Nordqvist A, Petersson CJ, Redlund-Johnell I: Mid-clavicle fractures in adults: End result study after conservative treatment. *J Orthop Trauma* 1998;12:572-576.

In this retrospective study of 225 consecutive midclavicular fractures treated nonsurgically, 185 patients were asymptomatic, 39 had moderate pain and a fair result, and one had a poor result. Nonunion occurred in seven patients and was associated with increased displacement. The authors suggested that the only indication for acute surgical management of a midclavicular fracture is skin compromise or neurovascular compromise.

Nowak J, Mallmin H, Larsson S: The etiology and epidemiology of clavicular fractures: A prospective study during a two-year period in Uppsala, Sweden. *Injury* 2000;31:353-358.

The authors found that the incidence of clavicular fractures was 50 per 100,000 (71 per 100,000 in males and 30 per 100,000 in females). In males, there was a greater incidence of comminution, and fractures occurred at a younger age.

Robinson CM: Fractures of the clavicle. Epidemiology and classification. *J Bone Joint Surg Br* 1998;80:476-484.

The authors report on a consecutive series of 1,000 clavicular fractures. They found that fractures were most common in males and that the most common mechanism was automobile accidents. Distal-third clavicular fractures occurred most often as a result of a fall and were more common in the elderly. The incidence of complications of union was greater in displaced diaphyseal and distal clavicular fractures. Displacement and comminution were risk factors for delayed union and nonunion.

Shen WJ, Liu TJ, Shen YS: Plate fixation of fresh displaced midshaft clavicle fractures. *Injury* 1999;30: 497-500.

This is a report of the results of ORIF of 251 acute midshaft clavicular fractures. The nonunion rate was 3%. There were only five infections. Twenty-eight percent had numbness distal to the incision and 171 (68%) had the plate removed. The satisfaction rate was 94%.

Simpson NS, Jupiter JB: Clavicular nonunion and malunion: Evaluation and management. *J Am Acad Orthop Surg* 1996;4:1-8.

This is a good review article about clavicle nonunion and malunion. The authors emphasize the fact that these types of problems are relatively uncommon. They discuss the reconstructive options for the infrequent cases in which nonunion or malunion results in clinically significant pain and dysfunction.

Webber MC, Haines JF: The treatment of lateral clavicle fractures. *Injury* 2000;3:175-179.

The authors reviewed the results of nonsurgical treatment of 15 displaced type II distal-third clavicular fractures. They found that nonsurgical treatment was not warranted and recommended early surgical intervention.

Wirth MA, Rockwood CA Jr: Acute and chronic traumatic injuries of the sternoclavicular joint. *J Am Acad Orthop Surg* 1996;4:268-278.

This is an excellent review of sternoclavicular joint injuries.

Wu CC, Shih CH, Chen WJ, et al: Treatment of clavicular aseptic nonunion: Comparison of plating and intramedullary nailing techniques. *J Trauma* 1998;45:512-516.

In this retrospective review of surgical treatment of clavicular nonunions, ORIF with intramedullary rod fixation had a lower complication rate and an increased rate of union.

Classic Bibliography

Acus RW III, Bel RH, Fisher DL: Proximal clavicle excision: An analysis of results. *J Shoulder Elbow Surg* 1995;4:182-187.

Eskola A, Vainionpaa S, Ptiala H, et al: Outcome of clavicular fracture in 89 patients. *Arch Orthop Trauma Surg* 1986;105:337-338.

Longia GS, Ajmani ML, Saxena SK: Study of diaphyseal nutrient foramina in human long bones. *Acta Anat (Basel)* 1980;107:399-406.

Chapter 22

Scapular Fractures

Kirk L. Wong, MD

Matthew L. Ramsey, MD

Gerald R. Williams, Jr, MD

Introduction

Fractures of the scapula are relatively uncommon, accounting for 1% of all fractures, 3% of shoulder girdle injuries, and 5% of fractures involving the shoulder. Because scapular fractures occur in high-energy situations, the patient often presents with associated injuries of the ipsilateral limb, shoulder girdle, and thoracic cage. In polytrauma patients, scapular fractures frequently are overlooked or neglected because other life-threatening injuries are present.

In most cases, scapular fractures can be treated nonsurgically with short-term immobilization followed by functional treatment. Traditionally, indications for surgical treatment have included glenoid rim fractures associated with instability and combined fracture patterns such as ipsilateral clavicle and scapular neck fracture— the so-called floating shoulder. More recently, however, surgical treatment of displaced intra-articular glenoid fractures without associated glenohumeral instability has been emphasized increasingly. In contrast, recent literature suggests that not all ipsilateral clavicle and scapular neck fractures may require surgical stabilization. This chapter reviews the pertinent anatomy, classification schemes, treatment recommendations, and results of treatment for scapular fractures, with particular emphasis on information gained in the last 5 years.

Anatomy

The scapula is suspended from the lateral end of the clavicle by the coracoclavicular and acromioclavicular ligaments. These two ligamentous complexes provide the only rigid attachment of the scapula to the axial skeleton. Goss described the superior shoulder suspensory complex (SSSC) as consisting of a bony and soft-tissue ring at the end of a superior and inferior bony strut. The ring is composed of the glenoid process, the coracoid process, the coracoclavicular ligaments, the distal clavicle, the acromioclavicular joint, and the acromial pro-

cess. The superior strut is the middle clavicle; the inferior strut is the lateral scapular body and spine. This complex maintains a stable relationship between the scapula and the axial skeleton (Fig. 1).

Absent from this original description of the SSSC was the coracoacromial ligament. This ligament has recently been shown to be an important stabilizer of the glenoid process in scapular neck fractures. In most scapular neck fractures, the fracture line is medial to the base of the coracoid process, thereby creating a medial (ie, proximal) fragment, consisting of the acromion, scapular spine, and scapular body, and a lateral (ie, distal) fragment, consisting of the glenoid and coracoid processes (Fig. 2). Because the coracoacromial ligament is an important connection between the proximal and distal fragments of a scapular neck fracture, it should be included in the SSSC (Fig. 3).

A floating shoulder results when the distal fragment of a scapular neck fracture loses its attachments to the proximal fragment and to the axial skeleton via the clavicle. The addition of a clavicle shaft fracture to an ipsilateral scapular neck fracture without any additional fractures or ligament disruptions reduces the medial stability of a scapular neck fracture by only 30%. The combinations of fractures and ligament injuries that theoretically can produce a floating shoulder are discussed in the classification section.

Associated Injuries

Fractures of the scapula are usually the result of high-energy trauma, such as that caused by motor vehicle accidents. Consequently, there is a high prevalence—as much as 96% in one series—of associated injuries. Ipsilateral rib fractures are the most common associated injury, occurring in approximately 27% to 50% of patients. Other associated injuries include pulmonary injuries such as pulmonary contusions and hemopneumothorax (16% to 40% of patients), ipsilateral clavicle fractures (23% to 26%), and injuries to the brachial plexus and subclavian artery (12%). A high association of neurovascular in-

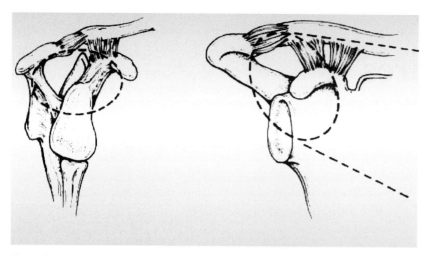

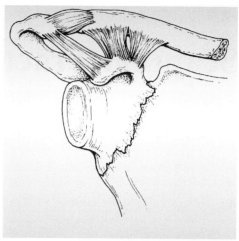

Figure 1 SSSC as described by Goss. *(Reproduced from Goss TP: Scapular fractures and dislocations: Diagnosis and treatment. J Am Acad Orthop Surg 1995;3:22-33.)*

Figure 2 Scapular neck fractures exiting medial to the coracoid base produce medial and lateral fragments connected by the coracoacromial ligament.

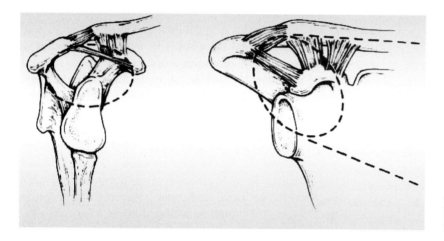

Figure 3 The coracoacromial ligament is an important stabilizer of the glenoid process and should be included in the SSSC.

juries with ipsilateral acromion and first rib fractures has been noted. Other life-threatening associated injuries are closed head trauma and intra-abdominal injuries.

Classification

Fractures of the scapula can be classified according to the location of the fracture, including the body, neck, glenoid fossa, acromion, spine, and coracoid. In the two largest series of scapular fractures reported, the distribution was as follows: scapular body fractures accounted for 35% to 43% of the fractures; neck, 26%; glenoid, 10%; acromion, 8% to 12%; spine, 6% to 11%; and coracoid, 5% to 7%.

Comprehensive classification systems for scapular fractures as a whole have been provided by the Orthopaedic Trauma Association, Ada and Miller, and Goss. All of these classification systems are based on the degree of displacement and/or fracture location. Other classification systems are focused on the specific site of injury, such as the glenoid fossa, scapular neck, coracoid, or acromion.

Coracoid Process

Fractures of the coracoid process in 67 consecutive patients were analyzed in a recent study. The authors simplified the classification into two types, based on the relationship between the fracture site and the coracoclavicular ligament. Type I fractures were proximal to the attachment of the coracoclavicular ligament and were commonly associated with injuries such as an acromioclavicular dislocation, fracture of the scapular spine or the acromion, or fracture of the lateral end of the clavicle. These "double disruptions" are best treated surgically to reconstruct a link between the clavicle and the scapula. Type II fractures that are distal to this ligament can be treated nonsurgically because the scapuloclavicular connection is maintained.

Acromion and Lateral Scapular Spine

Another classification by Ogawa and Naniwa for fractures of the acromion and the lateral scapular spine separated these fractures into two main categories. Type I fractures consist of the anatomic acromion and the extremely lateral scapular spine, and type II fractures are located in the more medial aspect of the spine and can extend to the spinoglenoid notch. Type I injuries occur as a result of an indirect force transmitted by the humeral head and glenoid that becomes a shearing force acting horizontally between the clavicle and the scapula. This mechanism of injury is commonly associated with acromioclavicular joint injuries, coracoid fractures, and distal clavicle fractures. In type II fractures, the mechanism is direct force from the posterior or posterolateral direction, and associated injuries are infrequent.

Glenoid

Ideberg and associates' classification of intra-articular glenoid fractures is not new, but it is the most widely used and deserves emphasis. Type IA involves the anterior portion of the glenoid rim, and type IB involves the posterior portion. Type II fractures involve a fracture line that runs from the glenoid fossa to the lateral border of the scapular body. Type III fractures are glenoid fossa fractures that extend into the superior border of the scapula. Type IV fractures involve a fracture line that runs from the fossa across the scapular body to exit along the medial border of the scapula. Type V fractures are a combination of type II, III, and IV fractures. Goss later added a type VI fracture, which is a severely comminuted fracture of the glenoid fossa (Fig. 4).

Scapular Neck

There are at least three types of combined injuries that can produce a floating distal fragment (floating shoulder) in cases of a scapular neck fracture: type I, purely osseous injuries; type II, purely ligamentous injuries; or type III, combined osseous and ligamentous injuries. The purely osseous floating shoulder injury patterns are a fracture of the scapular neck combined with a fracture of the coracoid base (type IA), or a fracture of the clavicle shaft and scapular spine or acromion (type IB) (Fig. 5, *A* and *B*). The purely ligamentous (type II) floating shoulder is characterized by a fracture of the scapular neck combined with disruption of the coracoacromial and coracoclavicular ligaments (Fig. 5, *C*). Combined osseous and ligamentous floating shoulder injury patterns include ipsilateral scapular neck fracture, clavicle shaft fracture, and coracoacromial and acromioclavicular ligament disruption (type IIIA); or ipsilateral scapular neck fracture, acromion or scapular spine fracture, and coracoclavicular and acromioclavicular ligament disruption (type IIIB) (Fig. 5, *D* and *E*).

Currently, there are no established criteria for the diagnosis of coracoacromial ligament disruption in cases of suspected floating shoulder. However, coracoclavicu-

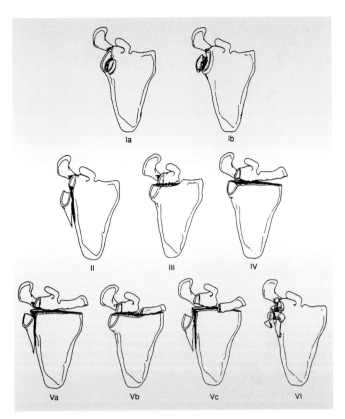

Figure 4 Ideberg classification of fractures of the glenoid cavity as modified by Goss. *(Reproduced from Goss TP: Scapular fractures and dislocations: Diagnosis and treatment. J Am Acad Orthop Surg 1995;3:22-33.)*

lar and acromioclavicular ligament injury can be inferred on the basis of displacement of the acromioclavicular joint. Furthermore, combined fracture patterns that potentially isolate the distal fragment from the proximal fragment and the axial skeleton can readily be identified radiographically. In the presence of these combined fracture patterns or in ipsilateral scapular neck and clavicle shaft fractures in which the distance between the tip of the coracoid process and the anteromedial acromion is deemed to be greater than the known length of the coracoacromial ligament, surgical stabilization is considered.

Evaluation

Fractures of the scapula usually are noted on the chest radiograph. Individuals with this injury usually complain of pain over the shoulder girdle. Physical findings such as localized swelling, crepitus with range of motion, and ecchymosis suggest an underlying scapular fracture. A thorough physical examination including neurologic assessment is important to document any deficit and to look for other associated osseous injuries. Initial radiographs of the shoulder should include three views: true AP, lateral projection in the plane of the scapula (Y view), and true axillary. If a coracoid fracture is sus-

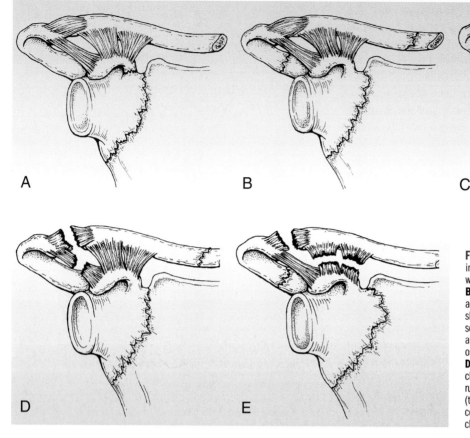

Figure 5 Purely osseous floating shoulders may include **A,** fractures of the scapular neck combined with a fracture of the coracoid base (type IA) or **B,** fractures of the clavicle and scapular spine or acromion (type IB). Purely ligamentous floating shoulders occur with **C,** combined fracture of the scapular neck and injury to the coracoclavicular and coracoacromial ligaments (type II). Combined osseoligamentous floating shoulders result from **D,** a scapular neck fracture combined with a clavicle shaft fracture, coracoacromial ligament disruption, and acromioclavicular capsule disruption (type IIIA) or **E,** scapular spine/acromion fracture, coracoacromial ligament disruption, and acromioclavicular capsule disruption (type IIIB).

pected, a Stryker notch view is helpful.

Because of the complex anatomy of the scapula and the overlying chest cavity, CT is sometimes necessary to precisely define these injuries. In certain situations, three-dimensional CT reconstructions can aid in preoperative planning for repair of complex fracture patterns. Appropriate software can subtract the image of the humeral head to reveal an unobstructed view of the scapula and glenoid fossa (Fig. 6).

Complications

Reports of complications following scapular fracture have been uncommon. Complications include glenohumeral arthritis from malunited intra-articular fractures, scapulothoracic dissociation, suprascapular nerve compression, and scapulothoracic crepitus from scapular body malunion. In addition, painful nonunion of a scapular body fracture recently has been reported.

Surgical Indications

Most scapular fractures can be treated successfully nonsurgically. However, certain fractures may be managed best by surgical reduction and stabilization. These include acromion or scapular spine fractures with downward tilting of the lateral fragment and subsequent sub-

acromial narrowing, coracoid fractures with extension into the glenoid fossa and articular step-off of 5 mm or more, anterior or posterior glenoid rim fractures associated with persistent or recurrent glenohumeral instability, and intra-articular glenoid fractures with more than 5 mm of residual displacement in the absence of glenohumeral instability. Consideration should be given to the degree of comminution and the ability to obtain sufficiently rigid fixation for early mobilization.

The surgical indications for floating shoulders, especially those involving ipsilateral clavicle and scapular neck fractures, are evolving. Reasonable indications at this time include scapular neck fractures with more than 3 cm of medial displacement.

Nonsurgical Treatment and Results

Most scapular fractures can be treated satisfactorily with a brief (1-week) period of sling immobilization followed by passive range-of-motion and pendulum exercises as comfort allows. Close radiographic follow-up ensures that loss of reduction is identified early. Most scapular fractures are sufficiently healed by 6 weeks to discontinue immobilization and allow active and active assisted range of motion. Maximal functional recovery generally takes 6 to 12 months.

Earlier studies found that nonsurgical treatment of scapular fractures was uniformly successful. One study followed 38 patients with fractures of the body, neck, or spine. Within 1 year, all patients had regained a full range of painless shoulder motion, and the fractures had united. In one of the largest series of scapular fractures treated nonsurgically, the authors found satisfactory outcomes in all patients. Yet another study followed patients in whom 50 scapular body, neck, and spine fractures were treated nonsurgically; the study found good functional results in all patients.

In contrast, more recent reports have indicated that the results of nonsurgical treatment of displaced scapular fractures involving the scapular neck or scapular spine are often poor. One analysis of 108 patients with scapular body, neck, and spine fractures treated nonsurgically found significant disability in patients with displaced scapular spine and neck fractures. Fifty percent of patients with comminuted scapular spine fractures had weakness with abduction, and 70% experienced pain at rest. Of 16 patients from this series with displaced scapular neck fractures, 20% had limited range of motion, 50% had pain, 40% had weakness with exertion, and 25% noted popping. Therefore, the authors recommended surgical fixation in comminuted scapular spine fractures and scapular neck fractures having more than 40° of angulation or 1 cm of translation.

Another study had similar results. Of 68 patients treated nonsurgically for fractures of the scapular body, neck, or spine with an average follow-up of 14 years, 50% of the patients with residual deformity of the scapula had significantly more clinical symptoms.

Surgical Approaches and Technique

Floating Shoulder

The approach for open reduction and internal fixation (ORIF) of floating shoulder depends on the age of the fracture and the injury pattern. In acute (7 days or less) displaced type IA fractures, surgical stabilization of the scapular neck through the utilitarian posterior approach described for type II glenoid fossa fractures is indicated. In acute type IB fractures, ORIF of the clavicle and scapular spine/acromion fractures will reduce the scapular neck fracture through ligamentotaxis. Type II floating shoulder is managed by ORIF of the scapular neck fracture through the utilitarian posterior approach.

Acute type IIIA floating shoulder is managed by ORIF of the clavicle. Ligamentotaxis through the intact coracoclavicular ligament usually will reduce the scapular neck. If reduction of the scapular neck does not occur, coracoclavicular ligament disruption can be inferred, and the scapular neck also should be fixed. Acute type IIIB floating shoulder is treated with ORIF

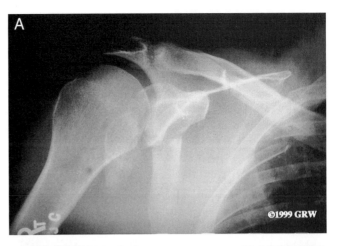

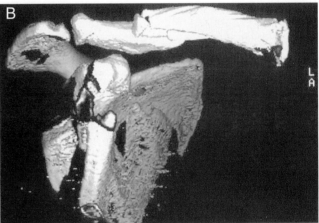

Figure 6 A, AP radiograph of scapular fracture. **B,** Three-dimensional CT reconstruction with the humerus digitally subtracted allows determination of the fracture pattern. *(Copyright © 1999 Gerald R. Williams, MD, Philadelphia, PA.)*

of the scapular spine/acromion. The intact coracoacromial ligament usually will reduce the scapular neck.

Glenoid Fossa Fractures

Available surgical approaches for ORIF of glenoid fossa fractures include the anterior deltopectoral, superior transdeltoid, and posterior approaches. Posterior approaches may be limited or extensile. The Judet posterior approach involves elevation of the entire infraspinatus muscle from the scapula. This approach provides excellent exposure of the posterior scapula; however, it often is not necessary. For more complicated fracture patterns, combined approaches may be necessary. The main factor in choosing the approach is the need for fixation along the lateral scapular border. The path of the axillary nerve makes placement of a plate along the anterior aspect of the lateral scapular border difficult. Therefore, if fixation along the lateral scapular border is contemplated, a posterior approach should be considered.

Type IA glenoid fossa fractures are exposed through an anterior deltopectoral approach. The fracture may be

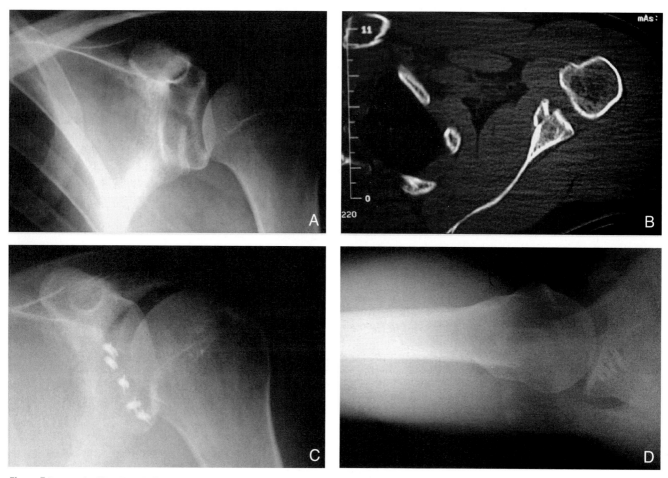

Figure 7 Preoperative AP radiograph **(A)** and CT scan **(B)** demonstrating a displaced anterior glenoid rim fracture in association with recurrent anterior subluxation. Postoperative AP **(C)** and axillary **(D)** radiographs following ORIF with suture anchors demonstrate anatomic reduction.

stabilized with a screw or with suture anchors (Fig. 7).

Type IB glenoid fossa fractures may be exposed through a limited posterior approach. The deltoid is split over the glenohumeral joint for a distance of 4 to 5 cm distal to the scapular spine. The fracture usually involves the posteroinferior glenoid. Therefore, the interval between the infraspinatus and teres minor is used without incising the infraspinatus tendon. The capsule is incised to see the reduction. The fracture is stabilized with an interfragmentary screw.

Type II glenoid fossa fractures most often require fixation along the lateral border of the scapular spine. Therefore, a utilitarian, extensile posterior approach is required. A curvilinear incision is made beginning at the base of the scapular spine, proceeding laterally along the scapular spine, and curving distally and medially at the posterolateral acromial border to parallel the lateral margin of the scapula. The posterior deltoid origin may be released from the scapular spine and retracted laterally. The infraspinatus tendon is incised and reflected medially; the dorsal portion of the teres minor and teres major (if needed) origins are reflected off the lateral scapular border. This allows access to most of the lateral scapular border for fixation (Fig. 8).

Type III glenoid fossa fractures theoretically may be approached superiorly, anteriorly, or posteriorly. Because fixation along the lateral scapular border is not necessary and because the deforming force on the displaced fragment is the conjoined tendon anteriorly, an anterior deltopectoral approach may be preferred. The subscapularis is reflected to expose the anterior scapular neck, but the capsule does not necessarily need to be incised. A neutralization plate can be placed on the anterior scapular neck. A percutaneously placed superior-to-inferior interfragmentary screw strengthens the fixation. Posterior comminution may require a supplemental or primary posterior approach (Fig. 9).

Type IV glenoid fossa fractures are uncommon. The transverse fracture line usually is associated with another, vertically oriented fracture line. In either case, the potential need for fixation on both the medial and lateral scapular borders favors the posterior approach.

Type V glenoid fossa fractures, which are a combination of types II, III, and IV, are the most surgically

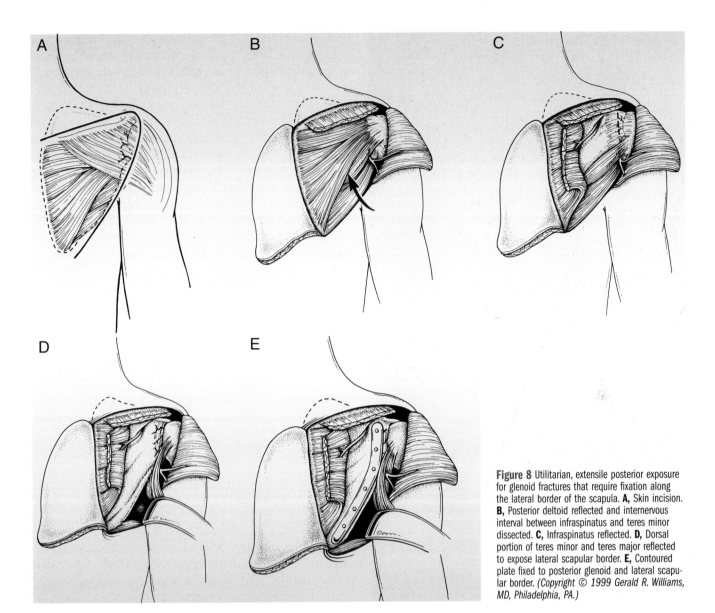

A B C

D E

Figure 8 Utilitarian, extensile posterior exposure for glenoid fractures that require fixation along the lateral border of the scapula. **A,** Skin incision. **B,** Posterior deltoid reflected and internervous interval between infraspinatus and teres minor dissected. **C,** Infraspinatus reflected. **D,** Dorsal portion of teres minor and teres major reflected to expose lateral scapular border. **E,** Contoured plate fixed to posterior glenoid and lateral scapular border. *(Copyright © 1999 Gerald R. Williams, MD, Philadelphia, PA.)*

demanding of all scapular fractures. The need for fixation along the lateral scapular border dictates a posterior approach. The utilitarian, extensile approach described for type II fractures is most useful. In addition to a plate along the lateral scapular border, some form of fixation of the transverse fracture line traversing the scapular body and exiting medially may be required. The goal is anatomic reconstruction of the articular surface (Fig. 10).

Type VI glenoid fossa fractures most often are not amenable to internal fixation because of the severe comminution. To some extent, the glenoid fragments may mold to the shape of the humeral head.

Surgical Treatment Results

Several recent investigators have reported successful results with ORIF for specific subgroups of scapular fractures. One study retrospectively reviewed 37 displaced scapular fractures that were treated with open reduction and stable fixation. With an average follow-up of 6.5 years, 79% of the patients achieved good to excellent results. The authors of another study evaluated 20 patients with displaced scapular fractures treated with surgical fixation. There were six scapular neck and six glenoid fractures. Ninety-five percent of patients had no or minimal pain at an average follow-up of 6.1 years.

The literature on fixation of ipsilateral clavicle and scapular neck fractures is confusing. The authors of one study reported good or excellent functional results in 14 of 15 patients treated with ORIF of both fractures. In two other studies, good or excellent results were achieved in 17 of 19 patients treated with ORIF of the clavicle alone.

More recently, the role of surgical fixation of these fractures has been questioned because of the lack of

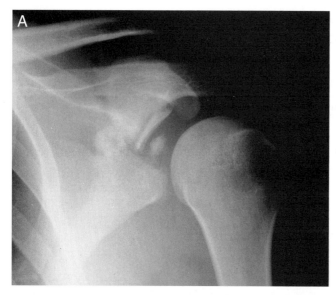

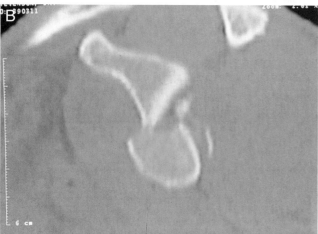

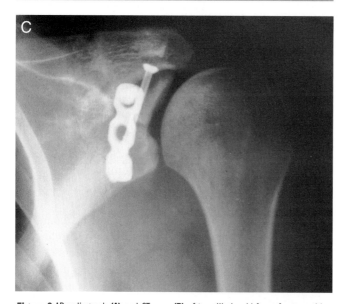

Figure 9 AP radiograph **(A)** and CT scan **(B)** of type III glenoid fossa fracture with posterior comminution. This was stabilized with an anterior neutralization plate and a superior-inferior interfragmentary screw placed percutaneously. Note the small area of posterior deficiency created by excision of the comminuted fragment **(C)**. *(Copyright © 1999 Gerald R. Williams, MD, Philadelphia, PA.)*

nonsurgical controls and the relatively small size of previous studies. The authors of one study reviewed 16 cases of ipsilateral fracture of the clavicle and scapular neck treated nonsurgically, with 13 patients available for follow-up. There were 10 displaced scapular fractures and 5 comminuted clavicle fractures. With a mean follow-up of 7.5 years, 92% of the patients achieved good to excellent results using the scoring method of Herscovici.

Another study of 15 patients with ipsilateral scapular neck and clavicle fractures demonstrated union in all but one patient. This patient had a clavicular nonunion from segmental bone loss after sustaining a gunshot wound to the clavicle. There were eight clavicle fractures with more than 10 mm of displacement and five scapular neck fractures with more than 5 mm of displacement or angulation greater than 45°. According to the scoring system of Herscovici, all of the patients achieved good to excellent results. Using the Rowe assessment method, all but one patient had an excellent or good result. The authors believe that nonsurgical treatment of these injuries is as good as or better than surgical treatment, especially in patients with less than 5 mm of fracture displacement. However, additional studies were recommended to further define indications for surgical fixation in severely displaced scapular fractures.

Glenoid fossa fractures with minimal displacement can be treated nonsurgically. Close radiographic monitoring is necessary to be certain that fracture displacement does not occur. Although the amount of step-off that would lead to pain, stiffness, and/or posttraumatic arthritis is not known, several authors suggest different criteria for surgical intervention. One author recommends 5 mm of step-off as the cut-off for surgical fixation for articular injuries and 10 mm for rim fractures to prevent recurrent glenohumeral instability. The authors of another article recommend anatomic reconstruction when articular step-off exceeds 2 mm. The authors of one study performed ORIF for nine intra-articular glenoid fractures with displacements of 4 to 8 mm. All of the patients were free from osteoarthritis at an average follow-up of 4 years (range, 2 to 10 years).

Summary

Scapular fractures are uncommon injuries that often result from high-energy trauma. Thorough evaluation is required to uncover concomitant injuries. Nonsurgical management is indicated in most, if not all, extra-articular scapular body fractures. Indications for surgery are evolving, and reported results are difficult to compare because of lack of standardization, particularly with respect to displacement. Despite these inconsistencies, surgical stabilization is indicated in glenoid rim fractures associated with persistent or recurrent instability, glenoid fossa frac-

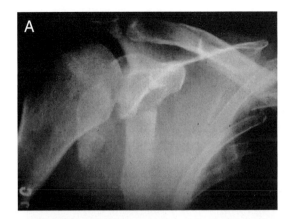

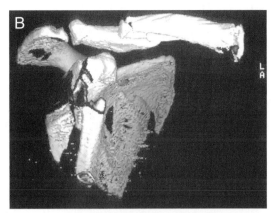

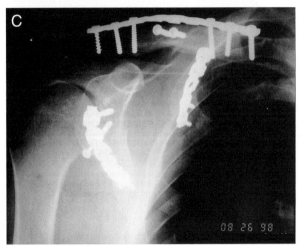

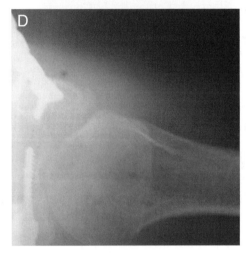

Figure 10 AP radiograph **(A)** and three-dimensional CT reconstruction **(B)** of type V glenoid fossa fracture associated with a clavicular shaft fracture. Stabilization of the scap-ula and glenoid was obtained through an extensile posterior approach. An anatomic reduction of the articular surface was achieved. **C** and **D,** Note the plate on the medial scapular border to control transverse body fracture.

tures with more than 5 mm of residual displacement, acromion or scapular spine fractures with downward tilting of the lateral fragment and subsequent subacromial narrowing, and coracoid fractures with extension into the glenoid associated with more than 5 mm of displacement. Surgical stabilization of scapular neck fractures is predicated on the presence of severe displacement of the distal fragment and/or associated ligamentous or osseous injury patterns that imply greater instability. The often satisfactory results reported for nonsurgical treatment demand that surgical treatment be skillfully performed. Surgical approaches are varied and fracture pattern-specific. Regardless of the method of treatment, the goal is to achieve enough stability for the patient to begin passive range of motion within the first week after injury.

Annotated Bibliography

Ebraheim NA, Mekhail AO, Padanilum TG, Yeasting RA: Anatomic considerations for a modified posterior approach to the scapula. *Clin Orthop* 1997;334:136-143.

The authors described a modified posterior approach to the scapula. For more superior exposure, an acromion osteotomy can be used. The suprascapular neurovascular bundle was identified on 20 cadavers to be 1.4 ± 0.1 cm from the gle-

noid rim. The circumflex scapular artery was 2.8 ± 0.5 cm from the inferior glenoid margin.

Edwards SG, Whittle AP, Wood GW: Nonoperative treatment of ipsilateral fractures of the scapula and clavicle. *J Bone Joint Surg Am* 2000;82:774-780.

The authors analyzed the results of nonsurgical treatment of 20 patients with ipsilateral scapular neck and clavicle fractures. Most of the clavicle fractures were displaced, but only five scapular fractures were displaced more than 5 mm. Nineteen fractures united uneventfully. All of the patients achieved good to excellent results. The authors believe that nonsurgical treatment of floating shoulder injuries, especially those that are minimally displaced, is appropriate because good results can be obtained without the risks associated with surgical fixation.

Ogawa K, Naniwa T: Fractures of the acromion and the lateral scapular spine. *J Shoulder Elbow Surg* 1997;6: 544-548.

The purpose of this study was to evaluate the validity of collectively handling fractures lateral to the spinoglenoid notch as fractures of the acromion and to ascertain the mechanism of injury. These fractures were separated into two groups, with type I consisting of those of the anatomic acromion and the extremely lateral scapular spine and type II comprising fractures descending to the spinoglenoid notch. Type I fractures usually are displaced significantly secondary to associated injury of the acromioclavicular ligament, coracoid, or distal clavicle. Thus, surgical reduction and fixation generally is required.

Ogawa K, Yoshida A, Takahashi M, Ui M: Fractures of the coracoid process. *J Bone Joint Surg Br* 1997;79: 17-19.

This study presents 67 patients with fractures of the coracoid, classifying them by the relationship between the fracture site and the coracoclavicular ligament.

Ramos L, Mencia R, Alonso A, Fernandez L: Conservative treatment of ipsilateral fractures of the scapula and clavicle. *J Trauma* 1997;42:239-242.

This is one of the two review articles evaluating the results of ipsilateral clavicle and scapular neck fractures treated nonsurgically. Of 16 patients with an average follow-up of 7.5 years, 92% achieved good to excellent functional results.

Classic Bibliography

Ada JR, Miller ME: Scapular fractures: Analysis of 113 cases. *Clin Orthop* 1991;269:174-180.

Armstrong CP, Van der Spuy J: The fractured scapula: Importance and management based on a series of 62 patients. *Injury* 1984;15:324-329.

Bauer G, Fleischmann W, Dussler E: Displaced scapular fractures: Indication and long-term results of open reduction and internal fixation. *Arch Orthop Trauma Surg* 1995;114:215-219.

Eyres KS, Brooks A, Stanley D: Fractures of the coracoid process. *J Bone Joint Surg Br* 1995;77:425-428.

Goss TP: Fractures of the glenoid cavity. *J Bone Joint Surg Am* 1992;74:299-305.

Goss TP: Double disruptions of the superior shoulder suspensory complex. *J Orthop Trauma* 1993;7:99-106.

Goss TP: Fractures of the glenoid neck. *J Shoulder Elbow Surg* 1994;3:42-52.

Goss TP: The scapula: Coracoid, acromial, and avulsion fractures. *Am J Orthop* 1996;25:106-115.

Gupta R, Sher J, Williams G, Iannotti JP: Nonunion of the scapular body: A case report. *J Bone Joint Surg Am* 1998;80:428-430.

Hardegger FH, Simpson LA, Weber BG: The operative treatment of scapular fractures. *J Bone Joint Surg Br* 1984;66:725-731.

Herscovici D, Fiennes AG, Allgower M, Ruedi TP: The floating shoulder: Ipsilateral clavicle and scapular neck fractures. *J Bone Joint Surg Br* 1992;74:362-364.

Ideberg R, Grevsten S, Larsson S: Epidemiology of scapular fractures: Incidence and classification of 338 fractures. *Acta Orthop Scand* 1995;66:395-397

Imatani RJ: Fractures of the scapula: A review of 53 fractures. *J Trauma* 1975;15:473-478.

Kavanagh BF, Bradway JK, Cofield RH: Open reduction and internal fixation of displaced intra-articular fractures of the glenoid fossa. *J Bone Joint Surg Am* 1993;75:479-484.

Leung KS, Lam TP: Open reduction and internal fixation of ipsilateral fractures of the scapular neck and clavicle. *J Bone Joint Surg Am* 1993;75:1015-1018.

McGahan JP, Rab GT, Dublin A: Fractures of the scapula. *J Trauma* 1980;20:880-883.

McGinnis M, Denton JR: Fractures of the scapula: A retrospective study of 40 fractured scapulae. *J Trauma* 1989;29:1488-1493.

Nordqvist A, Petersson C: Fracture of the body, neck, or spine of the scapula: A long-term follow-up study. *Clin Orthop* 1992;283:139-144.

Nordqvist A, Petersson C: Incidence and causes of shoulder girdle injuries in an urban population. *J Shoulder Elbow Surg* 1995;4:107-112.

Rikli D, Regazzoni P, Renner N: The unstable shoulder girdle: Early functional treatment utilizing open reduction and internal fixation. *J Orthop Trauma* 1995;9: 93-97.

Wilber MC, Evans EB: Fractures of the scapula: An analysis of forty cases and a review of the literature. *J Bone Joint Surg Am* 1977;59:358-362.

Chapter 23

Diaphyseal Fractures of the Humerus

David Ring, MD

Jesse B. Jupiter, MD

Introduction

Recent research has reemphasized the predictability of nonsurgical functional brace treatment of diaphyseal fractures of the humerus as well as highlighted the potential problems with surgical treatment. Given the excellent results of functional brace treatment, surgical treatment of fractures of the diaphyseal humerus must be carefully justified. For situations in which surgical treatment is indicated, the ability to obtain adequate fixation and address concomitant injuries of the radial nerve has been enhanced by descriptions of more extensile surgical exposures. Nonunion of the humerus is the most common cause of failure of fracture treatment. Recent outcome studies demonstrated the severe disability associated with unstable humeral nonunion. The unique problems associated with treatment of nonunion after prior intramedullary rod fixation have been defined, and suggestions have been made for dealing with poor bone quality and nonunions with bone defects.

Epidemiology

A recent study reported an incidence of approximately 14 diaphyseal humeral fractures per 100,000 population per year. The incidence increased with advancing age. In addition, there is a bimodal distribution similar to that seen with many other fractures, with a peak of predominantly young men injured in high-energy accidents and a second peak of predominantly elderly women injured in simple falls. More severe injuries with segmental fractures (3.3%), complex open fractures (< 1%), and bilateral fractures (none reported) are less common.

Associated Injuries

The best management of humeral fractures associated with radial nerve dysfunction is still disputed. Some authors, who emphasized the potential risk of the nerve being lacerated or entrapped, suggested early exploration. Most studies document recovery of the radial nerve in most patients, and nonsurgical treatment of the fracture with expectant management of the nerve injury still predominates in the literature. In some unusual cases with penetrating trauma or severe wounds, immediate nerve exploration may be indicated. When the nerve is explored, stable internal fixation of the fracture is recommended.

Some very complex fractures are associated with injury to the brachial artery. These are often near amputations. Prompt restoration of vascular supply to the arm is important because irreversible damage of skeletal muscle occurs within 6 hours. When definitive fixation of the humerus can be completed quickly, skeletal repair may precede vascular repair. Otherwise, the humerus is secured provisionally with an external fixator while the brachial artery is repaired. The forearm compartments should be released to avoid compartment syndrome after reperfusion.

Nonsurgical Treatment

The recent report of functional brace treatment of 922 patients with diaphyseal fractures of the humeral shaft reemphasizes the efficacy of this form of treatment (Fig. 1). Only 3% of fractures failed to heal, none had unacceptable deformity, and 98% of patients achieved full or near-full motion of the shoulder and elbow in a relatively short period after brace removal.

Functional bracing proved successful even for more difficult fractures that are sometimes considered for surgical treatment, including fractures of the distal or proximal third, segmental fractures, low-grade open fractures, low-velocity gunshot fractures, and fractures in obese patients. There were no infections. Sixty-six of 67 radial nerve palsies recovered spontaneously.

Contraindications to Functional Bracing

Given the excellent results of functional bracing, the role of surgical treatment must be carefully defined. Careful

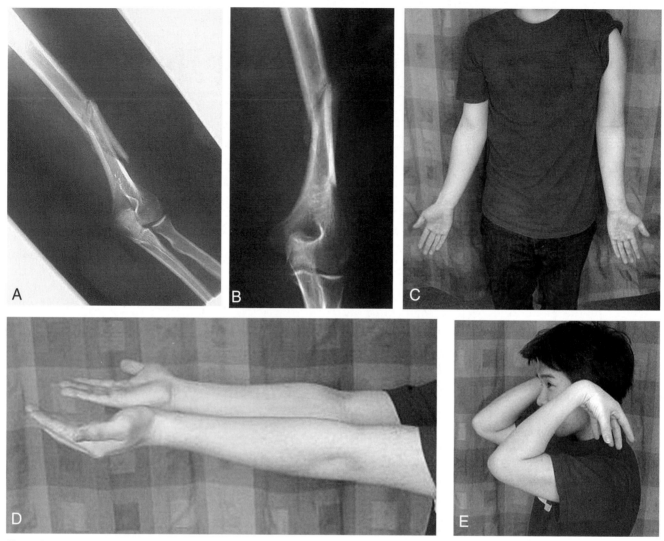

Figure 1 Functional bracing is the optimal treatment for most diaphyseal fractures of the humerus. A patient fractured his left humerus while snowboarding. **A,** Radiographs taken at the time of injury show a slightly angulated fracture of the distal third of the humeral diaphysis. **B,** Eight weeks after the injury radiographs showed established healing. The patient stated he had not been wearing the brace for a few days because he felt that he did not need it anymore. **C,** The slight angulation was noticeable, but it did not inhibit the patient's function. At only 8 weeks after the injury, extension **(D)** and flexion **(E)** were fully restored.

consideration of all of the proposed contraindications to functional bracing finds that few are absolute.

Failure to obtain or maintain adequate alignment may be an indication for surgical treatment; however, none of the 922 patients in a recent series had a manipulative reduction. Gravity alone restored adequate alignment in all patients. Furthermore, it remains unclear what constitutes inadequate alignment because, as a result of the global mobility of the shoulder, good upper extremity function is compatible with substantial varus or valgus deformity of the humerus.

The one fracture type that remains troublesome and merits close attention is the long oblique fracture of the proximal third of the diaphysis. In some cases the deltoid is attached to the distal fragment and, as the patient becomes more comfortable and more functional, the pull of the deltoid can increase deformity and motion at the fracture site and prevent healing. Muscle interposition also seems to be more common at this site. There are insufficient data to recommend surgical treatment, and in most patients these fractures probably will heal with proper functional bracing. If surgical treatment is necessary, the functional bracing will have helped patients return to daily functional tasks, facilitated resolution of edema in the limb, and allowed restoration of elbow function. Little if any ground is lost in the ultimate goal of restoring a functional limb.

Alcoholic patients and otherwise unreliable patients are said to be poor candidates for functional bracing, but they are equally poor candidates for internal fixation. Nonsurgical treatment at least avoids the potential complications of surgery.

Segmental fractures, low-velocity gunshot fractures, and fractures associated with low-grade open wounds are all well treated in a functional brace.

Multiple trauma is also a potential indication for surgical treatment, but this has not been defined clearly or substantiated. In fact, flexible intramedullary rod fixation—one of the most popular methods for treating fractures of the humerus in multiply injured patients—does not totally eliminate the need for brace wear in all patients and may not facilitate crutch ambulation. A more clearly defined situation in which surgical treatment of a fracture of the humerus might be useful is the patient with lower limb injury in whom the ability to bear weight on the upper extremity might facilitate mobilization. More stable internal fixation may be useful in this situation.

Given that bilateral upper extremity injuries can leave a patient dependent on others for basic daily tasks, surgical treatment of a humeral fracture might be useful when both upper limbs are injured. These decisions must be based on the specific injuries and needs of each individual patient.

The best indications for surgical treatment are fractures associated with substantial soft-tissue injury (such as severe open wounds, extensive burns, or vascular injuries), complex upper extremity injuries such as the so-called floating elbow (concomitant fracture of the diaphyseal humerus and forearm), and pathologic or impending pathologic fractures.

Technique of Functional Bracing

Considering the importance of functional bracing in the treatment of diaphyseal fractures of the humerus, it is worthwhile to review the details of the technique. The fracture is stabilized initially in a coaptation splint and sling. Although there is rarely any need to manipulate the fracture, the alignment is improved in most cases if the splint is molded into the deltoid insertion area to minimize varus angulation. Gravity also helps to restore alignment if the arm is kept dependent. Patients are instructed not to lean on or support the elbow during the early stages of healing in order to enhance restoration of normal alignment.

Once the acute symptoms have subsided and the swelling has decreased (usually within 1 week), a functional brace is fitted to the arm. Either a simple sling or a collar-and-cuff sling is used to support the arm below the elbow (Fig. 2). This sling is primarily for comfort and can be discontinued as soon as the patient is comfortable. Patients are shown how to adjust the brace and tighten the Velcro straps several times a day to accommodate the changes that occur as swelling subsides. The brace is worn at all times except during bathing.

During the first few weeks, patients should be monitored closely to ensure that they understand the need

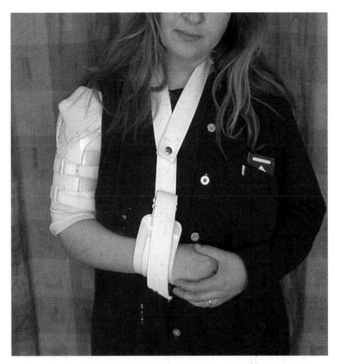

Figure 2 Treatment combines polypropylene fracture bracing with gravitational force to improve alignment. A collar and cuff is an alternative to a sling early on. Active elbow mobility is allowed when comfortable.

to keep the arm strictly dependent and how to adjust the brace. In addition, the brace often creates pressure areas, either at the distal limit (antecubital fossa) or proximal medial aspect, and these need to be addressed with brace modifications.

Patients begin pendulum exercises of the shoulder once the brace has been applied. Active elevation and abduction of the shoulder are prohibited until early healing is established both clinically and radiographically (usually about 8 weeks). The sling is removed for a few minutes several times a day for the patient to perform combined active and passive exercises of the elbow in an attempt to regain full range of motion of this joint as soon as possible. Once elbow extension is restored, or as soon as comfort allows, patients are weaned from the sling and active elbow motion is encouraged.

Patients should be seen frequently early on to ensure proper brace use, to check for pressure areas, and to monitor the exercise program. The brace is removed on clinical and radiographic union (usually between 8 and 12 weeks after the injury).

Surgical Treatment

When surgical treatment is indicated, the goal is to restore alignment and stability to (1) help rehabilitate complex upper extremity injuries by allowing immediate active functional use of the arm, (2) facilitate the care of

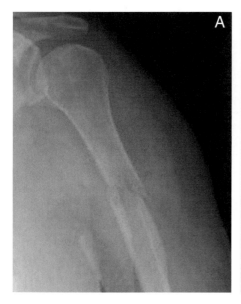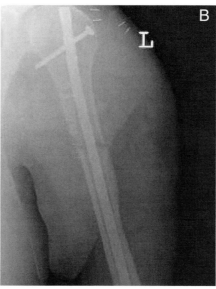

Figure 3 Pathologic fracture of the humerus represents the best indication for intramedullary rod fixation. **A,** This radiograph shows a pathologic diaphyseal fracture of the humerus. **B,** Intramedullary rod fixation helped relieve pain and restore function to the limb.

traumatic wounds, and (3) allow functional use, including weight bearing through the upper extremity. Narrow-diameter (flexible) intramedullary rods have had some enthusiastic advocates, but they may not always achieve these goals. Larger-diameter rods with locking screws have proved successful for impending and established pathologic fractures (Fig. 3) and fractures associated with severe burn injuries. Drawbacks of rigid intramedullary nailing include rotator cuff injury and difficulties associated with reconstruction should the fracture fail to heal. To date, studies that compare the results of intramedullary rod fixation with results of plate fixation have not demonstrated any advantage of rods in terms of union or function. However, intramedullary rod fixation is associated with a second procedure to remove the rod. Knowledge of extensive surgical exposures and proper plating techniques will help increase the chances of a good result.

Intramedullary Fixation

Narrow-Diameter (or Flexible) Intramedullary Rods

Narrow-diameter (or flexible) intramedullary rods have been used successfully for the fixation of fractures of the humerus in multiply injured patients. Adjuvant functional brace treatment is recommended after flexible nailing when the narrow-diameter intramedullary rods fail to achieve rotational stability. Support for narrow-diameter intramedullary fixation of the humerus reflects the appeal of the relative simplicity of this technique. Although there are proponents of this technique, problems have been reported in some series. In recent series, the rate of nonunion was as high as 8%, the reoperation rate as high as 100%, and the rate of rod migration as high as 34%. Attention to technical details is imperative for success.

Locking Intramedullary Rods

Enthusiasm for interlocked intramedullary fixation of the humerus followed the success of similar implants for diaphyseal fractures in the femur and tibia. As clinical experience with this type of humeral fixation has increased, it has been shown to have a number of problems.

Antegrade Insertion

Antegrade rod insertion is the most common form of intramedullary rodding of the humerus. A decade ago, several clinical studies promoted use of a specific nail for intramedullary fixation of the humerus through a proximal portal. Subsequent publications identified a number of problems associated with use of this implant. Because the distal locking mechanism of this nail is not rigid, nonunion rates upward of 22% and a 37% rate of shoulder problems have been reported.

The placement of an intramedullary nail into the humerus is technically demanding, with risk of injury to either the shoulder or elbow. The humerus can be quite narrow, and the potential exists for iatrogenic fragmentation or distraction of the fracture with nail insertion. Distraction at the fracture is very poorly tolerated in the humerus and can be a source of nonunion. Reaming the intramedullary canal introduces the danger of injury to the radial nerve and has been associated with segmental necrosis of the humerus.

In recent prospective randomized trials that compared large-diameter intramedullary rod fixation with plate and screw fixation for fractures of the humeral diaphysis, union rates were comparable. However, intramedullary rod fixation was associated with more shoulder pain, healing problems, nerve injuries, and reoperations than was plate fixation.

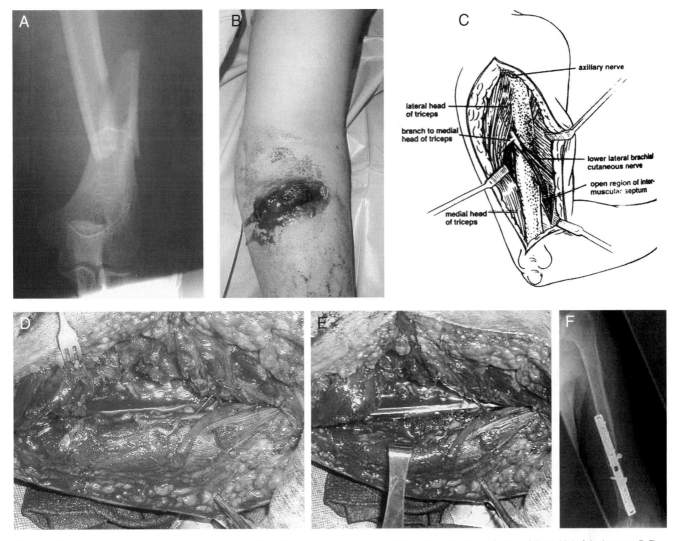

Figure 4 A 20-year-old man sustained complex trauma to the left arm in a motor vehicle collision. **A,** The radiograph shows a fracture of distal third of the humerus. **B,** The proximal humeral fragment broke through the skin in the anterior forearm. **C,** This illustration shows the extensive exposure of the posterior humerus and radial nerve that is possible through an extended lateral or modified posterior exposure. **D,** An extended lateral exposure was used to repair the fracture and explore the radial nerve. The nerve was found lacerated; the proximal end can be seen draped across the triceps. **E,** Plate fixation through the lateral approach provided stable fixation and the radial nerve was repaired. **F,** Ten months after surgery, the humerus had solidly healed.

Humeral nonunion after intramedullary rodding often is associated with additional problems. Removal of a well-seated rod can cause substantial injury to the rotator cuff and proximal humerus. In addition, motion of a loose nail can erode and thin the cortices along the entire length of the nail. When this is combined with the osteopenia associated with stress shielding and disuse of the limb, the quality of the bone is greatly diminished, and stable internal fixation can be difficult to achieve.

Retrograde Insertion
The prevalence of shoulder dysfunction after insertion of a large-diameter intramedullary nail has created interest in distal insertion sites. The early clinical reports of retrograde intramedullary nailing for diaphyseal humeral fractures have been favorable. Whether the nail is

introduced through an entrance hole in the supracondylar (metaphyseal) area or more distally in the olecranon fossa, potential exists for iatrogenic fracture. Recent biomechanical investigations have shown that the hole made for insertion creates a substantial stress riser that places the limb at risk of fracture below the rod with functional activities and weight bearing. Modification of nail designs to enhance their flexibility may extend the application of this approach.

Pathologic Lesions of the Diaphysis
Surgical fixation of pathologic lesions of the proximal humerus is performed for both impending fracture and for pathologic fracture. In the former instance the goal of internal fixation is to relieve pain and reduce fracture risk, allowing confident functional use of the up-

per extremity. This step can improve quality of life in severely ill patients with limited life expectancy. A larger-diameter rod with locking screws is preferred to provide skeletal stability and avoid direct exposure of the pathologic lesions. Concerns about rotator cuff function and secondary reconstruction are less important in this circumstance. The extent of the pathologic area is sometimes uncertain, and the rod can bridge most of the length of the humerus. Intramedullary fixation of established pathologic fractures is more demanding than that for impending fractures but may still be the best option (Fig. 3).

Placement of an intramedullary rod is relatively safe and simple in this situation because the integrity of the humerus is maintained, limiting the danger of injuring the radial nerve. Open plate fixation would involve dissection of the tumor—a situation that could lead to extensive blood loss or injury to the radial nerve. Lesions involving the distal third of the humerus are not as easily stabilized with intramedullary devices because the intramedullary canal terminates above the distal metaphysis.

Patients with primary bone tumors or metastases consistent with long survival should be treated with tumor resection and limb reconstruction where appropriate.

Plate and Screw Fixation

Plate and screw fixation remains the most predictable method for surgical treatment of diaphyseal fractures of the humerus. Numerous series, including recent prospective randomized trials, demonstrated a nonunion rate of 5%. Technical aspects of open reduction and internal fixation are critical for success. Failed plate fixation tends to be a result of inadequate surgical technique, usually involving fixation with plates of insufficient length. Recent descriptions of extensile surgical exposure should help surgeons avoid these errors.

Most authors recommend heavier plates. Using a plate with 4.5-mm screws, the goal of fixation is to use a minimum of three screws on either side of a transverse, short oblique, or spiral fracture in addition to interfragmentary compression screws (ie, a plate between six and eight holes in length).

For multifragmented fractures, a bridging-type plate is applied to span the area of comminution, preserving the muscular and periosteal attachments to the fragments. Indirect reduction techniques are used instead of techniques that involve extensive dissection and anatomic reduction of all of the fracture fragments to avoid devascularizing the fragments. A minimum of four screws should be placed into the main proximal and distal fragments beyond the area of fragmentation; this may necessitate a plate of nine or more holes. For fractures of the distal half of the humeral diaphysis, the application

of such long plates requires identification and mobilization of the radial nerve when a lateral or posterior exposure is used (Fig. 4).

Surgical Exposures

Anterolateral Exposure

The anterolateral exposure described by Henry represents the safest, most straightforward method for exposing fractures of the proximal third as well as many fractures of the middle third of the humerus. Proximally, the interval between the deltoid and pectoralis major is developed. At the distal aspect of the exposure the brachialis is split longitudinally, with one third taken laterally and two thirds medially, corresponding to the innervation of the brachialis by the radial and musculocutaneous nerves, respectively. The periosteum and muscular attachments to the humeral fracture fragments are preserved where possible. The insertion of the deltoid is very broad, and a portion of the insertion can safely be mobilized laterally to facilitate placement of a plate. As much as 80% to 90% of the humerus can be exposed using this exposure. The distal limit for plate application is the coronoid fossa of the distal humerus. The surgeon must also beware of the radial nerve as it passes anteriorly between the brachialis and brachioradialis distally.

A major drawback of this approach is that it can be difficult to address associated radial nerve laceration because exposure of the proximal aspect of the nerve lying posterior to the humerus can be very difficult. When there is a possibility of radial nerve injury, an extensile lateral exposure is recommended.

Posterior and Extended Lateral Approaches

The posterior exposure of the distal third of the humerus uses a midline split of the triceps. If the surgeon finds that more proximal exposure is needed to gain adequate fixation, the radial nerve should be identified and mobilized. If more proximal exposure is required, the entire triceps muscle can be mobilized off the lateral intramuscular septum instead of splitting the triceps. This exposure represents the intramuscular interval used by the modified posterior and extended lateral exposures. The difference between these exposures lies in the skin incision, which can be posterior, posterolateral, or directly lateral.

The modified posterior exposure of the humerus is performed through a midline posterior skin incision. A lateral skin flap is elevated. A cutaneous nerve is identified (one of the inferior lateral cutaneous nerves of the arm) and traced along the intramuscular septum to identify the radial nerve. Alternatively, the triceps is swept medially off the lateral intramuscular septum until the fat that surrounds the radial nerve is identified. Once the radial nerve is identified, the triceps can be mobilized medially above and below the nerve and the nerve mobilized from the surface of the humerus. Specific dissection of the nerve is not necessary except to identify it; it can be kept within the surrounding fat and muscle.

A cadaver study of exposure to the posterior humerus demonstrated the ability to gain access to 55% of the humerus through a standard posterior exposure without mobilizing the radial nerve, to 76% after mobilizing the radial nerve, and to nearly the entire humerus (94%) using the modified posterior exposure and mobilizing the radial nerve.

The extended lateral exposure was derived from the exposure used to harvest lateral arm flaps. A direct lateral skin incision is used, and a cutaneous nerve is traced to the radial nerve. Once the radial nerve is identified, either the posterior or anterior aspect of the humerus can be prepared for plate application. The main advantage of this approach is that the radial nerve can be traced extensively both proximally and distally in the wound. Consequently, the extended lateral exposure is ideal for the treatment of fractures associated with radial nerve injury (Fig. 4). If the radial nerve must be traced, the skin incision is extended along the posterior aspect of the deltoid proximally. Alternatively, it can be extended anteriorly in the deltopectoral interval.

Medial Exposure

The medial exposure of the humerus is best suited for fractures associated with vascular injuries and nonunions requiring a vascularized bone graft. The medial exposure also represents a good alternative in patients concerned about cosmesis (since the scar is on the less obvious inner aspect of the arm) and in obese patients because the adipose tissue tends to retract away from the wound with gravity. Through a direct medial skin incision the deeper structures are exposed while branches of the medial brachial cutaneous nerve of the arm are protected. The median nerve, brachial artery, and medial antebrachial cutaneous nerves are mobilized and protected, and the brachialis is elevated extraperiosteally from the surface of the humerus. Additional care must be taken to protect the musculocutaneous nerve proximally and the ulnar nerve distally. The humerus can be exposed from the medial epicondyle to the insertion of the pectoralis major.

Complex Fractures

Humeral fractures occurring as part of a more complex upper extremity injury and humeral fractures associated with severe soft-tissue injury are uncommon. In these instances, internal fixation of the humeral fracture is associated with a high rate of union; however, overall limb function often is compromised by associated soft-tissue

and/or neurovascular injury. Given the circumferential muscle envelope surrounding the humerus, open wounds severe enough to be rated Gustilo and Anderson type 3, particularly type 3B, often represent near amputations.

To optimize the results of treating these complex injuries, most fractures should be treated with stable plate and screw fixation to allow mobilization of joints and musculotendinous units while ensuring a high rate of union. Exceptions include high-velocity gunshot fractures and other severe soft-tissue injuries. In some cases the need for expediency may warrant the use of an external fixator, although plate fixation is appropriate for most fractures associated with vascular repairs.

Periprosthetic Fractures

Periprosthetic fractures of the humerus are uncommon. One recent series reported the results for nine patients. Functional brace treatment was successful in four of five patients even though all five were at the distal limit of the prosthesis, an area thought to be at particular risk for nonunion given the stress riser produced by the implant. Another series reported union in all four patients treated with a functional brace. Recommendations for surgical treatment include fractures associated with loose prostheses and fractures that fail to heal in a functional brace. Fractures distal to the humeral prosthesis can be treated with humeral stem revision to a long-stem implant and internal fixation with cerclage wires or cables. Alternatively, if the humeral prosthesis is well fixed and positioned, the fracture can be fixed with a hybrid plate and cerclage fixation.

Nonunion

The incidence of nonunion is uncertain. Approximately one half of nonunions represent failed nonsurgical treatment in which there is usually a persistent wide displacement suggesting soft-tissue interposition. The other half represent inadequate surgical fixation with either short plates or inadequate intramedullary implants.

Hypertrophic nonunions of the humerus, those that show some attempts at healing, are often stable, and patients may retain functional use of their upper limb although pain tends to be present. In contrast, atrophic nonunions, particularly synovial nonunions, are usually unstable. Such unstable nonunions can be extremely disabling, particularly in older patients because they have a diminished capacity for adapting to musculoskeletal problems. This instability was recently quantified in a group of older patients with unstable, atrophic nonunions. There was very severe, near complete disability of the upper extremity in many patients. Obtaining stable fixation of the osteopenic humerus is challenging in these

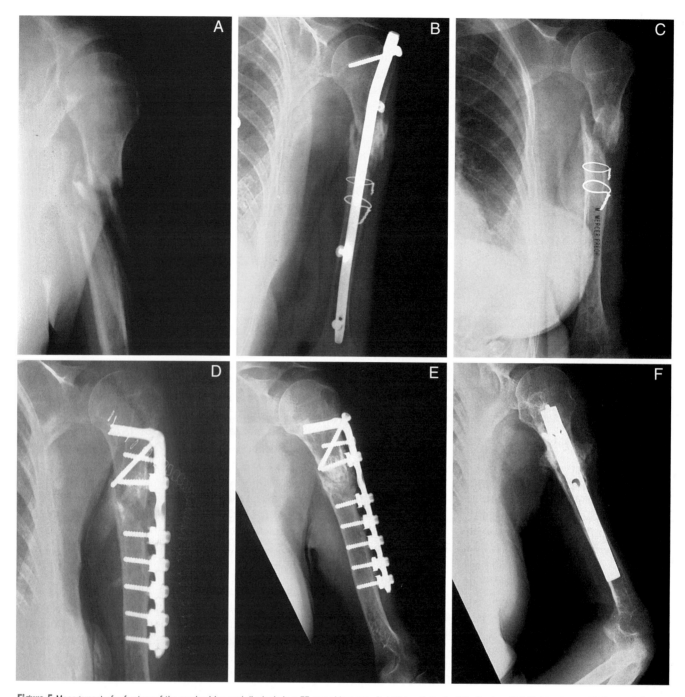

Figure 5 Management of a fracture of the proximal humeral diaphysis in a 77-year-old woman. **A,** Initial radiograph of the fracture. **B,** Initial treatment with intramedullary rod fixation and supplementary cerclage wires. **C,** The rod was prominent at the shoulder and was removed, but the fracture had not united and proved unstable. **D,** Surgical fixation was performed with a blade plate and screws reinforced by Schuhli nuts. **E, F,** AP radiographs 2 years later show good callus formation. Good function was restored.

patients. Combinations of fixation techniques that incorporate long plates, blade plates, Schuhli nuts (Synthes, Paoli, PA) and other screw enhancement techniques, and allograft struts in addition to autogenous bone graft can enhance the success rate (Fig. 5).

The most predictable treatment of nonunion of humeral diaphysis fractures has been plate and screw fixation with autogenous cancellous bone grafting. A recent study examined this specific problem after the failure of

locking (large-diameter) intramedullary nails. Exchange to a new intramedullary nail was successful in only 4 of 10 cases. Plate fixation achieved union in all of 9 patients but was technically very difficult because of compromised bone quality. In addition, shoulder dysfunction that related to the insertion and subsequent removal of an antegrade rod compromised the result in many cases.

Atrophic nonunions with bony defects after complex wounds, infection, multiple surgical attempts to gain union, or synovial nonunion represent a more challenging subset of nonunions. Whereas the humerus will tolerate substantial shortening, shortening can be difficult in the setting of an established nonunion, particularly if the surrounding soft tissues are scarred. Furthermore, the mobilization required to appose the fracture fragments would devascularize the fragments and impede healing. Vascularized fibular grafting remains a good option for large defects (6 cm or greater) and very scarred, dysvascular, and noncompliant soft-tissue envelope. The more straightforward treatment of bridge plating and autogenous bone grafting represents a good option when there is a well-vascularized muscular envelope and a small- to moderate-sized defect. Contouring the plate away from the bone at the site of the nonunion, the so-called wave plate osteosynthesis, may have some biologic and mechanical advantages.

Summary

The mainstays of treatment of diaphyseal humeral fractures are functional bracing and plate and screw fixation. While interest in intramedullary fixation is growing, associated problems have limited its indications. Any surgical treatment must be carefully considered given the good results of fracture bracing in closed fractures, low-grade open fractures, low-velocity gunshot fractures, segmental and mutifragmented fractures, and periprosthetic fractures. Malalignment is rarely a problem with nonsurgically treated fractures. Effective plate fixation requires familiarity with a variety of surgical exposures and confidence in handling the radial nerve. Unstable nonunions of the humerus are extremely disabling and merit surgical treatment.

Annotated Bibliography

Brumback RJ: The rationales of interlocking nailing of the femur, tibia, and humerus. *Clin Orthop* 1996;324: 292-320.

This article notes that the role of intramedullary locked nailing is much less well defined in the humerus than in the femur and tibia. The author states that "until good long-term studies can verify some advantage to the patient in terms of improved clinical outcome without undue risk, it is thought that humeral interlocking nailing should rarely be chosen as the method of fracture care."

Campbell JT, Moore RS, Iannotti JP, Norris TR, Williams GR: Periprosthetic humeral fractures: Mechanisms of fracture and treatment options. *J Shoulder Elbow Surg* 1998;7:406-413.

This series focuses on intraoperative fractures, but five postoperative fractures were included. Four were treated with a functional brace, and all healed.

Chapman JR, Henley MB, Agel J, Benca PJ: Randomized prospective study of humeral shaft fracture fixation: Intramedullary nails versus plates. *J Orthop Trauma* 2000; 14:162-166.

This study compares diaphyseal humeral fracture fixation with intramedullary nails and plates. Although healing problems were uncommon in both groups, shoulder problems and subsequent surgeries were more common among patients treated with intramedullary rods.

Farragos AF, Schemitsch EH, McKee MD: Complications of intramedullary nailing for fractures of the humeral shaft: A review. *J Orthop Trauma* 1999;13: 258-267.

This review details the disadvantages of intramedullary nail fixation of fractures of the humerus, including antegrade and retrograde insertion site problems, the problems of reaming in the humerus, neurovascular injury, iatrogenic comminution, fracture at the end of the implant, healing problems, and the difficulties of reconstructive surgery after intramedullary rod fixation.

Flinkkila T, Hyvonen P, Lakovaara M, Linden T, Ristiniemi J, Hamalainen M: Intramedullary nailing of humeral shaft fractures: A retrospective study of 126 cases. *Acta Orthop Scand* 1999;70:133-136.

This is a retrospective study of antegrade rodding with the Seidel nail. There was a 22% nonunion rate and shoulder dysfunction in 37%.

Gerwin M, Hotchkiss RN, Weiland AJ: Alternative operative exposures of the posterior aspect of the humeral diaphysis with reference to the radial nerve. *J Bone Joint Surg Am* 1996;78:1690-1695.

This study evaluated exposures of the posterior humerus. Only 15 cm of the humerus (55% of the total length) can be exposed through the standard posterior triceps splitting exposure. Mobilization of the radial nerve adds 6 cm of exposure for a total of 76%. Elevating the entire triceps off the lateral intramuscular septum and identifying and protecting the radial nerve exposes nearly the entire humerus (94% of the total length).

Habernek H: Letter: A locking nail for fractures of the humerus. *J Bone Joint Surg Br* 1998;80:557.

This letter retracts the author's 1991 articles suggesting good results with the Seidel nail and reporting that shoulder problems are actually very common. This "change of opinion" reemphasizes the caution with which the scientific literature must be interpreted, particularly when the early results of a new implant or technique are reported.

McCormack RG, Brien D, Buckley RE, McKee MD, Powell J, Schemitsch EH: Fixation of fractures of the shaft of the humerus by dynamic compression plate or intramedullary nail: A prospective randomised trial. *J Bone Joint Surg Br* 2000;82:336-339.

The results of this study were comparable for patients in whom nails and plates were used. More shoulder pain was noted in patients in the nail group.

McKee MD, Miranda MA, Riemer BL, et al: Management of humeral nonunion after the failure of locking intramedullary nails. *J Orthop Trauma* 1996;10:492-499.

This study reviews the surgical treatment of 21 ununited fractures of the humerus after intramedullary nailing. Treatment was more complex because of shoulder injury caused by nail removal and bone loss associated with motion of the loose rod. Exchange nailing resulted in healing in only 4 of 10 patients. Plate fixation and autogenous cancellous bone grafting was successful but was very challenging.

Mills WJ, Hanel DP, Smith DG: Lateral approach to the humeral shaft: An alternative approach for fracture treatment. *J Orthop Trauma* 1996;10:81-86.

The direct lateral exposure of the humerus is similar to the modified posterior exposure in that the radial nerve is identified and mobilized at the lateral intramuscular septum. The lateral skin incision facilitates exposure of the radial nerve posterior proximally and anterior distally and is, therefore, the favored exposure of humeral fractures with associated radial nerve palsies in which radial nerve repair may be necessary.

Otsuka NY, McKee MD, Liew A, et al: The effect of comorbidity and duration of nonunion on outcome after surgical treatment for nonunion of the humerus. *J Shoulder Elbow Surg* 1998;7:127-133.

An ununited fracture of the humerus healed in all 21 patients treated with plate fixation and autogenous cancellous bone grafting. Lack of correlation between patient-oriented outcome measures (SF-36) and physician-oriented measures was noted in patients with comorbid factors such as head injury, injury to the pelvis or lower limbs, preexisting severe mental or physical diseases, or secondary gain issues.

Remiger AR, Miclau T, Lindsey RW, Blatter G: Segmental avascularity of the humeral diaphysis after reamed intramedullary nailing. *J Orthop Trauma* 1997; 11:308-314.

These case reports of segmental necrosis of the humerus after reamed intramedullary nailing support clinical impressions that reaming of the humerus may be more detrimental to blood supply and healing than reaming of the femur and tibia.

Ring D, Jupiter JB, Quintero J, Sanders RA, Marti RK: Atrophic ununited diaphyseal fractures of the humerus with a bony defect: Treatment by wave-plate osteosynthesis. *J Bone Joint Surg Br* 2000;82:867-871.

In this multicenter series of 15 patients with ununited fractures of the humeral diaphysis with bone loss, good results were obtained with the use of wave plate osteosynthesis. A large autogenous cancellous graft will bridge the defect when protected with relative stability and a well-vascularized muscular envelope.

Ring D, Perey BH, Jupiter JB: The functional outcome of operative treatment of ununited fractures of the humeral diaphysis in older patients. *J Bone Joint Surg Am* 1999;81:177-190.

This series of 22 patients demonstrates that healing can be achieved in most cases in spite of poor bone quality, synovial nonunion, and bone loss. Specific techniques for fixation of poor quality bone including the use of longer plates, blade plates, and augmented screws are helpful. Successful union was associated with dramatic improvements in patient-oriented outcomes and independent functioning.

Rodriguez-Merchan EC: Compression plating versus Hackethal nailing in closed humeral shaft fractures failing nonoperative reduction. *J Orthop Trauma* 1995;9: 194-197.

This study compares the results of elastic narrow intramedullary nail fixation with plate and screw fixation and found comparable results. However, intramedullary nailing was associated with a 100% reoperation rate.

Rommens PM, Blum J, Runkel M: Retrograde nailing of humeral shaft fractures. *Clin Orthop* 1998;350:26-39.

The authors advocate retrograde insertion of a locked intramedullary nail for fixation of diaphyseal fractures of the humerus. They reported 4% fragmentation at the insertion site, 4% postoperative radial nerve palsy, and 7% nonunion.

Sarmiento A, Zagorski JB, Zych GA, Latta LL, Capps CA: Functional bracing for the treatment of fractures of the humeral diaphysis. *J Bone Joint Surg Am* 2000;82: 478-486.

Six hundred twenty of 922 patients with fractures of the humeral diaphysis treated with functional bracing were followed until healing. This included 155 open fractures (25%) (118% due to a low-velocity gunshot injury), 219 distal third diaphyseal fractures (35%), and six segmental fractures (1%). All fractures healed with acceptable angulation and, in spite of the relatively short follow-up time, 98% of the patients regained full or near-full motion of the shoulder and the elbow.

Shazar N, Brumback RJ, Vanco B: Treatment of humeral fractures by closed reduction and retrograde intramedullary Ender nails. *Orthopedics* 1998;21:641-646.

This article reports on the use of Ender nails for retrograde fixation of diaphyseal humeral fractures. Postoperative functional bracing is always used in conjunction with these elastic intramedullary nails, and postoperative weight bearing with crutches is not advised. Thus, the major advantages of surgical fixation in patients with multiple injuries are not realized. The nonunion rate is around 8%. The reoperation rate was 19% in this series.

Strothman D, Templeman DC, Varecka T, Bechtold J: Retrograde nailing of humeral shaft fractures: A biomechanical study of its effects on the strength of the distal humerus. *J Orthop Trauma* 2000;14:101-104.

A supracondylar (or metaphyseal) entry portal for retrograde intramedullary nail insertion was found to diminish the torque to failure to 71% and the energy to failure to 37% of an intact specimen. The numbers for the olecranon entry portal were 55% and 18%, respectively.

Svend-Hansen H, Skettrup M, Rathcke MW: Complications using the Seidel intramedullary humeral nail: Outcome in 31 patients. *Acta Orthop Belg* 1998;64:291-295.

This is one of several studies in which the initially good results reported with the Seidel nail were retracted.

Tytherleigh-Strong G, Walls N, McQueen MM: The epidemiology of humeral shaft fractures. *J Bone Joint Surg Br* 1998;80:249-253.

The authors reported treatment of 249 fractures of the diaphyseal humerus over a 3-year period. A bimodal distribution of young patients with high-energy injury mechanisms and older patients with low-energy mechanisms was observed. Multifragmented fractures, segmental fractures, and fractures with severe open wounds occurred in fewer than 10% of patients.

Wright TW, Cofield RH: Humeral fractures after shoulder arthroplasty. *J Bone Joint Surg Am* 1995;77:1340-1346.

Nine periprosthetic humeral fractures were reviewed. The authors suggest that the best initial treatment of periprosthetic fractures of the humerus is probably coaptation splinting followed by a functional orthosis. Surgical treatment is appropriate for fractures associated with loose prostheses and fractures that fail to heal in a functional orthosis.

Yang KH, Han DY, Kim HJ: Intramedullary entrapment of the radial nerve associated with humeral shaft fracture. *J Orthop Trauma* 1997;11:224-226.

Fracture of the humeral diaphysis associated with a radial nerve palsy remains a difficult and disputed management issue. As this case report illustrates, intramedullary fixation is risky in the presence of a radial nerve palsy because the nerve can be entrapped within the fracture site where it is susceptible to closed reaming or nail insertion.

Yokoyama K, Itoman M, Kobayashi A, Shindo M, Futami T: Functional outcomes of "floating elbow" injuries in adult patients. *J Orthop Trauma* 1998;12: 284-290.

This series of 14 patients with a floating elbow reflects the severity of these high-energy injuries. When both the humeral and the forearm fractures have stable fixation with plates and screws, good elbow motion should be more predictably obtained; however, due to the severity of the trauma and the associated injuries, the overall prognosis for the upper extremity is less certain.

Zinman C, Norman D, Hamoud K, Reis ND: External fixation for severe open fractures of the humerus caused by missiles. *J Orthop Trauma* 1997;11:536-539.

This study reports the use of external fixation for fractures of the humerus. Twenty-six soldiers with high-velocity gunshot fractures of the humerus were treated with radical débridement and external fixation. Injuries to nerves and blood vessels were common, and 11 fractures had delayed union or nonunion. However, the use of external fixation was credited with a recent improvement in the limb salvage rate with such severe injuries.

Classic Bibliography

Henry AK: *Extensive Exposure*, 2nd ed. London, England, Churchill Livingstone, 1973.

Section 5

Arthritis/ Arthroplasty

Section Editor:
Joseph P. Iannotti, MD, PhD

Chapter 24

Inflammatory Arthritis of the Shoulder

David N. Collins, MD

Introduction

Arthritis is the most common musculoskeletal manifestation of systemic inflammatory conditions that affect the shoulder. These processes include rheumatoid arthritis, spondyloarthropathies, disorders of connective tissue (systemic lupus erythematosus), and crystalline and deposition disorders. This chapter will focus on rheumatoid arthritis, the most prevalent inflammatory arthropathy, and its effect on the shoulder girdle.

Incidence

Rheumatoid arthritis affects 20 to 40 in 100,000 adult individuals; its incidence increases with age. Women outnumber men twofold to threefold. Although it is not commonly one of the first joints affected by rheumatoid arthritis, the shoulder rarely escapes involvement, especially with advancing disease. When present, rheumatoid arthritis usually occurs to some degree in both shoulders.

Pathogenesis

Rheumatoid arthritis is best described as a systemic autoimmune disorder without a known primary cause. Connective tissue throughout the body is at risk, although the major distinctive feature of the disease is chronic, often erosive, synovitis. The activities and interrelationships of heritable factors, autoimmunity, and infectious agents are being explored to uncover the etiology of rheumatoid arthritis.

Pathophysiology

The initial event leading to symptomatic rheumatoid arthritis appears to take place in the subsynovial microvascular network. The immune response to antigens leads to activation and proliferation of the synovial membrane layer. Synovial fluid production increases with higher concentrations of inflammatory cells and chemical mediators of inflammation. By the process of angiogenesis, the synovial membrane and its supporting structure sustain the membrane's expansion. Acquiring abrasive malignancy-like properties, this tissue, known as pannus, has no boundary. It spreads onto adjacent articular cartilage, tendons, tendon sheaths, and ligaments and has the capacity to invade periarticular bone.

Pathoanatomy

The entire shoulder girdle is susceptible to the rheumatoid process, which may result in involvement of the three diarthrodial joints as well as the biceps tendon, rotator cuff, and subacromial bursa. Resultant attenuation can lead to rupture, producing full-thickness rotator cuff defects. This phenomenon occurs in 10% to 50% of all patients and in one third of patients undergoing total shoulder arthroplasty. If the rotator cuff is not torn, most patients will exhibit cuff thinning or attenuation. The long head of the biceps tendon usually is ruptured. Most patients with Larsen radiographic grade 4 or 5 (osseous collapse) have extensive rotator cuff disease.

The acromioclavicular joint may become involved primarily or by inflammatory processes extending from the subacromial space. Within 15 years from the time of disease onset, more than two thirds of patients exhibit involvement of the acromioclavicular joint. Typical findings include inferior joint margin erosions; degenerative features including osteophytes and sclerosis without rheumatoid changes are rare.

Manifestions of rheumatoid arthritis in the glenohumeral joint predominantly involve the superior and lateral surfaces of the humeral head. The characteristic marginal osseous erosions found superior and medial to the greater tuberosity correspond to the insertion of the rotator cuff, the junction of the articular cartilage, and the most frequent site of rotator cuff tearing.

More than half of all patients will show definite glenohumeral joint involvement that is more minimal than severe. However, in one fourth, severe changes will exist bilaterally. Glenohumeral space joint narrowing occurs relatively late; it typically is seen after marked erosive destruction.

The relationship of acromioclavicular and glenohumeral involvement is unclear. Acromioclavicular involvement is more prevalent than glenohumeral involvement and is a clinical problem in up to one third of patients. It is possible for acromioclavicular joint symptoms to occur before glenohumeral joint changes, although the extent of acromioclavicular joint involvement generally correlates with glenohumeral involvement. Both joints are affected in more than 50% of patients. Solitary glenohumeral joint disease is the most uncommon type of articular involvement of the shoulder.

As the glenohumeral cartilage erodes, joint volume may diminish, resulting in contracture of the capsule and the musculotendinous cuff. If the cuff remains intact, mild to moderate concentric erosion of the glenohumeral joint occurs. In the presence of a dysfunctional cuff, imbalanced muscular forces may result in ascent of the humeral head. Progressive eccentric superior and medial glenoid wear will ensue, sometimes to the base of the coracoid process. Further abrasive entrapment of the musculotendinous cuff between the acromion, acromioclavicular joint, and humeral head may contribute to full-thickness tearing. Eventually, superior forces override all soft-tissue restraints, leading to containment only by the components of the coracoacromial archway. Even this final barrier of escape may succumb, leaving the humeral head superiorly dislocated and tenting the attenuated deltoid origin.

Clinical Evaluation

It would be quite rare to assess a patient for shoulder pain only to discover, via appropriate diagnostic tools, that the patient has rheumatoid arthritis. Instead, patients with known rheumatoid arthritis frequently come to the orthopaedist for evaluation of shoulder pain. The source of pain is elucidated by careful history taking, thorough examination of the cervical spine and affected shoulder girdle, and imaging. A lidocaine injection test may be invaluable for localizing the source of shoulder pain to a specific anatomic structure.

The effects of rheumatoid arthritis on the shoulder evolve insidiously and slowly. With a few exceptions, the physical findings are usually nonspecific and include decreased range of motion, weakness, crepitation, and atrophy. Synovial fluid from the glenohumeral joint may pass through a full-thickness defect in the rotator cuff into the subdeltoid and subacromial bursa where it may accumulate, simulating a mass.

The radiographic findings depend on the duration and extent of disease. Osteopenia, juxta-articular erosions,

and concentric loss of articular cartilage are common findings. The glenohumeral relationship may be altered in the superior direction as a result of imbalanced muscular forces or rotator cuff damage. End-stage findings may include obliteration of the acromiohumeral interval with formation of an acromiohumeral "articulation," large confluent cysts, humeral head collapse, and centralization of the glenoid. CT is used to characterize osseous morphology and glenohumeral relationships; it often is done in conjunction with preoperative planning for implant arthroplasty. Arthrography may be useful to confirm needle position during arthrocentesis and to assess the rotator cuff. Findings on MRI scans help to determine the volume and location of fluid about the shoulder, as well as the extent of rotator cuff disease.

Neer described three types of glenohumeral rheumatoid arthritis based on radiographic appearance. Not unlike osteoarthritis, the dry type is associated with joint space narrowing, subchondral cysts, and erosions with marginal osteophytes. Marginal erosions, sometimes quite extreme, characterize the wet type. The proximal humerus may acquire a pointed contour because of osseous prominence smoothing. Rapid destructive loss of cartilage and bone with centralization and distortion of the glenohumeral joint contour characterizes the wet and resorptive phases.

Nonsurgical Treatment

Significant osteoarticular damage will develop in most patients with active rheumatoid arthritis within the first 2 years after the onset of the disease. The intent of nonsurgical treatment, therefore, is to diminish or arrest the inflammatory components of the disease process in an attempt to reduce its morbidity and mortality. Nonsurgical treatment should seek to provide effective pain relief, maintain function, preserve the quality of life, and reduce irreversible joint damage. Nonsteroidal antiinflammatory drugs, glucocorticoids, and antirheumatic disease-modifying drugs used alone or in combination with each other are the cornerstones of nonsurgical management. Adjunctive instillation of steroids into affected joints, bursae, or tendon sheaths is extremely useful as a means of controlling acute inflammation. Immunosuppressants, biologic agents, and antibiotics are being investigated for their possible contributions to disease remission.

Physiotherapy should be used to establish and maintain a functional range of motion. Though perhaps somewhat less effective than isotonic methods, isometric strengthening exercises may be more suitable because of joint inflammation and destruction. Aggressive physiotherapy deters recovery of motion and power and should be avoided for the acutely inflamed shoulder.

Surgical Treatment

Surgical intervention should be considered when pain control can no longer be addressed effectively, even on a temporary basis, by nonsurgical means or when irreversible soft-tissue and osteoarticular alterations are anticipated. It is helpful to more precisely define the lesions responsible for pain with use of sophisticated imaging or, alternately, local anesthetic injection techniques.

The sternoclavicular joint rarely requires surgical treatment. When necessary, arthrotomy, synovectomy, débridement, and resection arthroplasty are performed. Care is taken not to render the articulation unstable.

The acromioclavicular joint may require surgical treatment as an isolated disorder. More often, it is treated in conjunction with a rotator cuff repair or glenohumeral joint implant procedure. An arthroscopic approach may be used for isolated involvement. Arthrotomy accompanied by débridement, synovectomy, and distal partial (1 to 1.5 cm) claviculectomy effectively address the rheumatoid disorders of this articulation.

The predominant signs and symptoms of rheumatoid arthritis are sometimes confined to the contents of the subacromial space. Isolated bursal hypertrophy may exist, but it is more often associated with a bursal-side partial-thickness rotator cuff tear. Bursectomy can be performed by arthroscopic or open techniques. Caution is advised regarding the surgical alteration of the coracoacromial archway because primary acromial spurring is rarely a contributing factor. Rendering the coracoacromial ligament dysfunctional or the anterior deltoid origin incompetent disables the natural mechanisms for blockage of superior ascent of the humeral head, commonly seen in rheumatoid arthritis.

Full-thickness rotator cuff tears, rarely isolated events in rheumatoid arthritis, should be considered with respect to involvement of the acromioclavicular and glenohumeral joints. As such, they often are treated concomitantly at the time of a glenohumeral joint or acromioclavicular joint procedure. Although comfort and function are successfully restored to almost 85% of all patients undergoing rotator cuff repair, the subset of patients with rheumatoid arthritis with rotator cuff tears has only recently been reported. Factors mitigating against a favorable outcome include attenuated soft tissue, osteoporosis, antimetabolic and corticosteroid medication, muscular weakness, dependence on the upper extremities for gait and mobilization assistance, and limited overall rehabilitation potential.

If the glenohumeral articular cartilage is reasonably well preserved and if concomitant lesions (eg, osteonecrosis) are absent, glenohumeral joint synovectomy via open or arthroscopic methods can be considered.

Lesions of the biceps tendon, subacromial bursa, and rotator cuff are addressed simultaneously.

Glenohumeral arthrodesis, for the most part, is considered only as a salvage procedure when a previous implant has failed or massive destruction precludes implant arthroplasty. Osteopenia may preclude effective stabilization. Rehabilitation and postoperative function may be challenged as a result of ipsilateral or peripheral joint involvement.

Resection arthroplasty remains an effective alternative to implant arthroplasty, but it has several major disadvantages. Pain relief is unpredictable in the presence of poor stability, power, and motion. These factors, as well as the disease status of ipsilateral joints, may render the upper extremity relatively useless.

When pain and dysfunction attributable to glenohumeral joint involvement persist despite optimum medical management and changes in the joint surface preclude synovectomy, implant arthroplasty is indicated. However, the timing of surgical intervention may be based on additional factors. Integrity of the rotator cuff is essential for maintenance of function. Earlier implant arthroplasty has been proposed as a means of preserving rotator cuff integrity. Implant arthroplasty arrests ascent of the humeral head, a cause of cuff impingement. Moreover, removal of glenohumeral cartilage from the joint during the procedure fosters termination of the intra-articular inflammatory process. Delays in surgery result in a greater degree of osteoarticular deformity, destruction, and soft-tissue involvement. Rotator cuff tears become more frequent and extensive, making successful repair a challenge.

Rheumatoid arthritis commonly involves multiple joints, some of which may be involved simultaneously and actively when shoulder surgery is being contemplated. Ipsilateral shoulder and elbow disease presents unique challenges in terms of surgical timing and technique. The order of joint replacement should be influenced mainly by the extent of clinical involvement, as opposed to the anticipated functional gains. The sequence of replacement does not appear to influence the result, ratings, or functional scores. Although it appears that ample pain relief may be obtained from single joint replacement, significant functional gains are not achieved until both joints have been replaced. Despite improving the function of the replaced joint, the arthroplasty leaves the function of the unreplaced joint unchanged. The results are acceptable but inferior to a single isolated joint involvement treated with joint replacement. The interval between replacements appears to have no impact on the results.

The structural quality of the bone in a patient with rheumatoid arthritis may be extremely poor, a factor to consider during the exposure and preparation of the humerus. Both the humerus and the glenoid are at risk for fracture during glenoid preparation. Osteoporosis often is accompanied by deficiencies of glenoid and humeral bone as a result of cystic and erosive changes, increasing the vulnerability to iatrogenic fracture. For this reason, some authors have advised maintenance of at least a 6-cm interval between the humeral components of ipsilateral shoulder and elbow arthroplasties or their respective cement mantles by the appropriate selection of implant length and the use of cement restrictors. Alternately, imminent fracture of the intercalary humeral segment may be averted by the extension of the cement column to achieve full humeral canal filling.

The timing and sequence of shoulder arthroplasty should be considered relative to involvement of weight-bearing joints. For patients who depend on the upper extremity for gait assistance, lower extremity arthroplasty preceding shoulder arthroplasty offers the benefit of eventual relief of weight-bearing demands on the upper extremity. Sometimes, however, the shoulder is involved to an extent that may preclude practical upper extremity support following lower extremity arthroplasty. In that event, lower extremity arthroplasty should follow shoulder arthroplasty by no less than 3 months. This allows for adequate reattachment of the subscapularis and rotator cuff, if repaired.

For special circumstances occurring more frequently in rheumatoid arthritis than in noninflammatory arthritis, hemiarthroplasty, rather than total shoulder arthroplasty, is a more suitable reconstructive option to consider. If erosion or cystic resorption of glenoid bone stock has made it insufficient to stably support a glenoid component, hemiarthroplasty is favored. Massive and irreparable rotator cuff tears invite superior glenohumeral instability following total replacement arthroplasty. The placement of a glenoid implant in this setting results in an unacceptably high glenoid loosening rate by a "rocking horse" mechanism. Occasionally, extreme medialization with associated soft-tissue contracture reduces joint volume to the extent that only a humeral component can be placed without overstuffing the joint. A significant downside of hemiarthroplasty is the potential development of symptomatic glenoid erosion, the most frequent reason for revision of painful hemiarthroplasty to total shoulder arthroplasty.

For patients with rheumatoid arthritis who are undergoing shoulder arthroplasty, particularly those who have been treated with immunosuppressive drugs for prolonged duration, intraoperative soft-tissue and osseous specimens should be sent for histologic analysis. Non-Hodgkin's lymphoma has been reported as a finding in one such patient who had no symptoms or signs of malignancy preoperatively.

Results

Recently, the radiologic patterns of disease described by Neer have been correlated with intraoperative findings with emphasis on the rotator cuff and glenoid. All shoulders in the study were Larsen grade 4 or 5; they included 45 wet shoulders, 92 resorptive shoulders, 20 dry shoulders, and 10 end-stage shoulders. Rotator cuff tears were seen in 25 dry shoulders, 12 resorptive shoulders, and 3 end-stage shoulders. The rotator cuff was thin in 50 resorptive shoulders. Deficiencies of the glenoid bone were found in all but 26 shoulders, 24 of which were the wet type. Larsen grade bore no correlation with the glenoid or the rotator cuff status. From these findings, the shoulder at risk appears to be the wet type shoulder. In this shoulder, a high incidence of cuff rupture and early radiographic progression precedes glenoid damage. For these shoulders, timely referral and early surgical intervention, sometimes synovectomy, is often appropriate. Five radiologic patterns of destruction have been identified and used for the assessment and selection of the optimal surgical treatment (Table 1).

Arthroscopic synovectomies afforded both pain relief and improved range of motion only for the nonprogressive type and pain relief only for the erosive type. For this group, pain relief and range of motion improvement could be obtained only with implant arthroplasty. Arthroscopic synovectomy provided neither pain relief nor range of motion in the collapse type. Implant arthroplasty provided pain relief without improvement of range of motion for collapse and erosion types. Total shoulder arthroplasty or hemiarthroplasty showed no difference regardless of the destructive pattern. Glenoid erosions were observed in 7 of 19 instances of hemiarthroplasty, with no difference between destructive patterns. Arthrosis-like shoulders rarely require surgery. Arthroscopic synovectomy should be considered when there are no destructive changes.

Longer-term follow-up of total shoulder arthroplasty averaging 7.7, 9.5, and 12.2 years is now available. Clinical results reveal excellent or satisfactory results in two thirds of patients with the potential to fully meet their recovery goals, and pain relief is sustained for more than 90% of patients. This finding is consistent regardless of Larsen grade, age, gender, rotator cuff status, and pre- or postoperative range of motion. With recovery of range of motion inversely correlated with the Larsen grade, normal or nearly normal range of motion is rarely achieved. Nevertheless, most patients will experience marked improvement in range of motion, enabling the hand and sometimes the arm to be placed to the level of the shoulder. An additional significant functional improvement is the ability to sleep comfortably on the affected side. Restoration of anatomic alignment by ideal humeral and glenoid component positioning has been shown to offer

TABLE 1 Radiographic Patterns of Destruction in the Rheumatoid Shoulder

Type of Disease	Radiographic Features	Treatment
Nonprogressive	Small, insignificant erosions only, even 15 to 20 years after disease onset	Arthroscopic synovectomy (+ pain, + motion)
Arthrosis-like	Typical arthritic features: osteophytes, joint space narrowing, sclerosis of subchondral bone	Nonsurgical
Erosive	Marginal lesions without collapse	Implant arthroplasty (+ pain, + motion)
Collapse	Coalescence of large subchondral cysts associated with collapse of the subchondral trabeculae	Implant arthroplasty (+ pain, - motion)
Mutilating	Severe bone destruction and bone absorption, often with a "cut off" appearance	Implant arthroplasty (+ pain, - motion)

significant improvements in certain comfort and functional parameters.

Superior subluxation of the humeral head of more than 5 mm as a result of thinning or tearing of the rotator cuff has been reported to occur in more than 50% of shoulders. This relationship to glenoid component loosening is well established, and there appears to be some correlation with humeral component loosening. Over time, glenoid loosening becomes more prevalent (50%), as does alteration of the position of a press-fit humeral component. In addition to thin or torn rotator cuffs, factors associated with loose components include female gender and glenoid deficiencies.

Radiolucent zones around metal or cement interfaces with bone have always been a source of concern and investigation. More recent studies reveal that there is likely to be progression of the extent and width of the zones, especially around the glenoid component. The development of radiolucent zones after 2 years of follow-up has been shown to occur in almost 50% of loose components. Even in this setting, not all patients will have severe pain, and fewer yet may require revision.

The need for revision of loose components may be infrequent for several reasons. Patients with rheumatoid arthritis usually place lower demands on their joints; those reliant on upper extremity support for gait and transfer assistance are exceptional considerations. A protective effect may exist as a result of ipsilateral joint involvement, which limits extremity use. Finally, scapulothoracic function generally is well preserved.

Today's shoulder surgeon is able to use modern humeral implants, some of which are designed speci-

fically for press-fit fixation, and to employ superior methods of glenoid preparation for the placement of anatomically designed glenoid components. It seems intuitive that when coupled with a complete understanding of the effects of rheumatoid arthritis on the shoulder, appropriately timed surgical intervention, and execution of the technical method of shoulder arthroplasty with utmost accuracy, results exceeding those in the most current reports will be realized.

Annotated Bibliography

Arredondo J, Worland RL, Sinnenberg RJ Jr, Qureshi GD: Non-Hodgkin's lymphoma as an unexpected diagnosis in a shoulder arthroplasty. *J Arthroplasty* 1999; 14:108-111.

This case report describes the occult occurrence of non-Hodgkin's lymphoma in an immunosuppressed patient with rheumatoid arthritis. It was diagnosed from intraoperative tissue sent for routine histologic examination.

Collins D, Harryman D, Wirth M: A prospective multi-center functional outcome study of arthroplasty in glenohumeral inflammatory arthritis. *J Shoulder Elbow Surg* 1999;8:186-187.

This prospective, relatively short-term follow-up study indicates that hemiarthroplasty and total shoulder arthroplasty both improved functional outcome for patients with rheumatoid arthritis. An intact rotator cuff, use of a glenoid component, and restoration of glenohumeral alignment gave the best results.

Cuomo F, Greller MJ, Zuckerman JD: The rheumatoid shoulder. *Rheum Dis Clin North Am* 1998;24:67-82.

The epidemiologic aspects of rheumatoid arthritis are discussed, along with pathology, differential diagnosis, clinical and radiographic findings, and treatment approaches.

Gill DR, Cofield RH, Morrey BF: Ipsilateral total shoulder and elbow arthroplasties in patients who have rheumatoid arthritis. *J Bone Joint Surg Am* 1999;81:1128-1137.

This study gives detailed results and analyses of 17 patients undergoing ipsilateral total shoulder and elbow arthroplasties, providing important guidelines regarding the timing and sequence of the operations.

Hirooka A, Wakitani S, Yoneda M, Ochi T: Shoulder destruction in rheumatoid arthritis: Classification and prognostic signs in 83 patients followed 5-23 years. *Acta Orthop Scand* 1996;67:258-263.

The natural course and possibility of making prognoses about shoulder joint destruction were studied in a series of patients. These findings may be valuable in selecting treatment for the rheumatoid shoulder.

Langenegger T, Michel BA: Drug treatment for rheumatoid arthritis. *Clin Orthop* 1999;366:22-30.

This review indicates that disease-modifying antirheumatic drugs may alter the course of rheumatoid arthritis. The early results of investigations of immune response–altering biologic agents hold promise.

Lehtinen JT, Belt EA, Lyback CO, et al: Subacromial space in the rheumatoid shoulder: A radiographic 15-year follow-up study of 148 shoulders. *J Shoulder Elbow Surg* 2000;9:183-187.

Significant collapse of the acromiohumeral space appears to take place during the progression from Larsen stage 3 to stage 4. Imaging surveillance and early orthopaedic intervention may improve the treatment of the rheumatoid shoulder.

Rozing PM, Brand R: Rotator cuff repair during shoulder arthroplasty in rheumatoid arthritis. *J Arthroplasty* 1998;13:311-319.

The evolution of an alternative surgical approach to total shoulder arthroplasty when rotator cuff repair is anticipated is described. The results are better when a good repair is obtained.

Sneppen O, Fruensgaard S, Johannsen HV, Olsen BS, Sojbjerg JO, Andersen NH: Total shoulder replacement in rheumatoid arthritis: Proximal migration and loosening. *J Shoulder Elbow Surg* 1996;5:47-52.

Factors associated with component loosening and proximal humeral migration were evaluated in a prospective study of 51 patients with 62 Neer mark II total shoulder arthroplasties. Average results were not significantly influenced by proximal humeral migration or component loosening.

Sojbjerg JO, Frich LH, Johannsen HV, Sneppen O: Late results of total shoulder replacement in patients with rheumatoid arthritis. *Clin Orthop* 1999;366:39-45.

The results of 62 shoulders in 51 patients followed for an average of 7.7 years are reviewed. Proximal humeral component migration led to a 42% glenoid component failure rate.

Stewart MP, Kelly IG: Total shoulder replacement in rheumatoid disease: 7- to 13-year follow-up of 37 joints. *J Bone Joint Surg Br* 1997;79:68-72.

A mean follow-up of 9.5 years of 58 Neer II total shoulder replacements in 49 patients is reported. Progressive component loosening was prevalent, but the need for revision was infrequent.

Torchia ME, Cofield RH, Settergren CR: Total shoulder arthroplasty with the Neer prosthesis: Long-term results. *J Shoulder Elbow Surg* 1997;6:495-505.

With an average follow-up of 12.2 years, this study provides valuable long-term information on glenoid loosening, press-fit humeral component loosening, and clinical results. The fate of glenoid radiolucent zones is carefully analyzed and raises concerns regarding durable component fixation.

Wakitani S, Imoto K, Saito M, et al: Evaluation of surgeries for rheumatoid shoulder based on the destruction pattern. *J Rheumatol* 1999;26:41-46.

In the presence of destructive changes, arthroscopic synovectomy does not effectively eliminate pain or restore range of motion. Implant arthroplasty is necessary to achieve these results.

Classic Bibliography

Figgie HE III, Inglis AE, Goldberg VM, Ranawat CS, Figgie MP, Wile JM: An analysis of factors affecting the long-term results of total shoulder arthroplasty in inflammatory arthritis. *J Arthroplasty* 1988;3:123-130.

Franklin JL, Barrett WP, Jackins SE, Matsen FA III: Glenoid loosening in total shoulder arthroplasty: Association with rotator cuff deficiency. *J Arthroplasty* 1988;3:39-46.

Larsen A, Dale K, Eek M: Radiographic evaluation of rheumatoid arthritis and related conditions by standard reference films. *Acta Radiol Diagn (Stockh)* 1977;18:481-491.

Matthews LS, LaBudde JK: Arthroscopic treatment of synovial diseases of the shoulder. *Orthop Clin North Am* 1993;24:101-109.

Neer CS II (ed): *Shoulder Reconstruction.* Philadelphia, PA, WB Saunders, 1990, pp 212-222.

Chapter 25

Management of Osteoarthritis of the Shoulder

John J. Brems, MD

Introduction

Primary glenohumeral osteoarthritis (OA) was most succinctly defined as limitation of glenohumeral movement, loss of articular joint space, and humeral head enlargement resulting from a ring of osteophytes. However, rotator cuff tears usually are not present in primary OA of the shoulder. Primary OA of the shoulder typically results in glenoid erosion, which usually is posterior and may result in posterior subluxation of the entire joint. Features of primary glenohumeral OA are described in Table 1.

Etiology and Pathophysiology

OA of the shoulder can be either primary or secondary. The exact etiology of primary OA is not known. However, it may be caused by remote or asymptomatic mechanical trauma that alters the biochemical milieu of the shoulder and ultimately causes a biochemical degradation of the articular cartilage. The exact cause of each instance of secondary OA must be identified because appropriate treatment may involve both orthopaedic and nonorthopaedic medical intervention.

The most common causes of secondary OA include trauma, instability, and prior joint surgery. Less common causes include infection, osteonecrosis, gout, Paget's disease, rheumatoid disease and its variants, and a number of metabolic conditions, including ochronosis, sickle cell disease, and epiphyseal dysplasias.

The final common pathway to OA is articular cartilage failure. The changes that result in this failure may be precipitated by biochemical, anatomic, traumatic, mechanical, pathologic, or metabolic alterations in the local environment of the cartilage. It is not entirely clear whether the initial injury is to the articular cartilage itself or whether the pathologic process begins with alteration of the mechanical properties of the subchondral bone. Changes in the physical and mechanical properties of the subchondral bone may alter its ability to respond to even normal physiologic forces.

With stiffening of the subchondral plate, changes in shear occur within the cartilage layer, which, in turn, initiate changes in the ultrastructure of the cartilage. Water is imbibed, and a host of cascading events occur throughout the cartilage substance, resulting in inability to tolerate applied forces. As the cartilage degrades, joint stability is compromised and periarticular osteophytes, which are a characteristic and defining radiographic feature, begin to form at the articular margins. Increasing friction within the affected joint induces mechanical destruction of the remaining cartilage. With less force absorbed and efficiently transferred as a result of the declining amount and quality of articular cartilage, the adjacent bone is subjected to more stress. The added stress results in the characteristic subchondral sclerosis seen in the medial humeral head and posterior glenoid where joint forces are greatest. Joint fluid is forced hydraulically through microscopic fissures in the subchondral bone, ultimately forming subchondral cysts seen on radiographs of osteoarthritic joints. The joint becomes more geometrically incongruent, resulting in painful loss of motion in the affected shoulder.

When a joint has been traumatized to a point beyond its ability for self-repair, degenerative joint disease (OA) is likely to occur with the passage of time. In the situation in which the initial assault to the articular cartilage is mechanical, an overt intra-articular fracture is not necessary to begin the cascade of cartilage destruction. Careless use of the arthroscope may damage the articular surface, thereby initiating the cascade of events that will lead to the development of degenerative disease many years in the future. Theoretically, even the use of a retractor to lever on the humeral head during instability surgery may damage the articular cartilage at a microscopic level and be responsible for development of OA decades later. With this very long interval between insult and disease, correlation of cause and effect is nearly impossible to establish.

Even the best anatomic reduction of an articular surface fracture is not truly anatomic at the microscopic or ultrastructural level. The subsequent mechanical forces

| **TABLE 1** | **Features of Primary Glenohumeral Osteoarthritis** |

Rotator Cuff

    Degeneration with fibrosis (especially the subscapularis)

    Tearing uncommon (< 5%)

Capsule

    Enlargement inferior, possibly posterior

    Contracture anterior

Joint Position

    Centered

    Posterior subluxation

Humeral Head

    Erosion central with flattening

    Increased size

    Peripheral osteophytes (especially inferior)

    Sclerosis

    Subchondral cysts

    Cartilage loss: superior, central, or complete

Glenoid

    Erosion central and posterior with flattening

    Peripheral osteophytes

    Sclerosis

    Subchondral cysts

    Cartilage loss: central or posterior

(Reproduced from Cofield RH, Becker DA: Shoulder arthroplasty, in Morrey BF (ed): Reconstruction Surgery of the Joints, ed 2. New York, NY, Churchill Livingstone, 1996, p 754.) © Mayo Foundation, Rochester, MN.

and joint motion over long spans of time are known to result in a much higher probability of OA than exists in a joint that never has sustained such injury because the cartilage that was damaged has little intrinsic ability for self-repair.

Joint instability is believed to be associated with the development of secondary OA, but the association of OA and instability of the shoulder is not as clear as it is with other joints. The physician must distinguish between laxity (asymptomatic joint looseness) and instability (symptomatic humeral head translation that may or may not be associated with joint laxity). Instability always is associated with some element of trauma. In the classic case of a TUBS (traumatic-unidirectional-Bankart-surgery) lesion, significant trauma results in dislocation or subluxation (instability). As the glenohumeral joint absorbs enough energy to dislocate, the cartilage is subjected to severe shear forces and sustains significant microscopic, if not macroscopic, injury. Arthroscopic inspection of the recently dislocated shoulder reveals striking evidence of cartilage injury that is not evident on routine radiographs. This is not to say that instability is merely a type of mechanical event that has been defined as being associated with the development of OA. Nearly 20% of individuals with untreated instability will develop OA in years to come. The relationship between instability and OA is better evaluated by studying the AMBRI (atraumatic-multidirectional-bilateral-rehabilitation-inferior capsular shift) syndrome. Although prevalence and incidence assessments are impossible to ascertain in asymptomatic individuals, it is generally accepted that individuals with symptomatic, untreated multidirectional instability (MDI) rarely develop OA. On the other hand, the incidence of OA is higher in patients who have undergone stabilization procedures for MDI.

The osseous elements of the shoulder confer relatively little intrinsic stability; consequently, the integrity of ligaments and neuromuscular control are paramount. If ligaments are tightened inappropriately or inaccurately, imbalance of joint forces occurs and OA follows. The critical importance of maintaining near-normal external rotation of the shoulder after surgical shoulder stabilization procedures has been documented, and a direct correlation has been established between the occurrence of OA and a significant loss of external rotation after stabilization procedures. Global balance of ligament tension remains a key treatment goal of instability management, whether it be surgical or nonsurgical. The natural history of untreated multidirectional shoulder instability does not necessarily lead to a high incidence of OA.

Surgical procedures that lead to altered joint mechanics and kinematics likely increase the probability of secondary OA. Mechanical joint disruptions associated with intra-articular fractures and the kinematic alterations provoked by rotator cuff muscle tears result in a higher incidence of secondary OA. Intra-articular fixation devices—staples, tacks, anchors, and the like—even when perfectly placed according to the surgeon's desires, may alter joint kinematics enough to result in secondary OA of the shoulder.

Clinical Presentation

There is no classic clinical presentation of the patient with OA. It is not uncommon for patients to have more complaints of limited motion and function than of pain.

Impairment of activities of personal care bring the patient to seek medical care as often as complaints of pain. Although the patients may be of any age, it seems that more patients in their 30s and 40s who underwent stabilization procedures are developing arthritis of the affected shoulder joint. When the association of instability repairs and the early development of advanced OA was first identified, the condition was called arthrosis of dislocation.

Patients with OA describe night pain that is characteristically positional but is unlike the night pain associated with rotator cuff tears, which is an unremitting, toothache-like pain that prevents sleep or causes severe sleep interruption. Patients with OA tend to learn to avoid lying on their affected shoulder and, once settled, can obtain quality sleep. Patients also report morning stiffness, often improved by a hot shower, and they note audible and palpable crepitus when reaching up to dress themselves. Patients also commonly mention the inability to wash their hair or to pass a belt or fasten a bra behind the back. Medical histories may reveal trials of oral anti-inflammatory medications, steroid injections, or physical therapy programs. A carefully obtained history including surgeries, medications, allergies, and social factors is important to determine whether the condition is primary or is secondary to some other pathologic process that may require concomitant treatment.

The physical examination of the shoulder must begin at the neck. Patients with OA of the shoulder have a very high incidence of associated, though asymptomatic, OA of the cervical spine. The most common levels for OA of the cervical spine are C5, C6, and C7—the same levels that provide the motor and sensory supply to the shoulder. Assessment of cervical spine motion in all planes is required. Any limitation of motion or provocation of ipsilateral limb symptoms requires radiographic evaluation at the very least.

The examination of the shoulder itself begins with observation of both shoulders. The astute physician will note muscular atrophy, muscle contours, and neck-to-shoulder distance. Significant differences in shoulder elevation occur with excessive scapular rotation on the affected side. There usually is asymmetry in the shoulder width when comparing affected and unaffected sides.

Assessment of range of motion is performed with the patient in both the supine and sitting positions. The American Shoulder and Elbow Surgeons determined the appropriate positions in which to make these measurements. Total shoulder elevation and external rotation are assessed with the patient supine to eliminate any contribution from the spine. Active elevation is recorded with the patient supine to diminish the impact of gravity. Finally, both elevation and external rotation strength are assessed with the patient either sitting or standing under

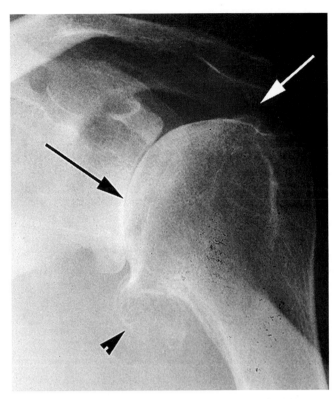

Figure 1 True AP radiograph demonstrating the characteristic features of OA. The black arrow points to the absent glenohumeral joint space. The black arrowhead identifies the large osteophyte at the inferior anatomic neck. The white arrow indicates the well-preserved subacromial space, which usually is consistent with integrity of the rotator cuff in this condition.

the influence of gravity. Any discrepancy in strength is noted and related to either pain or muscle weakness. The patient with advanced OA usually has limited motion in all planes. Crepitus is both audible and palpable and provokes pain. Although strength usually is maintained and rotator cuff tears are distinctly uncommon in primary OA, pain may be significant enough during muscle strength testing that a false-positive weakness may be noted. The examination is completed only when a neurologic assessment of motor and sensory integrity is performed.

Radiographic Studies

In the evaluation of OA, plain radiographs are usually sufficient to fully assess the extent of the disease. It is important to obtain appropriate projections in both the AP and axillary planes. The true AP view (Fig. 1) is obtained by having the patient turn the affected shoulder toward the radiographic film. When this is done properly, there is no overlap of the humerus on the glenoid, and the joint space is clearly seen. On this view, the physician can measure the extent of cartilage loss, assess humeral head sphericity, and note the presence and extent of anatomic neck osteophytes. However, the AP view will not allow assessment of the ring of osteophytes because

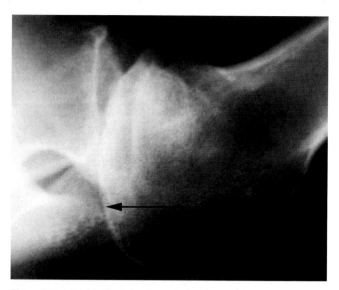

Figure 2 West Point (axillary) view demonstrating characteristic posterior glenoid wear. The arrow indicates the area where the central portion of the humeral head is articulating with the posterior rim of the glenoid. With time, the posterior glenoid erodes, altering the version of the joint.

the anterior extent is superimposed on the anterior neck. Usually only the inferior aspect of the osteophytic ring is evident. In the true AP view it is important to note the degree of medial glenoid bone loss because this information provides significant insight and predictive ability for glenoid resurfacing. The AP projection permits assessment of the subacromial humeral space as a rough measure of rotator cuff status. Interpretation of the greater tuberosity contour and sclerosis combined with the clinical assessment of strength should provide the physician with a very reasonable prediction of cuff integrity.

The axillary or West Point view is also important in the radiographic assessment of the shoulder, particularly in the evaluation of and preoperative planning for shoulder arthroplasty (Fig. 2). This projection permits evaluation of posterior glenoid bone status. The pathophysiology of glenohumeral OA typically results in significant posterior glenoid bone erosion, which often is the limiting factor when considering the possibility of glenoid resurfacing. This view also allows assessment of the longitudinal alignment of the limb and prediction of the potential for posterior shoulder instability. Knowledge of these issues can help the surgeon plan glenoid and humeral version modifications during joint replacement. When glenoid erosion is not well quantified on plain radiographs, a limited CT study provides additional needed information. At this time, no other imaging techniques have been found to provide additional benefits.

Nonsurgical Management

In designing treatment recommendations for a patient with OA, physicians should remember two important

points: that this is not a fatal condition, and that they are not treating a shoulder, they are treating a patient with a shoulder malady. Very often, a patient's symptoms will be less severe than the radiographs would imply or predict. It is important to treat the patient, not the radiograph!

Nonsurgical care should begin with patient education and an explanation of the condition. Often, educating a patient about his or her situation will diminish both anxiety and symptoms. Judicious use and trials of oral anti-inflammatory medications may provide dramatic relief of symptoms and improve quality of sleep. Activity modification emphasizing diminishing repetitive activities, especially those with the limb positioned near the terminal extent of the patient's motion arc, often will ameliorate symptoms. Intra-articular steroids should be used only with complete understanding that they typically offer little benefit and offer a source and site for potential infection that may forever preclude shoulder replacement. Physical therapy modalities should also be prescribed based on a complete understanding of the degree of joint incongruity as defined by the radiographs. Sending a patient to a physical therapist with the intent of improving range of motion in the face of a severely incongruent joint is ill advised and only makes the symptoms worse.

The Internet has offered individuals access to countless remedies of varying worth. The use of nutritional supplements, such as glucosamine, chondroitin sulfate, and shark cartilage, seems to be increasing, yet well-designed scientific studies assessing their efficacy are lacking. Prolotherapy has its proponents; also, the use of magnets has some yet-to-be-explained benefit for many patients with OA.

Surgical Management

When nonsurgical options have been exhausted and the patient's quality of life is compromised by OA, a number of surgical treatment options are available. These options include arthroscopic or open joint débridement, synovectomy, osteotomies, release of contractures, tendon lengthening, resection arthroplasty, interpositional arthroplasty, arthrodesis, and joint replacement.

There is very little in the literature to support the value of either open or arthroscopic joint débridement for OA of the shoulder unless it is confined to early changes in which the humeral head remains spherical and concentrically reduced within the normal glenoid. Of two studies of arthroscopic management of early OA, neither addressed the cartilage loss or loss of humeral sphericity. The authors of another study noted that arthroscopic débridement is of marginal value in more advanced clinical cases. The condition of 75% of their patients became worse following arthroscopic débridement. Another author made the same observations and no longer recommends arthroscopic management of glenohumeral OA. Retrieval of loose bodies in early OA has merit, but removal of periarticular osteophytes has not been shown to be of benefit. Arthroscopic synovectomy as treatment for synovial chondromatosis, pigmented villonodular synovitis, and removal of loose bodies with the hope of preventing OA has been described. In one recent study, a series of 45 patients was followed 2 years after arthroscopic débridement of grade IV osteochondral lesions of the humeral head and glenoid. Although the authors acknowledged that the therapeutic benefit of arthroscopic surgery was unclear in either altering or improving the natural course of the articular degeneration, carefully selected patients found at least temporary improvement in pain and function. The authors defined a good candidate for arthroscopic débridement as an individual with a congruent, well-centered joint, little or no osteophyte formation, mild or no subchondral sclerosis or cyst formation, and an osteochondral lesion that is no larger than 2 cm. Regaining and retaining a full arc of motion is critical for a favorable result. Neer described the few cases of open cheilectomy as dismal failures.

Arthrodesis is rarely if ever indicated as a treatment for OA. The only reason to consider arthrodesis is for management of painful paralysis about the shoulder, such as may occur in severe and permanent brachial plexus injury that renders the arthritic shoulder painful with no anticipated recovery of motor function. Treatment of persistent septic arthritis may require arthrodesis, although resection arthroplasty may be more appropriate. Although arthrodesis of the hip or knee may be more appropriate than arthroplasty in a young, vigorous individual, age alone is never a contraindication to shoulder arthroplasty if there are appropriate indications for the procedure. In those younger patients who have a particularly physically demanding occupation, arthrodesis may be appropriate. However, both the patient and physician must weigh the lifelong consequences of an arthrodesis against preservation of shoulder motion with an arthroplasty combined with a change in career.

Resection arthroplasty is rarely indicated for the management of shoulder OA. It is more commonly used as a salvage procedure for failed shoulder arthroplasty, especially for definitive management of severe postarthroplasty infection. In the geriatric patient with cuff tear arthropathy, resection arthroplasty may have a place; however, results of humeral head replacement have been more rewarding to patients.

Prosthetic arthroplasty—total shoulder replacement or humeral head replacement—remains the treatment of choice for management of OA. Although Neer was not the first surgeon to experiment with humeral head

replacement, he is credited with the initiation of modern shoulder replacement techniques. Because he was dissatisfied with the poor clinical outcomes of patients who sustained severe fractures of the proximal humerus, in 1951, he developed a technique for replacing the humeral head with a prosthesis. After recognizing the significant improvement of patients with this problem, he rapidly applied humeral head replacement to the management of OA.

For the next 20 years, few advances were made in shoulder replacement technology. During those 20 years, surgeons recognized that patients who had undergone replacement surgery had shoulder muscle fatigue and poor strength. The surgeons also became increasingly concerned with postprosthetic instability and the need to deal with the often incongruent and severely worn glenoid. Addressing these concerns, the first polyethylene glenoid component was designed and implanted in 1971. The concept behind development of the glenoid component was that it would provide a smooth articulating surface for the humeral component and it would lateralize the joint, thereby lengthening and strengthening the rotator cuff muscle sleeve. The next advance occurred in 1973, when a new humeral head was designed to mate with the glenoid component and a completely nonconstrained but fully conforming total shoulder system was available for general use.

Over the past 30 years, there has been an acceleration in the number of designs made available to the patient and surgeon, with more than a dozen shoulder replacement designs currently available. Advances have been made in both the anatomic design and the metallurgy and polymer chemistry of the components. Increased recognition of the critical importance of restoring proper myofascial sleeve tension while achieving stability and maintaining ability for external rotation has dramatically improved functional outcomes of total shoulder replacement over the last two decades. The original designs were fixed head-stem units that, when cemented, made it virtually impossible to treat subsequent glenoid disease. Nearly all contemporary shoulder replacement systems are based on modularity between the humeral stem and a variety of humeral head sizes. Glenoid configurations have changed and evolved similarly in the last decade. Although all glenoid components currently are polyethylene, metal-backed glenoid components were used until high failure rates and finite element analysis highlighted their inherent problems. The essential principles of soft-tissue balance, myofascial sleeve tension, restoration of version, and joint stability must remain the primary goals of the reconstructive shoulder surgeon.

Special Considerations

Total Shoulder Replacement Versus Humeral Head Replacement

In the treatment of OA, there is no absolute consensus regarding the issue of resurfacing the glenoid. Most surgeons note pain relief is more likely following glenoid resurfacing. There are some surgeons who believe that given a congruent glenoid, even if it is devoid of articular cartilage, humeral head replacement alone is sufficient. The decision to resurface the glenoid must also take into consideration the morphology of the glenoid, the degree of retroversion, and the quality of the host bone. Thus, the surgeon must consider the anticipated level of activity and forces that will be applied to the implanted device. It is intuitively less desirable to resurface a glenoid in a 50-year-old, very active farmer who manipulates 70 to 100 lb daily than it would be to resurface a glenoid in a 65-year-old sedentary office worker, given similar extent of OA in both patients.

The glenoid frequently has considerable posterior bone loss, resulting in excessive retroversion. This bone loss alters the humeral alignment such that its long axis is fixed posterior to the anatomically correct location. If the long axis has been situated in this nonanatomic position for some time, significant alteration of the muscle force vectors and muscle mechanics occurs. Therefore, the combination of excessive retroversion of the glenoid and humeral malalignment leads to significant posterior instability. Much of this problem may be corrected at the time of glenoid resurfacing by reaming the anterior glenoid in an effort to reestablish more anatomically correct version. With extensive posterior bone loss, bone grafting may be required to support the glenoid component. In some situations, the glenoid is so severely involved that grafting and reaming will not provide an adequate substrate, and humeral head replacement alone is performed.

There are few data regarding the relative advantages of keel design versus peg design for glenoid resurfacing. In preparing the glenoid with marginal posterior bone stock for pegged components, penetration of the posterior cortex should be carefully avoided. The surgeon should attempt to reestablish the anatomic joint line with respect to medial and lateral positions, thereby allowing anatomic reconstruction of rotator cuff muscle length-tension relationships.

The metal-backed glenoid components used in the past were quite bulky and resulted in significant lateralization of the anatomic joint center of rotation. There currently is no known reason to use metal-backed components, and in fact mathematical modeling seems to suggest reasons not to use this construct. The perceived advantage of metal backing is that it provides a substrate for cement-less, bone ingrowth applications. However, the older hooded glenoid components that were designed to offer superior stability in the face of cuff deficiency had a very high failure rate and should not be considered today.

Glenoid Lucent Lines and Glenoid Loosening

Although glenoid components of many designs have been in use for nearly three decades, the incidence and ramifications of lucent lines surrounding the component are unknown and frequently debated. Numerous incidence studies and meta-analyses have been performed by many authors. The reported prevalence of lucent lines varies from 30% to 90% at 10 years postoperatively, and in many studies their presence has been noted on radiographs taken within days of the procedure. Lucent lines have been classified according to location (around the keel, pegs, or screws) and by the width of the line; however, these classifications fail to define accurately or to predict clinically symptomatic loosening. The long-term implications of these lucent lines are unknown, but lessons learned from similar radiographic findings in the acetabulum, femur, and tibia are disconcerting. Perhaps because there is less force on the glenoid during normal use, symptoms are not present in the face of a frankly loose glenoid. Clinical experience suggests that a patient becomes symptomatic only when there is gross failure. Despite a high incidence of radiographic loosening and a significant number of lucent lines, clinical loosening remains distinctly uncommon. In a detailed meta-analysis involving 30 studies spanning 15 years of experience with metal-backed and all-polyethylene components implanted for a variety of diagnoses, the failure rate was only 2.0%. Using the Kaplan-Meier method of analysis, authors have estimated the probability of implant survival at 15 years to be 87%.

Meticulous glenoid preparation should be practiced. Numerous authors have recognized the critical importance of near-perfect mating of the glenoid surface to the component. There must be no rocking of the component in any plane before cement placement, and there must be perfect congruency between the face of the glenoid and the back of the glenoid component. Cement technique must be equally meticulous, with the cement placed in a very dry glenoid neck. The advantages of glenoid resurfacing, including less pain, less glenohumeral friction, better fulcrum, increased stability, and improved strength, must be weighed against the disadvantages. Glenoid resurfacing clearly increases the probability of component failure, requires increased surgical time and blood loss, and limits the intensity of allowed activities. Analysis of peer-reviewed articles that compare revision rates for total shoulder replacements with those for humeral head replacements indicates that the overall glenoid revision rate is 3.2%, compared with 1.8% for humeral components.

Cemented Versus Cementless Installation

In patients with OA, humeral metaphyseal bone stock is usually quite substantial, and press-fit, cementless installation can result in a stable joint if the humeral components are properly sized. Cement is unnecessary if there is immediate and substantial axial and rotational stability at the time of humeral component placement. However, degenerative cysts may occupy a significant portion of the proximal humeral metaphysis, rendering it incompetent to provide rotational stability. If metaphyseal bone is porotic, soft, or in any way insubstantial, methylmethacrylate should be used for secure component fixation. Although humeral loosening and other problems related to humeral cement are clearly rare, one author reported that 50% of cementless humeral components designed for cemented use shift or subside within 15 years.

Despite the concerns about glenoid lucent lines associated with methylmethacrylate, cemented fixation of the glenoid remains the technique of choice for most surgeons. A few investigators continue to study the application of cementless techniques; however, current US Food and Drug Administration guidelines require the use of methylmethacrylate for glenoid fixation. There is a paucity of peer-reviewed literature on the benefits of cementless glenoid components, and advantages and disadvantages have not yet been adequately defined.

Soft-Tissue Imbalance

The pathophysiology and pathomechanics of OA often result in posterior subluxation of the glenohumeral joint. This physical malalignment over time results in increased capacity and stretching of the posterior capsule. Simultaneously, the presence of osteophytes and loss of external rotation result in contracture and shortening of the subscapularis and anterior capsule. Addressing these concerns is necessary to maximize the benefit of total shoulder arthroplasty. Passive external rotation should be measured after the patient has been anesthetized so that pain will not adversely affect assessment. If external rotation is not 40° to 45°, capsular release and subscapularis lengthening must be considered. These techniques must be anticipated at the beginning of the procedure because they are a consideration when determining the surgical approach to the joint. Functional lengthening of the subscapularis can be achieved by releasing it from the lesser tuberosity and reattaching it at the humeral neck osteotomy (Fig. 3). In a humerus of average size, advancing the subscapularis insertion by 1 to 1.5 cm results in 20° to 30° of increased external rotation.

The volume of the posterior capsular pouch, the degree of posterior soft-tissue stretching, and posterior glenoid

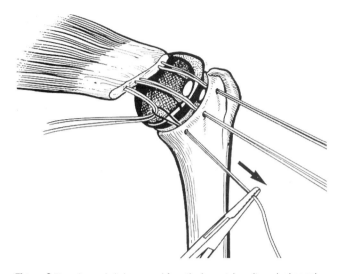

Figure 3 The subscapularis is removed from the lesser tuberosity and advanced medially to the site of the osteotomy. It is sutured to the bone with heavy suture or Dacron tapes to secure the repair.

wear act together to make the shoulder replacement posteriorly unstable. If appropriate compensatory anteversion of a humeral component that is fit with the proper size head results in excessive posterior translation or instability during trial reduction, plication of the posterior capsule becomes appropriate. It is not appropriate to enhance posterior stability by increasing the head size and overstuffing the joint. This latter technique results in severe rotator cuff imbalance and is a source of chronic pain, weakness, and overall dissatisfaction with the new joint.

Complications

Complications related to shoulder arthroplasty should be defined as perioperative (occurring during the hospitalization) or late (occurring anytime after discharge). Intraoperative and perioperative complications nearly always relate to deficiencies of surgical technique. The most common acute complications associated with shoulder arthroplasty include instabilities related to deficient bone or soft tissues, inadequate restoration of proper myofascial tension, incomplete contracture release, and general soft-tissue imbalance about the joint. With aggressive reaming, periprosthetic fractures may occur, and there always is risk of excessive blood loss and nerve injury. Meticulous surgical technique usually will provide protection against blood loss in excess of 300 mL and will make infraclavicular brachial plexus injuries distinctly rare. Proper position of the humeral head in an anatomic location above the greater tuberosity should preclude postoperative impingement. As with any operation, attention to detail should minimize the occurrence of these types of complications. Fortunately, with the judicious use of perioperative parenteral antibiotics, the incidence of primary wound infection should be much less than 1%.

Late complications are more common than those occurring in the perioperative period. Instability continues to occur late, often many years after the original procedure. The forces that resulted in the initial posterior subluxation often remain and over time cause further posterior instability. As the patient's age increases, rotator cuff tears become more likely; these can result in late weakness, pain, and superior instability, particularly if the coracoacromial arch was sacrificed during the original surgery. The same forces that initially caused glenohumeral OA may also be responsible for acromioclavicular joint arthrosis and anterior acromial osteophytes that cause extrinsic impingement.

The issues of late glenoid loosening and lucent lines have already been discussed. Periprosthetic fractures are rare events; this is fortunate because they are particularly difficult to treat. Because the modulus of elasticity of normal bone differs from that of the prosthesis, most fractures occur at the bone-prosthesis junction and are transverse, making them very unstable. Conversion to a long-stem prosthesis may be required. With previously cemented stems, treatment becomes significantly more difficult, and if the fracture cannot be treated adequately using closed techniques, application of plates or cortical allograft fixed with cerclage wires or bands may become the only reasonable options, though this is less than ideal.

Late infection is a concern with any prosthetic device. Hematogenous spread is rare, but when it does occur late, immediate and aggressive surgical treatment may save the joint. The literature relating to the lower extremities indicates that if a gram-positive organism is present, immediate and thorough débridement may be possible. With a gram-negative organism, there is universal agreement within the infectious disease community that retrieval of the components is necessary for adequate treatment. Most often, by the time the shoulder arthroplasty has become infected, the rotator cuff has been digested and is of very poor quality. Resection arthroplasty has provided two patients with such infections with sterile, nondraining wounds at 5 and 6 years, respectively, with remarkably functional limbs and minimal pain.

Results and Outcomes

Because the results of prosthetic joint replacement of the shoulder with symptomatic OA are so superior, there is no contemporary peer-reviewed literature comparing arthrodesis, resection arthroplasty, osteotomy, and synovectomy as treatments for OA. In one report, satisfactory results were reported from arthroscopic synovectomy in very early glenohumeral OA. Reports of satisfactory results from arthroscopic cheilectomy are lacking, and the procedure is not intuitively reasonable, for the reasons stated earlier. Therefore, this review is limited to the

outcomes of shoulder arthroplasty, both total shoulder replacement and humeral head arthroplasty alone.

Shoulder arthroplasty, whether total shoulder replacement or humeral head replacement alone, provides predictable improvement in pain. With appropriate physical therapy after surgery, most patients find dramatic improvement in their function and overall quality of life. Patients in most series report slightly improved pain scores and satisfaction with glenoid resurfacing, but the desire for less pain must be balanced with the ability to safely and securely implant the glenoid component. Results of humeral head replacement alone, although not quite as good in most series, tend to deteriorate at a faster rate than total shoulder replacements even though glenoid lucent lines are present in a significant number of patients. It was found that more than 50% of a well-reviewed group of patients had pain and that 26% had been converted from humeral head replacements to total shoulder replacements within 10 years of their index operation.

Concern for the longevity of glenoid components demands continued vigilance. Although meta-analysis and survivorship studies give reason for optimism, continuing study and search for improved designs and fixation methods are needed. It is difficult to completely evaluate outcomes data by review of the literature because, although there is a plethora of data, no series has evaluated the results of arthroplasty for the treatment of OA. Virtually all series comprise patients with a variety of diagnoses, the most common of which are inflammatory arthritides that are known to have higher failure rates. However, the literature has established the fact that both total shoulder replacement and humeral head replacement offer significant improvement in pain and overall patient satisfaction with minimal deterioration over time.

Annotated Bibliography

Arredondo J, Worland RL: Bipolar shoulder arthroplasty in patients with osteoarthritis: Short term clinical results and evaluation of birotational head motion. *J Shoulder Elbow Surg* 1999;8:425-429.

This is a prospective study of 43 patients with OA who underwent bipolar shoulder arthroplasty. The authors report early promising results with maintenance of birotational head motion for up to 6 years.

Cameron BD, Galatz LM, Ramsey ML, Williams GR, Iannotti JP: Non-prosthetic management of grade IV osteochondral lesions of the glenohumeral joint. *J Shoulder Elbow Surg* 2002;11:25-32.

Arthroscopic débridement, with or without arthroscopic capsular release, was evaluated in 61 patients. Average patient satisfaction score improved from 0.67 preoperatively to 6.28 at final follow-up, with 87% of patients saying they would have the surgery again.

Cofield RH, Becker DA: Shoulder arthroplasty, in Morrey BF, An KN (eds): *Reconstructive Surgery of the Joints*, ed 2. New York, NY, Churchill Livingstone, 1996, p 754

A comprehensive review of shoulder arthroplasty is presented.

Gartsman GM, Russell JA, Gaenslen E: Modular shoulder arthroplasty. *J Shoulder Elbow Surg* 1997;6:333-339.

One hundred consecutive modular shoulder arthroplasties were evaluated prospectively. This is a comprehensive analysis of shoulder arthroplasty comparing total shoulder replacement with humeral head replacement for benefit of pain and improved overall quality of living. There is a thorough discussion of complications and comparison of costs of the procedures.

Karduna AR, Williams GR, Williams JL, Iannotti JP: Glenohumeral joint translations before and after total shoulder arthroplasty: A study in cadavera. *J Bone Joint Surg Am* 1997;79:1166-1174.

This article provides a detailed biomechanical analysis of shoulder motion examined in cadaveric shoulders, both in their natural state and following shoulder arthroplasty. The purpose was to obtain a better understanding of those forces that may contribute to joint failure.

Levine WN, Djurasovic M, Glasson JM, Pollock RG, Flatow EL, Bigliani LU: Hemiarthroplasty for glenohumeral osteoarthritis: Results correlated to degree of glenoid wear. *J Shoulder Elbow Surg* 1997;6:449-454.

A series of 30 patients underwent hemiarthroplasty for primary or secondary OA. A retrospective analysis of outcome was correlated with degree of glenoid wear. The authors noted that whereas hemiarthroplasty is an effective procedure, it should be reserved for those patients with concentric glenoid wear only.

Lynch NM, Cofield RH, Silbert PL, Hermann RC: Neurologic complications after total shoulder arthroplasty. *J Shoulder Elbow Surg* 1996;5:53-61.

This is a detailed analysis of more than 400 shoulder arthroplasties performed during a 14-year period with attention directed to neurologic complications associated with this type of surgery. Risk factors for the development of nerve injuries and long-term follow-up are reviewed.

Rodosky MW, Bigliani LU: Indications for glenoid resurfacing in shoulder arthroplasty. *J Shoulder Elbow Surg* 1996;5:231-248.

These authors present a comprehensive review of the literature and discuss a meta-analysis of glenoid resurfacing. Indications, contraindications, and detailed radiographic data are presented. Current recommendations are given with an analysis of the current understanding of glenoid loosening and the interpretation of glenoid lucent lines.

Stone KD, Grabowski JJ, Cofield RH, Morrey BF, An KN: Stress analyses of glenoid components in total shoulder arthroplasty. *J Shoulder Elbow Surg* 1999;8:151-158.

Finite element analysis was performed to determine and characterize the stresses present at the bone-implant interface in cementless glenoid replacements. Mathematical modeling indicated that under conditions of concentric and eccentric loading, stress transfer to the subchondral bone was less in metal-backed cementless glenoid components.

Torchia ME, Cofield RH, Settergren CR: Total shoulder arthroplasty with the Neer prosthesis: Long-term results. *J Shoulder Elbow Surg* 1997;6:495-505.

This study of 113 total shoulder replacements reviews the long-term survival of total shoulder replacements. The probability of implant survival was 93% after 10 years in this study, although 44% of glenoids had radiolucencies and 49% of cementless humeral stems demonstrated a shift in position. A detailed analysis of complications is included.

Vaesel MT, Olsen BS, Sojbjerg JO, Helmig P, Sneppen O: Humeral head size in shoulder arthroplasty: A kinematic study. *J Shoulder Elbow Surg* 1997;6:549-555.

Glenohumeral kinematics following shoulder arthroplasty was studied in a cadaveric model. Alterations in the normal kinematics were studied by incorporating different head sizes on modular humeral components. The authors conclude that a slightly larger than normal head size is required during arthroplasty to reconstruct the kinematics of the normal glenohumeral joint.

Walch G, Boileau P: Prosthetic adaptability: A new concept for shoulder arthroplasty. *J Shoulder Elbow Surg* 1999;8:443-451.

Detailed anatomic studies of 65 cadaveric humeri provide the design rationale for a shoulder replacement system that respects normal anatomic offset between the anatomic humeral axis and the humeral neck. Eighty-six shoulders were studied following shoulder arthroplasty with this prosthetic system; 95% of patients with OA experienced excellent outcomes at up to 5 years' follow-up.

Weinstein DM, Bacchieri JS, Pollock RG, Flatow EL, Bigliani LU: Arthroscopic débridement of the shoulder for osteoarthritis. *Arthroscopy* 2000;16:471-476.

Early glenohumeral arthritis in 25 patients (19 men and 6 women) with an average age of 46 years was treated using arthroscopic débridement. At an average follow-up of 34 months (range, 12 to 63 months), results were rated as excellent in 8%, good in 72%, and unsatisfactory in 20%.

Classic Bibliography

Brenner BC, Ferlic DC, Clayton ML, Dennis DA: Survivorship of unconstrained total shoulder arthroplasty. *J Bone Joint Surg Am* 1989;71:1289-1296.

Friedman RJ, Hawthorne KB, Genez BM: The use of computerized tomography in the measurement of glenoid version. *J Bone Joint Surg Am* 1992;74:1032-1037.

Hawkins RJ, Angelo RL: Glenohumeral osteoarthrosis: A late complication of the Putti-Platt repair. *J Bone Joint Surg Am* 1990;72:1193-1197.

Johnson LL (ed): The glenohumeral joint, in *Diagnostic and Surgical Arthroscopy of the Shoulder*. St Louis, MO, Mosby-Year Book, 1993, pp 276-364.

Matthews LS, Wolock BS, Martin DF: Arthroscopic management of inflammatory arthritis and synovitis of the shoulder, in McGinty JB, Caspari RB, Jackson RW, Poehling GG (eds): *Operative Arthroscopy*. New York, NY, Raven Press, 1991, pp 573-581.

Neer CS, Morrison DS: Glenoid bone-grafting in total shoulder arthroplasty. *J Bone Joint Surg Am* 1988;70: 1154-1162.

Neer CS II: Replacement arthroplasty for glenohumeral osteoarthritis. *J Bone Joint Surg Am* 1974;56:1-13.

Neer CS II, Watson KC, Stanton FJ: Recent experience in total shoulder replacement. *J Bone Joint Surg Am* 1982;64:319-337.

Richman JD, Rose DJ: The role of arthroscopy in the management of synovial chondromatosis of the shoulder: A case report. *Clin Orthop* 1990;257:91-93.

Chapter 26

Osteonecrosis and Other Noninflammatory Degenerative Diseases of the Glenohumeral Joint

Lloyd Johnson III, MD

Leesa M. Galatz, MD

Osteonecrosis

Osteonecrosis, also known as avascular necrosis and aseptic necrosis, is a condition in which bone death occurs secondary to a compromise in its blood supply. The humeral head is second only to the femoral head in the incidence of osteonecrosis. This chapter will focus on the etiology, evaluation, types of treatment, and results of treatment of both posttraumatic and nontraumatic osteonecrosis. In addition, hemochromatosis and synovial chondromatosis will be reviewed.

Blood Supply of the Proximal Humerus

The anatomy of the blood supply to the humeral head is important in the etiology of osteonecrosis. The humeral head is supplied primarily by the anterolateral ascending branch of the anterior circumflex artery (Fig. 1). The anterior circumflex artery originates from the axillary artery 1 cm distal to the inferior border of the pectoralis major. Traveling between the short head of the biceps and the coracobrachialis, it reaches the inferior border of the subscapularis. The anterolateral branch provides some branches to the lesser tuberosity before crossing under the tendon of the long head of the biceps. It then runs proximally in the lateral aspect of the intertubercular groove, entering the humeral head at a constant position at the proximal end of the transition from the greater tuberosity to the intertubercular groove. The terminal intraosseous portion of this branch has been called the arcuate artery. Through the arcuate artery, almost the entire humeral head is perfused. The posterior circumflex artery provides a blood supply only to the posterior portion of the greater tuberosity and a small posteroinferior portion of the humeral head.

Etiology

Any disruption in the blood supply to the humeral head can result in osteonecrosis. Common causes include trauma, corticosteroid use, alcohol abuse, radiation,

Gaucher's disease, systemic lupus erythematosus, and sickle cell disease, which may be the most common cause worldwide (Fig. 2). Occasionally, no cause can be identified. Ongoing tobacco use is associated with a 4.7-fold increase in the rate of idiopathic osteonecrosis, with former smokers having a 3.3-fold increased risk.

Presentation and Evaluation

Evaluation begins with a review of the patient's symptoms and history. Patients should be asked if they have a history of previous fracture, steroid use, systemic illness, or alcohol abuse. Patients report shoulder pain that is worse with motion. Those with advanced collapse also may feel or even hear a click with shoulder range of motion. Night pain and pain at rest occur but are not as common as with other shoulder disorders. On examination, motion is decreased. Active motion may be limited by pain; passive motion can be limited by capsular contracture later in the disease process. Standard radiographs including an axillary view should be obtained. Bone scans have poor sensitivity for osteonecrosis, with only 29% of lesions producing increased uptake. MRI is a better alternative to assist in the diagnosis of early osteonecrosis. Consideration also should be given to screening radiographs of the hips, because 81% of patients with shoulder pathology will have coexistent hip pathology.

Radiographic Classification of Proximal Humerus Osteonecrosis

A modification by Cruess of the Ficat-Arlet classification of osteonecrosis of the femoral head is the most widely used system. In stage I, radiographs are normal, but the lesions can be detected on MRI or occasionally on bone scan. This is not classified as stage 0 because histopathologic changes are present. In stage II, the humeral head remains spherical, but it is sclerotic and exhibits evidence of bony remodeling. Stage III is marked by subchondral

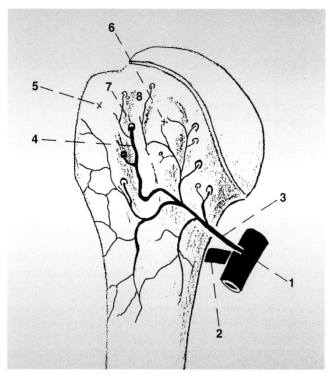

Figure 1 A, Graphic representation of the anterior aspect of the humeral head. 1 = axillary artery, 2 = posterior circumflex artery, 3 = anterior circumflex artery, 4 = anterolateral branch of the anterior circumflex artery, 5 = greater tuberosity, 6 = lesser tuberosity, 7 = constant site of entry of the anterolateral branch into bone, and 8 = intertubercular groove. *(Reproduced with permission from Gerber C, Schneeberger AG, Vinh TS: The arterial vascularization of the humeral head.* J Bone Joint Surg Am *1990;72:1486-1494.)*

collapse, resulting in the classic crescent sign. Although the head is aspherical and the cartilage may be distorted, there is no collapse of cartilage (Fig. 3). In stage IV, the articular surface has collapsed and signs of secondary osteoarthritis are present. Osteoarthritic changes in the glenoid mark the progression to stage V.

Treatment

Treatment of the patient with osteonecrosis should begin with nonsteroidal anti-inflammatory drugs and physical therapy for shoulder range of motion. It is also important to ensure that the patient does not have a coexistent problem such as rotator cuff tendinitis. An intra-articular injection of local anesthetic can be helpful in determining the etiology of the patient's pain. All offending agents such as steroids or alcohol should be stopped if possible; however, for some conditions, steroids may be the only available therapy. It has also been noted that the level of pain increases when patients with osteonecrosis stop taking steroids. One study has suggested that patients whose osteonecrosis has a traumatic etiology may not benefit from nonsurgical treatment as much as other patients.

Once nonsurgical therapy has failed, attention turns to surgical management. Surgical options include core decompression, hemiarthroplasty, and total shoulder arthroplasty. The decision to perform an arthroplasty should be based on patient function in addition to radiographic findings. In one study, the authors reported that at 3 years after diagnosis, 45% of patients with stage IV and 21% of patients with stage V osteonecrosis had adequate functioning and minimal pain so that they had not required an arthroplasty.

Core Decompression

Results of core decompression are mixed, but there is some suggestion that it may be helpful in earlier stages of the disease. One study reported on 63 shoulders with multiple etiologies that were treated for osteonecrosis with core decompression and followed for an average of 10 years. For stage I osteonecrosis, 94% were successful (score of greater than 24 on University of California at Los Angeles shoulder rating system). For stages II, III, and IV, the respective success rates were 88%, 70%, and 14%. Similar results have been found in a study of core decompression in patients with atraumatic osteonecrosis. All patients experienced immediate pain relief in the initial study. The authors recommended core decompression for stages I through III and arthroplasty for stage IV and higher.

The use of core decompression for treatment of patients with stage III osteonecrosis is controversial. Authors of one study reported that core decompression in this group was unsuccessful. However, their group included only five patients with stage III disease versus 23 patients in the study described earlier. One possible advantage of core decompression in a patient with stage III disease is that it may delay the need for a hemiarthroplasty. During core decompression, care must be taken to make the insertion site just lateral to the bicipital groove to avoid injury to the ascending branch of the anterior circumflex artery.

Arthroplasty

Either a hemiarthroplasty or a total shoulder arthroplasty (TSA) is indicated in patients with stage III, IV, or V osteonecrosis in whom nonsurgical management has failed. In patients with stage V disease, a TSA should be performed unless the patient has a relative contraindication such as an irreparable rotator cuff or glenoid destruction that is so severe that it would be impossible to obtain adequate fixation of the component. In stage III and IV disease, either a hemiarthroplasty or a TSA can be performed. In a recent review of 88 shoulders treated with either hemiarthroplasty or TSA, 79.5% had subjective improvement and 77.3% had only occasional or no pain at an average follow-up of 9 years. Inferior results in both American Shoulder and Elbow Surgeons (ASES) shoulder score and motion were noted in patients with traumatic osteonecrosis, whereas superior results were noted in patients with steroid-induced disease. Patients with steroid-induced osteonecrosis had an average of 75% of full forward elevation versus 50% in the trauma group. Complications included postoperative rotator cuff tears in 18%. Only one component required revision, although half had radiographic signs of loosening.

Other Surgical Options

One case report described treatment of symptomatic shoulder osteonecrosis with arthroscopic débridement. The patient had stage III osteonecrosis of one shoulder and stage IV of the other. The patient had loss of motion in addition to mechanical symptoms. Postoperatively, there was mild improvement of motion in addition to pain relief and mechanical symptoms.

Posttraumatic Osteonecrosis

Fracture is the most common cause of posttraumatic osteonecrosis. Either the injury or the surgical exposure can disrupt the blood supply and produce osteonecrosis. The rate of osteonecrosis is slightly higher in fractures treated with open reduction than in those treated with closed management. If during the surgical approach the remaining anastomotic network is intact, the anterior circumflex artery can be ligated medial to the intertubercular groove without producing osteonecrosis. Rates of osteonecrosis in proximal humerus fractures range from 3% to 25% for three-part fractures and are as high as 90% in four-part fractures. Osteonecrosis is suspected in patients with persistent pain after fracture healing. Although osteonecrosis may be demonstrated on plain radiographs, MRI may be needed for definitive diagnosis. Treatment is the same as outlined previously; however, patients with a traumatic etiology have not responded as well to nonsurgical therapy. In addition, their ASES shoulder score is lower, and they have less postoperative range of motion.

Sickle Cell Disease

Sickle cell disease and other hemoglobinopathies are believed to represent the most common causes of osteonecrosis worldwide. Radiographic evidence of humeral head osteonecrosis has been noted in 5.6% to 28% of patients with sickle cell disease. Shoulder function is decreased in 64% of these patients. Bilateral involvement is noted in 44%. When all patients with sickle cell disease are examined, only 53% have normal shoulder function. Many patients with normal radiographs but abnormal examination results are believed to have stage I osteonecrosis.

Evaluation of shoulder pain in a patient with sickle

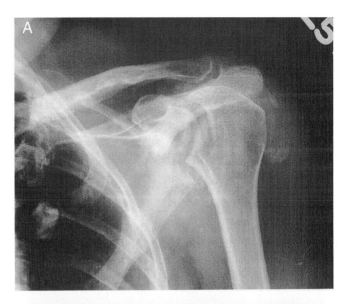

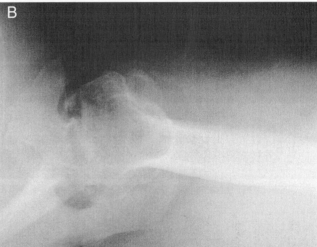

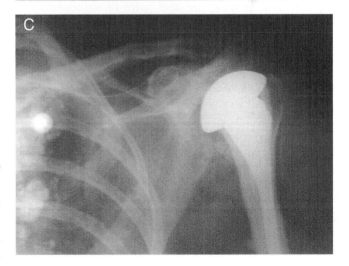

Figure 2 Radiographs of a 66-year-old woman several years after radiation for a left breast carcinoma. Findings at the time of surgery also included a massive irreparable rotator cuff tear. **A,** An AP radiograph of the left shoulder demonstrates significant bone loss involving the humeral head. **B,** An axillary radiograph also demonstrates severe bone loss. **C,** Although there was glenoid involvement, a hemiarthroplasty was performed because of the absence of a competent rotator cuff.

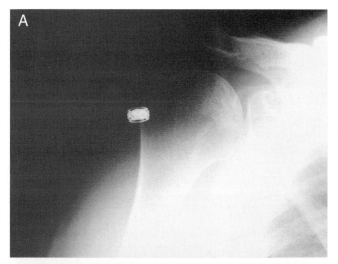

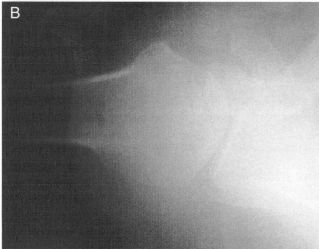

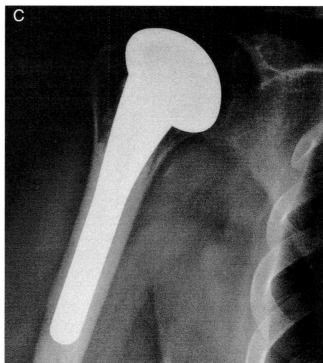

Figure 3 Radiographs of a 59-year-old woman with lupus erythematosus and steroid-induced osteonecrosis of the humeral head. **A,** AP radiograph of the shoulder demonstrates sclerosis and subchondral bone collapse. **B,** Axillary radiograph demonstrates subchondral bone collapse and flattening of the humeral head. **C,** Postoperative radiograph after hemiarthroplasty.

cell disease can produce a long list of differential diagnoses. In addition to the high rates of osteonecrosis, these patients have increased rates of bone infarctions, which can secondarily become infected resulting in osteomyelitis, and septic joints. Work-up should begin with plain radiographs. If these are normal, MRI should be considered to identify potential stage I osteonecrosis.

Treatment of patients with osteonecrosis and sickle cell disease is expected to become more common in orthopaedic practice as the life expectancy of these patients continues to increase. Mean life expectancy for patients with sickle cell disease has increased from 14 years in 1973 to 45 years in 1993. Treatment should proceed as with other patients who have osteonecrosis; however, the possibility of an increased risk of prosthetic loosening should be considered. In addition, some authors suggest periodic screening radiographs of all patients with sickle cell disease. Ultimately, treatment to correct the amino acid substitution may lie in gene therapy. A reversal of the osteonecrotic lesions has been reported in a child who received a bone marrow transplant for sickle cell disease.

Gaucher's Disease

Gaucher's disease (type I) is an autosomal-recessive disorder resulting from deficiency in the enzyme glucocerebroside hydrolase. As a result of this deficiency, sphingolipid accumulates in the macrophages of the reticuloendothelial system. Bone is affected as the sphingolipid-laden cells, known as Gaucher's cells, infiltrate the marrow. This infiltration can lead to osteonecrosis and painful bone infarctions, which can become secondarily infected. Osteonecrosis occurs most commonly in the hip and secondarily in the humeral head. In a study of enzyme replacement therapy, screening radiographs of 51 patients with type I Gaucher's disease showed that eight had proximal humerus osteonecrosis. One of the treatments of Gaucher's disease has been splenectomy. Historically, patients treated with splenectomy have shown a reversal of their systemic symptoms but a progression of their bone ailments. This study also demonstrated that patients who had undergone splenectomy had a tenfold greater risk for osteonecrosis of one of the major joints.

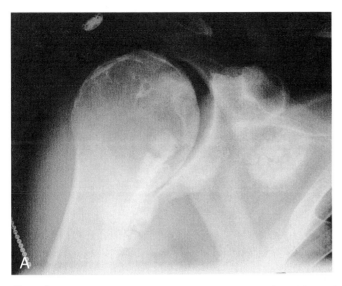 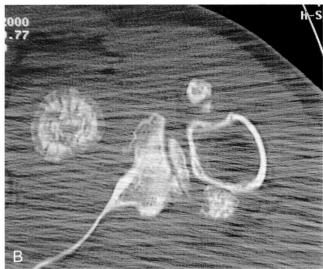

Figure 4 Imaging studies of a 49-year-old man in the late stages of synovial osteochondromatosis with secondary shoulder arthritis. **A,** An AP radiograph demonstrates several free bodies including several tracking down the biceps tendon sheath. In addition, there are significant degenerative changes involving the glenohumeral joint. **B,** A CT scan demonstrates multiple free bodies and secondary degenerative changes.

Treatment of advanced osteonecrosis secondary to Gaucher's disease in the humeral head includes arthroplasty. There is evidence, however, of increased risk of component loosening in these patients. Histologic analysis of the membrane from a loose cementless bipolar hip component showed that the tissue was packed with Gaucher's cells. Recent therapy with alglucerase, which is a replacement enzyme, has been shown to reverse some of the systemic effects of Gaucher's disease in the hematopoietic system, liver, and spleen. A case report of a patient receiving alglucerase also has shown a return to normal appearance in radiographs and MRI scans. Although it has not yet been studied, medical management with enzyme replacement appears to improve arthroplasty results by decreasing prosthetic loosening.

Hemochromatosis

Hemochromatosis is an autosomal-recessive disorder in which a general body overload of iron stores results in tissue damage. The classic patient with hemochromatosis is a Caucasian male with bronze diabetes and associated heart and liver damage. The incidence of this disease is 1 in 200 in Caucasians, and it occurs 10 times more frequently in men. Women are relatively protected by the iron loss during menstruation, lactation, and pregnancy. Hemochromatosis has been associated with an increased risk of arthropathy. Approximately 64% of patients with hemochromatosis have arthropathy, with the hands and the wrists most commonly involved. Hip and shoulder involvement is also common. On radiographs, there is a high incidence of chondrocalcinosis in addition to the usual findings in osteoarthritis. MRI is

unable to demonstrate the intra-articular iron stores. Treatment of the underlying condition has involved phlebotomy to diminish the total body stores of iron. Although this procedure has stabilized the progression of the diabetes and cardiac manifestations, it has not stopped the progression of arthropathy.

Pathologic examination of proximal femur specimens has shown findings consistent with osteoarthritis in most; however, in 42% there was a split in the cartilage at the tidemark, which is the boundary between the uncalcified and calcified cartilage. This is the area of greatest stress concentration. It has been proposed that there is an abnormal cartilage matrix secondary to the iron causing chondrocyte toxicity. This abnormal matrix increases the stiffness of the cartilage, leading to calcification and fragmentation in the region of greatest stress, the tidemark. There also is an increased incidence of pathologically demonstrated osteonecrosis in patients with hemochromatosis compared to patients with osteoarthritis (26% versus 19%). Patients with hemochromatosis also are at increased risk for infections with *Yersinia enterocolitica*, which has been demonstrated to have caused an infection of a total hip prosthesis in one of these patients. Treatment of the patient with shoulder arthropathy secondary to hemochromatosis is the same as that for other causes of shoulder arthropathy.

Synovial Osteochondromatosis

Synovial osteochondromatosis is a rare, benign condition in which the synovium undergoes osteocartilaginous metaplasia. This condition is generally monoarticular. The knee is the most commonly affected joint, followed by the hip, elbow, and shoulder. Patients present with a feeling of crepitation in the shoulder, which later leads to pain and loss of motion. The calcification of the synovium eventually produces loose bodies, which can be demonstrated on plain films. CT can be helpful in differentiating between other causes of loose bodies in the shoulder because it demonstrates the calcification of the synovium. In addition to the loose bodies, these patients can have multiple secondary rotator cuff tears and subsequent shoulder arthritis (Fig. 4). This entity has been classified into three phases. In the early stage, all disease is intrasynovial. In the transitional stage, loose bodies develop. In the late stage, there are only multiple loose bodies with no intrasynovial disease. Treatment includes synovectomy and removal of loose bodies. Rotator cuff tears should be repaired. Osteoarthritis can be treated with arthroplasty. Rare transformation to chondrosarcoma has been reported.

Annotated Bibliography

Osteonecrosis

Basamania CJ, Jaramillo JC, Wirth MA, Rockwood CA Jr: Abstract: Treatment of posttraumatic versus atraumatic avascular necrosis of the shoulder. *64th Annual Meeting Proceedings.* Rosemont, IL, American Academy of Orthopaedic Surgeons, 1997, p 51.

The authors report that nonsurgical treatment of patients with osteonecrosis with a traumatic etiology was not as successful as in patients with osteonecrosis with a different etiology.

Cushner MA, Friedman RJ: Osteonecrosis of the humeral head. *J Am Acad Orthop Surg* 1997;5:339-346.

This review article contains an excellent discussion of the stages of osteonecrosis of the humeral head.

Hattrup SJ, Cofield RH: Osteonecrosis of the humeral head: Relationship of disease stage, extent, and cause to natural history. *J Shoulder Elbow Surg* 1999;8:559-564.

Associated factors such as corticosteroid use, trauma, Gaucher's disease, sickle cell disease, and radiation necrosis, in addition to the need for prosthetic replacement surgery, status of the shoulder that had not been operated on, and prognostic factors were evaluated in 150 patients (200 shoulders) with osteonecrosis of the humeral head.

Sickle Cell Disease

Hernigou P, Bernaudin F, Reinert P, Kuentz M, Vernant JP: Bone-marrow transplantation in sickle-cell disease: Effect on osteonecrosis: A case report with a four-year follow-up. *J Bone Joint Surg Am* 1997;79:1726-1730.

This is the case report of a 13-year-old patient with humeral head osteonecrosis and sickle cell disease with frequent and severe crises. Ultimately, the patient required bone marrow transplantation. After transplantation, shoulder radiographs and MRI were normal.

Gaucher's Disease

Rodrigue SW, Rosenthal DI, Barton NW, Zurakowski D, Mankin HJ: Risk factors for osteonecrosis in patients with type 1 Gaucher's disease. *Clin Orthop* 1999;362:201-207.

This is a retrospective review of 51 patients with Gaucher's disease. Fifteen of the 51 had at least one site of osteonecrosis; eight had involvement of the humeral head. This study also showed that patients who had undergone a splenectomy as treatment of Gaucher's disease had a tenfold increased rate of osteonecrosis.

Hemochromatosis

Montgomery KD, Williams JR, Sculco TP, DiCarlo E: Clinical and pathologic findings in hemochromatosis hip arthropathy. *Clin Orthop* 1998;347:179-187.

This is a review of 19 total hip arthroplasties in 15 patients with hemochromatosis. At 10-year follow-up, a revision secondary to acetabular loosening was required in one hip. In this study, the prevalent split in the cartilage at the tidemark was noted.

Synovial Osteochondromatosis

Hardy P, Decrette E, Jeanrot C, Colom A, Lortat-Jacob A, Benoit J: Arthroscopic treatment of bilateral humeral head osteonecrosis. *Arthroscopy* 2000;16:332-335.

This is a case report that describes postoperative improvement in pain and function following arthroscopy for stage III and IV osteonecrosis. Follow-up occurred from 5 months to 2 years following surgery.

Hattrup SJ, Cofield RH, Osteonecrosis of the humeral head: Relationship of disease stage, extent, and cause to natural history. *J Shoulder Elbow Surg* 1999;8:559-564.

In this review of 200 patients with humeral head osteonecrosis, 97 shoulders required arthroplasty. However, the study showed that some patients with severe disease may have good functioning without surgical intervention.

Hattrup SJ, Cofield RH: Osteonecrosis of the humeral head: Results of replacement. *J Shoulder Elbow Surg* 2000;9:177-182.

In this review of 127 shoulders in 114 patients treated with arthroplasty for humeral head osteonecrosis, 79.5% had postoperative improvement and 77.3% had no pain or only occasional pain. Patients with a traumatic etiology had inferior results whereas those with steroid-related disease had superior results. Radiographic loosening was common but rarely required revision.

Ko JY, Wang JW, Chen WJ, Yamamoto R: Synovial chondromatosis of the subacromial bursa with rotator cuff tearing. *J Shoulder Elbow Surg* 1995;4:312-316.

The authors reported on a patient with multiple rotator cuff tears associated with synovial chondromatosis who underwent a partial synovectomy, rotator cuff repair, removal of loose bodies, and subacromial decompression. At 2-year follow-up, the patient had full range of motion with no pain or radiographic evidence of recurrence.

LaPorte DM, Mont MA, Mohan V, Pierre-Jacques H, Jones LC, Hungerford DS: Osteonecrosis of the humeral head treated by core decompression. *Clin Orthop* 1998;355:254-260.

In this report of 63 shoulders in 43 patients in whom nonsurgical therapy had failed and core decompression for proximal humerus osteonecrosis was necessary, the authors stressed the importance of avoiding injury to the ascending branch of the anterior circumflex artery. Success rates for stages I, II, III, and IV osteonecrosis were 94%, 88%, 70%, and 14%, respectively. The authors recommended core decompression for stages I through III osteonecrosis.

L'Insalata JC, Pagnani MJ, Warren RF, Dines DM: Humeral head osteonecrosis: Clinical course and radiographic predictors of outcome. *J Shoulder Elbow Surg* 1996;5:355-361.

In this review of 65 shoulders in 42 patients with osteonecrosis of the humeral head, 35 shoulders required surgery. Five underwent core decompression for stage III disease, and all had progression of disease. The authors recommend that core decompression should not be performed for stage III osteonecrosis.

Mont MA, Maar DC, Urquhart MW, Lennox D, Hungerford DS: Avascular necrosis of the humeral head treated by core decompression: A retrospective review. *J Bone Joint Surg Br* 1993;75:785-788.

This is a review of 30 shoulders that had undergone core decompression. All stage I and II shoulders had a good result. Seven of 10 stage III shoulders had a good result even if the disease had advanced radiographically. The authors recommended core decompression for stages I through III osteonecrosis.

Mont MA, Payman RK, LaPorte DM, Petri M, Jones LC, Hungerford DS: Atraumatic osteonecrosis of the humeral head. *J Rheumatol* 2000;27:1766-1773.

This is a report of 127 shoulders with atraumatic osteonecrosis. Results were good for core decompression in stages I through III. Arthroplasty should be used for stage IV. The authors report that bone scans are not a good screening test and that there is a high incidence of coexistent femoral head disease.

Classic Bibliography

Barton NW, Brady RO, Dambrosia JM, et al: Dose-dependent responses to macrophage-targeted glucocerebrosidase in a child with Gaucher's disease. *J Pediatr* 1992;120:277-280.

Chung SM, Ralston EL: Necrosis of the humeral head associated with sickle cell anemia and its genetic variants. *Clin Orthop* 1971;80:105-117.

Cruess RL: Experience with steroid-induced avascular necrosis of the shoulder and etiologic considerations regarding osteonecrosis of the hip. *Clin Orthop* 1978; 130:86-93.

Cruess RL: Steroid-induced avascular necrosis of the head of the humerus: Natural history and management. *J Bone Joint Surg Br* 1976;58:313-317.

David HG, Bridgman SA, Davies SC, Hine AL, Emery RJ: The shoulder in sickle-cell disease. *J Bone Joint Surg Br* 1993;75:538-545.

Eustace S, Buff B, McCarthy C, MacMathuana P, Gilligan P, Ennis JT: Magnetic resonance imaging of hemochromatosis arthropathy. *Skeletal Radiol* 1994; 23:547-549.

Faraawi R, Harth M, Kertesz A, Bell D: Arthritis in hemochromatosis. *J Rheumatol* 1993;20:448-452.

Finch SC, Finch CA: Idiopathic hemochromatosis: An iron storage disease: Iron metabolism in hemochromatosis. *Medicine* 1955;34:381-430.

Gerber C, Schneeberger AG, Vinh TS: The arterial vascularization of the humeral head: An anatomical study. *J Bone Joint Surg Am* 1990;72:1486-1494.

Hirota Y, Hirohata T, Fukuda K, et al: Association of alcohol intake, cigarette smoking, and occupational status with the risk of idiopathic osteonecrosis of the femoral head. *Am J Epidemiol* 1993;137:530-538.

Laing PG: The arterial supply of the adult humerus. *J Bone Joint Surg Am* 1956;38:1105-1116.

Milgram JW: Synovial osteochondromatosis: A histopathological study of thirty cases. *J Bone Joint Surg Am* 1977;59:792-801.

Milner PF, Kraus AP, Sebes JI, et al: Osteonecrosis of the humeral head in sickle cell disease. *Clin Orthop* 1993;289:136-143.

Murphy FP, Dahlin DC, Sullivan CR: Articular synovial chondromatosis. *J Bone Joint Surg Am* 1962;44:77-86.

Nissim, JA: The role of protein in iron metabolism: A clue to primary haemochromatosis. *Guys Hosp Rep* 1966;115:183-209.

Perry BE, McQueen DA, Lin JJ: Synovial chondromatosis with malignant degeneration to chondrosarcoma: Report of a case. *J Bone Joint Surg Am* 1988; 70:1259-1261.

Platt OS, Brambilla DJ, Rosse WF, et al: Mortality in sickle cell disease: Life expectancy and risk factors for early death. *N Engl J Med* 1994;330:1639-1644.

Porcellini G, Campi F, Brunetti E: Osteoarthritis caused by synovial chondromatosis of the shoulder. *J Shoulder Elbow Surg* 1994;3:404-406.

Schlegel TF, Hawkins RJ: Displaced proximal humeral fractures: Evaluation and treatment. *J Am Acad Orthop Surg* 1994;2:54-78.

Sennara H, Gorry F: Orthopedic aspects of sickle cell anemia and allied hemoglobinopathies. *Clin Orthop* 1978;130:154-157.

Tauber C, Tauber T: Gaucher disease: The orthopaedic aspect: Report of seven cases. *Arch Orthop Trauma Surg* 1995;114:179-182.

van Wellen PA, Haentjens P, Frecourt N, Opdecam P: Loosening of a noncemented porous-coated anatomic femoral component in Gaucher's disease: A case report and review of literature. *Acta Orthop Belg* 1994;60: 119-123.

Chapter 27

Proximal Humeral Malunions, Posttraumatic Arthritis, and Postcapsulorrhaphy Arthritis

Joseph P. Iannotti, MD, PhD

Brian T. McDermott, MD

Proximal Humeral Malunions and Posttraumatic Arthritis

Fractures of the proximal humerus are common and can be expected to be more prevalent as life expectancy and associated osteoporosis increase. Most of these fractures are treated nonsurgically with good outcomes. Unfortunately, in an occasional patient the treatment, either surgical or nonsurgical, results in malunion or posttraumatic arthritis. These patients usually have severe pain with loss of motion and function of the shoulder.

Treatment of proximal humeral malunion or posttraumatic arthritis is made difficult by disruption of normal anatomic relationships, joint incongruity, soft-tissue scarring, rotator cuff defects, postsurgical changes, and/or neurologic impairment. For the patient with symptoms, nonsurgical treatment options to reduce pain and improve function do not exist; therefore, surgical reconstruction often is necessary.

A thorough preoperative evaluation of the patient should be completed to determine the causative factors for the malunion. Determination of the causative factors will help direct surgical treatment.

Etiology

Malunion results from either inadequate reduction of the displaced fragments or loss of fixation following closed reduction, closed reduction and percutaneous pinning, or open reduction and internal fixation (ORIF). Although malunions sometimes occur following ORIF, they occur more commonly after closed treatment. The higher incidence of malunion with closed treatment may be secondary to the acceptance of a displaced fracture and unsatisfactory fracture configuration. Nonsurgical treatment of a displaced proximal humeral fracture may be a selected option in patients who are poor candidates for surgery or are severely injured. The malunion seen after internal fixation usually is secondary to inadequate fragment fixation obtained in the cancellous bone of the proximal humerus.

Other causes of proximal humeral malunions include inadequate immobilization, inadequate length of immobilization, or soft-tissue interposition at the fracture site. Excessively aggressive rehabilitation can result in loss of fracture fragment position or fixation.

Posttraumatic arthritis has many causes, the most common of which are osteonecrosis of the humeral head or a proximal humeral malunion with intra-articular incongruity greater than 2 mm. Osteonecrosis is more prevalent after displaced three- and four-part fractures. Less common causes of posttraumatic arthritis include chronic unreduced dislocations, recurrent dislocations, and other malunions or nonunions of the proximal humerus or glenoid.

Evaluation

The evaluation of all patients with proximal humeral malunion or posttraumatic arthritis begins with a thorough and detailed history. Patients typically have pain, stiffness, and loss of function. It is useful to determine the patient's primary symptoms and functional limitations. This information helps define the goals of surgical treatment and provides the basis on which to judge the outcome of treatment. A summary of the previous treatments should include the type and duration of immobilization. If surgical treatment was performed, the surgical notes should describe the initial fracture pattern, type of hardware used (if any), soft-tissue repairs, and complications (intraoperative).

The physical examination should determine scapular and proximal humeral deformities, muscular atrophy, and previous surgical scars. Passive range of motion (ROM) should be assessed, with special attention given to abduction, forward flexion, and external rotation, with the arm by the side. A decrease in passive ROM may represent capsular contracture, soft-tissue or bony impingement, resistance secondary to pain, or a combination of these factors. The influence of pain on loss of motion may not be understood fully until an examination under anesthesia is performed.

Evaluation of the integrity of the rotator cuff is essential. Soft-tissue injuries, including rotator cuff tears, are not uncommon after a proximal humeral fracture. Strength testing of the cuff musculature should be performed. Resistance to external rotation and the external rotation lag sign are used to assess strength of the posterior cuff, and the lift-off test and abdominal compression test are used to assess subscapularis strength. Weakness revealed by strength testing does not necessarily indicate a tear. The weakness may be secondary to displacement or malunion of the tuberosities, resulting in a decrease in mechanical advantage and strength. Severe loss of passive rotational motion also results in inaccurate measurement of rotator cuff strength. An MRI study may be helpful but is less reliable when distorted anatomy is present. Therefore, the integrity of the cuff cannot be ascertained fully until the cuff is visually inspected intraoperatively.

A careful and detailed neurologic examination must be performed. Neurologic injury is very common in proximal humeral fractures, especially in the elderly, with up to 50% having an electromyogram-diagnosed injury. Neurologic injuries are more common with fracture-dislocations. The brachial plexus should be examined meticulously, with special attention given to axillary, suprascapular, and musculocutaneous nerves. Sensation over the lateral border of the deltoid is not a reliable indication of axillary nerve injury; therefore, a motor examination should be performed as well. Patients who have undergone previous surgeries may experience symptoms of intraoperative nerve injury.

Imaging studies can be critical to understanding the pathology present. Good-quality, plain radiographs of the involved shoulder, including at least an AP view in the plane of the scapula and an axillary view, are required for all patients. Supplemental rotation films can be completed as needed on an individual basis. Three-dimensional studies can be helpful to evaluate the extent of soft-tissue and bony injuries. CT scanning and three-dimensional reconstruction are particularly useful in assessing bony detail. In addition to evaluating articular surface incongruity, CT scanning can help identify the special relationship between the greater and lesser tuberosities, humeral head, and shaft. Studies have shown that CT more clearly identifies bony malposition than do plain radiographs. MRI is good for evaluation of soft-tissue injuries. Rotator cuff tears, labral tears, muscular atrophy, and early osteonecrosis of the humeral head are particularly well visualized. Scanograms can help identify the proper length of the humerus. Knowing the proper length of the humerus is helpful during reconstruction with prosthetic arthroplasty to determine soft-tissue balancing.

Preoperative assessment should determine if there is articular incongruity as a result of posttraumatic arthri-

tis, osteonecrosis with head collapse, or humeral head split fractures. If this is found to be the case, then hemiarthroplasty is indicated. Isolated tuberosity or surgical neck malunion without joint incongruity is treated by osteotomy and internal fixation. Combined tuberosity and neck malunions often will require hemiarthroplasty if both tuberosities and the surgical neck require osteotomy.

Types of Malunions

Greater Tuberosity Malunions
Two-part greater tuberosity malunions primarily involve two patterns: the greater tuberosity can be displaced superiorly or posteriorly, depending on the dominant deforming force supplied by the tendinous insertions of the rotator cuff. In some cases, the fragment is displaced both superiorly and posteriorly. If the supraspinatus is the dominant deforming force, the fragment will be pulled superiorly. This situation is visualized easily on an AP view of the shoulder. The superiorly displaced fragment will lead to loss of abduction and forward flexion by impingement against the acromion. This secondary impingement can occur with as little as 5 mm of superior displacement. If the displacement is large, it probably indicates a coexistent rotator cuff tear. The rotator cuff tear may be caused by the secondary impingement or result from the initial traumatic event. If the displacement is greater than 1 cm, it may lead to a symptomatic nonunion.

When the posterior elements of the rotator cuff are the major deforming force, the tuberosity will be pulled posteriorly. Posterior displacement may be difficult to view on an AP radiograph alone; therefore, an axillary view or CT scan is beneficial. With a posteriorly displaced greater tuberosity, the fragment will impinge against the glenoid during attempted external rotation, resulting in loss of motion. In addition to the loss of ROM, the muscles of the rotator cuff lose their mechanical advantage as their point of insertion is moved proximally, and the patient can experience weakness in elevation and external rotation.

Lesser Tuberosity Malunions
An isolated lesser tuberosity fracture is rare. It is difficult to diagnose on an AP view alone, and an axillary view or CT scan is helpful. The deforming force is from the subscapularis, resulting in the fragment being pulled anteromedially. This displacement usually leads to loss of internal rotation and subcoracoid impingement secondary to the fragment's medial malposition over the articular surface. Stiffness is very common following this fracture. Another possibility is an avulsion fracture of the lesser tuberosity. Lesser tuberosity avulsion frac-

tures usually result in negligible loss of overhead function but also result in clinically significant weakness of internal rotation and subscapularis function.

Surgical Neck Malunions

Most often, malunions of surgical neck fractures are seen with anterior angulation and a varus deformity. A significant amount of varus deformity (30°) can be tolerated without much functional loss as long as the joint is supple. For every degree of varus angulation, there usually is an equal loss of elevation. The deforming forces in this injury are the pull of the pectoralis major and rotator cuff. The pectoralis pulls the shaft anteriorly while the rotator cuff abducts the humeral head. With this deformity, the greater tuberosity is rotated with the articular surface, leading to abutment of the greater tuberosity against the glenoid with attempted forward flexion or abduction. In most cases, varus malunion of a surgical neck fracture results in maintenance of normal rotational motion with the arm by the side.

Three- and Four-Part Malunions

Three- and four-part malunions are complex problems, which can result in severe deformities and significant complications. In three-part malunions, either the greater or lesser tuberosity is displaced along with the surgical neck. If the greater tuberosity is left intact, the head will be externally rotated and abducted secondary to the intact superior and posterior portion of the rotator cuff. The shaft will be pulled anteromedially by the pectoralis, and the lesser tuberosity will retract medially. Fractures in which the greater tuberosity is displaced will result in the articular surface being internally rotated by the pull of the subscapularis. The greater tuberosity is posterosuperiorly displaced by the intact cuff, and the humeral shaft again is retracted anteromedially. Malunions of this magnitude often lead to severe loss of function and motion along with pain. They also are associated with an increased incidence of posttraumatic degenerative arthritis and osteonecrosis of the humeral head.

Four-part malunions are challenging to treat. In these malunions, both tuberosities and the surgical neck are displaced. These malunions are associated with significant soft-tissue injures and adhesions, joint incongruity, and an increased chance of osteonecrosis. Frequently, the head is quite distorted and the displacement of the tuberosities is large. Patients with four-part malunions typically have severe pain and disability secondary to restricted ROM, osteonecrosis, soft-tissue injuries, and contractures.

Malunions of Fracture-Dislocations

Malunions of fracture-dislocations are another complex problem. The humeral head is dislocated from the glenoid fossa and often is in a subcoracoid position or along the posterior glenoid. The humeral head is wedged against the glenoid and often is scarred into this position. If the head is located anteriorly, it may be scarred to the neurovascular structures. Osteonecrosis of the humeral head is expected in these injuries.

Treatment

Prior to the institution of treatment, an overall assessment of the patient should be performed. Nonsurgical treatment may be appropriate for those who have mild disability or low functional demands, are a poor surgical risk, or are unable (or unwilling) to cooperate with a postoperative rehabilitation program. Conversely, patients who are young, have severe pain and disability, or are unable to function with limited use of one upper extremity should be considered for surgical treatment.

Nonsurgical Treatment

Nonsurgical treatment includes a limited array of options, but the mainstay is physical therapy. The goal of physical therapy is to strengthen the shoulder musculature and help maintain or improve ROM. By increasing the strength of the shoulder, it is hoped that the patient will gain ROM and increase functionality of the arm. In conjunction with physical therapy, nonsteroidal anti-inflammatory drugs (NSAIDs), rest or avoidance of provocative activities, ice, or intra-articular steroid injections may help control pain. Pain management specialists can be of great value in controlling chronic pain.

Surgical Treatment

Surgical treatment for malunion and posttraumatic arthritis is challenging. The goals of a painless stable joint with functional ROM and strength are difficult to achieve. Multiple studies have shown that surgical treatment of an acute fracture is less technically demanding and has better results than surgical treatment of a malunion or posttraumatic arthritis. The authors of one study compared acute and chronic arthroplasties in the treatment of three- and four-part proximal humeral fractures. They found the results of the acute group were far superior to those of the chronic group. Only 14% (2 of 14) of the chronic group were found to have good results. Surgical treatment can be separated into three types of surgery: humeral head–conserving treatment, humeral head–replacing treatment, and glenohumeral arthrodesis.

Humeral head–conserving treatment is most appropriate for malunions that have an intact articular surface and humeral head blood supply. This situation is seen most often in two-part and some three-part proximal humeral malunions. Treatment consists of osteotomies with internal fixation, soft-tissue reconstruction, and lysis

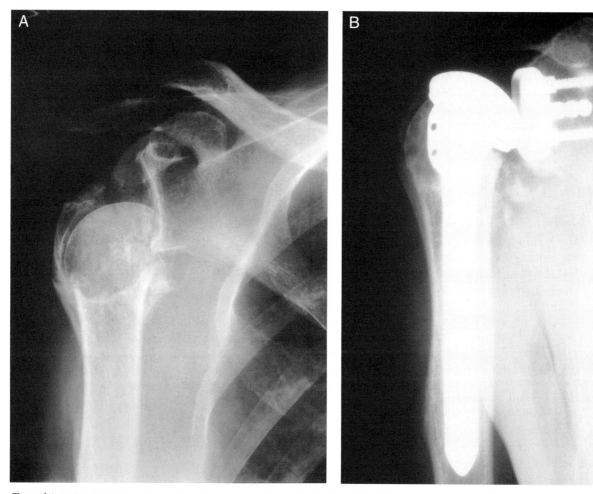

Figure 1 A, A valgus impact four-part malunion with secondary posttraumatic arthritis requiring total shoulder arthroplasty. In this patient the tuberosities did not require osteotomy because they healed in a satisfactory position in relation to the humeral shaft. **B,** Head height was corrected by placing the humeral prosthesis above the height of the greater tuberosity.

of adhesions. In the case of a greater tuberosity malunion with minimal superior displacement (5 mm) and symptoms related predominantly to impingement, subacromial decompression with exostectomy and lysis of adhesions may be sufficient. Most tuberosity malunions are treated with osteotomy and interfragmentary suture, but if the fragment is large enough and has good bone quality, interfragmentary screw fixation can be achieved. After osteotomy, surgical neck malunions are usually fixed with a blade plate. Some authors have had good results treating surgical neck malunions and loss of motion with an open release of adhesions and soft-tissue contractures and trimming of any bony prominences. After ORIF for treatment of malunion, active ROM should be avoided until clinical healing has occurred.

Humeral head–replacing treatment is used when there is evidence of humeral head osteonecrosis and/or significant articular surface incongruity secondary to head-split fracture or posttraumatic arthritis. This is seen most often with three-part, four-part, and fracture-dislocation malunions. In most cases of four-part malunion, both

tuberosities will require osteotomy to allow placement of the humeral head prosthesis in the correct height and version. In some cases, the tuberosities are healed in a satisfactory position in relation to the humeral shaft and do not require osteotomy (Fig. 1). If the head is not centered and humeral length is not maintained, function will be impaired. A review of 23 patients who underwent late reconstruction with prosthetic arthroplasty for proximal humeral malunion showed 95% relief from pain but a lower return of functionality than has been reported for acute fracture reconstruction. The authors of another study reported satisfactory results in 68% of a similar patient population. They defined a satisfactory result as slight or no pain, at least 90° of active forward elevation, and functional use of the arm that is at least 50% that of the normal side. Many other authors have confirmed these results of good pain relief but inferior functional return as compared with acute humeral head replacement. This loss of functionality is probably the result of adhesions and retraction of the tuberosities and soft tissues. The decision whether to use hemiarthroplasty or

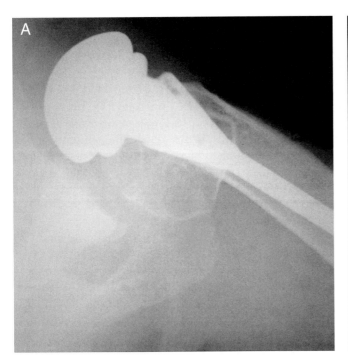

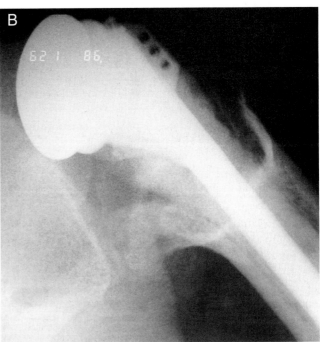

Figure 2 A and **B,** Axillary views of two different patients, demonstrating anterior dislocation of the humeral prosthesis because of a posteriorly displaced greater tuberosity malunion that was not osteotomized.

total shoulder arthroplasty is based on the function of the rotator cuff and glenoid surface. When the glenoid surface shows signs of arthritis and the cuff is intact, a glenoid-resurfacing replacement is used. In the presence of a nonfunctional rotator cuff, a hemiarthroplasty is performed without glenoid resurfacing.

Postoperative rehabilitation after hemiarthroplasty and tuberosity reconstruction must allow for tuberosity healing. Displacement or nonunion of the tuberosities often results in a poor outcome (weakness, pain, dislocation). Limited goals rehabilitation using a postoperative brace during the first several weeks after surgery should be initiated. The brace should be removed only for hygiene, dressing, and daily therapy, which consists of pendulum exercises and supine active-assisted ROM in forward flexion. Active ROM and rotational exercises are delayed until the tuberosities are healed (6 to 8 weeks).

Arthrodesis of the glenohumeral joint is used less frequently since the advances in prosthetic arthroplasty. Malunions or posttraumatic arthritis in the presence of deltoid denervation and rotator cuff deficiency or with superimposed infections may be treated with arthrodesis. Arthrodesis offers better function than resection arthroplasty.

Complications

Many complications are associated with the treatment of proximal humeral malunions and posttraumatic arthritis. Intraoperative complications include infection, nerve in-

jury, and disruption of the remaining blood supply to the humeral head, resulting in osteonecrosis. Dissection is difficult in the presence of scar tissue and malunion, and it is important to know the position of the surrounding neurovascular structures. In no case is this knowledge more critical than in the anterior fracture-dislocation with adhesion to the neurovascular bundle. Deep infection following surgical treatment in the shoulder is rare because of high vascularity and protective musculature. If infection does occur, aggressive irrigation, débridement, hardware removal, and parenteral antibiotics are indicated.

Postoperative complications including stiffness (most common), instability, nonunion or malunion following osteotomies, failed hardware, and myositis ossificans also can result in disability. Myositis ossificans is seen most commonly after surgical reconstruction of fracture-dislocations. Hardware failure can result from inadequate fixation, poor purchase in osteoporotic bone, and early postoperative motion. As the hardware displaces, it may cause impingement or become loose, causing articular cartilage or nerve damage. Dislocation or subluxation will occur in many cases of hemiarthroplasty and tuberosity reconstruction for malunions (Fig. 2). The instability occurs if the tuberosities fail to heal to the shaft, if there is asymmetric capsular contracture, persistent tuberosity malunion, or with nonanatomic positioning of the humeral head height or version. In some cases, more than one of these factors may play a role.

Postcapsulorrhaphy Arthritis

Etiology

The incidence of arthritis following some anterior procedures for the treatment of glenohumeral instability has been reported to be up to 80% in surgically treated shoulders. In a 1983 study, the so-called dislocation arthropathy was described. A positive correlation between the severity of the arthritis and the loss of external rotation regardless of the method of treatment was found. Postcapsulorrhaphy arthritis can occur from an error in diagnosis or surgical treatment. For example, if a patient with multidirectional instability is believed to have only anterior instability and has an anterior stabilization procedure that results in asymmetric and excessive tightening of the anterior capsule, the humeral head will likely subluxate posteriorly. This subluxation results in increased pressure and wear of the posterior glenoid and humeral head, resulting in arthritis. The same problem would occur if the posterior capsule were tightened asymmetrically in the face of anterior laxity. The goal of surgical treatment for instability should be to establish a balance of capsular tension on all sides of the joint.

Another cause of postcapsulorrhaphy arthritis is the use of hardware during capsulorrhaphy. Studies have shown that the use of metal, such as screws, staples, or pins, during capsulorrhaphy increases the incidence of glenohumeral arthritis. The hardware may become loose or may be placed improperly, thus damaging the glenohumeral articular surface. The use of newer biodegradable devices may decrease this problem.

Multiple studies have shown that recurrent dislocations, humeral head (Hill-Sachs) or glenoid rim bony defects, and a history of instability have no influence on the incidence of arthritis. One study of patients with primary anterior dislocations showed that 16% of patients with only one documented dislocation had radiologic evidence of arthritis (35% of these were moderate to severe). These cases of arthritis were caused not by surgery but by the dislocation. These findings were no different than findings in patients who had multiple dislocations and no surgery. Positive risk factors for arthritis include a first dislocation at an older age, delayed reduction of a shoulder dislocation, and displaced articular fractures.

Evaluation

Often, patients with postcapsulorrhaphy arthropathy are young; in one report, the average age was 38 years. It is therefore necessary to define the patient's current and anticipated activity levels because this information will influence treatment decisions, including whether to use prosthetic arthroplasty. As motion becomes increasingly restricted, the loss of shoulder function also increases, and activities of daily living become more difficult.

The type of capsulorrhaphy previously performed must be known when planning a second procedure. It is important to know if the capsulorrhaphy was a tightening of the capsule alone (eg, capsular shift), a shortening of the musculotendinous unit (eg, Putti-Platt procedure), or surgery to alter the bony anatomy (eg, Bristow procedure). If only the capsule was involved, a capsular release should be appropriate. In the patient with a shortened musculotendinous unit, a subscapularis lengthening often is needed. For the patient whose bony anatomy has been altered, as by a Bristow procedure, osteotomy of the transferred coracoid along with soft-tissue releases may be required.

Evaluation of the degree of loss of motion is critical to both surgical decision making and prognosis. Severely limited passive external rotation (< 25°) is common in patients with postcapsulorrhaphy arthropathy. Severe loss of external rotation is more often associated with more severe posterior glenoid erosion. In addition, extensive soft-tissue releases, anteroinferior capsulotomy, and subscapularis lengthening often are required with more severe loss of rotation.

Imaging studies are essential in evaluating a patient with postcapsulorrhaphy arthritis. Plain radiography should include at minimum an AP view of the shoulder in the scapular plane and an axillary view. The AP view allows evaluation of the glenohumeral joint space and arthritic changes, whereas the axillary view gives information on the anterior-posterior relationship of the humeral head within the glenoid fossa and the degree of glenoid erosion. Both views are helpful for determining the presence and status of hardware. CT may be beneficial in helping to define humeral head position, glenoid version, or glenoid bone loss.

Treatment

Treatment of patients with substantially restricted motion of the shoulder following anterior capsulorrhaphy is dictated by the severity of the pain, degree of functional impairment, the extent of arthritic changes, and the degree of loss of motion.

Nonsurgical Treatment

Nonsurgical treatment is appropriate for patients with mild pain, mild degenerative changes of the glenohumeral joint, and more than 30° of external rotation or loss of less than 20° to 30° of external rotation compared with the opposite side. There also must be no evidence of hardware-related problems. Nonsurgical treatment includes NSAIDs, physical therapy, or intra-articular steroid injections. Although a substantial increase in ROM is not to be expected, the mild decrease in pain may be sufficient for the patient to be satisfied. The authors of one study reported a 64% success rate (7 of 11 patients) when treating arthritic glenohumeral joints after anterior capsulorrhaphy nonsurgically with NSAIDs and physical therapy. The authors of another study reported similar findings when treating arthritic glenohumeral joints nonsurgically after Bristow procedures, with 50% (5 of 10 patients) reporting fair or better results.

Surgical Treatment

Unfortunately, not all patients with postcapsulorrhaphy arthritis can be successfully treated nonsurgically. The most commonly used surgeries in the face of glenohumeral arthritis following capsulorrhaphy are arthroscopic or open anteroinferior capsular release, prosthetic arthroplasty, and arthrodesis.

Release of the anterior structures alone, capsule and/or subscapularis lengthening, is most commonly done in the presence of mild arthritic changes and significant loss of external rotation compared with the opposite shoulder. In one study, the authors performed a subscapularis release in patients with mild to severe arthritic changes (6 of 10 were severe). All patients had a dramatic decrease in pain with no need for analgesics and increased external rotation of 27° on average at 3.5 years follow-up. In patients with 0° of external rotation or less at 6 months following anterior shoulder capsulorrhaphy, some authors recommend an anterior release to help prevent glenohumeral arthritis.

In patients with moderate to severe arthritic changes, prosthetic arthroplasty is the procedure of choice despite the young age of these patients. If the glenoid articular cartilage is of sufficient quality, a humeral head replacement alone may be considered. Component positioning may be difficult secondary to bone loss or alterations in soft-tissue tensioning. The authors of one study reported a high incidence of posterior glenoid wear in these shoulders. To compensate, the authors place the humeral component in 5° to 10° less retroversion than usual. Their decision to use a glenoid-resurfacing component is based on the glenoid bone stock and shape. Patients with posterior glenoid bone loss and a nonconcentric articulation were treated with glenoid resurfacing. Preservation of deltoid function as well as myofascial balancing is crucial to a well-functioning arthroplasty. Several authors report excellent pain relief and return of a functional range of motion following prosthetic arthroplasties.

Arthrodesis has extremely limited indications in the current age of shoulder surgery. In patients with postcapsulorrhaphy arthritis, it should be restricted to management of a superimposed septic arthritis, painful paralysis about the shoulder, or a patient who chooses to return to strenuous lifting activities.

Annotated Bibliography

Proximal Humeral Malunions and Posttraumatic Arthritis

Beredjiklian PK, Iannotti JP: Treatment of proximal humerus fracture malunion with prosthetic arthroplasty. *Instr Course Lect* 1998;47:135-140.

The authors provide a thorough discussion of proximal humeral malunions and the use of arthroplasty for treatment. A basic classification system is developed that allows proximal humeral malunions to be divided into bony and soft-tissue anomalies.

Beredjiklian PK, Iannotti JP, Norris TR, Williams GR: Operative treatment of malunion of a fracture of the proximal aspect of the humerus. *J Bone Joint Surg Am* 1998;80:1484-1497.

The authors performed a retrospective review of 39 patients managed surgically for a malunion of the proximal humerus. They reported satisfactory results in 27 patients (68%). Treatment of articular incongruity with arthroplasty was successful in 74% of the patients.

Bosch U, Skutek M, Fremerey RW, Tscherne H: Outcomes after primary and secondary hemiarthroplasty in elderly patients with fractures of the proximal humerus. *J Shoulder Elbow Surg* 1998;7:479-484.

The authors compared the results of acute versus chronic arthroplasties for three- and four-part proximal humeral fractures. The authors found significantly better results among the acute reconstructions.

Connor PM, Flatow EL: Complications of internal fixation of proximal humeral fractures. *Instr Course Lect* 1997;46:25-37.

The authors present a detailed description of the complications encountered when ORIF is performed in the patient with a proximal humeral fracture.

Gerber C, Hersche O, Berberat C: The clinical relevance of posttraumatic avascular necrosis of the humeral head. *J Shoulder Elbow Surg* 1998;7:586-590.

The authors retrospectively review 25 patients with posttraumatic osteonecrosis of the humeral head. They discovered that patients did better if the fracture healed in an anatomic or nearly anatomic position. The result in the patient who has anatomic healing of the fracture is similar to that in a patient who has a shoulder arthroplasty performed for a complex humeral fracture.

Muldoon MP, Cofield RH: Complications of humeral head replacement for proximal humeral fractures. *Instr Course Lect* 1997;46:15-24.

The authors present a detailed discussion of the complications that can be seen when performing shoulder arthroplasty in the face of proximal humeral fractures.

Norris TR, Green A, McGuigan FX: Late prosthetic shoulder arthroplasty for displaced proximal humerus fractures. *J Shoulder Elbow Surg* 1995;4:271-280.

This article presents a retrospective review of 23 patients who underwent a shoulder arthroplasty for failed treatment of three- or four-part proximal humeral fractures. Shoulder pain was reduced in 95% of patients. Average active forward elevation increased 24°, and external rotation increased 21°.

Siegel JA, Dines DM: Proximal humerus malunions. *Orthop Clin North Am* 2000;31:35-50.

The authors present a thorough discussion of the subject of proximal humeral malunions. Their discussion includes etiology, evaluation, treatment, and current results.

Wiater JM, Flatow EL: Posttraumatic arthritis. *Orthop Clin North Am* 2000;31:63-76.

The authors present a detailed review of posttraumatic glenohumeral arthritis. They discuss etiology, preoperative evaluation, treatment, complications, and reported results of treatment.

Zyto K, Kronberg M, Brostrom L-A: Shoulder function after displaced fractures of the proximal humerus. *J Shoulder Elbow Surg* 1995;4:331-336.

The authors assessed the functional outcome of three- and four-part proximal humeral fractures with a 3-year follow-up. The functional outcome of the three-part fractures was much better than that of the four-part fractures. The three-part fractures had better ROM, no evidence of osteonecrosis, and less disability.

Postcapsulorrhaphy Arthritis

Bigliani LU, Weinstein DM, Glasgow MT, Pollock RG, Flatow EL: Glenohumeral arthroplasty for arthritis after instability surgery. *J Shoulder Elbow Surg* 1995;4:87-94.

The authors reviewed 17 patients who underwent prosthetic arthroplasty for glenohumeral arthritis after instability surgery. They report 77% satisfactory results and 23% unsatisfactory results. ROM significantly improved. Previous surgery had distorted the anatomy, and special techniques were required to correct soft-tissue contracture and compensate for posterior glenoid bone loss.

Brems JJ: Arthritis of dislocation. *Orthop Clin North Am* 1998;29:453-466.

The author presents a complete discussion of postcapsulorrhaphy arthritis, which he calls arthritis of dislocation. The nonsurgical and surgical factors that can lead to this condition are reviewed and preoperative workup and surgical and rehabilitation approaches are discussed.

Hovelius L, Augustini BG, Fredin H, Johansson O, Norlin R, Thorling J: Primary anterior dislocation of the shoulder in young patients: A ten-year prospective study. *J Bone Joint Surg Am* 1996;78:1677-1684.

The authors performed a prospective study on 247 primary anterior dislocations. Patients were divided into three different treatment groups. The authors found that the type and duration of the initial treatment had no effect on the rate of recurrence. Recurrent dislocation necessitating surgical treatment had developed in 23%. An equal amount of glenohumeral arthritis was seen in patients with one versus multiple dislocations.

Kiss J, Mersich I, Perlaky GY, Szollas L: The results of the Putti-Platt operation with particular reference to arthritis, pain, and limitation of external rotation. *J Shoulder Elbow Surg* 1998;7:495-500.

The authors review the results of 90 Putti-Platt procedures with an average follow-up of 9 years. The redislocation rate was 9%. The incidence of osteoarthritis was 73%, with 30% being moderate to severe. They conclude that the incidence and severity of arthritis, pain, and limitation of external rotation are significantly increased after the Putti-Platt procedure.

van der Zwaag HM, Brand R, Obermann WR, Rozing PM: Glenohumeral osteoarthrosis after Putti-Platt repair. *J Shoulder Elbow Surg* 1999;8:252-258.

The authors reviewed the results of 66 Putti-Platt procedures at a mean follow-up of 22 years. The redislocation rate was only 3%. Osteoarthritic changes of the glenohumeral joint were found in 61%, with 26% being moderate to severe. The rate of arthritis is increased in patients who have undergone a Putti-Platt procedure and is correlated with the length of time since surgery.

Warner JJ, Johnson D, Miller M, Caborn DN: Technique for selecting capsular tightness in repair of anterior-inferior shoulder instability. *J Shoulder Elbow Surg* 1995;4:352-364.

The authors propose a technique to help prevent overtightening or undertightening of the capsule when performing an anterior capsulorrhaphy in the presence of anterior instability. They state that their approach decreases the loss of external rotation that is commonly seen with anterior capsulorrhaphies.

Classic Bibliography

Banas MP, Dalldorf PG, Sebastianelli WJ, De Haven KE: Long-term follow-up of the modified Bristow procedure. *Am J Sports Med* 1993;21:666-671.

Brav EA: An evaluation of the Putti-Platt reconstruction procedure for recurrent dislocation of the shoulder. *J Bone Joint Surg Am* 1955;37:731-846.

Craig EV: Open reduction and internal fixation of greater tuberosity fractures, malunions, and nonunions, in Craig EV (ed): *Master Techniques in Orthopaedic Surgery: The Shoulder.* New York, NY, Raven Press, 1995, pp 289-307.

Cofield RH, Kavanagh BF, Frassica FJ: Anterior shoulder instability. *Instr Course Lect* 1985;34:210-227.

Dines DM, Warren RF, Altchek DW, et al: Posttraumatic changes of the proximal humerus: Malunion, nonunion, and osteonecrosis. Treatment with modular hemiarthroplasty or total shoulder arthroplasty. *J Shoulder Elbow Surg* 1993;2:11-21.

Flatow EL, Cuomo F, Maday MG, Miller SR, McIlveen SJ, Bigliani LU: Open reduction and internal fixation of two-part displaced fractures of the greater tuberosity of the proximal part of the humerus. *J Bone Joint Surg Am* 1991;73:1213-1218.

Frich LH, Sojbjerg JO, Sneppen O: Shoulder arthroplasty in complex acute and chronic proximal humeral fractures. *Orthopedics* 1991;14:949-954.

Hawkins RJ, Angelo RL: Glenohumeral osteoarthrosis: A late complication of the Putti-Platt repair. *J Bone Joint Surg Am* 1990;72:1193-1197.

Hawkins RJ, Bell RH, Gurr K: The three-part fracture of the proximal part of the humerus: Operative treatment. *J Bone Joint Surg Am* 1986;68:1410-1414.

Leach RE, Corbett M, Schepsis A, Stockel J: Results of a modified Putti-Platt operation for recurrent shoulder dislocations and subluxations. *Clin Orthop* 1982;164:20-25.

Lombardo SJ, Kerlan RK, Jobe FW, Carter VS, Blazina ME, Shields CL Jr: The modified Bristow procedure for recurrent dislocation of the shoulder. *J Bone Joint Surg Am* 1976;58:256-261.

Lusardi DA, Wirth MA, Wurtz D, Rockwood CA Jr: Loss of external rotation following anterior capsulorrhaphy of the shoulder. *J Bone Joint Surg Am* 1993;75:1185-1192.

MacDonald PB, Hawkins RJ, Fowler PJ, Miniaci A: Release of the subscapularis for internal rotation contracture and pain after anterior repair for recurrent anterior dislocation of the shoulder. *J Bone Joint Surg Am* 1992;74:734-737.

Morrey BF, Janes JM: Recurrent anterior dislocation of the shoulder: Long-term follow-up of the Putti-Platt and Bankart procedures. *J Bone Joint Surg Am* 1976;58:252-256.

Neer CS II: Displaced proximal humeral fractures: Part I. Classification and evaluation. *J Bone Joint Surg Am* 1970;52:1077-1089.

Neer CS II: Displaced proximal humeral fractures: Part II. Treatment of three-part and four-part displacement. *J Bone Joint Surg Am* 1970;52:1090-1103.

Neer CS, Foster CR: Inferior capsular shift for involuntary inferior and multidirectional instability of the shoulder: A preliminary report. *J Bone Joint Surgery Am* 1980;62:897-908.

O'Driscoll SW, Evans DC: Long-term results of staple capsulorrhaphy for anterior instability of the shoulder. *J Bone Joint Surg Am* 1993;75:249-258.

Regan WD Jr, Webster-Bogaert S, Hawkins RJ, Fowler PJ: Comparative functional analysis of the Bristow, Magnuson-Stack, and Putti-Platt procedures for recurrent dislocation of the shoulder. *Am J Sports Med* 1989;17:42-48.

Samilson RL, Prieto V: Dislocation arthropathy of the shoulder. *J Bone Joint Surg Am* 1983;65:456-460.

Sidor ML, Zuckerman JD, Lyon T, Koval K, Schoenberg N: Classification of proximal humerus fractures: The contribution of the scapular lateral and axillary radiographs. *J Shoulder Elbow Surg* 1994;3:24-27.

Weaver JK, Derkash RS: Don't forget the Bristow-Latarjet procedure. *Clin Orthop* 1994;308:102-110.

Wredmark T, Tornkvist H, Johansson C, Brobert B: Long-term functional results of the modified Bristow procedure for recurrent dislocations of the shoulder. *Am J Sports Med* 1992;20:157-161.

Young DC, Rockwood CA Jr: Complications of a failed Bristow procedure and their management. *J Bone Joint Surg Am* 1991;73:969-981.

Zuckerman JD, Matsen FA: Complications about the glenohumeral joint related to the use of screws and staples. *J Bone Joint Surg Am* 1984;66:175-180.

Chapter 28

Shoulder Arthroplasty: Complications and Revision

Stephen B. Gunther, MD

Tom R. Norris, MD

Introduction

Shoulder arthroplasty has become a widely accepted and commonly performed procedure in the United States and many other developed countries. Arthritis, fracture, nonunion, malunion, tumor, and rotator cuff arthropathy are conditions that can be treated with shoulder arthroplasty. The number of shoulder arthroplasties performed in the United States has increased in each of the past 5 years. In 1998, 17,500 humeral head and total shoulder arthroplasties were performed, and more than 20,000 were performed both in 2000 and 2001. However, shoulder arthroplasties still represent only one tenth the number of total hip or total knee replacements performed each year. Surgeons doing only one or two shoulder replacements per year perform up to 85% of the procedures. Hence, the potential for complications in these settings is significantly higher than in centers in which surgeons routinely perform the procedure.

The number of complications requiring revision surgery is likely to increase along with the increase in shoulder arthroplasties. Even though the incidence of complications varies depending on the initial diagnosis, several types of complications can occur with any shoulder arthroplasty. This chapter reviews common complications and provides a logical approach to revision shoulder arthroplasty.

Complications

Numerous complications occur in association with shoulder arthroplasty (Table 1). The timing of complications is most easily divided into those occurring intraoperatively, those occurring during the early postoperative period, and those occurring years later. Meticulous attention to detail in preoperative planning, surgical technique, and rehabilitation can minimize the risk of these complications.

Implant Loosening

The predisposition to component loosening depends on many factors, including implant design, materials, method of fixation, bone stock, rotator cuff deficiency, joint mechanics, and the presence of infection. The load transmitted across the glenohumeral joint during active shoulder elevation is significant, approximating 90% of body weight when the arm is abducted 90°. An anatomic reconstruction ideally maintains normal excursion of the joint and preserves the original center of rotation. Small changes in anatomic version, radius of curvature, and offset change the center of rotation. This change adversely alters the range of motion and contact stress across the articular surface and, thus, may predispose to implant loosening. Recently, there has been more emphasis on re-creation of the original glenohumeral geometry to minimize the risk of component loosening and wear.

Any factors that cause abnormal joint motion or contact stresses predispose to mechanical loosening and implant failure. Therefore, it is critical to correct bony deformity and balance soft tissues. Asymmetric glenoid arthritis, posttraumatic deformity, and malunions of the proximal humerus should be realigned if possible. Rotator cuff tears should be repaired if possible. Capsular laxity and capsular contractures should be addressed with plication or release to balance the soft tissues.

Component loosening is a relatively common complication. Prosthetic loosening had been believed to occur almost exclusively in glenoid implants. However, recent evidence with 10-year follow-up has demonstrated subsidence in more than 50% of the noncemented humeral stems in one series involving implants that were designed for use with cement. Late onset of pain as well as radiographic parameters of progressive radiolucent lines or shift in component alignment should be evaluated on a longitudinal basis for both the glenoid and the humeral stem. With better cementing techniques, early postoperative radiolucent lines have become less common in shoulder implants than the 30% to 80% originally reported. However, standardized radiographic technique and clinical parameters must be used to evaluate implant loosening. To date, only fluoroscopically posi-

TABLE 1	Complications That Occur in Association With Shoulder Arthroplasty

Common Complications of Hemiarthroplasty

Instability

Implant loosening/subsidence

Implant malposition

Tuberosity nonunion/malunion

Progressive glenoid arthritis

Common Complications of Total Shoulder Arthroplasty

Instability

Rotator cuff tear

Implant loosening

Implant wear

Fracture

Less Common Complications of Shoulder Arthroplasty

Infection

Nerve injury

Rotator cuff impingement

Heterotopic ossification

Bone loss/osteolysis

Stiffness

TABLE 2	Causes of Instability

Implant malrotation

Incorrect humeral height

Capsular laxity from previous instability

Asymmetric capsular contractures

Rotator cuff tear

Bone deformity/bone loss

Neurologic injury

tioned radiographs are reproducible in follow-up studies demonstrating progressive lucent lines.

Implant Wear

Implant fatigue, surface wear, and debris associated with osteolysis have not been extensively studied in the literature. Hip and knee arthroplasty re-search has proven a correlation between osteolysis and polyethylene debris, with a macrophage-induced destruction of periprosthetic bone. New data have characterized both the size and shapes of polyethylene wear debris and the cytokine response to these particles. Although the scope of the problem does not seem to compare to that of knee and hip reconstructive surgery, early reports parallel findings of particulate debris and subsequent soft-tissue response.

There is recent evidence of both surface wear and fatigue failure in retrieved glenoid specimens. Surface wear is noted on low-power magnification as abrasion, burnishing, and scratching, and fatigue failure produces component fracture, delamination, and pitting (Fig. 1). Hip implants sustain mostly wear, and knee implants are more predisposed to fatigue failure; shoulder implants develop both surface wear and fatigue failure. Both hylamer and the thin polyethylene with metal backing have been shown to wear more rapidly and should be avoided.

Instability

Instability is another relatively common complication of shoulder arthroplasty (0% to 18% for unconstrained prostheses), especially in patients with predisposing bone or soft-tissue deficiencies. Any deficiency in structures that maintain glenohumeral joint stability must be addressed (Table 2). These include implant malalignment, capsuloligamentous imbalance, rotator cuff dysfunction, bony deficiency, and neurologic injury. Anterior instability is associated with subscapularis rupture unless proven otherwise (Fig. 2). Other contributing factors include relative anteversion of the humeral component, anteversion of the glenoid component, an oversized humeral head, or anterior deltoid dehiscence. Posterior instability can be caused by posterior capsular laxity, excessive retroversion of the humeral or glenoid component, or rotator cuff dysfunction. Superior instability is caused by rotator cuff dehiscence as well as coracoacromial arch insufficiency from previous surgery. Inferior instability may be caused by setting the humeral prosthesis too low or by axillary nerve injury. Inferior instability must also be differentiated from transient inferior subluxation caused by posttraumatic deltoid atony, which commonly occurs with fractures of the proximal humerus.

Fractures

Fractures of the humerus or glenoid during or after surgery are rare complications, but they may be difficult to treat. Predisposing factors, such as deficient or osteopenic bone, scar, malunions, and rheumatoid arthritis, make adequate surgical exposure important. Inadequate surgical

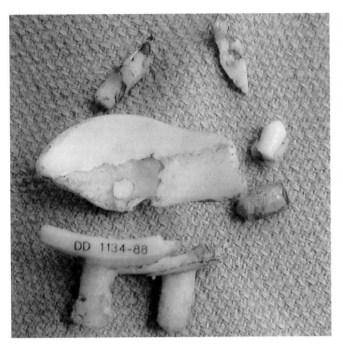

Figure 1 Glenoid implant wear and fatigue fracture.

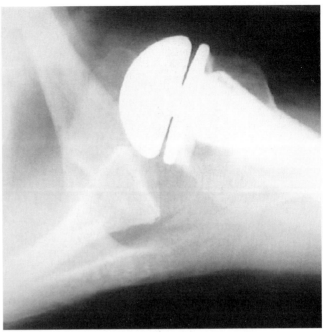

Figure 2 Axillary radiograph of anterior instability following hemiarthroplasty.

exposure, overzealous reaming, forceful humeral impaction with increased hoop stresses, or excessive torque may cause intraoperative fractures. These intraoperative fractures are best addressed at the time of surgery.

The type of surgical fixation depends on the fracture pattern, fracture location, and implant stability as well as timing. Most intraoperative fractures should be treated with immediate fixation. Treatment of periprosthetic fractures with long stems and cerclage cables has permitted postoperative rehabilitation without additional protection (Fig. 3). Alternatively, periprosthetic fractures can be reduced and stabilized with plate fixation of the humeral shaft in order to avoid removing the humeral prosthesis. Plate fixation around a prosthesis is not as secure as struts and cables. Failure of fixation within the fracture site leads to a nonunion and further patient disability (Fig. 4). Postoperative fractures may be treated nonsurgically if they occur distal to a well-fixed, functional shoulder replacement, especially if the patient has limited goals. Alternatively, surgical fixation permits early mobilization with favorable results.

Infection

Infection after total shoulder arthroplasty can be devastating, but it is rare (0% to 4%). Similar factors predispose patients to total joint infections in shoulders and other joints. Diabetes mellitus, rheumatoid arthritis, and lupus erythematosus all compromise the immune system. Immunosuppressive medications such as those used in chemotherapy, systemic steroids, and multiple local steroid injections also increase the risk of infection. Prophylactic antibiotics are used on a routine basis. Antibiotic-impregnated cement may be added as a supplement in high-risk patients and with revisions. As with other joint replacements, the choice of treatment depends on timing, the virulence of the infecting organism, the general health of the patient, and implant stability. Options for treatment are antibiotic suppression, irrigation and débridement, immediate or delayed exchange arthroplasty, resection arthroplasty, and arthrodesis.

Nerve Injuries

Nerve injuries, including neurapraxia and nerve lacerations, have been reported (0% to 2%). Most nerve injuries related to shoulder arthroplasty are neurapraxias of the brachial plexus related to traction. Direct nerve injury to peripheral nerves such as the axillary nerve and musculocutaneous nerve may be related to blunt retraction or laceration. The use of methotrexate, the long deltopectoral approach, and shorter duration of surgery have been correlated with neurologic complications. Most of these injuries have not interfered with long-term outcome of the primary arthroplasty procedure.

Rotator Cuff Tears and Impingement

Postoperative tearing of the rotator cuff occurs in approximately 3% to 4% of patients with total shoulder replacements. Most intraoperative tears can be prevented by careful retraction of the supraspinatus tendon during humeral cutting and broaching. Preoperative and

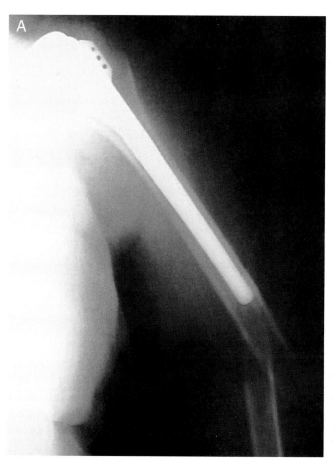
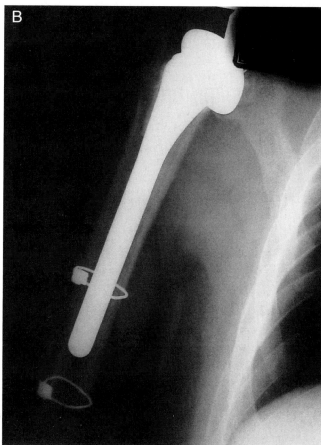

Figure 3 A, Periprosthetic humerus fracture. **B,** Revision arthroplasty with long-stem implant and cable fixation.

intraoperative rotator cuff tears should be repaired if possible. A massive irreparable tear should preclude glenoid resurfacing because of the relatively high risk of glenoid loosening, which is caused by the rocking horse phenomenon associated with superior migration of the humeral head. Postoperative tearing of the rotator cuff is treated preferentially with repair. Tears that do not cause significant pain or dysfunction can be managed nonsurgically. Most surgeons favor repair of acute perioperative tears with adequate tissue. Rotator cuff impingement also may cause shoulder pain in arthroplasty patients and may be treated by either arthroscopic or open acromioplasty.

Revision Surgery

Preoperative Planning

A general approach to revision shoulder arthroplasty should incorporate a basic understanding of complications, a detailed history and physical examination of the patient, and appropriate laboratory testing and radiographic examination. A complete preoperative evaluation is vital in this patient population because the cause of shoulder pain is sometimes difficult to discern and multiple factors often complicate clinical results.

The history begins with documentation of any preexisting shoulder pathology and any previous surgery. The quality of tissues at the time of the prior arthroplasty procedure should be noted. The surgeon must be prepared to remove the prosthesis and should understand the type of prosthesis, its size and mode of fixation, and presence of bone ingrowth. It is also important to elicit any recent history of trauma, instability, or infection.

On physical examination, the physician should note any atrophy and should carefully document both active and passive range of motion. Rotator cuff tears may result in atrophy and weakness. Capsular contractures or an overstuffed joint (humeral component set too high or humeral head too large) causes stiffness. Stability testing should include not only anterior and posterior laxity but also inferior and superior laxity. Any clunking or catching in the joint may represent a loose polyethylene glenoid or fractured component. The examination also should incorporate a thorough evaluation of nerve and muscle function. Electromyographic testing is useful in documenting neuromuscular damage.

The radiographic evaluation should begin with serial radiographs. The full list of potential radiographic and laboratory tests is shown in Table 3. Plain radiographs should

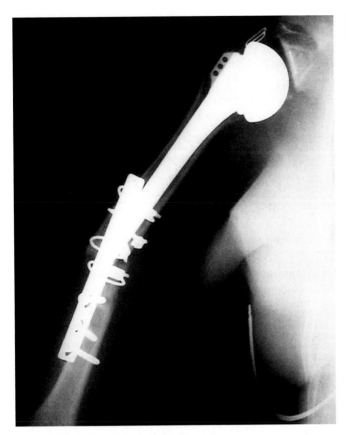

Figure 4 Failed periprosthetic fracture fixation.

TABLE 3	Potential Radiographic and Laboratory Tests

Radiographic Evaluation

Plain radiographs

Fluoroscopy

Arthrography

CT scan

Indium-labeled white blood cell scan

Nonradiographic Evaluation

Complete blood cell count

Erythrocyte sedimentation rate

C-reactive protein

Aspiration-culture

Electromyogram

be assessed for humeral height, offset, and humeral head size. An oversized humeral head or a humeral component set too high may cause stiffness and increased contact stress on the glenoid. Conversely, an undersized humeral head may cause instability or abutment of a humeral collar on the glenoid. A humeral component set too low may cause inferior instability and loss of abduction strength. Therefore, the surgeon should determine preoperatively whether the patient's anatomy has been distorted.

Motion and stability should also be measured to gauge the biomechanical forces across the glenohumeral joint. For example, a shoulder with posterior subluxation will increase the contact force and shear force on the posterior glenoid and thus cause asymmetric posterior wear (Fig. 5). Also, a stiff shoulder with an overstuffed joint may cause early glenoid wear. Determining these anatomic and biomechanical factors preoperatively is critical to restoring normal anatomy and kinematics during the revision.

Fluoroscopy may be used as an adjunct to evaluate implant version and loosening. Because the patient can be perfectly positioned in the plane of the scapula using fluoroscopy, a true AP image of the glenohumeral joint may be obtained. At this point, rotation of the arm denotes version of the humeral implant in relation to the scapula. Multiple images may be useful in evaluating possible loose components. An arthrogram may be obtained

along with the fluoroscopic examination to rule out a rotator cuff tear or fistula. Arthroscopic evaluation has recently been shown to be more accurate than arthrography in delineating glenoid loosening from other painful causes of failure. Arthroscopy can also be a useful adjunct to other studies in the evaluation and treatment of rotator cuff tears, biceps tendon pathology, impingement lesions, adhesions, and capsular contracture.

Routine laboratory tests (complete blood cell count, erythrocyte sedimentation rate) and aspiration can be helpful in evaluating infection, although clinical parameters are essential because neither laboratory findings nor aspiration are highly accurate in the setting of a low-grade infection. An indium-labeled white blood cell scan may be helpful in some cases. Finally, preoperative planning should include choice of revision instrumentation (Table 4). The surgeon may also consider preoperative blood donation, intraoperative cell salvage, preparation of the iliac crest for autogenous bone grafting, and supplemental allograft bone and tendon.

Surgical Technique

The patient should be examined under anesthesia for motion and stability. The most common surgical approach is the deltopectoral approach. This approach may be extended distally by incising the pectoralis major insertion if necessary. In some revisions with extensive scarring and contractures, it may even be beneficial to elevate the anterior deltoid from the clavicle and acromion initially to protect the deltoid muscle from injury during retraction. The coracoid is an important landmark at the top of the deltopectoral interval. Adjuvant procedures such as acromioplasty and distal clavicle resection may be benefi-

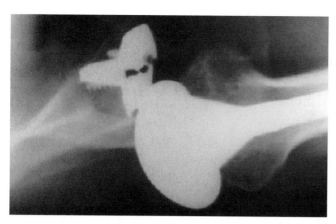

Figure 5 Posterior prosthetic subluxation.

TABLE 4 | Revision Instrumentation and Materials

Implant removal instrumentation

Long-stem humeral implants

Cable and fracture fixation systems

Autograft bone instrumentation

Allograft bone

Allograft tendon

cial for impingement, just as capsular releases may be necessary to eliminate soft-tissue contracture.

Preoperative anterior instability or excessive external rotation indicates a probable subscapularis tendon tear. An internal rotation contracture may represent subscapularis shortening and capsular contractures. There are several techniques for lengthening a contracted subscapularis tendon. Coronal z-lengthening may be performed on a thick, healthy tendon, but sub-sequent weakness and dehiscence have been reported. Subscapularis recession from the lesser tuberosity to the edge of the prosthesis is an alternative, but it also may result in subsequent weakness or failure. Extensive circumferential release of the subscapularis muscle and tendon both from the anterior capsule and from the scapular neck at the subcoracoid level can be extremely helpful. This extensive release may obviate the need for other forms of lengthening. A lesser tuberosity osteotomy with medial transfer may be done to shorten the tendon. If primary repair or transfer is insufficient, reconstruction of the subscapularis may be necessary. Achilles tendon allograft, quadriceps tendon autograft, and pectoralis major tendon transfer are all potential options.

Prostheses should be evaluated for instability, component loosening, wear, and reactive synovitis. Loose components should be revised to a larger press-fit prosthesis with impaction grafting or a cemented prosthesis. Malpositioned components and those with excessive wear may also require revision. Progressive glenoid arthritis requires conversion of hemiarthroplasty to a total shoulder replacement if there is sufficient rotator cuff to center the humeral head. Some glenoid revisions with large cavitary or segmental cortical defects require grafting with autograft or allograft bone. Replacement of a new polyethylene glenoid component may be possible only as a staged procedure if there is extensive bone loss.

The humeral components should be matched to the original humeral head size and anatomic offset to avoid overstuffing the joint and impinging on the rotator cuff (Fig. 6). The superior margin of the humeral head should lie approximately 5 to 8 mm above the greater tuberosity, and the humeral head should directly face the glenoid when the arm is in neutral rotation. The soft-tissue structures must also be balanced to create a stable glenohumeral articulation. Capsular contractures should be released and a patulous capsule plicated instead of oversizing the humeral head for stability.

The surgeon must consider revising the humeral component in certain situations. For example, a humeral head that lies lower than the greater tuberosity may lead to impingement of the greater tuberosity on the acromion. A humeral head that lies more than 1 cm above the greater tuberosity is associated with a complex of potential impingement pain, rotator cuff rupture, and stiffness from overstuffing the joint. A bipolar shoulder in which the head frequently locks in a varus position may exacerbate this problem. Altered version predisposes to asymmetric wear and instability. Therefore, humeral malalignment is best corrected by humeral component revision with realignment instead of merely changing humeral head size.

Revision surgery for instability is difficult and has produced mixed results. Anterior instability is almost invariably associated with subscapularis rupture. This is addressed by subscapularis repair, pectoralis transfer under the conjoined tendon, or allograft reconstruction. It may require a change in humeral component version and humeral head size as well. Posterior instability may be caused by posterior capsular laxity, glenoid component retroversion, or excessive humeral component retroversion. Component revision and posterior capsular plication may be necessary. Also, posterior glenoid bone deficiency may require bone grafting if the version cannot be corrected by reaming the high anterior cortex. Rotator cuff tears, which contribute to instability, should be repaired.

Inferior instability may be a result of either deltoid dysfunction or inappropriate humeral height. Humeral height is most often misjudged during humeral head replace-

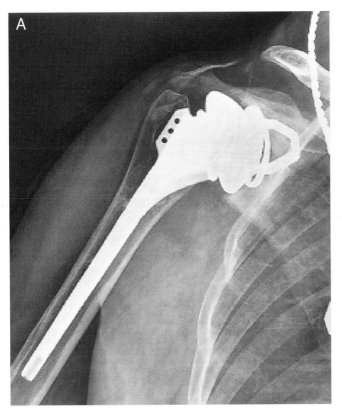 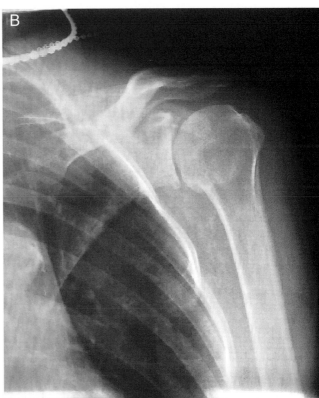

Figure 6 A, Overstuffed total shoulder arthroplasty with excessive lateral offset. **B,** Contralateral shoulder.

ment in the treatment of fractures. The humeral head height must match the glenoid. Superior instability from rotator cuff tears or coracoacromial arch insufficiency from previous surgery may be managed with rotator cuff repair if possible and coracoacromial ligament repair or allograft reconstruction if necessary. When the rotator cuff is not repairable, glenoid replacement should be avoided because of the relatively high risk of loosening. The coracoacromial ligament thus should be maintained to prevent subsequent anterior-superior instability (humeral head escape). The Reverse prosthesis holds promise for the nonfunctional rotator cuff in revisions.

Revision for infection is not common. Most previous reports describe resection arthroplasty, but chronic antibiotic suppression and exchange arthroplasty similar to other joint replacements may also be beneficial. Fractures should be fixed at the time of surgery with a long-stem implant and supplemental fixation. Some postoperative periprosthetic fractures may be treated with a fracture brace if the components are stable and well aligned.

Summary

Although shoulder arthroplasty is successful in relieving pain and facilitating function in most patients, many different complications may occur. Anatomic reconstruction of the glenohumeral joint and appropriate soft-tissue balancing are important goals of primary joint replacement. Revision surgery should begin with a thorough preoperative evaluation of potential complications and full preparation of the surgical environment. Surgery should be tailored to the area of deficiency, and rehabilitation should match the expectations of the surgeon and the patient.

Annotated Bibliography

Complications

Campbell JT, Moore RS, Iannotti JP, Norris TR, Williams GR: Periprosthetic humeral fractures: Mechanisms of fracture and treatment options. *J Shoulder Elbow Surg* 1998;7:406-413.

This retrospective review of 21 periprosthetic humeral fractures demonstrates five mechanisms of fracture. The authors classify these fractures, and they suggest revision with long-stem intramedullary implants and cerclage fixation for fractures at the tip of the prosthesis. They recommend surgical fixation for unstable shaft fractures to allow continued rehabilitation without further protection.

Freedman KB, Williams GR, Iannotti JP: Impingement syndrome following total shoulder arthroplasty and humeral arthroplasty: Treatment with arthroscopic acromioplasty. *Arthroscopy* 1998;14:665-670.

This is a retrospective review of six patients with refractory impingement syndrome following shoulder arthroplasty who were treated with arthroscopic acromioplasty. Five of the six patients were completely satisfied with the procedure.

Gunther SB, Graham J, Norris TR, Ries MD, Pruitt L: Retrieved glenoid components: A classification system for surface damage analysis. *J Arthroplasty* 2002;17: 95-100.

Polyethylene glenoid implants from 10 consecutive shoulder arthroplasty revisions were analyzed for surface damage and fatigue failure. A classification scheme was designed for wear analysis of glenoid components. Both surface wear and subsurface fatigue failure mechanisms were shown to contribute to glenoid polyethylene failure.

Hersch JC, Dines DM: Arthroscopy for failed shoulder arthroplasty. *Arthroscopy* 2000;16:606-612.

This article describes the rationale, technique, and results of arthroscopic evaluation and treatment of failed shoulder arthroplasties in 10 patients.

Klimkiewicz JJ, Iannotti JP, Rubash HE, Shanbhag AS: Asceptic loosening of the humeral component in total shoulder arthroplasty. *J Shoulder Elbow Surg* 1998;7: 422-426.

This is a case report of aseptic loosening of a glenoid implant 3 years after total shoulder arthroplasty with a metal-backed glenoid implant. Ultra-high molecular weight polyethylene debris was demonstrated and postulated to be a causative factor in failure of the glenoid prosthesis.

Lynch NM, Cofield RH, Silbert PL, Hermann RC: Neurologic complications after total shoulder arthroplasty. *J Shoulder Elbow Surg* 1996;5:53-61.

This retrospective review of 417 total shoulder replacements found neurologic complications in 4% of patients. The long deltopectoral approach, the use of methotrexate, and shorter operations were found to be significant risk factors. Neurologic recovery was rated good in most patients (11 of 16).

Norris TR, Lipson SR: Management of the unstable prosthetic shoulder arthroplasty. *Inst Course Lect* 1998; 47:141-148.

This chapter describes the predisposing factors to the development of prosthetic instability as well as the rationale and conceptual basis of treatment.

Pearl ML, Kurutz S: Geometric analysis of commonly used prosthetic systems for proximal humeral replacement. *J Bone Joint Surg Am* 1999;81:660-671.

Four second-generation prosthetic implants for press-fit total shoulder replacements were compared with respect to their ability to match the superoinferior and mediolateral dimensions of the articular surface in 21 cadaveric humerii. None of the prosthetic systems replicated articular geometry, and they displaced the center of rotation a mean of 14.7 mm.

Torchia ME, Cofield RH, Settergren CR: Total shoulder arthroplasty with the Neer prosthesis: Long-term results. *J Shoulder Elbow Surg* 1997;6:495-505.

In this report of long-term outcome with 113 total shoulder replacements (Neer prosthesis) between 1975 and 1981, there was 93% implant survival at 10 years and 87% survival at 15 years.

Wirth MA, Agrawal CM, Mabrey JD, et al: Isolation and characterization of polyethylene wear debris associated with osteolysis following total shoulder arthroplasty. *J Bone Joint Surg Am* 1999;81:29-37.

Periprosthetic tissue from three revision total shoulder replacements was analyzed for wear associated with osteolysis. Polyethylene particles were characterized to be less round and more fibrillar than particulate debris from four revision total hip specimens.

Wirth MA, Rockwood CA Jr: Complications of total shoulder replacement arthroplasty. *J Bone Joint Surg Am* 1996;78:603-616.

This is a comprehensive review of complications in total shoulder arthroplasty surgery. The authors reviewed 41 series in the literature involving 1,858 total shoulder arthroplasties from 1975 through 1995. They noted that the average follow-up in these studies was only 3.5 years, and only five studies reported an average follow-up of 5 years or more. There were two survivorship analyses. The authors discussed this literature and their experience with the multiple complications encountered in shoulder arthroplasty surgery.

Revision Surgery

Gartsman GM, Roddey TS, Hammerman SM: Shoulder arthroplasty with and without glenoid resurfacing for patients with osteoarthritis. *J Bone Joint Surg Am* 2000; 82:26-34.

Forty-seven patients with glenohumeral osteoarthritis were randomly assigned to either hemiarthroplasty or total shoulder arthroplasty. Total shoulder arthroplasty provided superior pain relief at an average of 35 months follow-up, but it was associated with an increased cost of $1,177 per patient. None of the total shoulder arthroplasty patients required a second procedure, and three of the 25 hemiarthroplasty patients required a second procedure to resurface the glenoid.

Petersen SA, Hawkins RJ: Revision of failed total shoulder arthroplasty. *Orthop Clin North Am* 1998;29: 519-533

This article describes the pathogenesis of failed shoulder arthroplasty, preoperative evaluation, and surgical techniques for revision surgery.

Sperling JW, Cofield RH: Revision total shoulder arthroplasty for the treatment of glenoid arthrosis. *J Bone Joint Surg Am* 1998;80:860-867.

In this comprehensive review article on revision shoulder arthroplasty surgery, 18 shoulders in 17 patients were reviewed. The authors' findings indicated that most of the patients with painful glenoid arthrosis following hemiarthroplasty have pain relief and improved motion following revision to a total shoulder replacement.

Classic Bibliography

Bonutti PM, Hawkins RJ, Saddemi S: Arthroscopic assessment of glenoid component loosening after total shoulder arthroplasty. *Arthroscopy* 1993;9:272-276.

Cofield RH, Edgerton BC: Total shoulder arthroplasty: Complications and revision surgery. *Inst Course Lect* 1990;39:449-462.

Neer CS II, Kirby RM: Revision of humeral head and total shoulder arthroplasties. *Clin Orthop* 1982;170: 189-195.

Section 6

Elbow Trauma, Fracture, and Reconstruction

Section Editor:
Shawn W. O'Driscoll, PhD, MD

Athletic Injuries and the Throwing Athlete: Elbow

Stephen Fealy, MD

Joel T. Rohrbough, MD

Answorth A. Allen, MD

David W. Altchek, MD

Mark C. Drakos, BA

Introduction

Injuries to the elbow joint in throwing athletes can best be characterized as medial tension injuries, lateral compression injuries, extension overload injuries, and tendinopathies. Most injuries progress from an initial valgus extension overload injury.

Functional Anatomy and Biomechanics

The throwing motion and the tennis groundstroke produce significant tensile forces medially and compressive forces laterally at the radiocapitellar joint line. The largest resultant force that the elbow experiences is during the acceleration phase of throwing when the elbow extends to 30° of flexion. These tensile forces peak at the medial elbow during the late cocking and early acceleration phases of throwing as the elbow moves from flexion to extension at speeds that have been estimated to reach 3,000°/s. Incomplete healing of the medial collateral ligament (MCL) will lead to attenuation of the normal ligamentous anatomy and architecture. Attenuation of the MCL complex (medial tension) will permit secondary compression at the radiocapitellar (lateral) joint. This cycle, because of the repetitive nature of throwing, will ultimately yield chondromalacia about the elbow and the possible formation of loose bodies.

Medial Collateral Ligament Complex

The MCL complex is composed of the anterior oblique, the posterior oblique, and the transverse ligaments. The MCL complex, particularly the anterior band, is the primary constraint against valgus stress.

The humeral attachment of the MCL arises from the anteroinferior surface of the medial epicondyle. The humeral origins of both the anterior and posterior bundles are posterior to the axis of motion and are more taut in flexion than in extension.

Lateral Collateral Ligament Complex

Whereas the MCL complex is composed of discrete bands, the lateral collateral ligament (LCL) complex consists of a complex of ligamentous fibers. The LCL originates from the inferior surface of the lateral epicondyle, near the axis of rotation. The proximal fibers of the ulnar part of the LCL cannot be separated from the rest of the complex. The ligament extends into the annular ligament in a fan-shaped expansion. The LCL and the annular ligament continue to insert onto the ulna, with the main part of the lateral ulnar collateral ligament inserting onto the tubercle of the supinator crest. The fibers become noticeable with varus or external rotational forces. Because the ligament is near the axis of rotation, it remains taut throughout the range of elbow flexion-extension with little change in the distance between the ligament origin and insertion. The main function of the complex is to provide external rotational and varus stability to the elbow joint.

Incompetence of this complex permits posterolateral rotatory instability, thereby creating posterolateral rotation of the ulnohumeral joint and posterior subluxation of the radial head. The lateral pivot shift test of the elbow, during which valgus and external rotation torques are applied to the forearm, results in subluxation of the elbow that reduces during flexion and a reproduction of the patient's mechanical symptoms. Patients with posterolateral rotatory instability have painful mechanical symptoms such as clunking, locking, or snapping, particularly when the elbow moves from supination and extension to pronation and flexion.

Ulnar Nerve

It is important to realize that dislocating or snapping ulnar nerve symptoms actually may be correctly attributed to a snapping medial head of the triceps. The inverse holds true as well. Both causes should be entertained in the differential diagnosis.

Lateral Elbow Pain

Osteochondritis Dissecans

Osteochondritis dissecans is a common cause of lateral elbow pain in throwing athletes and gymnasts between the ages of 10 and 15 years. The pain frequently is insidious and progressive in nature and is relieved with rest in most cases.

Patients may present with advanced disease, including swelling and a flexion contracture. Clicking, catching, or locking of the affected elbow, usually caused by an unstable flap or a loose body, are common symptoms.

Typical radiographs of patients with osteochondritis dissecans show a localized area in the capitellum with rarefaction and crater formation. In some patients, typical AP radiographs are normal, but AP views of the distal humerus with the elbow in 45° of flexion show irregularities, flattening, and/or fragmentation consistent with osteochondritis dissecans. On MRI, a discrete area of low signal intensity on T1 images indicates early osteochondritis dissecans, whereas T2 images may appear normal.

Whether the necrotic segment ultimately becomes a loose body is largely determined by the nature of ongoing stresses and whether the overlying articular cartilage is intact. According to one study, if the overlying articular cartilage remains intact, the segment may be absorbed and replaced with new bony tissue. Other studies have determined that an involved segment is exposed to shear stresses that lead to fragmentation and loose bodies once the mechanical support of the overlying articular cartilage is gone.

Osteochondritis dissecans of the elbow appears to be distinct from the less common Panner's disease, which is similar in both clinical and radiographic presentation. Panner's disease is an osteochondrosis of the capitellum that is self-limited and occurs in children between the ages of 4 and 8 years. Long-term sequelae or residual deformity usually is not involved in the natural history of Panner's disease, unlike osteochondritis dissecans of the elbow.

Initial treatment of patients with osteochondritis dissecans is rest with cessation of the offending activities. Treatment is directed according to presenting symptoms, radiographic findings, and status of the involved segment. The method of surgical treatment for osteochondritis dissecans often depends on whether the involved segment is attached, partially attached, or completely detached. Some authors recommend conservative care for 3 to 6 weeks or until the pain is resolved for intact capitellar lesions where the overlying articular cartilage is intact. The concomitant use of a brace to serve both as protection and as a deterrent from vigorous use is recommended. A gradual and progressive therapy program is begun once symptoms subside. The

goal of therapy is an ultimate return to sports. It has been reported that the best long-term results occur in patients with intact cartilage, but these patients and their families should be counseled about the possibility of sequelae.

Nonsurgical measures often are unsuccessful in patients with documented large chondral fragments and loose bodies, and in those with persistent symptoms. Surgery is indicated for these patients. Surgical management involves either an excision of a loose lesion and removal of loose bodies or reattachment of an osteochondral fragment. The role of subchondral penetration or débridement of the defect after fragment excision is unclear. Loose bodies in the elbow joint are removed arthroscopically. Some authors recommend attempting to reattach large osteochondral fragments if possible; reattachment may need to be done through an arthrotomy. Headless stainless steel screws, Kirschner wires, Herbert screws, and/or biosynthetic screws and pins may be used.

In one study, 31 patients with osteochondritis dissecans of the elbow were studied for an average of 23 years. These patients were treated with fragment excision and loose body removal. At follow-up, nearly half of the patients complained of loss of motion and pain with exertion. In more than half of the patients, radiographs showed osteoarthritic changes that had a clinical correlation with a symptomatic decrease in range of motion. The authors did not recommend reattachment of the fragment or drilling of the involved area. Other authors recommended that drilling or curetting the base of the lesion was the ideal treatment of the involved segment. They noted that loose bodies are associated with a poor outcome and therefore should be removed. In situ fixation of nondisplaced lesions with Herbert screws in six patients had successful results, with radiographic evidence of a normal joint and a full return to sports within 1 year. In a recent study, encouraging results were reported for seven patients who underwent a closed-wedge osteotomy of the capitellum to treat osteochondritis dissecans and were followed over a 7-year period. Revascularization of the capitellum was found within 6 months of the osteotomy.

Lateral Epicondylitis

Lateral and medial epicondylitis are common injuries that are associated with specific sports and occupational trades (Table 1). Lateral epicondylitis (tennis elbow) is the most common reason that patients seek medical help for elbow pain. The condition affects approximately 50% of all recreational tennis players and frequently occurs during the fourth decade of life. Patients have pain with resisted wrist extension or during a ten-

TABLE 1 | Common Activities Leading to Epicondylitis

	Lateral	Medial
Recreational	Tennis (groundstrokes)	Golf
	Racquetball	Rowing
	Squash	Baseball (pitching)
	Fencing	Javelin throwing
		Tennis (serving)
Occupational	Meat cutting	Bricklaying
	Plumbing	Hammering
	Painting	Typing
	Raking	Textile production
	Weaving	

(Reproduced from Jobe FW, Ciccotti MG: Lateral and medial epicondylitis of the elbow. J Am Acad Orthop Surg 1994;2:1-8.)

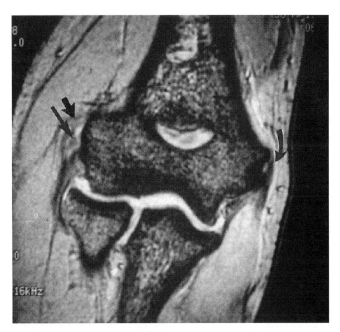

Figure 1 Coronal gradient-recalled MRI scan of a 58-year-old tennis player with diffuse elbow pain shows abnormal signal at the origin of the ECRB tendon (long straight arrow) with retraction off the lateral epicondyle. The extensor carpi radialis longus tendon origin (short straight arrow) is hyperintense but not disrupted. Abnormal signal at the origin of the common flexor tendon (curved arrow) indicates concomitant medial epicondylitis or flexor tendinosis. *(Reproduced with permission from Potter HG: Imaging of posttraumatic and soft tissue dysfunction of the elbow. Clin Orthop 2000;370:9-18.)*

nis backhand stroke. Pain often is localized 5 mm distal and anterior to the lateral humeral epicondyle, and symptoms are exacerbated as the elbow is brought into extension. Patients frequently are able to continue playing during initial bouts of lateral elbow pain. Risk factors for developing lateral epicondylitis include heavy racquets, inappropriate grip size, racquets that are too tightly strung, and poor backhand technique. It is important to differentiate lateral epicondylitis from degenerative arthritic changes in the radiocapitellar joint, which can mimic tennis elbow.

Lateral epicondylitis most often involves the extensor carpi radialis brevis (ECRB) and is frequently an overuse injury. The extensor digitorum communis, extensor carpi radialis longus, and extensor carpis ulnaris also may be involved. The initial pain is believed to be caused by microtears of the ECRB origin. Continued play without rest compromises the weakened muscle-tendon unit, causing microtears, which will heal through fibrosis and granulation tissue. Patients with chronic lateral epicondylitis have evidence of mucoid and/or hyaline degeneration of the tendon origin, which can be easily seen on MRI (Fig. 1). Furthermore, normal ECRB tendon fibers may be disrupted through angiofibroblastic hyperplasia. A palpable defect may be felt in the extensor origin in chronic injuries.

Radiographs of the affected elbow are routinely normal, but they may show evidence of calcific deposits in the extensor tendon origin. An edema pattern may or may not be seen in the extensor origin and surrounding tissues.

Nonsurgical Treatment
Fatigue of the wrist extensors is believed to be a contributing factor in the development of lateral epicondylitis. Therefore, treatment involves a coordinated rehabilitation protocol. Therapy should begin with activity modification and exercises, including active and passive range-of-motion routines three to five times per day. Exercises should begin with wrist exercises with and without resistance, progress to a forearm supination and pronation program, and then finish with the use of light weights in an effort to gain strength. Rotator cuff-strengthening exercises also should be done to maintain a balanced strength pattern in the involved extremity. A combination of ice and nonsteroidal anti-inflammatory medications is used in conjunction with the exercise. Treatment is focused on alleviating symptoms while maintaining motion of the elbow joint and is recommended for the noncompetitive athlete who has significant pain. More than three corticosteroid injections per patient are not recommended.

Counterforce bracing limits extensor muscle belly expansion, thereby limiting the muscle contractile tension. It is believed that the forearm support band limits extensor muscle fatigue by distributing the force created by wrist extension throughout the muscle belly rather than focusing it to the extensor origin. Evaluation of 50 normal volunteers with and without a forearm support band before and after a fatiguing exercise indicated that the forearm support band did not limit fatigue in the wrist extensors but rather increased the rate of fatigue in normal subjects.

Several studies have documented outcomes following nonsurgical treatment of lateral epicondylitis. Data suggest that symptoms will recur in less than 20% of patients.

Surgical Treatment

If a thorough and coordinated rehabilitation protocol fails to alleviate the patient's symptoms within 2 to 4 months, surgery should be considered. Several different surgical procedures for lateral epicondylitis have been described, including release of the extensor aponeurosis and débridement with repair of the defective tendon. Current surgical techniques for medial or lateral epicondylitis involve removing the pathologic portion of the tendon involved, repairing the resultant defect, and reattaching any elevated tendon edge back to the epicondyle.

Outcomes studies evaluating the results of surgery for lateral epicondylitis demonstrate that 85% to 90% of patients return to full activities. Of these patients, 10% have some pain with aggressive activities, and about 2% report no improvement. In 1,140 of 1,200 patients treated over a 10-year period, the success rate was 95%. Other authors recently reviewed their results in studies of failed lateral epicondylitis and revision surgery. Findings at revision surgery included residual tendinosis of the ECRB tendon in 34 of 35 elbows. In 27 of these elbows, the pathologic changes in the ECRB tendon had not been addressed originally, and in seven elbows the damaged tissue had not been completely excised. Salvage surgery included excision of pathologic tissue in the ECRB tendon origin combined with excision of excessive scar tissue and repair of the extensor aponeurosis when necessary. Based on a 40-point functional rating scale, 83% of the elbows (29 of 35) had good or excellent results at an average follow-up of 64 months (range, 17 months to 17 years). According to this study, failure of surgical treatment for tennis elbow can be prevented by resection of pathologic tissue usually present in the ECRB tendon, although successful results have been reported with surgical release as well.

Radial Nerve Entrapment

Radial nerve entrapment always should be included in the differential diagnosis of lateral epicondylitis. Radial nerve entrapment is a more difficult diagnosis to establish than lateral epicondylitis; as a result, approximately 5% of patients are estimated to be misdiagnosed as having lateral epicondylitis when the correct diagnosis is radial nerve entrapment.

Patients typically have elbow pain that radiates distally during active pronation and supination. Some may have weakness in extension of the elbow and/or wrist but no sensory deficits. Patients will have pain in the lateral epicondyle that is easily confused with lateral epicondylitis. Wrist drop or finger drop may be present, or atrophy of forearm musculature may be apparent. Nerve dysfunction may be confirmed with either an electromyogram or a nerve conduction test.

Although the ligamentous arcade of Fröhse is the primary inciting cause of nerve entrapment, ganglions and synovitis at the radiocapitellar joint and misguided screws used during radial head fixation may also injure the nerve. Soft-tissue entrapment of the posterior interosseous nerve (PIN) occurs at the arcade of Fröhse (the midportion of the supinator muscle as the PIN exits the supinator) or at the leash of Henry (radial recurrent vessels under the brachioradialis and extensor carpi radialis longus).

Treatment for radial nerve entrapment involves rest and a course of activity modification. Surgical decompression of the nerve at the radial tunnel may be indicated if nonsurgical measures fail.

Radiocapitellar Overload Syndrome

Radiocapitellar overload syndrome is an attritional injury that is the result of chronic medial instability. It is seen in conjunction with valgus insufficiency and posteromedial impingement. Recurrent lateral compression at the radiocapitellar joint produces articular cartilage wear and degeneration of the joint. Patients with radiocapitellar overload syndrome frequently will have loose bodies in the elbow and often may have flexion contractures. The pathology is essentially the same as that seen in primary osteoarthritis of the elbow. These patients often are throwing athletes who are near the end of their careers. Treatment is limited and will usually entail arthroscopic débridement and contracture release.

Medial Elbow Pain

Medial Epicondylitis

Medial epicondylitis is less common than lateral epicondylitis, but it has similar clinical and histologic characteristics. It is a type of tendinitis, which most commonly is precipitated by a microtear of the flexor-pronator muscle group, involving primarily the pronator teres and flexor carpi radialis; the flexor carpi ulnaris (FCU) also may be involved. Medial epicondylitis is seen most often in patients who play golf, but it also is seen in those who participate in throwing and racquet sports. In golfers with medial epicondylitis, the affected elbow is often on the arm engaged in the follow-through phase of motion. In tennis players, injury can result from both forehand groundstrokes and serving. Tennis players who place excessive topspin on their forehand groundstroke are more likely to develop medial epicondylitis than those who do not. Topspin on a forehand groundstroke is achieved through forced pronation, which aggravates the pronator muscle origin.

Patients with medial epicondylitis have pain localized slightly distal and anterior to the medial epicondyle; acute symptoms are common. Impaired grip strength and pain with resisted pronation and wrist flexion also occur. Ulnar neuritis and MCL injury should be considered in the differential diagnosis of medial epicondylitis.

As with lateral elbow conditions, nonsurgical measures remain the mainstay of treatment for medial epicondylitis. The initial goal of nonsurgical treatment should be relief of pain, followed by guided protocols with an end point of return to activities. Nonsurgical modalities such as ice, oral anti-inflammatory agents, counterforce bracing, and steroid injections may be used with varying degrees of success. Corticosteroid injections were found to provide short-term pain relief in more than 50% of patients with medial epicondylitis, but recurrence of symptoms was found nearly half of the time.

Surgery should be considered for patients in whom at least 10 weeks of nonsurgical therapy has failed. Thirty-five patients with medial epicondylitis in whom nonsurgical treatments had failed were evaluated. Of these patients, 97% had good or excellent results and 98% reported subjective satisfaction after the surgical procedure.

Medial Collateral Ligament Injuries and Physeal Injuries in Children

The physis is the weakest link in the medial elbow and often will be the first structure to fail. An MCL tear or MCL attenuation rarely is seen in children. It is essential to compare the injured elbow with the contralateral elbow both clinically and radiographically. Radiographs often show a widened physis medially, and MRI will confirm an intact MCL. Physeal injuries can be treated successfully with a course of rest that may require several months before resolution of symptoms.

Medial Collateral Ligament Injuries in Adults

Injuries to the MCL in the nonthrowing athlete usually can be managed nonsurgically with rehabilitation and activity modification. Modalities such as phonophoresis, electrical stimulation, and iontophoresis frequently are used during the acute phase to decrease swelling. Rehabilitation for the nonelite athlete should be a coordinated program that focuses on strengthening the medial-side flexor-pronator muscle mass as well as the shoulder musculature. Throwing, beginning with soft toss, often does

not begin until 3 months after therapy has begun. Patients who undergo a therapy program must be counseled that they may not be able to return to the same level of throwing despite aggressive rehabilitative efforts. However, certain individuals can successfully return to throwing if their pitching technique is modified to adapt to the injury. Namely, the throwing mechanisms are specifically evaluated to determine the point in the motion that precipitates the injury, and the throwing motion is modified accordingly. For patients with MCL injuries, continued pitching with an unstable elbow often leads over time to the development of severe posteromedial olecranon impingement and arthritic changes in the joint.

Although elite athletes may be able to compensate for the pain associated with MCL tears, they rarely are able to perform at the same competitive level because of continued medial-side valgus laxity. MCL injuries in the throwing athlete are most commonly the result of years of throwing and overuse, resulting in chronic microtrauma. MCL injury is common in baseball pitchers.

Clinical Presentation
In a recent study of 91 adult patients undergoing MCL reconstructions, one third could not recall an acute injury. Throwing athletes with a chronic injury have episodic medial elbow pain. Patients with chronic MCL incompetence may develop ulnar neuritis over time; this neuritis may be accompanied by ulnar nerve irritability and/or posterior elbow pain caused by olecranon impingement. The throwing athlete with an acute injury usually admits to a prodromal moment of seemingly innocuous medial pain. The next episode usually is accompanied by a pop, and further hard throwing is impossible. Patients with acute MCL tears often have ecchymosis at or just distal to the medial joint line within 2 days of injury. Evaluation of the throwing athlete with medial elbow pain should consist of a complete history, including the duration of symptoms; the phase of throwing during which pain occurs (most MCL injuries will cause pain during the acceleration phase); the location of pain (possible choices include the medial epicondyle, the area between the epicondyle and sublime tubercle, over the ulnar nerve, the sublime tubercle, or the posterior olecranon); whether ulnar nerve symptoms are present and, if so, during what activities and how often; and whether the athlete can throw at normal velocity. A source of confusion is the fact that many athletes will be able to throw in a modified fashion despite an injured MCL. The examiner should test for the reproduction of symptoms during resisted forearm pronation.

The valgus stress test is used to assess MCL stability (Fig. 2). This test is a difficult clinical maneuver that often is impossible to accomplish in large patients because the

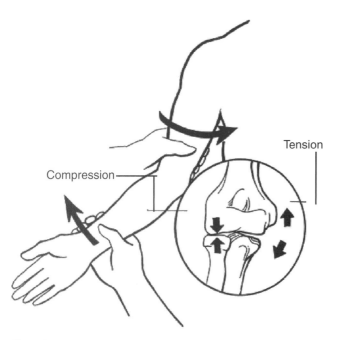

Figure 2 Valgus stress test. *(Reproduced with permission from Azar FM, Andrews JR, Wilk KE, Groh D: Operative treatment of ulnar collateral ligament injuries in the elbow in athletes. Am J Sports Med 2000;28:16-23.)*

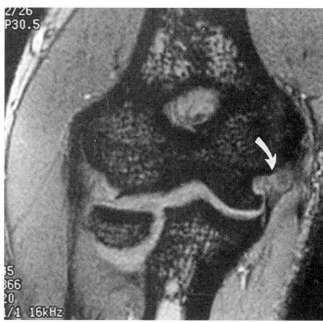

Figure 3 Coronal gradient-recalled MRI showing subacute MCL tear in a 24-year-old throwing athlete. Avulsion of the anterior bundle of the MCL (arrow) from the humeral origin is shown. *(Reproduced with permission from Potter HG: Imaging of posttraumatic and soft tissue dysfunction of the elbow. Clin Orthop 2000;370:9-18.)*

humerus must be stabilized, and it is difficult to stabilize the humerus at angles of elbow flexion greater than 30°. This test is performed with the patient in a sitting or supine position. The examiner uses one hand to provide a lateral post for the distal humerus and to control humeral rotation; with the opposite hand, the patient's forearm is maximally pronated and the elbow flexed, with a valgus force placed across the elbow. The test is positive for MCL injury when (1) the applied valgus stress reproduces symptoms of medial elbow pain, and (2) valgus laxity is greater than that of the contralateral elbow. The diagnosis is more likely to be confirmed by the first criterion than the second because the amount of abnormal laxity produced is often too small to be seen.

A provocative maneuver recently described in the literature, the moving valgus stress test, reproduces the patient's medial elbow pain and symptoms by rapidly extending the elbow from a starting position of full flexion while maintaining a constant valgus torque. The milking maneuver is also an effective test to evaluate patients with MCL insufficiency.

The final step of the physical examination is an extension test to detect whether posterior (olecranon) impingement is present. If the history and examination findings are suspicious for MCL injury, then radiographs and an MRI scan are performed.

Imaging

Radiographs of patients with MCL injuries are generally normal. Stress radiographs have historically been used to confirm the diagnosis of MCL laxity. Side-to-side differences of 0.5 mm obtained with a 150-N force applied to a 25° flexed elbow have been believed to be diagnostic of MCL laxity; however, recent studies show that this is not clinically significant and is difficult to interpret reliably. The following radiographic findings may be present in chronic MCL injuries: (1) calcifications in the MCL; (2) medial spurs on the humerus and ulna at the joint line, adjacent to the MCL; (3) spurs on the posterior olecranon tip, usually medial and occasionally fragmented; and (4) loose bodies in the olecranon fossa.

A CT arthrogram of an elbow with an MCL tear may reveal the classic T-sign consistent with undersurface tears that correspond with the anterior bundle of the MCL. MRI may be performed without contrast agents, using a 1.5 T scanner and an elbow coil with 3-mm coronal sections through the MCL. In addition to providing information about the ligament, MRI can reveal possible acute or chronic injury to the articular surfaces; the most common sites are the medial olecranon tip and underlying humeral trochlea (Fig. 3).

Reconstruction

The indication for reconstruction is medial elbow pain caused by incompetence of the MCL that prevents the athlete from throwing at his or her normal level. Surgical reconstruction of the MCL is reserved for those patients in whom a course of rehabilitation has failed and in whom evidence based on clinical history, physical examination, and imaging studies indicates that the MCL is the cause of symptoms. MCL reconstruction may be indicated for patients with either partial or complete ligament tears.

Surgical treatment of the torn MCL in a throwing athlete involves reconstruction with a tendon graft. Direct repair should be considered only in the presence of an acute traumatic avulsion, such as in weight lifters. Reconstruction of the MCL with a free tendon autograft is the most widely accepted surgical model today. This procedure is accomplished through transection of the flexor/pronator origin and includes routine transposition of the ulnar nerve. The current technique was developed in 1996. The goals were to perform a tendon graft reconstruction of the MCL in bone tunnels through a muscle-splitting safe zone approach without routinely transposing the ulnar nerve.

The arthroscope is introduced through a lateral portal into the anterior compartment. Diagnostic arthroscopy of the anterior compartment is used to evaluate the articular surfaces and the synovium and to identify loose bodies. If the diagnosis of MCL incompetence is still in doubt, an arthroscopic stress test may be performed. With the elbow at 90° of flexion, the forearm is in pronation and valgus stress is applied. In the normal elbow a maximum of 1 to 2 mm of medial opening will be observed. Greater than 3 mm of opening between the coronoid and the medial humerus will be observed if the MCL is incompetent.

Once the arthroscopy has been completed, the arm is released from the arm holder and placed on the hand table below it. An incision is created from the distal third of the intramuscular septum across the medial epicondyle to a point 2 cm beyond the sublime tubercle of the ulna. While exposing the fascia of the flexor pronator, care should be taken to identify and preserve the antebrachial cutaneous branch of the median nerve, which frequently crosses the surgical field. At this point MCL laxity can be confirmed by observing the separation of the joint surfaces by 3 mm or more with valgus stress.

The tunnel positions for the ulna are exposed (Fig. 4). The humeral tunnel position is located in the anterior half of the medial epicondyle in the anterior position of the existing MCL. The upper border of the epicondyle, just anterior to the intramuscular septum, is then exposed.

With the elbow reduced, the horizontal incision in the MCL is repaired using a No. 2-0 absorbable suture. The graft is then passed through the ulnar tunnel, generally from anterior to posterior. Final graft tensioning is performed by again placing the elbow through a full range of motion with varus stress placed on the elbow. Once the surgeon is satisfied with graft tension, the two sets of graft sutures are tied over the bony bridge on the humeral epicondyle (Fig. 5). Closure is performed by approximating the FCU fascia and subcutaneous and subcuticular closure. The elbow is then placed in a plaster splint at 60° of flexion.

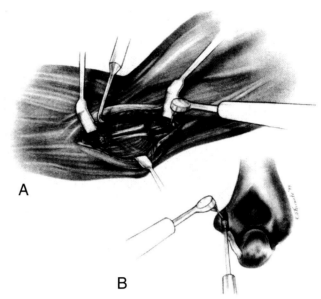

Figure 4 A, Creation of the ulnar tunnel using a curved curet to connect the ulnar holes. **B,** Creation of the single humeral tunnel using a burr and creation of the exit holes for the two suture bundles using the central burr. *(Reproduced with permission from Altchek DW, Hyman J, Williams R, et al: Management of MCL injuries of the elbow in throwers. Tech Should Elbow Surg 2000;1:73-81.)*

The most important potential complications are ulnar nerve injury, antebrachial cutaneous nerve injury, and fracture of the ulnar tunnel. If necessary, ulnar nerve transposition can be performed to avoid injury. The antebrachial cutaneous nerve should be identified and protected if a medial skin incision is used; the nerve is less at risk with a posterior incision. If the bridge of the ulnar tunnel is less than 1 cm, there is a risk of fracture. This risk can be minimized with proper exposure of the ulna and careful use of a small curette to connect the tunnels.

Postoperative Management
The elbow is first placed in a postoperative splint for 1 week. Then the sutures are removed, and the elbow is placed in a hinged brace. Initially, motion is allowed between 45° of extension and 90° of flexion. Over the following 5 weeks, motion is gradually advanced to full motion.

At this point, formal physiotherapy is begun. Any residual losses of elbow motion are corrected, and gradual strengthening of forearm and shoulder musculature is commenced. At 12 weeks, the strengthening program becomes more vigorous, and activities such as bench pressing light to moderate weights are allowed. At 4 months, the throwing program begins with short tossing. Generally, athletes do not throw in competitive situations until the ninth month.

Evaluation of Treatment
In a study of 56 patients who underwent MCL reconstruction, 68% (including 12 of 16 professional baseball

A
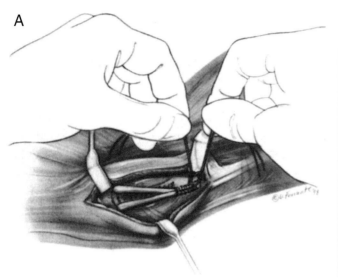

B
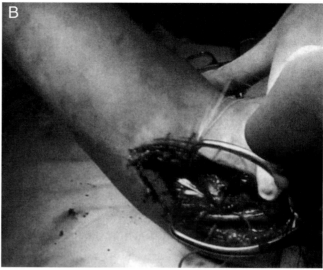

Figure 5 A, The anterior limb is passed into the humeral tunnel and the sutures from both limbs are tied over the bone bridge, securing the graft. **B,** Intraoperative photograph after completed reconstruction. *(Reproduced with permission from Altchek DW, Hyman J, Williams R, et al: Management of MCL injuries of the elbow in throwers. Tech Should Elbow Surg 2000;1:73-81.)*

players) had returned to their previous level of competition at a mean follow-up of 6.3 years. Because of a 21% incidence of ulnar nerve complications, the procedure has been modified to use a muscle-splitting approach without transposition of the nerve. In a recent study, the results of 78 MCL reconstructions and 13 MCL repairs, all with concomitant subcutaneous ulnar nerve transposition were reported. Seventy-four percent of these patients were available for follow-up; 79% of them returned to their previous level of competition. Ten patients in this group had preoperative ulnar nerve symptoms that resolved postoperatively in nine patients. It is conceivable that the lower incidence of ulnar nerve complications in this group was attributable to the subcutaneous transposition versus the submuscular transposition in the earlier study.

Valgus instability becomes clinically significant when there is a complete tear of the anterior bundle of the MCL; partial tears of the anterior bundle do not produce significant instability. Valgus instability was arthroscopically evaluated (via the anterolateral portal) using a serial cutting model in a cadaver study. Ulnohumeral joint opening could not be appreciated until the entire anterior bundle was sectioned. There was 1 to 2 mm of ulnohumeral joint opening present arthroscopically when a valgus force was placed on the elbow after the entire anterior bundle was sectioned. Complete sectioning of all bundles of the MCL complex yielded 4 to 10 mm of opening (Fig. 6). The greatest degree of ulnohumeral joint opening was found between 60° and 75° of elbow flexion with forearm pronation.

The "safe zone" for MCL exposure through an FCU muscle-splitting incision has been described. This study demonstrated that enough exposure could be obtained

through this muscle split and that MCL reconstruction could be performed without ulnar nerve transposition or flexor pronator muscle takedown. This technique was further augmented in 1995 with the use of suture anchors. Unfortunately, one third of the patients had a poor outcome because of an inability to tension the graft and suboptimal healing of the reconstruction to a suture anchor.

Ulnar Neuropathy

The ulnar nerve plays a distinct role in elbow problems of the throwing athlete. Ulnar neuropathy can occur secondary to many of the common pathologic conditions on the medial side of the elbow. Sources of injury to the ulnar nerve have been divided into three basic groups: compression, friction, and traction.

Compression neuropathy can develop secondary to space-occupying lesions such as bony spurs, scar tissue, thickening of the arcuate ligament, calcifications of the MCL, or hypertrophy of the medial head of the triceps. The path of the ulnar nerve about the elbow places it at risk for compression at several anatomic sites. These include the arcade of Struthers, the medial intermuscular septum, the cubital tunnel itself, the fascial origin of the flexor digitorum superficialis, and the confluence of the two heads of the FCU.

Friction neuropathy includes those insults associated with variable amounts of subluxation or dislocation of the ulnar nerve over the medial epicondyle. Instability of the ulnar nerve has been estimated to occur frequently (at a rate of 16%) within the general population. Most studies of MCL reconstructions in the literature report a

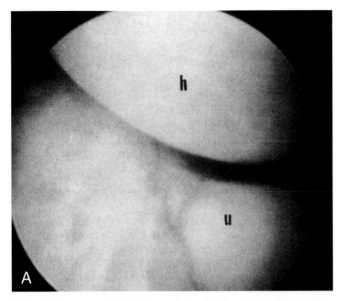
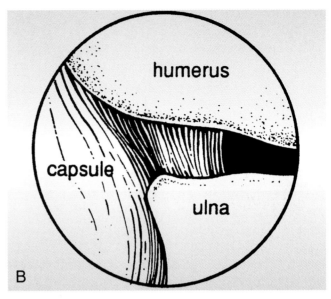

Figure 6 Complete sectioning of the anterior bundle allowed for ulnohumeral joint opening. **A,** 1 mm of articular opening is seen between the humerus (h) and the ulna (u) when viewed through the anterolateral portal. **B,** An illustration demonstrating medial joint line opening after the anterior bundle is completely sectioned. *(Reproduced with permission from Field LD, Altchek DW: Evaluation of the arthroscopic valgus instability test of the elbow. Am J Sports Med 1996;24:177-181.)*

significant number of patients with preoperative ulnar nerve symptoms. One study has reported 40% of throwing athletes with symptoms of ulnar nerve entrapment.

Clinical Presentation

The athlete with ulnar neuropathy typically will have numbness and tingling in the fourth and fifth fingers associated with medial elbow pain that radiates distally. Specific historic features include snapping at the medial elbow (which is indicative of a subluxating nerve), at the medial head of the triceps, or both.

Physical examination findings often include a positive Tinel's sign over the cubital tunnel or the two heads of the FCU. Neuromuscular weakness and sensory loss usually are not prominent features. Reproduction of symptoms with maximal elbow flexion and wrist extension (the elbow flexion test) can be helpful. Careful observation of and gentle palpation over the epicondylar groove during flexion and extension should help identify subluxation of the nerve or triceps. Several recent reports have described subluxation of the medial head of the triceps as more common than previously believed. Examination findings will typically consist of two palpable snaps when triceps subluxation is occurring in conjunction with ulnar nerve subluxation. In such instances, the ulnar nerve typically dislocates at 90° of flexion, while the medial head of the triceps dislocates at approximately 110°.

Treatment

Athletes with isolated ulnar neuropathy should be treated nonsurgically initially. However, results of non-surgical treatment are not as good in throwing athletes as in the general population, and surgical treatment is usually necessary.

The literature on surgical treatment of ulnar neuropathy shows comparable results in the general population regardless of the technique used. Decompression alone should be reserved for mild injuries in which clear evidence of an offending compressive lesion is present. Transposition is performed in more severe compression in which there is nerve instability.

Anterior Elbow Pain

Anterior elbow pain is most often the result of stretching or tearing of the anterior capsule, the distal biceps, or the brachialis muscles. This clinical picture may be seen after a posterior elbow dislocation or after a fall on an arm locked in extension and subsequently forced into hyperextension. Climbers frequently sustain pulls of the brachialis insertion because of the repetitive pulling involved in the sport.

Pronator Teres Syndrome

Diffuse anterior elbow pain that radiates distally into the forearm may be the result of median nerve entrapment, also known as pronator teres syndrome. The median nerve is compressed between the two heads of the pronator teres. Compression of the median nerve underneath the lacertus fibrosus or by the ligament of Struthers may produce a similar clinical picture and always should be included in the differential diagnosis. Cervical radiculopathy at the C6-7 level also may mimic pronator teres syndrome and should be included in the differential diagnosis.

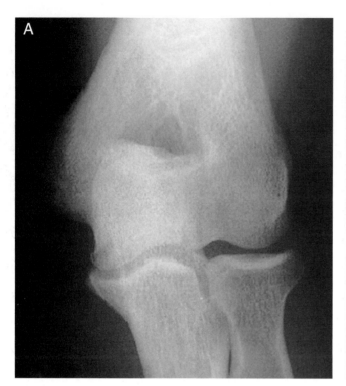
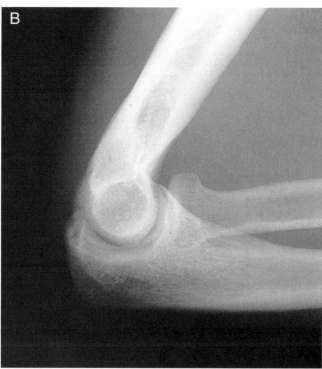

Figure 7 A, AP radiograph of the elbow of a baseball pitcher demonstrating posteromedial impingement and chondromalacia at the olecranon. Note medial spurs at the ulnohumeral joint. **B,** Lateral radiograph demonstrating chondromalacia at the proximal pole of the olecranon in a baseball pitcher with posteromedial impingement. *(Reproduced with permission from DiGiovine NM, Jobe FW, Pink M, et al: Electromyographic analysis of the upper extremity in pitching. J Shoulder Elbow Surg 1992;1: 15-25.)*

Symptoms may include paresthesias with or without a sustained decrease in sensation in the median nerve distribution distally. Thenar muscles are weak, but muscles of the anterior interosseous nerve (flexor pollicis longus, flexor digitorum profundus, and pronator quadratus) may be spared. Phalen's test and the carpal tunnel test will be negative in these patients. Electromyographic evaluation may not be diagnostic despite clinical supporting evidence, but it may become positive 4 to 6 weeks after the onset of median nerve entrapment. If nonsurgical measures including activity modification fail to alleviate the patient's symptoms, surgical release of the humeral head of the pronator teres and the superficialis bridge is indicated.

Distal Biceps Injuries

Avulsion injuries or tears of the distal biceps insertion into the radial tuberosity have received much attention in recent years. These injuries are the result of a sudden overload to the elbow when in midflexion. The diagnosis should be suspected based on the history, which often includes ecchymosis in the antecubital fossa a few days after the injury. Physical examination reveals pain and weakness on resisted supination and, to a lesser extent, flexion. The tendon is not palpable, although the bicipital aponeurosis can be if it is intact. MRI can be diagnostic.

The tendon should be repaired in young, healthy patients who perform manual labor as a vocation or who are active in sports. The distal biceps can be repaired through a two-incision muscle-splitting approach or a one-incision technique.

Posterior Elbow Pain

Posterior elbow pain is less common than lateral or medial elbow pain and is often a secondary effect of medial-sided instability. Posterior elbow pain in the pediatric population frequently is attributed to triceps apophysitis, which is an injury through the physeal plate. This injury, similar to Osgood-Schlatter disease, is the result of repetitive overload. Patients with triceps apophysitis have pain on resisted extension of the elbow. Patients with chronic pain may develop a large separation at the olecranon ossification center that is bridged by a fibrous rather than a bony union. These patients frequently require open reduction and internal fixation with autologous bone grafting to obtain bony union of the olecranon.

Posteromedial Impingement/Valgus Extension Overload Syndrome

Although posteromedial impingement is a clinical characteristic of posterior elbow pain, it is the result of chronic valgus overload that attenuates the MCL. Posteromedial

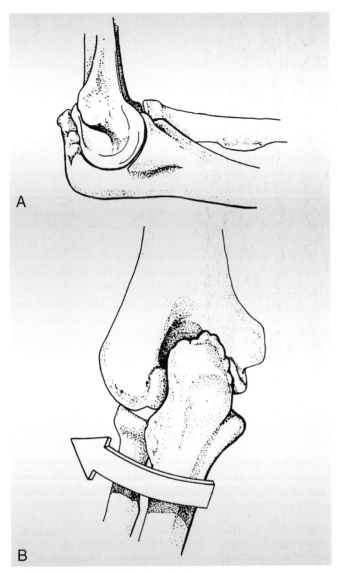

Figure 8 Posterior medial impingement. **A,** Lateral view of the elbow shows medial olecranon osteophytes with impingement along the humeral medial trochlear groove. **B,** Posterior view of the elbow showing the extent of posterior and posteromedial osteophytes as the elbow impinges into the olecranon fossa. Arrow indicates direction of dynamic stress generated in valgus extension overload syndrome and the resulting impingement of the olecranon process in olecranon fossa. *(Reproduced with permission from Wilson FD, Andrews JR, Blackburn TA, McCluskey G: Valgus extension overload in the pitching elbow. Am J Sports Med 1983;11:83-88.)*

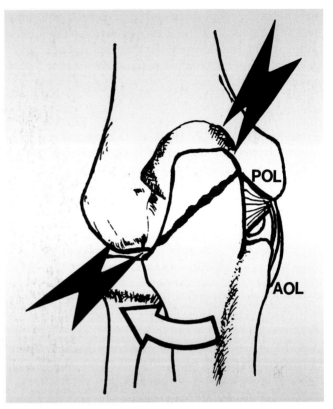

Figure 9 Pathomechanics of an oblique-type olecranon stress fracture. Illustration of posterior elbow showing impaction of olecranon into olecranon fossa and coronoid process in intercondylar notch (black arrows) to resist valgus stress (open arrow) during acceleration phase of pitching. AOL, anterior oblique band of MCL; POL, posterior oblique band of MCL. *(Reproduced with permission from Suzuki K, Minami A, Suenaga N, Kondoh M: Oblique stress fractures of the olecranon in baseball pitchers. J Shoulder Elbow Surg 1997;6:491-494.)*

impingement frequently is categorized as a medial elbow problem. It has been pointed out that valgus extension injuries can be thought of as either medial tension or lateral compression injuries along a continuum. These injuries are common in throwing athletes. Patients have pain in the elbow posteriorly with full extension; the pain worsens when a valgus load is applied to the joint. Posteromedial impingement may have the same clinical appearance as triceps tendinitis. Posteromedial impingement is confirmed using the valgus stress test.

An evaluation of professional pitchers found that chronic valgus attenuation produces valgus subluxation of the elbow during throwing, which can lead to both medial and lateral changes. This recurrent medial valgus load leads to lateral compression at the radiocapitellar joint that, in turn, can lead to chondromalacia and lesions of the capitellum. Fragmentation of osteochondral lesions of the capitellum produces loose bodies similar to those seen in osteochondritis dissecans. It has been reported that bony lesions also could be seen, specifically at the posteromedial olecranon (Fig. 7). Results from other studies noted that the space of the olecranon fossa in pitchers is compromised by both this hypertrophied humerus and chronic valgus angulation from the pitching motion. In these patients, the posteromedial olecranon impinges on the trochlea as the arm is brought into extension. This repetitive event is believed to produce chondromalacia, secondary osteophyte formation, and, potentially, loose bodies at the posteromedial olecranon (Fig. 8).

A nonsurgical treatment plan for patients with valgus extension injuries of the elbow has been outlined thoroughly. The two primary goals of this program are to achieve relief of pain and inflammation and to increase strength of the elbow with attention to forearm musculature. An elegant electromyographic evaluation of pitchers with MCL injuries demonstrated that a counterintuitive firing pattern of the flexor-pronator muscle mass occurs during the throwing motion. Thus, specific physical therapy programs are needed to strengthen the flexor-pronator muscles.

Stress Fractures

Stress fractures about the elbow are rare injuries most commonly seen in throwing athletes in the middle third of the olecranon. Stress fractures involving the olecranon are different than olecranon tip fractures, which are isolated to the proximal third of the olecranon. Much of the original information regarding olecranon stress fractures was gathered from observations of javelin throwers. The sudden and forceful hyperextension moment at the end of the javelin throw was believed to create a scenario in which the tip of the olecranon was forced into the olecranon fossa. Stress fractures of the olecranon now are believed to be the result of triceps overload. There has been debate as to whether olecranon tip fractures and stress fractures are the same entity, but it appears that they are distinct diagnoses. Clinically, tip fractures are more often the result of a sudden forceful throw, whereas the etiology of stress fractures is more insidious. Also, stress fractures are associated with posterior elbow pain over a longer period.

Stress fractures frequently are not evident on plain films, but the diagnosis can be confirmed with nuclear or CT imaging studies. Radiographically, the stress fracture may be transverse or oblique. Transverse olecranon stress fractures occur through the physis and frequently are seen in adolescents. These fractures are believed to occur as a result of direct triceps overload. Oblique stress fractures are believed to be the result of a valgus extension overload mechanism that causes repeated posteromedial impingement (Fig. 9). Athletes with olecranon stress fractures also may have an element of medial-sided instability that has contributed to their posterior elbow pain. The clinical examination should determine which phase of throwing produces the patient's symptoms. The milking maneuver is helpful in differentiating between olecranon and MCL pathology.

Nonsurgical treatment usually is effective in treating stress fractures, but surgical intervention may be indicated if immobilization fails to achieve bony union. Olecranon stress fractures must be observed serially during nonsurgical treatment because displacement requiring surgical fixation may occur.

Annotated Bibliography

Lateral Elbow Pain

Boyer MI, Hastings H II: Lateral tennis elbow: "Is there any science out there?" *J Shoulder Elbow Surg* 1999; 8:481-491.

This thorough review of the literature on the diagnosis and treatment of lateral epicondylitis indicates that there is a paucity of peer-reviewed published data of acceptable scientific quality and that there are many myths surrounding this common clinical syndrome. It provides a sound pathoetiology of the condition as well as a review and discussion of treatment modalities.

Field LD, Savoie FH: Common elbow injuries in sport. *Sports Med* 1998;26:193-205.

Elbow injuries are becoming more common in athletes who participate in sports that involve overhead arm motions. The authors reported on lateral epicondylitis, which occurs in more than 50% of athletes who use overhead motions, as well as on medial epicondylitis, which often occurs in golfers and tennis players. They state that nonsurgical treatment should be attempted first, followed by surgery if the patient does not respond to an extensive nonsurgical program.

Grundberg AB, Dobson JF: Percutaneous release of the common extensor origin for tennis elbow. *Clin Orthop* 2000;376:137-140.

This study examined 32 elbows (30 patients) with surgical intervention for tennis elbow. A percutaneous incision was made just distal to the lateral epicondyle, and the common extensor origin was released. Twenty-nine elbows had good or excellent results at a follow-up of 6 to 61 months (average, 26 months).

Kiyoshige Y, Takagi M, Yuasa K, Hamasaki M: Closed-wedge osteotomy for osteochondritis dissecans of the capitellum: A 7- to 12-year follow-up. *Am J Sports Med* 2000;28:534-537.

This article presents a 7- to 12-year follow-up of seven young baseball players diagnosed with osteochondritis dissecans of the capitellum. After surgical treatment with a closed-wedge osteotomy, six patients were able to return to their preinjury level of activity. There was minimal osteoarthritic change on radiographic examination and the treatment was recommended as useful for osteochondritis dissecans of the capitellum.

Kraushaar BS, Nirschl RP: Tendinosis of the elbow (tennis elbow): Clinical features and findings of histological, immunohistochemical, and electron microscopy studies. *J Bone Joint Surg Am* 1999;81:259-278.

This excellent review of lateral epicondylitis pathogenesis includes histologic, immunologic, and electron microscopic studies as well as clinical correlations and treatment options.

Kuklo TR, Taylor KF, Murphy KP, Islinger RB, Heekin RD, Baker CL Jr: Arthroscopic release for lateral epicondylitis: A cadaveric model. *Arthroscopy* 1999;3:259-264.

This study was designed to assess the safety and efficacy of an arthroscopic approach to release of the ECRB tendon. Ten fresh frozen cadaveric upper limbs were operated on with either a 2.7-mm or a 4.0-mm 30° arthroscope. Subsequently, the elbow was dissected with the arthroscope still in place to determine the distances to the neurovascular structures of the elbow. This intervention appeared to be a safe, reliable, and reproducible procedure for refractory lateral epicondylitis.

Peterson RK, Savoie FH III, Field LD: Osteochondritis dissecans of the elbow. *Instr Course Lect* 1999;48:393-398.

This is an excellent and comprehensive review of the topic.

Ruch DS, Cory JW, Poehling GG: The arthroscopic management of osteochondritis dissecans of the adolescent elbow. *Arthroscopy* 1998;14:797-803.

This is a retrospective analysis of 12 adolescents who underwent arthroscopic débridement alone followed by early range of motion. Follow-up at an average of 3.2 years indicated that average flexion contracture improved from 23° preoperatively to 10° postoperatively. Eleven patients had minimal mechanical symptoms postoperatively and were highly satisfied.

Takahara M, Ogino T, Sasaki I, Kato H, Minami A, Kaneda K: Long term outcome of osteochondritis dissecans of the humeral capitellum. *Clin Orthop* 1999; 363:108-115.

The long-term outcome of osteochondritis dissecans of the capitellum was examined in 53 patients. Seven of 14 patients treated nonsurgically and 18 of 39 patients treated by surgical removal of the loose fragment were found to have poor outcomes and residual elbow symptoms associated with activities of daily living. These outcomes may be the result of advanced lesions, osteoarthritis, and a large osteochondral defect.

Medial Elbow Pain

Azar FM, Andrews JR, Wilk KE, Groh D: Operative treatment of ulnar collateral ligament injuries of the elbow in athletes. *Am J Sports Med* 2000;28:16-23.

Ninety-one males between the ages of 15 and 39 years underwent a subcutaneous ulnar nerve transposition with stabilization of the nerve via fascial slings of the flexor pronator mass. This intervention was determined to be an effective treatment, with most athletes returning to their preinjury level of activity in less than 1 year.

Callaway GH, Field LD, Deng XH, et al: Biomechanical evaluation of the medial collateral ligament of the elbow. *J Bone Joint Surg Am* 1997;79:1223-1231.

This study evaluated the biomechanical and anatomic constraints of the MCL of the elbow under valgus stresses. It was found that the anterior band of the anterior bundle of the MCL was the primary constraint to valgus rotation at 30°, 60°, and 90° of elbow flexion. At 120° of flexion the anterior and posterior bands of the anterior bundle were primary corestraints. The posterior bundle was found to be a secondary constraint at 30° only. The clinical relevance is discussed with special attention to mechanism of injury and treatment implications.

Eygendaal D, Olsen BS, Jensen SL, Seki A, Sojbjerg JO: Kinematics of partial and total ruptures of the medial collateral ligament of the elbow. *J Shoulder Elbow Surg* 1999;8:612-616.

Angular displacement, increases in medial joint opening, and translation of the humeral head were identified and quantified in eight cadaveric elbows with respect to varying degrees of flexion. It was found that valgus instability should be evaluated at 70° to 90° of elbow flexion and that partial ruptures of the anterior bundle of the MCL could not be accurately evaluated based on medial joint opening.

Field LD, Altchek DW: Evaluation of the arthroscopic valgus instability test of the elbow. *Am J Sports Med* 1996;24:177-181.

In this study, seven fresh-frozen cadaveric elbows were used to establish a relationship between the extent of MCL injury and arthroscopic evidence of valgus instability, the amount of humeral joint opening, and the elbow position that maximizes visualization of this opening. It was found that the entire anterior bundle of the MCL must be sectioned before a measurable and reproducible medial joint opening can occur.

Hamilton CD, Glousman RE, Jobe FW, Brault J, Pink M, Perry J: Dynamic stability of the elbow: Electromyographic analysis of the flexor pronator group and the extensor group in pitchers with valgus instability. *J Shoulder Elbow Surg* 1996;5:347-354.

The authors examined the relative contributions of eight muscles surrounding the elbow, including the flexor pronator and extensor groups. They studied 26 pitchers with MCL insufficiency using high-speed cinematography and electromyography and compared them to uninjured pitchers. They found that the muscles on the medial side of the elbow do not assume the role of the MCL during the fastball pitch.

Miller TT: Imaging of elbow disorders. *Orthop Clin North Am* 1999;30:21-36.

This article presents an excellent discussion of the different imaging modalities (radiography, MRI, CT, and sonography) and their respective roles in evaluating elbow abnormalities.

O'Driscoll SW: Classification and evaluation of recurrent instability of the elbow. *Clin Orthop* 2000;370:34-43.

This article is an excellent review of the classification of elbow instability. In addition, it presents a thorough evaluation of the different tests used to assess elbow instability.

Potter HG: Imaging of posttraumatic and soft tissue dysfunction of the elbow. *Clin Orthop* 2000;370:9-18.

This article discusses the current problems and challenges facing a radiologist when identifying elbow pathologies. A thorough evaluation is presented on radiographs, MRI with and without contrast, CT imaging with three-dimensional reformations, and ultrasound.

Smith GR, Altchek DW, Pagnani MJ, Keeley JR: A muscle-splitting approach to the ulnar collateral ligament of the elbow: Neuroanatomy and operative technique. *Am J Sports Med* 1996;24:575-580.

The authors presented a more limited muscle-splitting approach to repair or reconstruction of the ulnar collateral ligament of the elbow than the standard lifting off of the tendon of the common flexor bundle at its origin on the medial epicondyle. They stated that the muscle-splitting approach is less traumatic and affords a safe and simple approach.

Timmerman LA, Schwartz ML, Andrews JR: Preoperative evaluation of the ulnar collateral ligament by magnetic resonance imaging and computed tomography arthrography: Evaluation in 25 baseball players with surgical confirmation. *Am J Sports Med* 1994;22:26-32.

This study evaluated 25 patients with medial elbow pain and found that MRI and CT were accurate in the detection of complete MCL tears. For partial MCL tears, the sensitivity and specificity of MRI were 57% and 100%, respectively. The sensitivity and specificity for CT arthrography of partial MCL tears were 86% and 91%, respectively. Five of seven patients who underwent CT arthrography had a T-sign consistent with an undersurface tear of the MCL.

Ulnar Neuropathy

Ciccotti MG, Jobe FW: Medial collateral ligament instability and ulnar neuritis in the athlete's elbow. *Instr Course Lect* 1999;48:383-391.

The authors review both MCL injuries and ulnar neuropathy, presenting a well-organized approach to diagnosis and treatment. Treatment recommendations are based on the authors' experiences.

Posner MA: Compressive neuropathies of the ulnar nerve at the elbow and wrist. *Instr Course Lect* 2000;49:305-317.

This excellent review of ulnar neuropathy presents the pathophysiology, diagnosis, treatment options, and results currently represented in the literature.

Spinner RJ, Goldner RD: Snapping of the medial head of the triceps and recurrent dislocation of the ulnar nerve: Anatomical and dynamic factors. *J Bone Joint Surg Am* 1998;80:239-247.

This article presents 17 patients with snapping of the medial head of the triceps as well as ulnar nerve instability. The pathomechanics and diagnostic pitfalls are well described. Most patients were managed surgically with good results.

Posterior Elbow Pain

Moskal MJ, Savoie FH III, Field LD: Arthroscopic treatment of posterior elbow impingement. *Instr Course Lect* 1999;48:399-404.

The authors summarize the nature of posterior elbow impingement and its evaluation, nonsurgical management, surgical techniques, and rehabilitation. Results were predominantly positive, and the authors concluded that this procedure, although technically challenging, is particularly valuable because of increased visualization and decreased soft-tissue trauma.

Suzuki K, Minami A, Suenaga N, Kondoh M: Oblique stress fracture of the olecranon in baseball pitchers. *J Shoulder Elbow Surg* 1997;6:491-494.

This article presents two case reports of olecrenon stress fractures with oblique fracture lines. The pathomechanics of this type of injury and its association with pitching in adolescent athletes are discussed.

Functional Anatomy and Biomechanics

DaSilva MF, Williams JS, Fadale PD, Hulstyn MJ, Ehrlich MG: Pediatric throwing injuries about the elbow. *Am J Orthop* 1998;27:90-96.

This article presents an excellent review of the anatomy and biomechanics during throwing of the elbow joint. It also discusses the diagnosis, treatment, rehabilitation, and prevention of pediatric throwing injuries of the elbow in contrast to adult injuries.

Maloney MD, Mohr KJ, el Attrache NS: Elbow injuries in the throwing athlete: Difficult diagnoses and surgical complications. *Clin Sports Med* 1999;18:795-809.

This article provides an excellent discussion of the challenges presented to accurate diagnosis and effective management of the injured elbow in throwing athletes. Anatomy, biomechanics, and a myriad of conditions that affect the elbow of the throwing athlete are reviewed, as well as the potential complications associated with surgical management.

Rettig AC: Elbow, forearm and wrist injuries in the athlete. *Sports Med* 1998;25:115-130.

This article is an excellent overview of the wide variety of soft-tissue, bone, tendon, ligament, and nerve injuries sustained by athletes in the elbow, forearm, and wrist in their respective competitive activities.

Classic Bibliography

Andrews JR, Timmerman LA: Outcome of elbow surgery in professional baseball players. *Am J Sports Med* 1995;23:407-413.

Bauer M, Jonsson K, Josefsson PO, Linden B: Osteochondritis dissecans of the elbow: A long-term follow-up study. *Clin Orthop* 1992;284:156-160.

Conway JE, Jobe FW, Glousman RE, Pink M: Medial instability of the elbow in throwing athletes: Treatment by repair or reconstruction of the ulnar collateral ligament. *J Bone Joint Surg Am* 1992;74:67-83.

Field LD, Callaway GH, O'Brien SJ, Altchek DW: Arthroscopic assessment of the medial collateral ligament complex of the elbow. *Am J Sports Med* 1995;23:396-400.

Glousman RE, Barron J, Jobe FW, Perry J, Pink M: An electromyographic analysis of the elbow in normal and injured pitchers with medial collateral ligament insufficiency. *Am J Sports Med* 1992;20:311-317.

Miller CD, Jobe CM, Wright MH: Neuroanatomy in elbow arthroscopy. *J Shoulder Elbow Surg* 1995;4:168-174.

Miller CD, Savoie FH III: Valgus extension injuries of the elbow in the throwing athlete. *J Am Acad Orthop Surg* 1994;2:261-269.

Nuber GW, Diment MT: Olecranon stress fractures in throwers: A report of two cases and a review of the literature. *Clin Orthop* 1992;278:58-61.

Chapter 30

Acute, Recurrent, and Chronic Elbow Instabilities

Shawn W. O'Driscoll, PhD, MD

Elbow instability has received much attention in the past few years, principally because its etiology and diagnosis are so much better understood. The mechanism by which an elbow dislocates has been clarified, and the relationship between the bony and soft-tissue constraints is also becoming clearer.

Key advances have occurred in the following areas: understanding of the mechanism of acute dislocations, reduction of a dislocated elbow, diagnosing recurrent elbow instability, biomechanics of the coronoid in fracture-dislocations, radial head replacement, and diagnosing chronic valgus instability.

Constraints to Elbow Instability

It is helpful to consider the static constraints of the elbow as a fortress resisting breakdown, with three primary constraints: the ulnohumeral articulation, medial collateral ligament (MCL), and lateral collateral ligament (LCL), especially the ulnar portion or the lateral ulnar collateral ligament (LUCL) (Fig. 1). Secondary constraints include the radial head, common flexor and extensor origins, and the capsule. Muscles that cross the elbow joint and produce compressive forces at the articulation are dynamic stabilizers.

A stable elbow is one in which the three primary constraints are intact. If the coronoid is fractured or lost, the radial head becomes a critical stabilizer. Therefore, the radial head must not be removed from dislocated elbows in which the coronoid is fractured unless secure fixation of the coronoid and ligaments can be achieved. The LCL is the primary constraint to posterolateral rotatory instability. One cadaver study showed that division of the ulnar part of the LCL near its origin, but not its insertion, resulted in this instability pattern.

Acute Elbow Instability

The three different patterns of acute instability of the elbow are posterolateral rotatory, valgus, and varus-

posteromedial rotatory. Posterolateral rotatory instability is the most common type and typically presents as a dislocation, a fracture-dislocation, or a fracture-subluxation. Acute subluxations without fracture often go undiagnosed. The only evidence that such an episode of instability has occurred might be the radiographic presence of a small flake fracture involving just the tip of the coronoid. These injuries occur from shearing of the coronoid beneath the trochlea as a result of posterolateral rotatory subluxation and can be considered analogous to the bony Bankart lesion from traumatic anterior instability of the shoulder. However, an isolated coronoid fracture that involves more than approximately 2 mm of the coronoid is cause for concern. This type of fracture likely represents varus-posteromedial rotatory instability, which appears to have a strong propensity to premature posttraumatic arthritis.

Acute valgus instability can occur after a traumatic event or as a culmination of long-standing chronic valgus overload. Traumatic valgus instability implies rupture of the MCL and, usually, a fracture of the radial head. It is a distinct problem, separate from dislocation. If the radial head is excised, the elbow is at high risk of remaining permanently unstable in valgus. Acute rupture of the MCL can occur in overhead athletes such as baseball pitchers but is usually the culmination of chronic valgus overload.

Finally, varus-posteromedial rotatory instability has been recognized only recently. A corollary of posterolateral rotatory instability, it occurs during axial loading of the elbow in flexion. The combination of varus and internal rotation moments during axial loading of the flexed elbow produces a fracture of the anteromedial coronoid and disruption (usually avulsion) of the LCL. The coronoid fracture may be large and comminuted or small and involving only the segment between the tip and sublime tubercle. The significance of this injury is that it results in ulnohumeral joint incongruity, which can lead to premature posttraumatic arthritis.

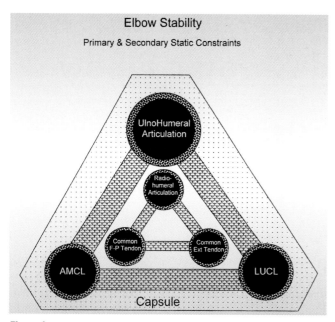

Figure 1 The static and dynamic constraints can be thought of as analogous to the defenses of a fortress. There are three primary static constraints to elbow instability: the ulnohumeral articulation, the anterior medial collateral ligament (AMCL), and the LCL, especially the LUCL. The secondary constraints include the radial head, common flexor and extensor tendon origins, and the capsule. Dynamic stabilizers include the muscles that cross the elbow joint and produce compressive forces at the articulation. *(Reproduced with permission from the Mayo Foundation, Rochester, MN.)*

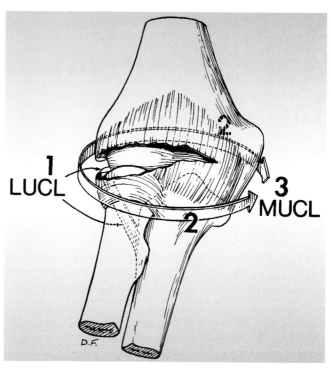

Figure 2 Soft-tissue injury progresses in a circle from lateral to medial in three stages. MUCL = medial ulnar collateral ligament.*(Reproduced with permission from O'Driscoll SW, Morrey BF, Korinek S, An KN: Elbow subluxation and dislocation. Clin Orthop 1992;280:186-197.)*

Etiology and Mechanism of Elbow Dislocation and Fracture-Dislocation

Simple dislocations (dislocations without fractures) typically result from falls on the outstretched hand and often occur during sports participation. Fracture-dislocations may occur from falls or from going over the handlebars of a bicycle or snowmobile, but most commonly occur during motor vehicle accidents. There are essentially two distinct mechanisms for these dislocations and fracture-dislocations. Most commonly the elbow displaces in posterolateral rotation. As the body approaches the ground, the elbow extends to place the hand on the ground. Elbow flexion begins immediately after contact with the ground, resulting in eccentric loading of the triceps, principally the medial head, which produces an external rotation moment at the ulnohumeral joint. Contraction of the adductors and internal rotators of the abducted shoulder causes internal rotation of the humerus against the forearm and hand, which are stabilized by the ground. As the body rotates internally with respect to the hand (the forearm rotates externally on the humerus), more internal rotation torque develops. When the mechanical axis is medial to the elbow, a valgus moment results. This clinical mechanism has been reproduced in cadaver elbows and has been captured by video analysis of actual elbow dislocations.

This pattern of dislocation is associated with a progressive soft-tissue (and/or bony) disruption that starts laterally and progresses around anteriorly and posteriorly to the medial side in a circle of disruption termed the "Horii circle" (Fig. 2). There are three stages in which the pathology correlates with the degrees of instability, and these have been confirmed experimentally (Table 1). The final stage is subdivided according to whether part or all of the MCL and the common flexor/pronator origin are disrupted.

In most cases, the elbow dislocates instead of fractures because the coronoid and radial head are rotated away from the distal humerus before sufficient axial load occurs to cause a fracture. Understanding this concept is key to understanding how the different patterns of fracture-dislocations fit into the overall mechanism of elbow dislocations. If the coronoid and radial head fail to rotate sufficiently away from the trochlea and capitellum (ie, into external rotation and valgus position), the tip of the coronoid and possibly the margin of the radial head will be fractured, an injury otherwise known as the terrible triad.

A second mechanism is responsible for fracture-subluxations and fracture-dislocations that apparently has not been recognized until just recently but is of great importance. Varus-posteromedial rotation injuries, which occur during flexion of the axially loaded elbow, cause disruption of the LCL and fracture of the anteromedial coronoid. The key to considering this diagnosis is recog-

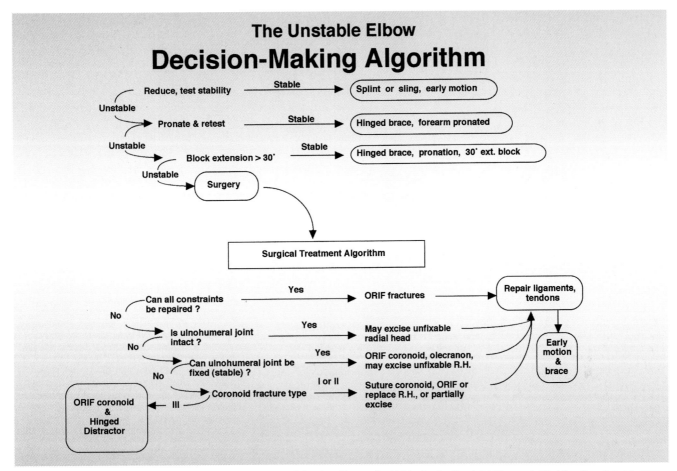

Figure 3 Decision-making algorithm for acute dislocations and fracture-dislocations. The term "stable" implies functional stability, meaning that the elbow does not apparently subluxate in the functional arc of motion and appears reduced on plain radiographs. ORIF, open reduction and internal fixation; RH, radial head. *(Reproduced with permission from the Mayo Foundation, Rochester, MN.)*

nition of the isolated coronoid fracture; for example, a coronoid fracture without a radial head fracture (especially in the absence of apparent dislocation). This injury may appear benign, but has a predisposition to rapid posttraumatic arthritis because of the persistent slight incongruity of the medial ulnohumeral joint.

Evaluation

Acute Elbow Dislocations

The elbow must be evaluated for stability after reduction of the dislocation. A decision-making algorithm approach has been proposed both for indications for surgery and for treatment options during surgery (Fig. 3). The elbow is gently moved through a range of motion in order to assess instability. If the elbow appears to subluxate or dislocate, it is placed in a splint or sling for 3 to 7 days and repeat AP and lateral radiographs are obtained. If the elbow subluxates or dislocates in extension or is incongruent on the radiograph, it should be placed in pronation and reassessed. If stability is restored, a hinged brace or cast brace with the forearm in full pronation is applied. An

TABLE 1	Stages of Soft-Tissue Disruption

Stage 1   Disruption of the LUCL

Stage 2   Disruption of the other lateral ligamentous structures and the anterior and posterior capsule

Stage 3   Disruption of the medial portion of the LCL (MUCL)

   3A   Partial MUCL disruption

   3B   Complete MUCL disruption

   3C   Distal humerus stripped of soft tissues
         Severe instability results in dislocation or subluxation

extension block of 30° is sometimes necessary. If the elbow requires an extension block of more than 30° to 45°, surgery should be considered. Extension blocks should be eased gradually, so that the brace permits full motion after 3 weeks. At each follow-up examination, the elbow should be reevaluated in exactly the same manner.

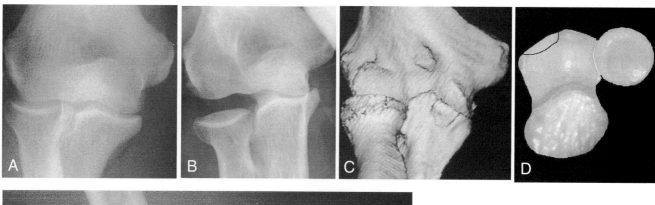

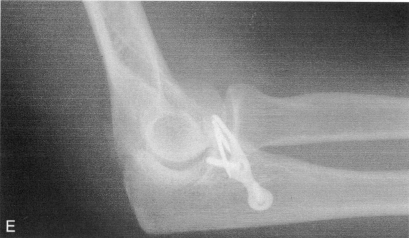

Figure 4 Varus-posteromedial rotatory instability involves an anteromedial coronoid fracture and disruption of the LCL. It may be subtle (A), but stress radiographs reveal varus opening and what appears to be medial narrowing (B). This latter finding is due to rotatory ulnohumeral subluxation, in which the medial trochlea subluxates anteriorly onto the coronoid fracture surface, giving the impression of narrowed joint space (wedge sign). CT scan with three-dimensional reconstruction reveals the anteromedial location of the fracture (C), which is illustrated schematically (D). These fractures require anatomic reduction and rigid fixation (E), and the LCL must be repaired. (Reproduced with permission from the Mayo Foundation, Rochester, MN.)

The elbow should be carefully studied radiographically before and after reduction to rule out subtle fractures of the coronoid and radial head in particular. Impaction fractures of the posterior (nonarticular) surface of the capitellum occur as a result of posterolateral rotatory subluxation of the elbow and are analogous to the Hill-Sachs lesion of the shoulder. In one study, nine patients suspected of having posterolateral rotatory instability and nine asymptomatic subjects underwent MRI, and the symptomatic patients had exploratory surgery. Tears of the ulnar part of the LCL were noted in all symptomatic patients. The anterior fibers of the LCL, including the annular ligament, were intact. Arthroscopic examination will confirm excessive opening of the ulnohumeral articulation and posterior subluxation of the radial head with supination stress applied to the elbow.

Instability may need to be assessed with the patient under general anesthesia. This assessment is easiest to perform and interpret when the arm is in the overhead position. The elbow is examined for valgus, varus, and posterolateral rotatory instability. Valgus testing is performed with the elbow fully pronated so that posterolateral rotatory instability is not mistaken for valgus instability. This mistake occurs because the ulna and radius as a unit rotate away from the humerus in response to valgus stress when the LCL is disrupted.

Forced pronation prevents rotation of the ulna and radius by using the intact medial soft tissues as a hinge or fulcrum, akin to the periosteum being used for this purpose during the reduction of a supracondylar fracture in a child. Varus testing is easiest to perform with the shoulder in full internal rotation. Both valgus and varus testing are performed with the elbow in full extension and several degrees of flexion to about 30° to unlock the olecranon from the olecranon fossa. Posterolateral rotatory instability is diagnosed using the lateral pivot-shift test of the elbow. Severe soft-tissue disruption can lead to false-negative test results. A positive test is characterized by a clunk seen and felt during reduction of the ulna and radius onto the humerus. With severe soft-tissue disruption, the elbow can sometimes remain dislocated even when flexed past 90°. To avoid this potential problem, the examiner's thumb can prevent the elbow from fully dislocating, or the degree of subluxation during pivot-shift testing can be limited.

In some circumstances, stress radiographs are indicated. Valgus and varus views, along with supination and pronation views, detect posterolateral rotatory instability and help determine if the medial side opens up with pronation (indicating disruption of the medial soft tissues). It is essential to keep the forearm locked in full pronation when testing for valgus instability because the elbow can subluxate into posterolateral rotatory displacement if the forearm is permitted to supinate. This position will be misinterpreted as valgus instability (false-negative test).

Acute Fracture-Dislocations and Fracture-Subluxations

The most important fracture-dislocation, discussed earlier, is a dislocated elbow with fractures of the coronoid and radial head. The injury usually occurs because of posterolateral or varus-posteromedial rotatory instability, but instead of the tissue disruption occurring through the anterior capsule, it traverses the radial head and coronoid. This injury is analogous to the pathoanatomic variations in perilunate injuries in the wrist, in which the presence of a Mayfield spiral fracture predicts that injuries passing through the scaphoid usually spare the scapholunate ligament, and vice versa. This injury, with rare exceptions, should be treated surgically. Evaluation of this injury consists of accurate radiographs, lateral tomograms or fine-cut CT and sagittal reconstructions.

Varus-posteromedial rotation injuries may be characterized by a minimally displaced anteromedial coronoid fracture or a comminuted coronoid fracture and obvious LCL disruption. Coronoid fractures that appear benign usually are mistakenly interpreted to be of no real major significance and are erroneously treated nonsurgically. Patients with isolated coronoid fractures should be evaluated for potential instability or joint incongruity. The AP radiograph may reveal a wedge sign (Fig. 4). Lateral tomograms may reveal a positive converging circles sign. The circular outlines of the trochlea and ulna converge anteriorly at the coronoid fracture site. Examination under anesthesia with stress radiographs (varus and pronation with axial loading of the elbow) usually will confirm the instability pattern. This type of injury requires anatomic reduction and rigid fixation of the coronoid and repair of the LCL.

Treatment

Reduction and Postreduction Management

The initial treatment of a dislocation that is not complicated by the presence of fractures is closed reduction, done in supination to clear the coronoid under the trochlea in order to minimize additional trauma to the medial soft tissues that have not yet been disrupted. Essentially, the deformity is recreated to make reduction possible and easy. The elbow is briefly splinted for 3 to 5 days after reduction, and then motion is begun unless subluxation or dislocation occur. Careful examination throughout the comfortable range of motion and AP and lateral radiographs initially and every 5 to 7 days for the first 3 weeks will detect any subluxation or

dislocation. If subluxation or dislocation is detected clinically or radiographically, a change of treatment is warranted. In a recent study, active motion and muscle strengthening were commenced under supervision on the day of injury. All 20 patients studied experienced a rapid return of normal function, although one patient had a redislocation. These data suggest that neither immobilization nor splinting are necessary.

Treatment is dictated by the stage or degree of instability as described in Table 1. Valgus stability following reduction is present when the forearm is fully pronated in stages 1 to 3A. Treatment is with immediate unlimited flexion and extension in a cast brace applied with the forearm in full pronation. A cast brace is not necessary if elbow stability, usually a result of the dynamic stabilizing effects of the muscles crossing the elbow joint, is noted in all positions of forearm rotation. In stage 3B or 3C instability, the elbow is unstable in extension and a cast brace (usually in neutral rotation) is applied with an extension block that is gradually extended during the healing phase so that extension beyond the point of instability is prevented. A total of 3 to 6 weeks of protected motion is adequate. Type 3B and 3C dislocations are not pronated because medial soft-tissue disruption is sufficient to permit opening of the medial side with forearm pronation.

Fractures

The coronoid is the most important part of the anterior force-bearing surface of the elbow and is important for stability. Coronoid fractures in the presence of elbow instability usually require reduction and internal fixation. If these fractures are small and involve only the tip of the coronoid, a pull-down suture works well. If the anteromedial or medial coronoid is involved, or if the fractures are large, these fractures should be treated with anatomic reduction and rigid internal fixation or by protection with a hinged external fixator. The critical fracture involves the anteromedial coronoid, which together with the usual LCL disruption, permits chronic ulnohumeral joint incongruity. Aggressive diagnosis and treatment of these fractures is important. Malunions or nonunions of the coronoid sometimes cause persistent instability, making reduction, fixation, or reconstruction necessary.

Fractures of the radial head associated with an elbow dislocation or subluxation are best managed with internal fixation where possible. If the radial head is too comminuted for stable internal fixation and has to be excised, prosthetic replacement with a metal radial head is indicated if the elbow has been unstable. As reported in the literature, the novel concept of a bipolar radial head permits accommodation of radiohumeral tracking while accepting some degree of error in component position and/or orientation, a complication that is not well tolerated by rigid radial head prostheses. Axial and translational stability of the radius, especially with rotatory subluxation of the elbow, might not necessarily be restored to normal because of the bipolar articulation.

Fractures of the olecranon usually do not cause clinical instability if less than 50% of the joint surface is involved. However, there is a measurable decrease in stability that is proportional to the percentage of the olecranon that is lost or fractured. Fractures that involve the joint surface anteriorly toward the coronoid or insertion of the collateral ligaments on the ulna are an important cause of elbow instability. An unstable elbow associated with a fracture of the olecranon should be treated by open reduction and internal fixation of the olecranon. This can be done by plating the ulna posteriorly with a six- to eight-hole 3.5 dynamic compression or reconstruction plate bent at an angle of approximately 70° to 80° between the last two holes at the tip of the olecranon. Specialized congruent precontoured plates designed specifically for the olecranon are available. This procedure permits excellent fixation on the proximal fragment and acts as a buttress to prevent anterior subluxation.

Acute Ligament Repair

Instability that does not permit early protected motion in a hinged brace is a clear indication for acute ligament repair. This instability usually occurs when associated fractures are present. In such cases, the ligament(s) may have been avulsed and can be repaired directly to bone with heavy sutures. Sometimes the tissue can be repaired but not strongly enough to stabilize the joint. When this occurs the repair is augmented by passing a heavy absorbable suture (No. 2 polydioxane) through the same course as for a ligament reconstruction and fixing it to the normal ligament attachments on the epicondyle and ulna.

Disruption of both collateral ligaments (and often the common flexor and extensor origins as well) is common in simple dislocations, although the MCL may be intact in fracture-dislocations. Stress radiographs performed under anesthesia can be used to determine the functional integrity of the MCL. Although the MCL generally has been believed to heal uneventfully, a recent study brings this concept into question. Fifty patients underwent a closed reduction of a posterolateral elbow dislocation, and the elbow was immobilized for 3 weeks. At long-term follow-up, 24 of 41 patients had valgus instability on stress radiographs, and 21 had osteoarthritis that correlated with the medial instability. Thus, valgus instability of the elbow after a dislocation may be much more common, and more serious, than previously believed. Although an earlier study failed to demon-

strate a difference in outcome between elbow dislocations treated surgically and those treated nonsurgically, the data from this 1987 study must be interpreted with the understanding that the study took place before the authors were aware of or able to diagnose the most common form of recurrent instability of the elbow, posterolateral rotatory instability.

Complications

The two main complications of simple dislocations (no fractures) are contractures and recurrent instability. Stiffness can be minimized by starting early motion. According to results of a long-term study of 52 patients with dislocations not complicated by associated fractures, 60% of patients had some symptoms, including pain or stress pain in 45% and significant flexion contractures of more than 30° in 15%, at final follow-up. Stiffness was directly related to the duration of immobilization and was predictable if the elbow was immobilized for 3 weeks or longer.

Recurrent Elbow Instability

When soft-tissue healing after elbow subluxation, dislocation, or fracture-dislocation is inadequate, recurrent instability can develop, which is almost always posterolateral rotatory instability. It can also be iatrogenic and is caused by violation of the LCL complex during release for treatment of tennis elbow and other lateral elbow surgery. The condition also can result from chronic soft-tissue stretching occurring secondary to connective tissue disorders or repetitive overload such as occurs in patients with long-standing cubitus varus deformity from childhood supracondylar malunions.

The etiology of recurrent instability has recently become better understood. The condition is probably more common than previously believed, and according to results from two long-term studies, symptoms of recurrent instability were reported in 15% and 35% of patients studied, although the instability usually could not be demonstrated on examination. (These examinations were performed prior to publication of the concept of posterolateral rotatory instability.)

Evaluation

Posterolateral rotatory subluxation is the most common cause of recurrent elbow instability. The ulnar part of the LCL is usually detached or attenuated. The MCL is usually intact, although why the LCL is less likely to heal than the MCL is not clear. Symptoms include recurrent painful clicking, snapping, clunking, or locking of the elbow occurring in the extension half of the arc with the forearm in supination. A history of trauma or surgery is likely unless the patient has a connective tissue disorder

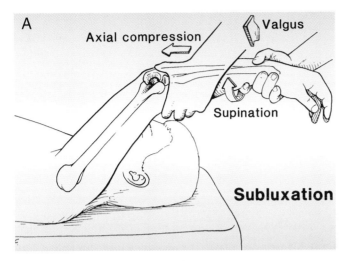

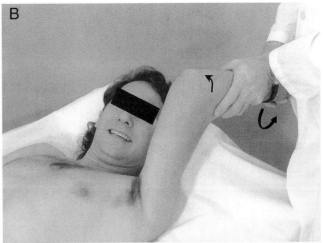

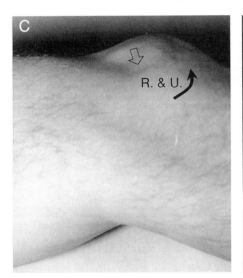

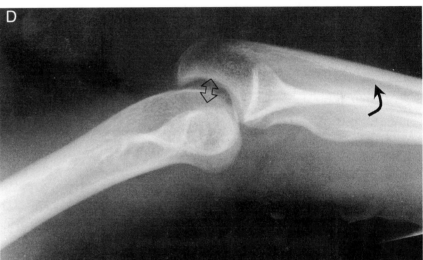

Figure 5 A, The lateral pivot-shift test of the elbow for posterolateral rotatory instability is performed with the patient supine and the arm overhead. A supination/valgus moment is applied during flexion causing the elbow to subluxate maximally at about 40° of flexion. **B,** This maneuver creates apprehension in the patient and is highly sensitive. **C,** If the patient is able to relax adequately, or is under general anesthesia, the elbow can be observed to subluxate so that the radius and ulna (R and U) rotate off the humerus (dark arrow). The skin is sucked in (hollow arrow) behind the radial head. Further flexion produces a palpable visible clunk as the elbow reduces if the patient is able to relax enough to permit that part of the examination. Unfortunately, the subluxation/reduction maneuver usually is not possible in the awake patient. **D,** A lateral stress radiograph taken during the lateral pivot-shift test reveals the radius and ulna to have supinated away from the humerus (dark arrow) leaving a gap in the ulno-humeral articulation (hollow arrow) and the radial head posterior to the capitellum. *(A and D are reproduced with permission from O'Driscoll SW, Bell DF, Morrey BF: Posterolateral rotatory instability of the elbow. J Bone Joint Surg Am 1991;73:440-446. B and C are reproduced with permission from Frymoyer JW (ed): Orthopaedic Knowledge Update 4. Rosemont, IL, American Academy of Orthopaedic Surgeons, 1993, pp 335-352.)*

or chronic stretching due to crutch-walking. Recurrent instability is typically caused by a previous dislocation, but can result from an injury as subtle as a sprain after a fall onto the outstretched hand. Radial head excision and lateral release for tennis elbow (due to violation of the ulnar part of the LCL) are other causes.

There are four principal physical examination tests for posterolateral rotator instability: the posterolateral rotatory apprehension test, lateral pivot-shift test (Fig 5, *A*), posterolateral rotatory drawer test, and stand-up test. The examination is best performed with the patient supine and the affected extremity overhead. The wrist and elbow are grasped in the same way as the ankle and knee when

examining the leg. The elbow is supinated with a mild force at the wrist, and a valgus moment is applied to the elbow during flexion. This action results in a typical apprehension response with reproduction of the patient's symptoms and a sense that the elbow is about to dislocate (Fig. 5, *B*). The actual subluxation and the clunk that occurs with reduction usually can be reproduced only with the patient under general anesthesia or occasionally after injecting local anesthetic into the elbow joint. The lateral pivot-shift test performed in that manner results in subluxation of the radius and ulna off the humerus, which causes a prominence posterolaterally over the radial head and a dimple between the radial head and the capitellum

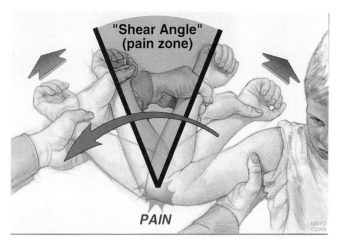

Figure 6 Moving valgus stress test for symptomatic partial tears of the MCL. A moderate valgus torque is applied to the fully flexed elbow, which is then quickly extended. A positive test is indicated by reproduction of the patient's pain as the elbow passes between 120° and 90°. Occasionally the position of maximum pain will extend past 90° down toward 70°. A positive test is confirmed when the same response, albeit usually to a lesser extent, is elicited by reversing the movements. *(Reproduced with permission from the Mayo Foundation, Rochester, MN.)*

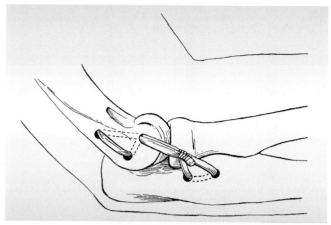

Figure 7 Reconstruction of the LUCL for posterolateral instability or recurrent dislocations. The tendon graft is fixed to the ulna near the tubercle on the supinator crest (which is felt by stressing the elbow in varus or supination) just at and distal to the annular ligament. The tendon graft is then passed through the isometric point on the lateral epicondyle (this point is usually more anterior than might be thought), out through a proximal hole posteriorly, and back into bone distally to reemerge at the isometric origin. It is then overlapped and sutured to itself. The capsule is imbricated and closed beneath the tendon graft to prevent it from rubbing on the side of the joint. *(Reproduced with permission from Gino Maulucci, Ontario, Canada, ©1992.)*

(Fig. 5, *C*). As the elbow is flexed to approximately 40° or more, reduction of the ulna and radius together on the humerus occurs suddenly with a palpable visible clunk. It is the reduction that is apparent. The third test is the posterolateral rotatory drawer test, which is a rotatory version of the drawer or Lachman test of the knee. With the patient supine and the arm overhead with the elbow flexed 40° to 90°, the forearm and arm are grasped exactly as though the elbow is a knee. The ulna and radius are translated off the humerus posterolaterally, pivoting around the intact MCL. The final test is the stand-up test. The patient's symptoms are reproduced when attempts are made to stand up from the sitting position by pushing on the seat with the hand at the side and the elbow fully supinated. A lateral stress radiograph obtained prior to feeling the clunk can be helpful to demonstrate the rotatory subluxation (Fig. 5, *D*).

Because consistent performance of the clinical tests for posterolateral rotatory instability requires experience, diagnostic imaging can be helpful.

Valgus Instability

Chronic valgus overload with rupture or attenuation of the MCL is diagnosed using patient history, physical examination, and stress radiographs. Patients with a history of repetitive valgus loading typically have medial elbow pain and may have actually heard or felt a pop at the time of ligament rupture. Tenderness over the MCL just anterior to the ulnar nerve and distal to the epicondyle can be confirmed with physical examination. Valgus stress may or may not be painful. The milking maneuver and the moving valgus stress test (Fig. 6) are valuable aids in establishing the diagnosis of a partial

tear. The milking maneuver is performed by positioning the affected elbow in supination and 90° or more of flexion, then pulling on the thumb with the other hand by reaching around behind the forearm of the involved limb.

Valgus stress radiographs are no longer considered as diagnostic as before. In one study, asymptomatic pitchers were shown to have apparently pathologic amounts of valgus opening of the medial ulnohumeral joint with stress. However, a normal stress radiograph does not rule out symptomatic ligament attenuation or partial tearing. The diagnosis thus depends more on the history and physical examination. The arthroscopic valgus stress test, which also has been considered specific for MCL injuries, may need to be validated in light of this new knowledge. MRI usually will show signal changes in the ligament and may also reveal changes in the overlying common flexor-pronator tendon origin. CT arthrography was shown in one study to reveal a T-sign in patients with partial tears of the undersurface of the MCL at its ulnar insertion. The T-sign refers to leakage of the contrast dye under the MCL so that it takes the shape of the letter T.

Treatment

Ligament Reconstruction

The avulsed LUCL is reattached or reconstructed with an autograft or allograft tendon, such as that of the palmaris longus or the semitendinosus (Fig. 7). The reconstruction technique currently used involves isometric placement of the origin on the lateral epicondyle and fixation to bone at either end. Surgery is performed in young patients so that violation of the epiphyseal plate on the lateral side of the humerus is prevented. With valgus or posterolateral rotatory instability, the anterior band of the MCL must also be reconstructed. Early motion in a cast brace can begin during the first week after surgery, with the forearm in full pronation (unless the anterior band of the MCL also was reconstructed). An extension block is sometimes used. In patients with severe instability or in revision cases, the elbow is sometimes immobilized in a cast for 3 weeks. In children, and in those patients who have previously undergone prolonged immobilization for up to 6 weeks without developing contractures, immobilization might be continued for 6 weeks.

Valgus Instability

The treatment for MCL injuries includes at least two sustained attempts at rehabilitation, including evaluation and retraining of motion in the presence of any abnormalities in the throwing mechanics. This evaluation includes focusing on the torso and lower extremities, concentrating on finding stiffness or weakness. After failure of nonsurgical treatment, the anterior band of the MCL is reconstructed using a palmaris longus tendon graft. Previous techniques for MCL reconstruction that involved transposition of the ulnar nerve were complicated by ulnar neuritis and neuropathy. In a recent study, the original technique has been modified to use a muscle-splitting approach without transposition of the ulnar nerve. Of 83 patients, only 5% had ulnar nerve symptoms, all of which were transient and resolved with nonsurgical management. Not only does this new technique have fewer complications, but also has a better success rate compared with the results of prior procedures.

Chronic Elbow Instability

Chronic instabilities present as either chronic dislocations or fracture-subluxations that are persistently unstable. Chronic dislocations are common in some underdeveloped countries, while persistent instability resulting from fracture-subluxations unfortunately is common even in countries with advanced medical care. Treatment of a chronic dislocation includes open reduction and removal of scar tissue to restore motion. Two options exist for providing stability: reconstruction of the MCL and LCL or maintenance of stability with a hinged external fixator while the periarticular soft tissues heal. If more than 50% of the joint surface itself is destroyed, interposition arthroplasty is performed as well. In one study of eight chronic elbow dislocations treated with open reduction and radial head excision or tricepsplasty if necessary, 63% had poor outcomes. Treatment of a fracture-subluxation that is persistently unstable is more challenging. These injuries are

managed similarly to chronic dislocations, but the bony surfaces must be reconstructed along with the ligaments. The most important structure is the coronoid, with the radial head a close second. Stability can be maintained temporarily with a hinged external fixator. Unfortunately, the results of these reconstructions are not as satisfactory, perhaps because the joint surfaces are often damaged. Loss of cartilage, and often some subchondral bone, compromises the congruity that is so intrinsic to this articulation and, thereby, compromises stability. As mentioned earlier, fracture-dislocations involving both the radial head and coronoid have a poor prognosis; the prognosis is even less promising with chronic injury. However, early clinical results from aggressive ligament reconstruction in combination with internal fixation in complex fracture-dislocations of the elbow have been very promising. The role of hinged external fixators is evolving.

Annotated Bibliography

Acute Elbow Instability

Azmi I, Razak M, Hyzan Y: The results of treatment of dislocation and fracture: Dislocation of the elbow: A review of 41 patients. *Med J Malaysia* 1998;53(suppl A): 59-70.

Of eight chronic elbow dislocations treated by open reduction and excision of radial head or tricepsplasty if necessary, 63% had poor outcomes.

Feldman DR, Schabel SI, Friedman RJ, Young JW: Translational injuries in posterior elbow dislocation. *Skeletal Radiol* 1997;26:134-136.

The authors describe the radiographic signs of an impaction fracture of the capitellum. Fracture results from a posterolateral rotatory subluxation or dislocation of the elbow.

Judet T, Garreau de Loubresse C, Piriou P, Charnley G: A floating prosthesis for radial-head fractures. *J Bone Joint Surg Br* 1996;78:244-249.

This article discusses the bipolar radial head prosthesis, which permits accommodation of radiohumeral tracking while accepting some degree of error in component position and or orientation.

McKee MD, Bowden SH, King GJ, et al: Management of recurrent, complex instability of the elbow with a hinged external fixator. *J Bone Joint Surg Br* 1998;80: 1031-1036.

In this multicenter study, 16 patients with recurrent complex elbow instability were managed using a hinged external fixator after a mean of 2.1 unsuccessful surgical procedures (range, 1 to 6 procedures). The fixator was applied at a mean of 4.8 weeks (range, 0 to 9 weeks) after the injury and remained on the elbow for a mean of 8.5 weeks (range, 6 to 11 weeks). There were 1 poor, 3 fair, 10 good, and 2 excellent results. It is important to differentiate between recurrent and persistent instability. Patients in whom the elbow is persistently unstable after surgery are at high risk of unsatisfactory outcomes, even when managed with a hinged external fixator, due to the high percentage of patients developing posttraumatic arthritis.

O'Driscoll SW, Jupiter JB, King GJ, Hotchkiss RN, Morrey BF: The unstable elbow. *J Bone Joint Surg Am* 2000;82:724-738.

This article presents the state-of-the-art thinking on the unstable elbow including how to manage each component of the bony and soft-tissue injuries. Salvage options are presented for those elbows that cannot be rendered stable. Most importantly, a decision-making algorithm is presented to determine when surgery is indicated and what surgical steps are necessary, especially for fracture-dislocations.

Popovic N, Gillet P, Rodriguez A, Lemaire R: Fracture of the radial head with associated elbow dislocation: Results of treatment using a floating radial head prosthesis. *J Orthop Trauma* 2000;14:171-177.

This article discusses the use of the bipolar radial head prosthesis to increase stability after a fracture-dislocation.

Ross G, McDevitt ER, Chronister R, Ove PN: Treatment of simple elbow dislocation using an immediate motion protocol. *Am J Sports Med* 1999;27:308-311.

This study emphasizes the importance of commencing active rehabilitation early, but under close supervision. Functional outcomes were essentially normal in all 20 patients, though one patient experienced a redislocation. Splinting or immobilization were not necessary.

Recurrent Elbow Instability

Cohen MS, Hastings H II: Rotatory instability of the elbow: The anatomy and role of the lateral stabilizers. *J Bone Joint Surg Am* 1997;79:225-233.

Pure rotational laxity was evaluated in cadaver elbows before and after sequential release of the lateral soft tissues. The common extensor tendon and the LCL complex (including the annular ligament) were interdependent in stabilizing the elbow. True posterolateral rotatory instability, a three-dimensional displacement, was not studied in the model.

Eygendaal D, Olsen BS, Jensen SL, Seki A, Sojbjerg JO: Kinematics of partial and total ruptures of the medial collateral ligament of the elbow. *J Shoulder Elbow Surg* 1999;8:612-616.

Selective transection of the MCL produced an increase in medial joint opening only after complete transection of the anterior part of the MCL and was maximum between 70° to 90° of flexion. Valgus instability should be evaluated at 70° to 90° of flexion. Detection of partial ruptures in the anterior bundle of the MCL based on medial joint opening and increased valgus movement was not possible in cadavers, although such partial tears might clinically be associated with attenuation that permits medial opening with valgus stress.

Eygendaal D, Verdegaal SH, Obermann WR, van Vugt AB, Poll RG, Rozing PM: Posterolateral dislocation of the elbow joint: Relationship to medial instability. *J Bone Joint Surg Am* 2000;82:555-560.

Fifty patients had a closed reduction of a posterolateral elbow dislocation and were immobilized for 3 weeks. At long-term follow-up, 24 of 41 patients had valgus instability on stress radiographs and 21 had osteoarthritis that correlated with the medial instability ($P = 0.001$). Persistent valgus instability of the elbow after a dislocation may be much more common, and more serious, than previously believed.

Faber KJ, King GJ: Posterior capitellum impression fracture: A case report associated with posterolateral rotatory instability of the elbow. *J Shoulder Elbow Surg* 1998;7:157-159.

This impaction fracture occurs as a result of posterolateral rotatory subluxation of the elbow and is analogous to the Hill-Sachs lesion of the shoulder.

Imatani J, Ogura T, Morito Y, Hashizume H, Inoue H: Anatomic and histologic studies of lateral collateral ligament complex of the elbow joint. *J Shoulder Elbow Surg* 1999;8:625-627.

Histologic examination of the LCL complex of the elbow confirmed that the ulnar part of the LCL blends with the annular ligament and more distally adheres closely to the supinator, extensor, and anconeus muscles. It represents a thickening of the capsuloligamentous complex.

O'Driscoll SW: Classification and evaluation of recurrent instability of the elbow. *Clin Orthop* 2000;370:34-43.

Posterolateral rotatory instability (PLRI) is the most common pattern of elbow instability, particularly that which is recurrent. PLRI can be considered a spectrum consisting of three stages according to the degree of soft-tissue disruption. Patients typically have mechanical symptoms. There are four principle physical examination tests: posterolateral rotatory apprehension test, lateral pivot-shift test, posterolateral rotatory drawer test, and the stand-up test. A lateral stress radiograph can show the rotatory subluxation.

O'Driscoll SW, Spinner RJ, McKee MD, et al: Tardy posterolateral rotatory instability of the elbow due to cubitus varus. *J Bone Joint Surg Am* 2001;83:1358-1369.

The authors describe delayed onset of posterolateral rotatory instability resulting from chronic cubitus varus malunions due to supracondylar fractures in childhood.

Olsen BS, Sojbjerg JO, Nielsen KK, Vaesel MT, Dalstra M, Sneppen O: Posterolateral elbow joint instability: The basic kinematics. *J Shoulder Elbow Surg* 1998;7:19-29.

The lateral pivot-shift test for PLRI was evaluated on cadaver elbows. As expected, releasing the LUCL from its ulnar insertion did not create laxity because the fibers of this structure can still resist force through their interconnections with the remainder of the LCL complex. However, releasing the LCL at the humeral origin, which is usually what happens with an elbow dislocation, did result in a positive lateral pivot-shift test. Ligament sectioning studies such as this are easily misinterpreted because the location of the release is important.

Potter HG, Weiland AJ, Schatz JA, Paletta GA, Hotchkiss RN: Posterolateral rotatory instability of the elbow: Usefulness of MR imaging in diagnosis. *Radiology* 1997; 204:185-189.

Because consistent performance of the clinical tests for PLRI require experience, it will be helpful to have accurate MRI scans of the LCL complex in patients suspected of having such instability.

Chronic Elbow Instability

Thompson WH, Jobe FW, Yocum LA, Pink MM: Ulnar collateral ligament reconstruction in athletes: Muscle-splitting approach without transposition of the ulnar nerve. *J Shoulder Elbow Surg* 2001;10:152-157.

This article discusses the muscle-splitting approach without transposition of the ulnar nerve in the treatment of elbow instability. In 83 cases, only 5% had ulnar nerve symptoms, all of which were transient and resolved with nonsurgical management. Interestingly, not only does this new technique have fewer complications, but the success rate was also better than for prior procedures.

Classic Bibliography

Josefsson PO, Gentz CF, Johnell O, Wendeberg B: Surgical versus non-surgical treatment of ligamentous injuries following dislocation of the elbow joint: A prospective randomized study. *J Bone Joint Surg Am* 1987;69:605-608.

Josefsson PO, Johnell O, Gentz CF: Long-term sequelae of simple dislocation of the elbow. *J Bone Joint Surg Am* 1984;66:927-930.

Mehlhoff TL, Noble PC, Bennett JB, Tullos HS: Simple dislocation of the elbow in the adult: Results after closed treatment. *J Bone Joint Surg Am* 1988;70: 244-249.

O'Driscoll SW, Bell DF, Morrey BF: Posterolateral rotatory instability of the elbow. *J Bone Joint Surg Am* 1991;73:440-446.

O'Driscoll SW, Horii E, et al: Anatomy of the ulnar part of the lateral collateral ligament of the elbow. *Clin Anat* 1992;5:296-303.

O'Driscoll SW, Morrey BF, Korinek S, An KN: Elbow subluxation and dislocation: A spectrum of instability. *Clin Orthop* 1992;280:186-197.

Osborne G, Cotterill P: Recurrent dislocation of the elbow. *J Bone Joint Surg Br* 1966;48:340-346.

Chapter 31

Elbow Stiffness

Scott P. Steinmann, MD

Introduction

Elbow stiffness is common with arthritis or after injury. The high degree of congruency of the joint, the proximity of muscle to the capsule, and the high likelihood of comminuted fractures all are factors that contribute to the propensity of the elbow for stiffness. Increased motion at the shoulder or wrist compensates partially for elbow stiffness. Whereas the shoulder helps to position the hand for maximum reach at the surface of a sphere of motion, the elbow contributes to motion within the sphere. Full elbow motion allows for self-contact and contact with the immediate environment. However, most activities of daily living can be performed if the elbow can move through a 100° arc of flexion from 30° to 130° and a 100° arc of rotation from 50° of supination to 50° of pronation. Specific sport or work activities may require full, or almost full, elbow motion. Most individuals will not seek treatment until loss of motion exceeds a 30° flexion contracture unless there is pain at the end points of motion or a vocation, hobby, or sport requires full motion. A loss of flexion generally causes more significant disability than does a loss of extension.

Etiology

Many elbow contractures occur as a result of trauma or arthritis. Rare causes include congenital conditions such as arthrogryposis, congenital dislocation of the radial head, or paralytic conditions such as cerebral palsy. A person with a head or burn injury is also at risk for development of an elbow contracture.

Injury about the elbow often involves trauma to the brachialis muscle as it crosses the anterior capsule. This close association allows for damaged muscle tissue to scar and tether normal capsular motion. The susceptibility of the elbow for comminuted fractures of the articular surface leads to an increased risk of stiffness after injury. Almost half of all distal humeral fractures have intra-articular involvement, and many of these are com-

minuted fractures. The unique architecture of the elbow articulation is a contributing factor in the development of comminuted fragments without soft-tissue attachments. Healing in an incongruent joint or with an avascular fragment can cause limitation of motion. In a study of 200 cases of posttraumatic stiffness, 20% were caused by supracondylar or intercondylar fractures, 20% by elbow dislocations, 38% by fracture-dislocations, and 10% by radial head fractures.

Classification

Elbow stiffness can be classified into extra-articular or extrinsic causes and intra-articular or intrinsic causes. The extrinsic contracture is simply a stiff elbow with no identifiable intra-articular pathology and with relatively normal articular surfaces and alignment. Extrinsic contracture can involve the skin (such as is seen after a burn), the muscle, or the capsule. Elbow trauma can result in capsular scarring or formation of heterotopic bone in the muscle, which ultimately will limit motion.

An intrinsic contracture involves intra-articular adhesions or intra-articular malunion. It can occur after an intra-articular fracture, bony avascular changes with loss of cartilage, or significant articular malalignment after trauma. It is rare for a patient to present with a pure intrinsic contracture. By the time elbow stiffness occurs after intra-articular trauma, the loss of motion will have been of such long standing that it will eventually result in a capsular contracture. Insidious onset of contracture typically results from an inflammatory arthropathy, a tumor such as osteoid osteoma, or osteochondritis dissecans.

Evaluation

Obtaining an adequate history of the elbow stiffness, particularly to determine the length of time of elbow contracture, is an important aspect of patient evaluation. The patient's priorities, such as improvement of motion or relief of pain, and factors such as work capacity and

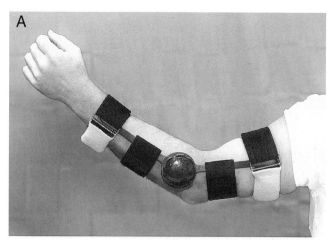

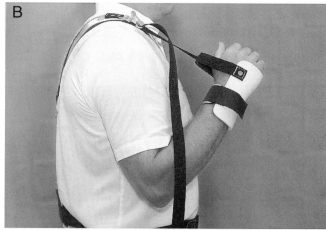

Figure 1 **A,** Patient-oriented static splint for prevention and treatment of elbow flexion contractures. This splint can be used for both flexion and extension; however, for flexion past 100°, a flexion-dedicated orthosis is best. **B,** Patient-oriented static splint for prevention and treatment of elbow flexion contractures. Full flexion is possible.

demands on the elbow and motivation for improvement, should be addressed and understood by the surgeon. Any vocation or activity that is important to the patient and places physical demands on the elbow also should be considered. Prior treatments, including surgical intervention, should be noted, along with any complications from treatment, including infections.

Physical examination should include an examination of the entire upper extremity. Normal shoulder and wrist function should be documented and any injuries to, or prior afflictions of, these joints should be recorded. The soft-tissue envelope of the elbow should be examined to check for prior skin incisions, evidence of prior infection, or scarring. Elbow motion (active and passive, flexion and extension) should be recorded. Range of pronation and supination should be noted, along with any abnormalities from the forearm to the wrist that might inhibit normal active motion. Contractures of recent onset have the potential for a greater response to a splinting treatment regimen.

Elbow stability should be assessed. It is quite possible for loss of flexion or extension to be present with concomitant collateral ligament injury. A neurologic examination of the upper extremities should reveal the condition of the ulnar, median, and radial nerves. Ulnar nerve function should be examined closely. Sensory changes in the hand, loss of grip strength or pinch, tenderness, or the presence of Tinel's sign along the tract of the nerve should also be watched for and documented. The ulnar nerve is in proximity to the joint capsule, putting it at risk for injury in patients with an inflammatory arthropathy. Additionally, surgical interventions to relieve elbow stiffness can be complicated by a postoperative ulnar neuropathy and, therefore, the preoperative condition of the nerve should be carefully recorded. If there is any question of neurologic dys-

function, a nerve conduction velocity study and electromyography can be performed.

Radiographic studies should always include AP, lateral, and oblique views of the elbow. In most cases these views will be adequate for diagnosing and planning a treatment program. When examining the radiographs, careful attention should be paid to the bony outline of the coronoid and radial head. The ulnohumeral articulation should be examined for evidence of subluxation. The radial head should directly oppose the capitellum on all radiographic views. If bony fragments are seen in the soft tissue, the radiographs should be inspected for the presence of an occult fracture. Additional radiographic assessment is best achieved with trispiral tomography or CT. MRI offers little additional information in the diagnosis or preoperative planning.

The elbow should be examined for heterotopic ossification, which can be a result of direct injury, a burn, or closed head injury. The incidence is less than 10% in fracture-dislocations of the elbow. However, if the patient has an associated head injury with elbow trauma, the risk of heterotopic ossification approaches 90%. There is no role for bone scintigraphy or laboratory testing of alkaline phosphatase in determining the timing of surgical excision of heterotopic bone. Radiographs should be obtained regularly to assess maturation of the heterotopic bone, which usually occurs during the first few months after injury. Excision of heterotopic bone at 4 to 6 months after elbow injury has not been associated with a greater recurrence rate. In pediatric patients, however, heterotopic ossification has been noted to spontaneously resolve, particularly in those with a resolving central nervous system injury. Such a patient may be observed for a longer period. Postoperative prophylaxis after excision of heterotopic bone has involved use of indomethacin or low-dose radiation (700 cGy); it is only recommended in high-risk cases because of concerns over radiation exposure.

Nonsurgical Treatment

Nonsurgical treatment of elbow stiffness is most successful when done within the first 3 months after the onset of the particular elbow affliction. The hallmark of nonsurgical treatment is to avoid the initial development of stiffness after insult to the elbow. The surgeon should watch for the development of loss of motion after injury so that proper rehabilitative measures can be instituted.

The cornerstone of nonsurgical treatment of the stiff elbow is the judicious application of a splinting/range-of-motion regimen. The role of manipulation under anesthesia remains unclear and is a controversial topic. Physical therapy should involve both active and passive exercises. There is no evidence to suggest that passive exercises cause heterotopic ossification in the elbow. On the other hand, aggressive therapy that can cause increased stiffness and pain should be avoided.

The adjustable static type of splint is preferable because it can move through a full range of motion but can be locked in an infinite number of positions (Fig. 1). A turnbuckle splint is the most common type. The goal of treatment is to achieve a plastic deformation of the soft tissue through stress relaxation. Splinting is done on a 21-hour program; the patient is allowed out of the splint for 1-hour periods in the morning, at noon, and at night. Flexion and extension are alternated at 2- to 3-hour intervals. Alternatively, shorter periods of use (15 to 30 minutes) can be attempted to prevent the discomfort associated with prolonged stretching. As the patient gradually gains motion, the brace is progressively moved to a greater range of motion and locked until the patient is comfortable and tolerates the new position. At night the splint is locked in the position most needed for either flexion or extension. As motion increases and flexion increases to greater than 100°, two types of splints are usually needed, one for flexion and one for extension. Dynamic splints generate continuous tissue tension and have been noted anecdotally to be less well tolerated and possibly a cause of inflammation.

Surgical Treatment: Extrinsic Contracture

Arthroscopic Release

If a splinting program is unsuccessful after 2 to 3 months, surgical treatment may be indicated. Surgical release of the elbow may be done using either an open or an arthroscopic technique; whether one technique is better than the other has not been determined. Arthroscopic treatment has been used as a treatment option

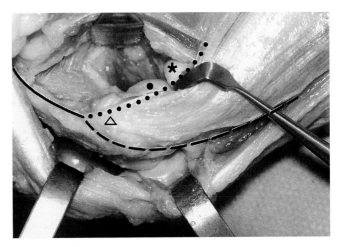

Figure 2 Lateral exposure-anterior interval. The dissection is continued anteriorly between the extensor carpi radialis longus anteriorly and the extensor carpi radialis brevis/extensor digitorum communis posteriorly (dotted line). This allows for exposure and release of the anterior capsule. Triangle = lateral epicondyle; asterisk = radial head; large dot = capitellum. Solid line is the lateral humerus at the interval between triceps and extensor carpi radialis longus; dashed line is Kocher's interval.

since the early 1990s, and there is a current surge of interest in its use.

There are potential risks to neurovascular structures during arthroscopic release. All three major nerves about the elbow are at risk: the radial and ulnar nerves are particularly prone to injury, with the median nerve being somewhat protected behind a layer of brachialis muscle.

Based on relative risk to the neurovascular structures, arthroscopic technique has been classified into three categories: (1) capsular detachment from the humerus (least effective, but minimal risk); (2) capsulotomy (reasonably effective, but moderate risk); and (3) capsulectomy (most effective, but highest risk). Current data and experience suggest that the efficacy of an arthroscopic release is high, although its safety remains to be confirmed. The use of retractors during elbow arthroscopy has been credited with an increase in the number of capsulectomies performed without permanent nerve injury and is essential for some elbow arthroscopic procedures.

Once an adequate field of vision is established, a synovectomy can be performed and loose bodies and osteophytes removed. A detailed description of capsulectomy technique is beyond the scope of this chapter.

Satisfactory results have been reported in several studies. In an early study, the average amount of flexion contracture after arthroscopic release decreased 35°. In a study of 25 patients with posttraumatic or degenerative arthrofibrosis, at 18 months follow-up all patients experienced increased motion and decreased pain. In another study of 24 patients with a stiff arthritic elbow, an arthroscopic modification of the Outerbridge-Kashiwagi procedure was performed with all patients having

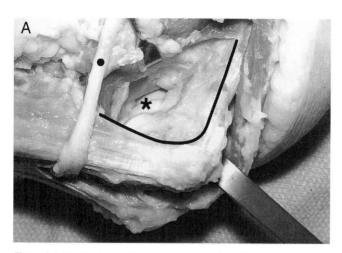

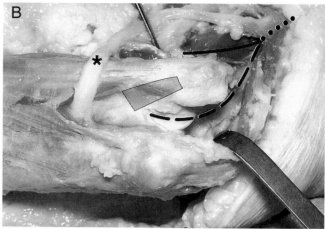

Figure 3 A, Medial release of the elbow. Anterior portion of flexor pronator group is released from the humerus. The middle portion of the flexor pronator group is left intact to preserve the anterior band of the medial collateral ligament. This allows for release of the capsule. Solid line shows dissection of the flexor pronator group (under anterior retractor); asterisk = trochlea; large dot = ulnar nerve transposed. **B,** The ulnar nerve (asterisk) is identified and transposed. The triceps is elevated off the humerus. The posterior capsule and posterior band of the medial collateral ligament can be released (dashed line) distally up to the anterior band (shaded) of the medial collateral ligament. Dotted line represents medial edge of humerus; solid line is anterior dissection of flexor pronator group.

a significant decrease in pain and an average increase in the arc of motion of 81°. In yet another study, the benefits of arthroscopy were documented in 25 patients, with an average improved elbow range of motion of 41°. Although arthroscopic débridement of stiff elbows can be an effective treatment, the learning curve is quite steep. Until a surgeon becomes proficient in the technique, an open release may be a safer surgical treatment option.

Open Capsular Release

Open capsular release has been reported more often in the literature than arthroscopic release, and several studies both in the United States and abroad have demonstrated its effectiveness. There is no generally agreed upon surgical technique for open release, although lateral and medial approaches are most common, with the lateral approach being more popular. The anterior approach has fallen out of favor because of the need to carefully dissect, identify, and protect most of the major neurovascular structures about the elbow and because it does not allow access to posterior structures.

The medial approach has been shown to be an effective method of mobilizing the stiff elbow in patients with associated medial heterotopic bone or ulnar neuropathy. It can be an ideal method of resecting isolated medial collateral ligament calcification. The lateral approach involves a reflection of the origin of the extensor carpi radialis longus and the distal fibers of the brachioradialis from the humerus to gain access to the superolateral capsule (Fig. 2). The triceps can be elevated from the posterior aspect of the humerus to gain access to the olecranon fossa for removal of osteophytes and excision of the posterior capsule. This method

allows for excision of the lateral half of the anterior capsule to the level of the coronoid. Access to the medial capsule is difficult. In one study, the mean total gain in the arc of flexion/extension was 45°.

In some cases, combined medial and lateral approaches are appropriate (Fig. 3). After a posterior incision is made, medial and lateral flaps are created, similar to the approach for a total elbow arthroplasty. If flexion to less than 90° is possible preoperatively, the ulnar nerve should be transposed to prevent postoperative neuropathy. If the preoperative arc of motion is limited to less than 110°, then the ulnar nerve should probably be transposed. With a flexion arc of greater than 110°, the ulnar nerve may not need to be transposed but might benefit from decompression. If the ulnar nerve is to be transposed, an incision through the capsule at the floor of the cubital tunnel beneath the ulnar nerve will release the posterior band of the medial collateral ligament and the posteromedial capsule (Fig. 3).

Postoperative Therapy

After arthroscopic or open surgical release of the stiff elbow, a structured postoperative therapy protocol is essential to maintaining the arc of motion achieved in the operating room. An understanding of the pathophysiology of joint contractures is helpful for the surgeon treating a patient with joint stiffness. The evolution of joint stiffness and the principles of continuous passive motion (CPM) have been reported in the literature. Essentially, there are four stages of stiffness after injury or surgery: bleeding, edema, granulation tissue, and fibrosis. Stage I, bleeding, occurs within minutes to hours after injury and results in distention of the joint capsule and swelling of the periarticular tissues. High hydrostatic

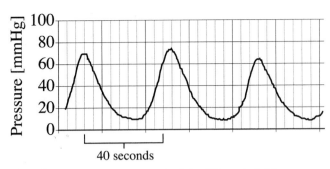

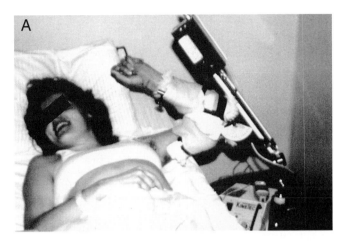

Figure 4 An intra-articular pressure tracing during CPM reveals that the pressure oscillates in a regular sinusoidal fashion. *(Reproduced with permission from O'Driscoll SW, Giori NJ: Continuous passive motion (CPM): Theory and principles of clinical application.* J Rehabil Res Dev *2000;37:179-188.)*

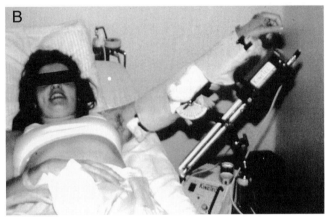

Figure 5 A and **B,** Photographs taken on the same day of surgery in a young patient with posttraumatic arthritis and stiffness of the elbow treated by distraction interposition arthroplasty and immediate commencement of a full range of motion on a CPM machine. Pain was controlled with an axillary indwelling catheter for brachial plexus block anesthesia. This particular machine does not permit a full range of motion of the elbow; this can be accomplished by augmenting the motion with wedges placed alternately beneath the wrist or elbow to enhance flexion or extension, respectively. *(Reproduced with permission from O'Driscoll SW, Giori NJ: Continuous passive motion (CPM): Theory and principles of clinical application.* J Rehabil Res Dev *2000;37:179-188.)*

pressures in the joint and stiff tissues will result in pain and an increased resistance to motion. Stage II, edema, occurs over hours or days, with inflammatory mediators causing blood vessels to leak plasma, contributing to a swollen and less compliant soft tissue surrounding the joint. Stage III, formation of granulation tissue, occurs over days to weeks. This loosely organized tissue becomes increasingly solid with the deposition of solid, extracellular matrix. Stage IV, fibrosis, occurs as the granulation tissue matures, forming rigid scar tissue.

Prevention of stiffness, therefore, entails the goal of minimizing the early accumulation of fluid in the periarticular soft tissues. This is accomplished by squeezing away from the joint area the fluid that has collected. CPM applied to a joint raises and lowers the hydrostatic pressure, resulting in a "pumping effect" that forces fluid out of the periarticular soft tissue (Fig. 4). The maximum benefit of CPM occurs in the first few days after surgery or injury. These basic principles of CPM can be applied to the elbow. Ideally, motion should be started as soon as possible (Fig. 5). If CPM is not started the first day, the arm should be elevated in full extension with the elbow above the shoulder for 36 hours. The patient should be evaluated to document any alterations in upper extremity nerve function, in particular, the status of the ulnar nerve. After normal function is noted, an indwelling axillary nerve block is performed and the arm placed in a CPM machine. It is important to remove all circumferential dressings and maintain a single elastic sleeve, which will prevent shear and stress to the skin and wound. The CPM should be through a full range of motion to maximize the wringing out or squeezing of the blood and edema fluid from the periarticular soft tissues. CPM should occur 24 hours a day, with only bathroom breaks allowed. Ideally, the patient remains in the hospital for 3 days and is discharged with a CPM machine for home use over a 3- to 4-week period. During this time, the patient should alternate between full flexion and full extension when using the machine. In

the patient in whom a delayed ulnar neuropathy develops, immediate transposition is recommended.

Surgical Treatment: Intrinsic Contracture

Surgical treatment of intrinsic elbow contracture typically involves detaching the lateral or medial collateral ligament complex and pivoting the joint open on the intact opposite ligament. The decision to resurface the joint with an interposition tissue is made if less than half the articular cartilage is remaining or if significant recontouring of the joint surface is necessary.

The choices of interposition tissue have historically included autologous fascia or dermal graft. Currently, allograft Achilles tendon has been used with success. Achilles tendon allograft is advantageous because it is associated with less morbidity. A tail of the graft can be

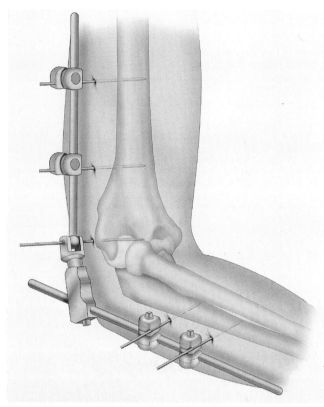

Figure 6 Degenerative joint disease II hinged fixator (Howmedica, Rutherford, NJ). Approximate placement of distraction device into the lateral humerus and ulna. The amount of distraction can be adjusted with a set-screw. The pin of the axis of rotation in the capitellum is temporary and must be removed.

maintained on each side to reconstruct the collateral ligaments if necessary.

After interposition arthroplasty, an elbow distraction device usually is applied. Several types are available; success depends on replicating the natural center of rotation, an area of less than 4 mm (Fig. 6).

The results of treatment of elbow contractures vary according to the duration of the stiffness as well as its etiology. A general survey of the literature would suggest an 80% expectation of achieving a functional arc of motion (30° to 130° flexion). Recent reports of arthroscopic release have been very encouraging, though studies will be required to document a difference in efficacy or safety.

Summary

Prevention is the best treatment for elbow stiffness occurring after trauma or surgery. A heightened awareness when caring for patients after elbow surgery or injury is necessary to identify and arrest the development of stiffness should it occur. Arthroscopic or open surgical techniques can be used to achieve an improvement in motion. Full release of all tight or impinging structures, both medial and lateral in the elbow joint, is required if the best results are to be obtained. The time-honored technique of CPM with adequate analgesia through a full range of motion help optimize results.

Annotated Bibliography

Fox RJ, Varitimidis SE, Plakeseychuk A, Vardakas DG, Tomaino MM, Sotereanos DG: The compass elbow hinge: Indications and initial results. *J Hand Surg Br* 2000;25:568.

The compass hinge was used in 11 patients with degenerative disease, contracture, or instability. Stability was not achieved if the coronoid fracture was not reconstructed. Pin tract infection occurred in 5 of 11 patients. Two patients sustained dislocations while wearing the hinge.

Kelly EW, Morrey BF, O'Driscoll SW: Complications of elbow arthroscopy. *J Bone Joint Surg Am* 2001;83: 25-34.

A large study of 473 elbow arthroscopies was conducted in 449 patients at a single institution. A serious complication (joint space infection) occurred after four (0.8%) of the arthroscopic procedures. Minor complications, such as superficial infection, minor contracture, and transient nerve palsy, occurred after 50 (11%) of the procedures. Although there were no permanent nerve injuries, the risk to neurovascular structures is emphasized, particularly in patients with rheumatoid arthritis.

Mansat P, Morrey BF: The column procedure: A limited lateral approach for extrinsic contracture of the elbow. *J Bone Joint Surg Am* 1998;80:1603-1615.

Thirty-seven patients were treated with the column approach for elbow stiffness. The average arc of flexion-extension improved 45°. The extensor carpi radialis longus and distal fibers of the brachioradialis were released from the humerus to gain access to the anterior joint capsule.

O'Driscoll SW, Giori NJ: Continuous passive motion (CPM): Theory and principles of clinical application. *J Rehab Res Develop* 2000;37:179-188.

Four stages of stiffness are discussed, along with the proper application of CPM.

O'Driscoll SW, Shankland SW, Beaton D: Patient adjusted static elbow splints for elbow contractures: A preliminary report. *J Shoulder Elbow Surg* 1996;5:S73.

Patients whose conditions did not respond to physical therapy were treated with static elbow splints. The average arc of motion improved from 73° to 103°.

Phillips BB, Strasburger S: Arthroscopic treatment of arthrofibrosis of the elbow joint. *Arthroscopy* 1998;14: 38-44.

Twenty-five patients with arthrofibrosis were treated by arthroscopic débridement. The supine position was used, with the elbow held in 90° of abduction and 90° of flexion in a balanced suspension device. The average improvement in the arc of motion was 41°.

Classic Bibliography

Bonutti PM, Windau JE, Ables BA, Miller BG: Static progressive stretch to reestablish elbow range of motion. *Clin Orthop* 1994;303:128-134.

Cullen JP, Pellegrini VD Jr, Miller RJ, Jones JA: Treatment of traumatic radioulnar synostosis by excision and postoperative low-dose irradiation. *J Hand Surg Am* 1994;19:394-401.

Duke JB, Tessler RH, Dell PC: Manipulation of the stiff elbow with patient under anesthesia. *J Hand Surg Am* 1991;16:19-24.

Gallay SH, Richards RR, O'Driscoll SW: Intraarticular capacity and compliance of stiff and normal elbows. *Arthroscopy* 1993;9:9-13.

Garland DE, Hanscom DA, Keenan MA, Smith C, Moore T: Resection of heterotopic ossification in the adult with head trauma. *J Bone Joint Surg Am* 1985;67:1261-1269.

Gates HS III, Sullivan FL, Urbaniak JR: Anterior capsulotomy and continuous passive motion in the treatment of post-traumatic flexion contracture of the elbow: A prospective study. *J Bone Joint Surg Am* 1992;74:1229-1234.

Green DP, McCoy H: Turnbuckle orthotic correction of elbow-flexion contractures after acute injuries. *J Bone Joint Surg Am* 1979;61:1092-1095.

Hastings H II, Graham TJ: The classification and treatment of heterotopic ossification about the elbow and forearm. *Hand Clin* 1994;10:417-437.

Jones GS, Savoie FH III: Arthroscopic capsular release of flexion contractures (arthrofibrosis) of the elbow. *Arthroscopy* 1993;9:277-283.

Mih AD, Wolf FG: Surgical release of elbow capsular contracture in pediatric patients. *J Pediatr Orthop* 1994;14:458-461.

Moore TJ: Functional outcome following surgical excision of hterotopic ossification in patients with traumatic brain injury. *J Orthop Trauma* 1993;7:11-14.

Morrey BF: Posttraumatic contracture of the elbow: Operative treatment, including distraction arthroplasty. *J Bone Joint Surg Am* 1990;72:601-618.

Morrey BF, Askew LJ, An KN: A biomechanical study of normal functional elbow motion. *J Bone Joint Surg Am* 1981;63:872-876.

Timmerman LA, Andrews JR: Arthroscopic treatment of posttraumatic elbow pain and stiffness. *Am J Sports Med* 1994;22:230-235.

Chapter 32

Elbow Arthritis

Scott P. Steinmann, MD

Introduction

Rheumatoid arthritis is the most common cause of elbow arthritis, with many patients having bilateral disease and involvement of many joints. Posttraumatic arthritis can potentially affect people of all age groups and can be a major source of disability at the elbow. Osteoarthritis tends to affect mainly males, particularly those in occupations involving repetitive manual labor.

Rheumatoid Arthritis

Rheumatoid arthritis of the elbow can severely limit a patient's functional activities. Twenty percent to 50% of patients affected by rheumatoid arthritis have elbow involvement. An isolated presentation of arthritis is unusual, occurring in less than 10% of patients.

Initially, a patient may present with a synovitis that will result in pain and distention of the joint capsule. The patient will find that a flexed position of the elbow is the most comfortable. With time, a contracture will ensue and if the synovitis progresses, erosion of the articular cartilage will occur. The synovitis will gradually affect both the bony structures and soft-tissue support of the joint. Bony destruction may continue after the articular cartilage has been lost by erosion into the subchondral bone with the gradual onset of joint instability. The ligamentous support of the elbow joint can become weakened by the chronic inflammation, resulting in gross varus/valgus instability, but instability is usually caused by bony loss.

A synovitis can also distend through the joint capsule into the forearm or upper arm. Pockets of inflamed synovium may invade the soft-tissue envelope of the elbow and produce compression of the ulnar or radial nerves, inducing a neuropathy. The synovium very often produces cysts in the bone of the distal humerus and proximal ulna. On occasion this synovitic invasion of the bone can be quite extensive, resulting in large cysts that can weaken the bone and cause intra-articular fracture and further joint destruction.

Evaluation

Rheumatoid arthritis has been classified into four stages. Stage I is characterized by a mild to moderate amount of synovitis with no radiographic changes. In stage II there is a chronic synovitis, with mild arthritic changes and loss of joint space evident on radiographs. Stage III is characterized by active synovitis with joint articular destruction (type A) and more advanced loss of subchondral bony architecture (type B). Stage IV involves extensive damage with loss of bone and gross instability. During the initial examination, an overall assessment of the function of major joints should be done to determine the patient's individual vocational needs.

Nonsurgical Treatment

The nonsurgical treatment of elbow arthritis is similar to that of arthritis of any other major joint. The mainstay of initial treatment involves the use of nonsteroidal anti-inflammatory medications. Care should be taken to observe patients for gastrointestinal side effects, a known complication of nonsteroidal anti-inflammatory therapy. In patients who cannot tolerate standard medication, cyclooxygenase-II inhibitors may offer some advantages. In the presence of more recalcitrant disease, an immunosuppressive agent may be indicated. Antimalarial agents, methotrexate, or gold salts can be used. These more potent medications can cause serious side effects such as thrombocytopenia, liver or renal failure, and pulmonary toxicity. Therefore, careful laboratory monitoring of blood cell counts and liver and kidney function should be done in patients treated with these medications. Newer immunosuppressive agents such as leflunomide, etanercept, or infliximab can affect the patient's ability to mount a response to infection; therefore, these patients should be monitored closely for any sign of sepsis. Oral corticosteroids are commonly used as a part of medical management. Patients on oral medication should be observed for the systemic effects of chronic steroid therapy. Intra-articular injection of corticosteroids can be helpful for the patient who is undergoing a painful episode of joint synovitis. In addition to medication, static splints can be used when symptoms are severe, along with use of cold or heat. A hinged splint is sometimes helpful if instability is a major symptom. An occupational therapist can recommend assistive devices that can improve the patient's ability to perform daily activities.

Surgical Treatment

Surgical treatment for rheumatoid arthritis is indicated after nonsurgical treatment has failed. Options include synovectomy, interposition arthroplasty, and joint replacement. Synovectomy is usually entertained as a surgical option early during the course of the disease, with arthroplasty being the most definitive treatment in later stages. The functional and radiographic presentation of the joint and the lifestyle demands of the patient are deciding factors for choice of surgical treatment.

Synovectomy

Synovectomy has proved to be an effective treatment in elbow arthritis. Patients typically have a painful synovitis distending the joint, limiting function and range of motion. The articular surface of the elbow joint may be partially eroded, but the subchondral bone is intact, maintaining structural stability. Open surgical synovectomy with resection of the radial head has been an accepted surgical practice for many years, with favorable results reported. Radial head excision provides easy access to the medial joint for extensive synovectomy. Recently, the need for radial head excision has been questioned. Proponents of radial head excision believe that it improves the rotation of the forearm and eliminates painful contact between the radial head and the capitellum. However, in some patients who have undergone radial head excision, advanced destruction has been noted at the ulnohumeral articulation, a condition possibly related to increased joint loading and valgus stress. Some experienced elbow surgeons believe the radial head should rarely be resected during synovectomy. Results of open synovectomy have been well documented. Many studies report that up to 90% of patients achieve excellent results during the first few years after surgery. Late follow-up at 5 to 10 years demonstrates a deterioration in these results with time, with an overall success rate ranging from 60% to 75%.

Arthroscopic synovectomy has recently been used with greater frequency. This technique does offer the ability to do a more complete synovectomy if the surgeon is familiar with the technique of elbow arthroscopy. As joint destruction continues in the later stages of the disease, bony landmarks in the joint that provide spatial orientation during arthroscopic surgery are blurred, making it more difficult to ascertain the location of vital structures such as the nerves. Complications of nerve resection that occur at the time of arthroscopic synovectomy have been reported. Although arthroscopy in the later stages of rheumatoid arthritis is potentially helpful to the patient, its role needs to be balanced against the higher risk of neurovascular complications. As more experience is gained in advanced techniques of arthroscopic synovectomy of the elbow, minimal morbidity and more rapid return of motion may occur.

Interposition Arthroplasty

Interposition arthroplasty has been used in an attempt to resurface the arthritic elbow. Different materials have included fascia, dermis, and allograft Achilles tendon. Although primarily described for treatment of osteoarthritis or posttraumatic arthritis, interposition arthroplasy has also been used to treat inflammatory arthritis of the elbow. The results, however, have not been promising. In one study, 28 patients had results inferior to those of patients treated with a total elbow arthroplasty. Additionally, extensive bone loss was associated with interposition arthroplasty, making later reoperation difficult or impossible. The overall indications for interposition arthroplasty are limited because many patients with rheumatoid arthritis have multiple joint involvement and therefore place lower demands on the elbow. Such patients are usually ideal candidates for total elbow arthroplasty because loosening and mechanical concerns are lessened.

Joint Replacement Arthroplasty

The indications for total elbow arthroplasty include intolerable pain that cannot be managed with conservative options. Such patients usually have contractures that limit their daily activities. Contraindications include active sepsis, a neuropathic joint, muscle weakness or paralysis, the need for soft-tissue coverage, a young, active patient, or severe bone loss. Total elbow arthroplasty has become a more common procedure over the past 10 years. Early designs had a high failure rate, with loosening and dislocation identified as major problems. Advances in design have improved with two general types of implants: linked and unlinked prostheses.

Unlinked or unconstrained prostheses rely on an intact soft-tissue envelope to maintain surface contact of the humeral and ulnar components for stability. Linked or semiconstrained implants have a "loose hinge" that allows several degrees of varus-valgus deformity and rotational laxity.

Pain relief after elbow arthroplasty is excellent and is comparable to the results of hip or knee arthroplasty. Ninety percent of patients achieve significant pain relief and improvement in function. Motion is also improved

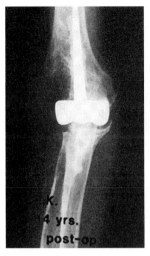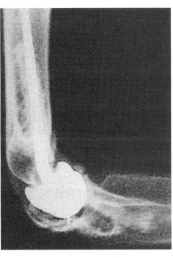

Figure 1 Unlinked (nonconstrained) total elbow arthroplasty. Patients with adequate bone stock and soft tissues for stability can be treated with a nonconstrained arthroplasty, such as the capitellocondylar (Ewald) prosthesis. This is the oldest elbow prosthesis still in use and is reported by the originator to have excellent long-term results. *(Reproduced with permission from Ewald FC, Simmons ED Jr, Sullivan JA, et al: Capitellocondylar total elbow replacement in rheumatoid arthritis. J Bone Joint Surg Am 1993;75:498-507.)*

considerably, with a functional range achieved in most patients. Improvements in extension are somewhat greater with a linked implant than with an unlinked implant. In patients with bone loss or significant soft-tissue contracture, a linked prosthesis allows for release of all contracted tissue and immediate postoperative motion. An unlinked device requires careful attention to soft-tissue balancing and requires adequate bone stock to support the prosthesis. Implantation of an unlinked prosthesis requires exact technique with a need to achieve precise positioning and maintain proper soft-tissue tension. Instability has been reported in 5% to 20% of unlinked prostheses.

Although insertion of unlinked prostheses can be challenging, use of the unlinked capitellocondylar prosthesis has shown satisfactory results. The results of 202 capitellocondylar prostheses were reported after 2 to 15 years of follow-up. Pain relief and function were excellent (Fig. 1). Revision surgery was necessary in only 5% of cases because of loosening, dislocation, or infection. This definitive study demonstrates that an experienced surgeon can implant the device with the potential for excellent long-term results.

The laxity in the loose hinge, linked implant allows for some of the forces across the elbow joint to be absorbed by the static (ligamentous) and dynamic (muscle) soft-tissue constraints rather than the prosthesis-bone interface as in a purely constrained or hinged device. Although a linked design might be expected to loosen more often than an unlinked design, this has not been the reported experience. In one study, a 95% Kaplan-Meier survival at 7 years was reported in 58 patients with rheumatoid arthritis using a linked Coonrad-Morrey

implant (Fig. 2). No instances of aseptic loosening were documented. In a study of total elbow arthroplasty in 24 patients with juvenile rheumatoid arthritis, 96% of patients had mild pain at postoperative evaluation and in the patients with 18 linked devices, there was no evidence of radiographic loosening. Because of these results, many would consider a linked implant to be indicated in most patients requiring arthroplasty for the treatment of rheumatoid arthritis.

The failure of elbow arthroplasty in the treatment of rheumatoid arthritis is related to factors such as infection, aseptic loosening, instability, and bearing surface wear. In patients with wear of a bushing in a linked device, reoperation and bushing replacement can offer satisfactory results if osteolysis is not yet severe. In the other modes of failure, removal of the prosthesis is usually required. Options after implant removal include conversion to a resection arthroplasty or salvage and reimplantation with a new prosthesis. In a study of 14 rheumatoid arthritis patients with failed total elbow arthroplasty caused by infection, aseptic loosening or instability, all of the infected elbows were converted to resection arthroplasty and the noninfected failures converted to a linked device. Resection arthroplasty resulted in poor function. If a prosthesis is infected, it and all bone cement should be removed. In a well-fixed prosthesis, this might involve bivalving the bone. Antibiotic-impregnated cement beads should be implanted while the patient receives intravenous antibiotics. After 6 weeks or when the bone is healed, the antibiotic beads are removed and if there are no signs of acute inflammation, a new prosthesis can be implanted using antibiotic in the cement. In most cases, after the bone loss associated with revision arthroplasty surgery, only a linked prosthesis can usually be inserted.

Overall, prosthetic replacement for rheumatoid arthritis has demonstrated excellent results. The more common complications include instability in the patients with unlinked implants and potential ulnar neuropathy (1% to 3% permanent injury) in all arthroplasty patients. Although the rate of infection remains relatively low (2% to 5%), it is a major concern.

When to use a linked prosthesis versus an unlinked, resurfacing prosthesis is a subject of debate. If a significant loss of bone or ligamentous instability is evident, or a wide surgical release of soft tissues is required, then a semiconstrained device should be ideal. Clinical results indicate that loosening may not be more common in linked designs than with resurfacing, unlinked designs. The potential advantage of preserving bone stock is not true for all resurfacing implant designs. The precise technique for implantation of an unlinked design requires anatomic accuracy while making bone cuts, or instability may result.

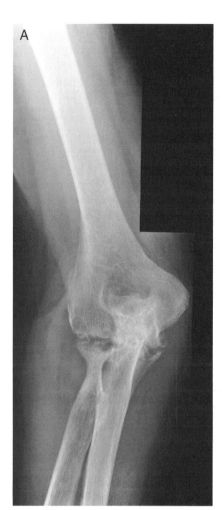

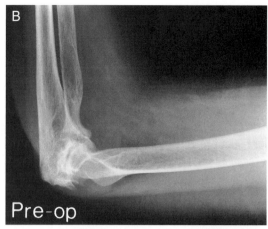

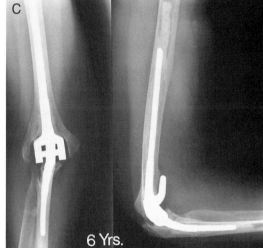

Figure 2 **A** and **B**, Type III rheumatoid involvement of the elbow. **C**, 6-year satisfactory result following replacement. *(Reproduced from Morrey BF, O'Driscoll SW: Elbow arthritis, in Norris TR (ed): Orthopaedic Knowledge Update: Shoulder and Elbow. Rosemont, IL, American Academy of Orthopaedic Surgeons, 1997, pp 379-386.)*

Posttraumatic Arthritis

Posttraumatic arthritis of the elbow is commonly seen after injury because of the high degree of constraint of the ulnohumeral articulation. Malunion, nonunion, and degenerative arthritis are common symptoms. Stiffness is often the initial complaint. Treatment is tailored to the individual, but is especially challenging for those with jobs involving manual labor.

Treatment

Arthroscopic treatment has recently been used in patients with mild degenerative changes after trauma. Débridement of joint surface irregularities due to prior fractures of the capitellum or radial head fractures can be done arthroscopically. Small articular malalignments can be made less prominent by shaving or burring. A supracondylar malunion healed in extension can be recontoured arthroscopically to reestablish greater flexion for the patient. If the articular trauma resulted in a significant extrinsic contracture of the joint, this can also potentially be released arthroscopically. Before extensive surgical procedures are performed, it is important

to analyze the patient's level of pain. If the patient has pain only at the extremes of motion (either flexion or extension), then impingement of a healed fracture fragment or an osteophyte is the probable cause. Débridement of the impinging structure would be beneficial. If the patient has pain through the arc of motion in addition to end-range pain, and if erosion or irregularity of the articulation are present, an interposition arthroplasty may be of benefit. Finally, if the patient complains of pain at rest or while sleeping, an inflamed synovium may be a significant source of pain and synovectomy may be warranted.

Radiographs obtained from patients with posttraumatic arthritis should be carefully examined for evidence of instability. An old coronoid fracture or malunion may be indicative of an incongruent joint. Likewise, if the radial head was removed at the time of initial fracture, then posterolateral instability may be a possibility. Resurfacing the joint with an interposition arthroplasty and placement of a hinged external fixation device will not be successful if underlying joint instability is not addressed. In a study of 10 patients treated with a Dynamic Joint Distractor (Howmedica, Rutherford, NJ) for post-

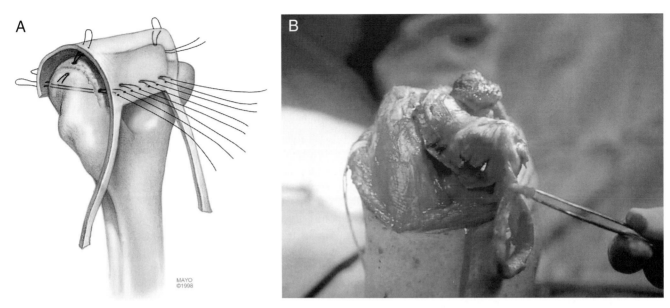

Figure 3 A, Interposition arthroplasty. Achilles tendon allograft is draped over the distal humerus. Sutures have been placed to secure it to the recontoured bony surface. Two tails are available to reconstruct the collateral ligaments. *(Reproduced with permission from the Mayo Foundation, Rochester, MN.)* **B,** Intraoperative view of Achilles tendon placed over recontoured distal humerus. Sutures have been placed through the humerus, securing the graft to the bone. A tail of graft can be seen on the right, held by forceps, which will be used to reconstruct the lateral collateral ligament.

traumatic arthritis, four patients had unstable elbows. After hinged external fixator removal, the elbow of only one of the four patients remained stable. In another study using the Compass Hinge (Smith & Nephew, Memphis, TN) in 11 posttraumatic patients, dislocation occurred in 2 of 11 patients (18%) while wearing the hinge and 2 of 3 unstable fractures remained unstable after the fixator was removed. The key to use of the hinged external fixator in patients with posttraumatic arthritis is to attempt to fix all bony defects or displacements at the time of surgery and to repair all ligamentous disruptions (Fig. 3). The hinged external fixator is used to protect the fragile stability of the joint that is achieved by restoring the bony and ligamentous anatomy. If the surgeon depends on the fixator to achieve stability after removal of the hinged device, subluxation eventually occurs.

Total elbow arthroplasty is a potential option for the patient with posttraumatic arthritis. Although excellent short-term results are possible, the durability of the prosthesis is of major concern. The use of the linked Pritchard-Walker prosthesis was studied in nine patients with posttraumatic arthritis. Improvement was not as successful as for patients with rheumatoid arthritis, in whom the functional rating was twice as great. In another study of total elbow arthroplasty patients, 18 had undergone an arthroplasty for posttraumatic arthritis. The 5-year survival rate was 53%. Of the 18 patients, there were two infections and five loose prostheses.

In yet another study, 38 active patients who had total elbow arthroplasty for posttraumatic arthritis were assessed, giving significant insight into the possible ben-

efits and complications associated with total elbow arthroplasty. At follow-up, all 38 prostheses were stable, with function restored to the elbow. No prosthesis was loose at an average follow-up of 5 years, which is a considerable improvement over prior reports. Complications were significant, with ulnar component fracture occurring in 12% and polyethylene bushing failure in 5%. Two patients (5%) developed an infection. The ulna fracturing and bushing wear associated with the prosthesis was believed to be directly related to the greater postoperative physical activity in these patients. The authors of the study recommended the implantation of a prosthesis only in patients willing to agree to postoperative limitations of no lifting of objects heavier than 4.5 kg or no lifting on a repetitive basis of any object heavier than 1 kg. Patients who develop a worn bushing or fracture of the ulnar component require surgery to replace the bushing or fractured ulnar stem. Obviously, the implantation of a prosthesis in a young patient should be done with caution and only if an individual seems capable of adhering to the necessary postoperative activity restrictions.

Allograft replacement of a severely destroyed elbow joint after trauma or tumor resection has been reported. In one study, all patients had radiographic changes suggestive of degenerative joint disease at 2-year follow-up. Complications occurred in 70% (16 of 23 patients). Allograft replacement is primarily a salvage procedure that should be considered only in the patient with significant bone loss, which is rare.

Total elbow arthroplasty has become a viable option

in elderly patients with a distal humeral nonunion. In a study of 36 patients with an average age of 68 years, a satisfactory result was achieved in 86%. Pain relief was significant, with 88% having severe or moderate pain preoperatively and 91% having no or only mild discomfort postoperatively. Complications, including infection, particulate synovitis, ulnar neuropathy, and worn polyethylene bushings, occurred in 18% of patients. In patients in whom repeat bone grafting and osteosynthesis are not successful, total elbow arthroplasty seems to be an effective treatment option.

Arthrodesis of the arthritic elbow joint is technically feasible but results often are not satisfying to the patient or surgeon. With the excellent results achieved in elderly patients after total elbow arthroplasty, arthrodesis is only a potential option in the young patient or as a salvage procedure in a patient with prior sepsis. Even in the manual laborer, an attempt should be made to avoid arthrodesis. There is no ideal position for elbow arthrodesis. If no other option is thought possible, an adjustable static splint can be worn for a period of time to allow the patient to select the desired position of fusion, or a cast can be used to hold the elbow in the desired position prior to committing to the arthrodesis.

Osteoarthritis

Osteoarthritis of the elbow joint has a consistent clinical presentation. The patients are almost all male, are around 50 years of age, and the dominant side is usually involved. Patients often describe a lifetime of manual work involving the affected extremity. Primary elbow arthritis is rare in women.

Patients often do not seek treatment until more than 30° of terminal extension is lost. Pain at the end point of motion is usually the primary reason to seek medical treatment, though patients may complain of elbow contracture and joint stiffness. Loss of pronation or supination is rare.

The patient may also present with painful catching or locking of the elbow, commonly seen in relatively young athletes and laborers who have a minimal loss of motion. This symptom often represents the early stages of the disease. At this point, radiographs or tomograms may reveal a loose body in the elbow. In the patient with moderate radiographic arthritis of the elbow, it is common to see many loose bodies on the radiographs or tomographs. Some of these ossific orbs are actually loose within the joint; however, others may appear loose but are actually embedded in scarred portions of the capsule.

In the patient with elbow pain, it is important to determine the nature of the pain. Minimal pain or pain only at the extremes of motion is a typical presentation

and probably represents impingement of osteophytes at the limitations of motion. Some of the osteophytes are mobile, as if nonunions. Pain through the arc of motion would signify articular cartilage degeneration or synovitis. Pain at night or pain at rest may be due to a synovitis, but this is a rare finding. The close association of the ulnar nerve to the posterior medial joint capsule allows the nerve to easily become affected by a synovitis or impinged by an osteophyte. Elbow pain is often a primary and initial complaint of patients with cubital tunnel syndrome. Many patients with degenerative disease of the elbow joint have a mild ulnar neuropathy. It is important to distinguish ulnar neuropathy from the mild arthritis seen on a radiograph.

Although primary degenerative arthritis is often evident after reviewing the patient's history, radiographs of the elbow will confirm the diagnosis. CT scans or trispiral tomography, if available, are a useful adjunct to locate osteophytes and loose bodies. In most cases, AP, lateral, and oblique radiographs will be sufficient. Peaking of osteophytes is commonly seen at the tips of both the olecranon and coronoid. Osteophytes are also noted on the lateral projections in the radial and coronoid fossae. The AP radiograph may be noted to have a rim of "fluffy" osteophytes filling the olecranon fossa.

Treatment

Initial treatment is with rest and nonsurgical measures. When these methods prove unsuccessful, patients usually request treatment for the loss of motion and for pain. Joint débridement, the initial treatment for elbow arthritis, involved splitting the triceps or elevation of the medial half of the triceps to approach the olecranon fossa. Fenestration of the fossa permits access to the tip of the coronoid to the anterior joint.

Removal of the radial head as an adjunct is almost never necessary. Removing the radial head may actually increase instability to the elbow and arthritic degeneration. This procedure does not predictably improve flexion of the joint. If further gains in flexion are desired, a column procedure or formal capsular release can be added to the procedure. Results of ulnohumeral arthroplasty for osteoarthritis of the elbow have generally been favorable.

In a study of 45 patients followed for a 6-year period, range of motion improved and pain relief was significant. The Mayo Elbow Performance Score increased from 54 to 83 points. Interestingly, 12 of the 45 patients developed ulnar nerve symptoms postoperatively, with 6 patients undergoing another operation to decompress or translocate the nerve. Postoperative ulnar neuropathy was more common in patients who had a stiff elbow before surgery. The overall rate of ulnar nerve dysfunction of 24% in this group of patients is a cause of concern. If a patient is

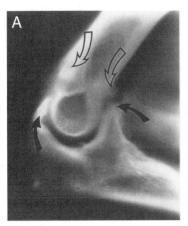
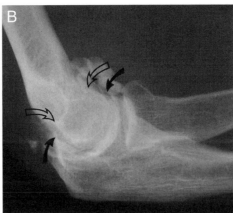
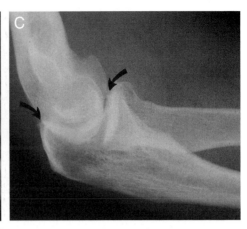

Figure 4 A, Lateral tomograms or CT reconstructions show the osteophytes on the olecranon and coronoid (solid arrows) as well as those in and around the olecranon and coronoid fossae (open arrows). **B,** Preoperative radiograph of an elbow with primary osteoarthritis. Multiple loose bodies are seen anteriorly and posteriorly. In addition, osteophytes (solid arrows) are seen on the olecranon and coronoid. The trochlea has osteophytes at the bottom of the olecranon and coronoid fossae (open arrows), so that the trochlea has become U-shaped rather than O-shaped. These must be removed to eliminate impingement and gain motion. **C,** Postoperatively, the osteophytes and loose bodies are not seen. *(Reproduced with permission from the Mayo Foundation, Rochester, MN.)*

undergoing surgery for a stiff elbow, they should be counseled on the potential risks of ulnar neuropathy. If a patient can flex the elbow only to 90°, then the ulnar nerve should be transposed at the time of surgery. If the elbow only can be flexed to 90° to 110°, the nerve probably should be decompressed or transposed. Overall, ulnohumeral arthroplasty offers satisfactory long-term results.

An interposition arthroplasty may act as a bridge between simple débridement and total elbow arthroplasty. In the young patient who has a severely degenerative joint, total elbow arthroplasty is not currently a viable option.

Arthroscopy has gained greater recognition as a treatment option for patients with osteoarthritis of the elbow. Arthroscopic surgery allows for the possibility of complete release of a tight capsule and débridement of all impinging osteophytes; this technique has been termed an osteocapsular arthroplasty. While using an open procedure such as the Outerbridge-Kashiwagi arthroplasty, it is difficult to address all tight capsular areas or bony osteophytes. Although osteophytes on the coronoid can be removed through the hole created in the olecranon fossa, osteophytes in the area of the radial fossa cannot be reached during an Outerbridge-Kashiwagi arthroplasty without a separate lateral approach. Arthroscopic osteocapsular arthroplasty offers the ability to inspect all areas of the anterior and posterior elbow joint and remove all potentially offending osteophytes (Fig. 4). One disadvantage of arthroscopic osteocapsular arthroplasty is the steep learning curve required to become proficient at the technique. Neurovascular structures, particularly the ulnar and radial nerves, are just a few millimeters away from the arthroscopic instruments during the surgical procedure. Participation in a surgical

skills course and practice in a cadaver laboratory are mandatory in order to learn the technique. Simple, brief arthroscopic removal of a few loose bodies is often not very beneficial to the patient.

The benefit of arthroscopy in the treatment of primary degenerative arthritis has been demonstrated in several studies. In one report, 35 athletes with degenerative changes in the elbow were treated with débridement. The majority of the patients felt better after surgery and 90% had improved pain relief and function. A study of 21 patients with posttraumatic or degenerative arthritis undergoing arthroscopic débridement demonstrated improvements in motion and a decrease in pain relief. Another study described the arthroscopic equivalent of an Outerbridge-Kashiwagi arthroplasty in 12 patients. All patients had improvement in their symptoms. In a second study, the arthroscopic Outerbridge-Kashiwagi arthroplasty approach was used in 24 patients and a significant decrease in pain and an average increase in the arc of motion of 81° were reported. Although excellent results were reported in these studies, arthroscopic fenestration of the olecranon fossa is usually not necessary in most patients. Through standard anterior and posterior portals, adequate débridement and burring of osteophytes is possible.

Annotated Bibliography

Rheumatoid Arthritis

Connor PM, Morrey BF: Total elbow arthroplasty in patients who have juvenile rheumatoid arthritis. *J Bone Joint Surg Am* 1998;80:678.

Twenty-four elbow replacements in patients with juvenile rheumatoid arthritis (average age, 36 years) were studied. The Mayo Elbow Performance Score increased from 31 points preoperatively to 90 points postoperatively. The flexion-extension arc improved from only 62° preoperatively to 90° postoperatively. None of the semiconstrained implants had evidence of loosening at the most recent follow-up.

Ferlic DC, Clayton ML: Salvage of failed total elbow arthroplasty. *J Shoulder Elbow Surg* 1995;4:290-297.

The authors revised 14 total elbow arthroplasties: three because of infection, six because of aseptic loosening, four because of instability, and one because a bearing mechanism failed. The infected elbows were converted to resection arthroplasties. The aseptic failures were successfully salvaged with implantation of a linked prosthesis. The noninfected elbows were successfully revised, resulting in pain relief.

Gill DR, Morrey BF: The Coonrad-Morrey total elbow arthroplasty in patients who have rheumatoid arthritis: A 10 to 15-year follow-up study. *J Bone Joint Surg Am* 1998;80:1327-1335.

Forty-one patients were examined with at least a 10-year follow-up. Forty-five of the 46 total elbow arthroplasties were not painful or were only mildly painful. There was an increase in the flexion arc of 13°. Bushing wear occurred in 11 patients. The rate of survival of the prosthesis was 92%.

Gschwend N, Simmen BR, Matejovsky Z: Late complications in elbow arthroplasty. *J Shoulder Elbow Surg* 1996;5:96-96.

This article presents a discussion of elbow replacement for rheumatoid and posttraumatic conditions. The satisfactory use of a semiconstrained implant for rheumatoid arthritis was demonstrated. The results in the elbows with posttraumatic conditions were not as satisfactory.

Hildebrand KA, Patterson SD, Regan WD, MacDermid JC, King GJW: Functional outcome of semiconstrained total elbow arthroplasty. *J Bone Joint Surg Am* 2000; 82:1379.

The results of total elbow arthroplasty with the Coonrad-Morrey prosthesis were reviewed in 51 elbows. The Mayo Elbow Performance Score for the group with inflammatory arthritis (90 points) was significantly higher than that of the group with a traumatic or posttraumatic condition (78 points). An ulnar nerve dysfunction was presented in 26% of elbows, and 23% had an intraoperative fracture. Progressive radiolucency was seen around the humeral prostheses in one elbow and around the ulnar prosthesis in eight elbows.

Lee BP, Morrey BF: Arthroscopic synovectomy of the elbow for rheumatoid arthritis: A prospective study. *J Bone Joint Surg Am* 1997;79:770-772.

Fourteen limited arthroscopic synovectomies for rheumatoid arthritis were performed without capsular release in 11

patients. Ninety-three percent achieved a short-term rating of excellent or good on the Mayo Elbow Performance Score. At later follow-up (42 months) only 57% maintained an excellent or good result. Four patients required total elbow arthroplasty.

Rozing PM: Souter-Strathclyde total elbow arthroplasty: A long-term follow-up study. *J Bone Joint Surg Br* 2000; 82:1129-1134.

Sixty-six Souter-Strathclyde prostheses were replaced in 59 patients. Twenty-four percent were revised, 9% for aseptic loosening, 4.5% for infection, and 4.5% for dislocation. Early complications included postoperative dislocation and ulnar neuropathy.

Posttraumatic Arthritis

Cheng SL, Morrey BF: Treatment of the mobile, painful arthritic elbow by distraction interposition arthroplasty. *J. Bone Joint Surg Br* 2000;82:233-238.

Thirteen patients with mobile, painful, arthritic elbows were treated with distraction interposition arthroplasty using fascia lata. Ten patients had posttraumatic arthritis. Of the four elbows that were unstable before surgery, only one remained stable following removal of the fixator.

Cobb TK, Morrey BF: Total elbow arthroplasty as primary treatment for distal humeral fractures in elderly patients. *J Bone Joint Surg Am* 1997;79:826-832.

Twenty-one elbows that had undergone total elbow arthroplasty were studied after acute distal humeral fracture. Twenty elbows had either an excellent or good result. No aseptic loosening occurred.

Dean GS, Hollinger EH, Urbaniak JR: Elbow allograft for reconstruction of the elbow with massive bone loss: Long-term results. *Clin Orthop* 1997;341:12-22.

Twenty-three patients had partial or total elbow joint allograft reconstruction. The majority were for posttraumatic disability. Complications occurred in 70%. This procedure is not recommended for routine use and is viewed as a salvage procedure.

Fox RJ, Varitimidis SE, Plakseychuk A, Vardakas DG, Tomaino MN, Sotereanos DG: The Compass Elbow Hinge: Indications and initial results. *J Hand Surg Br* 2000;25:568-572.

The Compass Elbow Hinge (Smith & Nephew, Memphis, TN) was used to treat 11 patients with degenerative disease, contracture, or instability. Dislocation occurred in 2 of 11 patients (18%). Pin-tract infections occurred in five patients. Two patients with unreconstructed coronoid fractures remained unstable after removal of the fixator. A hinged fixator cannot achieve stability without concomitant ligament or bony reconstruction.

Morrey BF, Adams RA: Semiconstrained elbow replacement for distal humeral nonunion. *J Bone Joint Surg Br* 1995;77:67-72.

Thirty-six patients, average age 68 years, had a semiconstrained elbow arthroplasty for distal humeral nonunion. Eighty-six percent had satisfactory results. Arthroplasty can be a safe treatment for this difficult clinical condition.

Schneeberger A, Adams R, Morrey BF: Semiconstrained joint replacement for posttraumatic arthritis. *J Bone Joint Surg Am* 1997;79:1211-1222.

Forty-one patients were treated with a semiconstrained implant for posttraumatic arthritis and followed for an average of 5.5 years. Eighty-three percent had a good or excellent result. Mechanical failure occurred in the form of ulnar component fracture in 12% and bushing failure in 5%. The procedure is contraindicated in patients who perform strenuous physical activity.

Osteoarthritis

Ljung P, Jonsson K, Larsson K, Rydholm U: Interposition arthroplasty of the elbow with rheumatoid arthritis. *J Shoulder Elbow Surg* 1996;5:81-85.

The authors examined 35 elbows at a median of 6 years following interposition arthroplasty. Humeral bone loss occurred in two thirds of the elbows and ulnar bone loss in one third. The long-term results of interposition were found to be inferior to total elbow replacement. Because of bone loss, reoperation for total elbow arthroplasty was made difficult or impossible.

O'Driscoll SW: Arthroscopic treatment for osteoarthritis of the elbow. *Orthop Clin North Am* 1995;26:691-706.

In this article, the author reviews the evaluation and arthroscopic treatment of primary degenerative arthritis of the elbow.

Ogilvie-Harris DJ, Gordon R, MacKay M: Arthroscopic treatment for posterior impingement in degenerative arthritis of the elbow. *Arthroscopy* 1995;11:437-443.

Arthroscopic débridement for degenerative arthritis of the elbow was performed on 21 patients. Postoperatively, all patients were rated as either excellent or good. There were no neurologic complications and no postoperative infections.

Oka Y, Ohta K, Saitoh I: Debridement arthroplasty for osteoarthritis of the elbow. *Clin Orthop* 1998;351:127-134.

Thirty-eight elbows were treated with open débridement after collateral ligament release. Both a medial and a lateral approach to the joint was used. Forty-two percent of patients had an ulnar neuropathy associated with the arthritis.

Classic Bibliography

Ewald FC, Simmons ED Jr, Sullivan JA, et al: Capitellocondylar total elbow replacement in rheumatoid arthritis. *J Bone Joint Surg Am* 1993;75:498-507.

Inglis AE, Pellicci PM: Total elbow replacement. *J Bone Joint Surg Am* 1980;62:1252-1258.

Kraay MJ, Figgie MP, Inglis AE, et al: Primary semiconstrained total elbow arthroplasty: Survival analysis of 113 consecutive cases. *J Bone Joint Surg Br* 1994;76: 636-640.

Morrey BF: Primary degenerative arthritis of the elbow: Treatment by ulnohumeral arthroplasty. *J Bone Joint Surg Br* 1992;74:409-413.

Morrey BF, Bryan RS, Dobyns JH, Linscheid RL: Total elbow arthroplasty: A five-year experience at the Mayo Clinic. *J Bone Joint Surg Am* 1981;63:1050-1063.

Redden JF, Stanley D: Arthroscopy fenestration of olecranon fossa in the treatment of osteoarthritis of the elbow. *Arthroscopy* 1993;9:14-16.

Tsuge K, Mizuseki T: Debridement arthroplasty for advanced primary osteoarthritis of the elbow: Results of a new technique used for 29 elbows. *J Bone Joint Surg Br* 1994;76:641-646.

Tulp NJ, Winia WP: Synovectomy of the elbow in rheumatoid arthritis: Long-term results. *J Bone Joint Surg Br* 1989;71:664-666.

Ward WG, Anderson TE: Elbow arthroscopy in a mostly athletic population. *J Hand Surg Am* 1993;18:220-224.

Chapter 33

Radial Head Fractures

Graham J.W. King, MD, MSc, FRCSC

Introduction

Radial head fractures are the most common fractures of the elbow. Although they sometimes occur in isolation, these fractures frequently are associated with dislocations of the elbow and with disruption of the medial collateral ligament (MCL), the lateral collateral ligament (LCL), or the interosseous ligament. The radial head is an important stabilizer of the elbow in the setting of these associated ligamentous injuries. Fractures of the coronoid, olecranon, and capitellum are commonly seen with radial head fractures and further impair elbow stability.

Although minimally displaced radial head fractures usually have a favorable functional outcome, displaced and comminuted fractures remain a challenge. Plain radiographs may be inadequate for decision making; in selected cases, CT is helpful to better characterize fracture size, displacement, and comminution. Internal fixation should be considered for displaced fractures, particularly those that block forearm rotation. There is increasing evidence to support the effectiveness of internal fixation for selected displaced radial head fractures. The most common clinical dilemma is encountered when deciding whether internal fixation of a radial head fracture is, or will be, sufficiently stable. An unstable or incongruent radial head following internal fixation often leads to a worse result than radial head excision or replacement. Recent biomechanical studies suggest that metallic radial head replacement is superior to radial head excision in the ligament-deficient elbow; however, clinical experience with metallic arthroplasty remains limited to medium-term follow-up.

Anatomy and Biomechanics

The radial head has a circular concave surface, or dish, that articulates with the capitellum (Fig. 1). The articulating surface is variably offset from the axis of the radial neck. The margin of the radial head that articulates with the radial notch of the ulna is slightly elliptical. The anterolateral third of the articular margin is

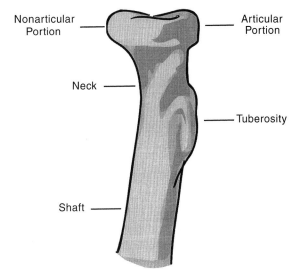

Figure 1 Anatomy of the proximal radius. The concave articulating surface of the radial head is variably offset from the axis of the radial neck. The margin of the radial head that articulates with the radial notch of the ulna is somewhat elliptical in shape. The portion of the radial head that does not articulate with the ulna is more rounded.

devoid of articular cartilage, allowing placement of internal fixation without impingement with the ulna during forearm rotation. With the forearm in neutral rotation, this safe zone is a 110° arc centered on a point 10° anterior to the midpoint of the lateral side of the radial head. The margin of this nonarticular portion has a more rounded shape. Placement of plates in this location often is required in the management of comminuted fractures involving the radial head and neck. The radial head is surrounded by the annular ligament; therefore, bulky internal fixation is poorly tolerated. Implants should be as low profile as possible to minimize soft-tissue adherence that may impede forearm rotation.

A better understanding of the lateral ligamentous anatomy of the elbow has resulted in improvements in surgical technique during radial head surgery. The lateral ulnar collateral ligament (LUCL) has been shown to be an important stabilizer against posterolateral rota-

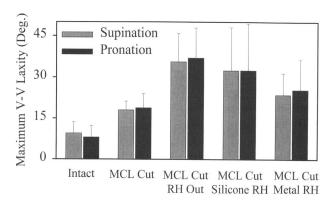

Figure 2 Stability contributed by the radial head. Graph of varus-valgus elbow laxity before and after MCL transection, radial head excision, and replacement with silicone and metallic radial head implants. Note that the metallic implant is more able than the silicone implant to improve elbow stability following radial head excision. RH = radial head. *(Adapted with permission from King GJ, Zarzour ZD, Rath DA, Dunning CE, Patterson SD, Johnson JA: Metallic radial head arthroplasty improves valgus stability of the elbow. Clin Orthop 1999;368:114-125.)*

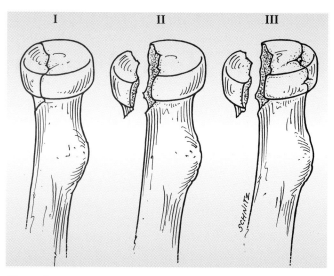

Figure 3 Mason classification. Type I, nondisplaced; type II, displaced wedge fragment(s); and type III, comminuted. *(Reproduced with permission from Morgan WJ: Fractures of the radial head. J Am Soc Surg Hand 2001;1:225-235.)*

tional instability of the elbow. Conventional surgical approaches through Kocher's interval between the extensor carpi ulnaris and the anconeus tend to expose the radial head too posteriorly to permit internal fixation of the commonly involved anterolateral portion of the radial head. In addition, iatrogenic injury to the LUCL is difficult to avoid unless the dissection is brought more anterior so that the radial collateral ligament (RCL) is divided at the midaxis of the radial head. Repair of the fascial interval between the anconeus and extensor carpi ulnaris has been shown to improve elbow stability.

Resisted isometric flexion has been estimated to generate forces across the elbow up to four times body weight. The radiocapitellar articulation may account for up to 60% of the load transfer across the elbow. Displaced fractures of the radial head result in a decreased residual surface area available for load transfer, and they increase posterolateral rotational stability of the elbow by virtue of a loss of capture of the articulating dish of the radial head with the capitellum. The radial head is also an important valgus stabilizer of the elbow, particularly in the setting of an incompetent MCL that is typically disrupted in the setting of a displaced radial head fracture. Recent biomechanical studies have demonstrated that the kinematics and stability of the elbow are altered by radial head excision, even in the setting of intact collateral ligaments. Radial head replacement with metallic prostheses has been shown to improve the valgus stability of the elbow (Fig. 2) and the axial stability of the forearm that have MCL and interosseous ligament disruption, respectively. Silicone radial head replacements were inferior to metallic implants in these studies.

Clinical Assessment

The mechanism of injury is commonly a fall on the outstretched hand. The radial head may fail under compressive axial or valgus loads, or, more commonly, a marginal shearing fracture may occur because of rotatory subluxation or dislocation of the elbow. Higher energy injuries are more likely to have an associated fracture of the capitellum, coronoid, or olecranon. Disruption of the MCL and/or LCL and the interosseous ligament, or a dislocation of the elbow and/or distal radioulnar joint also occurs with greater-impact forces. Inspection may reveal ecchymosis along the forearm and/or medial aspect of the elbow. The ligamentous structures of the wrist and forearm and the osseous structures of the elbow should be palpated carefully.

Imaging

AP, lateral, and oblique elbow radiographs usually provide sufficient information for diagnosis and treatment of radial head fractures. Because of a higher incidence of interosseous ligament injury, bilateral PA radiographs of both wrists in neutral rotation should be obtained to evaluate ulnar variance in patients with wrist discomfort and in those who have a comminuted radial head fracture. CT may be useful in selected cases to assist in quantifying fracture size, displacement, and comminution and to assist in preoperative planning.

Classification

Radial head fractures have been classified into three types: type I, nondisplaced; type II, displaced wedge fragment(s); and type III, comminuted (Fig. 3). A recent study demonstrated poor intraobserver and interobserver reproducibility of this classification based on plain radiographs. CT is helpful in preoperatively distinguishing between fracture types and in evaluating fracture size and displacement. A fourth type, a radial head fracture associated with an elbow dislocation was added later. A more recent development is a management-based classification with three types: I, nondisplaced or minimally displaced (< 2 mm); II, displaced but reconstructable; and III, unreconstructable as judged by radiographs or at surgery (Table 1). This latter classification has important implications with regard to treatment. The decision as to what fracture is reconstructable depends on surgical factors such as the surgeon's experience and implants available; patient factors such as osteoporosis; and fracture factors such as fragment size, comminution, and associated soft-tissue injuries. The ultimate decision as to whether a fracture is reconstructable often can be decided only during surgery.

Associated Injuries

Displaced radial head fractures are commonly associated with disruption of ligaments of the elbow or forearm. In one study, no patient with a minimally or nondisplaced fracture had an associated disruption of the MCL on stress radiographs. However, 71% of patients with a displaced shear fracture of the radial head or an impacted fracture of the radial neck had an MCL injury. All of the patients with a comminuted radial head fracture had disruption of the MCL of the elbow or the interosseous ligament of the forearm (91% and 9%, respectively).

A fracture of the capitellum may be seen as a chondral injury or a displaced fracture. Patients with an associated elbow subluxation or dislocation may also have a fracture of the coronoid (this combination of injuries—posterior dislocation of the elbow, radial head fracture, and coronoid fracture—is called the "terrible triad" with disruption of one or both collateral ligaments of the elbow). Larger coronoid fragments are associated with greater instability of the elbow. Fractures of the olecranon or proximal ulna may be seen, particularly with higher energy injuries such as those associated with a motor vehicle accident or a fall from a height.

Management

Radial head fractures should be managed based on patient factors such as age, bone quality, associated injuries, and activity level. Fracture factors that influence decision making include fracture size, displacement, and location and the presence of a block to forearm rotation. For example, an older patient with osteoporosis and a comminuted radial head fracture is a poor candidate for inter-

TABLE 1	Hotchkiss Classification of Proximal Radial Fractures*

Type I

Nondisplaced or minimally displaced fracture of head or neck

No mechanical block to rotation

Displacement < 2 mm or a marginal lip fracture

Type II

Displaced (usually > 2 mm) fracture of head or neck (angulated)

May have mechanical block to motion or be incongruous

Without severe comminution (technically possible to repair with ORIF)

More than a marginal lip fracture of the radial head

Type III

Severely comminuted fracture of the radial head or neck

Judged not reconstructable on basis of radiographic or intraoperative appearance

Usually requires excision for movement

All of these fractures may have associated injuries such as a coronoid fracture, elbow dislocation, or MCL or interosseous ligament tears

(Adapted with permission from Hotchkiss RN: Displaced fractures of the radial head: Internal fixation or excision. J Am Acad Orthop Surg 1997;5:1-10.)

nal fixation. Radial head arthroplasty is the preferred option for unreconstructable fractures in the setting of an associated injury to the MCL or interosseous ligament.

The initial management of a dislocated elbow associated with a radial head fracture is a gentle closed reduction of the elbow dislocation under intravenous sedation. Repeat radiographs following the reduction should be obtained to better evaluate the radial head fracture for further management. A careful assessment for an associated fracture of the coronoid is needed in patients with a radial head fracture, particularly in those patients with a history of an elbow dislocation. Small coronoid fragments are easily misinterpreted as fragments of the radial head. They can be distinguished by their typical triangular appearance and proximal location on the lateral radiograph resulting from their attachment to the anterior capsule. The presence of a coronoid fracture suggests an unstable elbow, for which surgical management is more likely to be required to achieve an optimal outcome.

Hotchkiss Type I Fractures

Currently, the best treatment for nondisplaced and minimally displaced radial head fractures and small marginal fractures, which do not cause a block to forearm rotation, is believed to be early active range of motion. Aspiration of the elbow hemarthrosis and injection of local anesthetic should be considered if there is sufficient pain to prevent evaluation of forearm rotation. Although these fractures are generally stable and subsequent displacement is un-

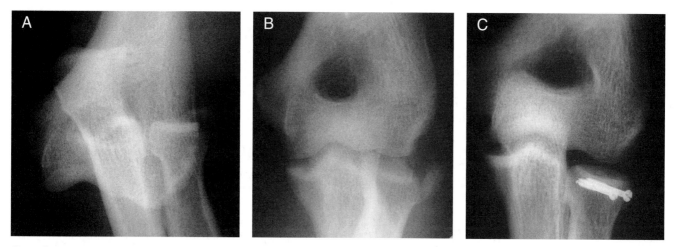

Figure 4 Hotchkiss type II fracture; ORIF with cannulated screws. AP radiograph **(A)** of a 23-year-old patient with a fracture-dislocation of the elbow. Residual displacement of a Hotchkiss type II radial head fracture can be seen following closed reduction of the elbow **(B)**. One year following ORIF of the radial head with 3.0-mm cannulated screws (Synthes, Missisauga, ON) and an LCL repair **(C)**. The patient returned to competitive wrestling.

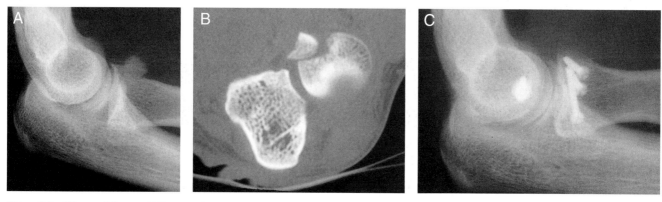

Figure 5 Hotchkiss type II fracture; ORIF with minifragment screws. AP radiograph **(A)** of a 43-year-old man involved in a motor vehicle accident. The patient had a block to supination that did not improve following injection of local anesthetic into the elbow. **B,** CT scan shows small extruded fragment of the radial head blocking forearm supination. **C,** Forearm rotation was restored following ORIF of the radial head with 2.0-mm cannulated screws (Synthes, Missisauga, ON).

common, careful clinical and radiographic follow-up is required. Active motion should be commenced within 1 week because of the frequent development of elbow stiffness with longer periods of immobilization. A collar and cuff are used for comfort between periods of active motion. The nighttime use of a static progressive extension splint should be considered if a flexion contracture is present 6 weeks after the injury.

The outcome of nondisplaced radial head fractures is generally favorable, with return of function within 12 weeks. Mild residual flexion contractures of 10° to 15° are not infrequent sequelae. Some patients develop arthrofibrosis and a more severe capsular contracture requiring arthroscopic or open débridement and release. Stiffness is more common in patients with associated injuries such as an elbow dislocation or coronoid fracture.

Hotchkiss Type II Fractures

These fractures are displaced 2 mm or more, involve a significant portion of the radial head, and can be man-

aged by open reduction and internal fixation (ORIF) (Fig. 4). They may have a mechanical block to motion or be incongruous. Small fragments that are extruded into the proximal radioulnar joint and block forearm rotation are included in this group if stable internal fixation can be achieved (Fig. 5). The decision to repair rather than excise or replace the radial head often can only be determined intraoperatively. ORIF of comminuted radial head fractures can be successful if stable internal fixation is achieved so that early motion can be initiated (Fig. 6). If comminution or osteoporosis prevents a congruous reduction and rigid fixation, radial head excision or replacement should be considered intraoperatively. Failed surgical reconstruction usually leads to significant stiffness and pain requiring further surgery, often with less than satisfactory outcomes.

Internal fixation is performed using small threaded wires; mini-Acutrak (Acumed, Beaverton, OR); Herbert; 1.5-, 2.0-, or 2.7-mm screws and plates; or 3.0-mm cannulated screws, depending on fragment size. If plate fixation

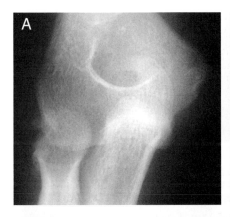

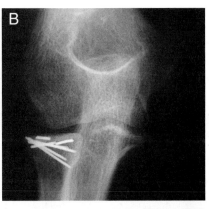

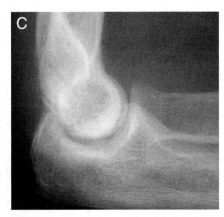

Figure 6 Hotchkiss type II fracture; ORIF with fine threaded wires. AP radiograph **(A)** of a 22-year-old woman who fell from a roof. Following closed reduction of the elbow, the patient underwent ORIF of a comminuted radial head fracture with 1.1-mm threaded wires. A lateral ligament repair was performed using sutures placed through drill holes in the lateral epicondyle **(B)**. The patient recovered a full arc of elbow motion and had no pain 6 months after the injury.

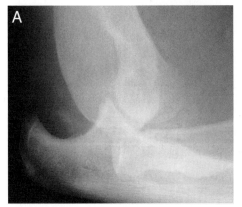

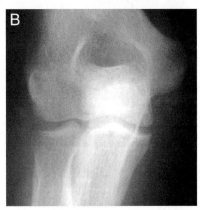

Figure 7 Hotchkiss type III fracture; fragment excision. Oblique radiograph of a 41-year-old man who fell off a scaffold and sustained a dislocation of the elbow and a radial head fracture **(A)**. During surgery, a comminuted segment of the radial head comprising approximately 20% of the articular surface could not be fixed and therefore was excised. Following repair of the lateral ligaments **(B and C)**, early motion was initiated, and the patient regained a functional arc of motion from 30° to 130°.

is used, the plate should be placed on the nonarticular portion of the radial head. This area, the lateral portion of the radial head with the forearm maintained in neutral rotation, can easily be found intraoperatively. Screws should be countersunk as far as possible to avoid impingement with the radial notch and annular ligament. Threaded Kirschner wires (K-wires) may be useful for small fragments not amenable to screw fixation. Smooth K-wires should be avoided because of their tendency to migrate during the postoperative period.

The clinical outcome of ORIF of the radial head has been good when an anatomic reduction and rigid internal fixation have been achieved and early motion has been initiated in the postoperative period. There has been a low incidence of nonunion, osteonecrosis, or stiffness requiring further surgery; however, the complication rate has been higher in patients with more comminuted fractures, particularly displaced fractures of the head and neck. The clinical and radiographic results in patients with nonsurgically treated displaced radial head fractures were inferior to those in a similar group of patients treated with ORIF in one study. The functional outcome and strength of patients treated with ORIF have also been reported to be superior to that of patients treated with radial head excision or silicone radial head replacement.

Hotchkiss Type III Fractures

Comminuted displaced radial head fractures, which cannot be managed reliably by ORIF, are treated with excision of the fragment(s), early or delayed radial head excision, or radial head replacement. These fractures are judged not reconstructable on the basis of radiographs or their intraoperative appearance. Early motion with delayed radial head excision may be considered in patients with comminuted fractures involving more than one third of the radial head provided they do not block forearm rotation and are not severely displaced. This approach may be useful in elderly, low-demand patients with injuries to the MCL or interosseous ligament and in patients with a delayed presentation. The radial head can be excised either open or arthroscopically if the patient remains symptomatic following healing of the fracture and any associated ligamentous injury.

Small fragments that block forearm rotation because of their extrusion into the proximal radioulnar joint or loose fragments that prevent reduction of the ulnohumeral joint are treated with open or arthroscopic fragment excision if ORIF is not technically feasible because of small fragment size, comminution, and osteoporosis (Fig. 7). Fractures that articulate with the proxi-

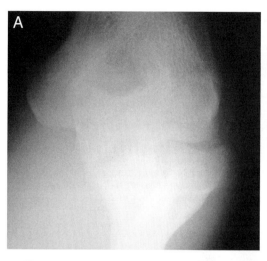

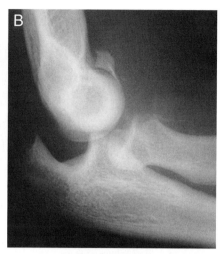

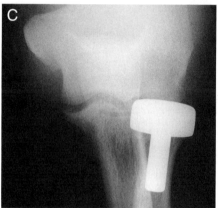

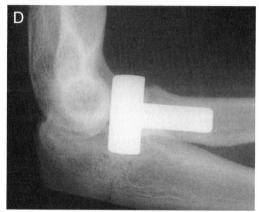

Figure 8 Hotchkiss type III fracture; radial head replacement. AP **(A)** and lateral **(B)** radiographs of a 34-year-old man who fell at high speed from an all-terrain vehicle. A comminuted fracture of the radial head, displaced fracture of the coronoid, and an elbow dislocation are noted. The comminuted radial head fracture could not be fixed and therefore was excised. Following suture repair of the coronoid, a modular metallic radial head arthroplasty (Evolve, Wright Medical Technology, Arlington, TN) was implanted and the lateral ligaments repaired using drill holes in the lateral epicondyle **(C** and **D)**. The elbow was stable for early postoperative motion.

mal radioulnar joint should be treated by radial head excision or replacement because a defect in that part of the radial head interferes with forearm rotation.

If radial head reconstruction is not possible, the presence of associated soft-tissue injuries and concomitant fractures should be considered because acute radial head excision is contraindicated in the setting of concomitant disruption of either the MCL or interosseous ligament. Intraoperative valgus stress views should be obtained using an image intensifier after radial head excision to ensure competency of the MCL of the elbow. Axial stress views to look for an interosseous ligament tear should also be obtained. If these intraoperative stress views are negative and there was no associated elbow dislocation and no clinical suspicion of a ligamentous injury, radial head excision without implant replacement may be considered. The outcome following primary radial head resection without replacement is controversial, with some authors reporting good clinical and radiographic results and others reporting a high incidence of pain, weakness, and degenerative arthritis, particularly at long-term follow-up.

Radial head replacement arthroplasty is indicated for displaced comminuted radial head fractures in which stable internal fixation is not achievable and there are associated soft-tissue or bony injuries (Fig. 8). Silicone implants have been used in the past; however, they are biomechanically inferior to metal and have a significant incidence of failure due to fracture and fragmentation with the production of silicone synovitis. Recent clinical series in which metallic implants were used had good results relative to earlier series in which silicone implants were used. Most metallic radial head implants that have been developed and used have a monoblock design. This design has made their clinical application difficult because of the need to subluxate the elbow to allow for insertion of these devices. Recently, modular metallic radial head prostheses with separate heads and stems have become available; these prostheses have allowed improved sizing options and easier implantation. Although the short- and medium-term results of metallic radial head implants are encouraging, the long-term outcome with respect to loosening, capitellar wear, and arthritis has not been reported.

Surgical Techniques

The patient is placed on the operating table in the supine position with a tourniquet in place. A sandbag placed beneath the ipsilateral scapula assists in positioning the arm across the chest. Prophylactic antibiotics are administered, and general or regional anesthesia is initiated. A posterior elbow incision just lateral to the tip of the olecranon is used, and a full-thickness lateral flap is developed on the deep fascia. This extensile incision decreases the risk of cutaneous nerve injury and provides access to the radial head, coronoid, MCL, and LCL if needed for the management of more complex injuries. The fascial interval between the anconeus and extensor carpi ulnaris (ECU) is identified and developed. The ECU is elevated slightly anteriorly off the LCL complex such that the RCL and annular ligament can be incised at the midaxis of the radial head, staying anterior to the LUCL (Fig. 9). The RCL and overlying extensor muscles are elevated anteriorly to expose the anterior half of the radial head. The LUCL is preserved to prevent the development of posterolateral rotatory instability. Disruption of the LCL complex and common extensor muscles from the lateral epicondyle is commonly noted in patients after an elbow dislocation, simplifying surgical exposure of the radial head.

An alternative approach for more uncomplicated fractures is to divide the common extensor and capsule/ligament complex as a single layer in the interval between the extensor carpi radialis longus and brevis. The landmarks for this approach are a line joining the lateral epicondyle and Lister's tubercle.

Fragment excision may be facilitated with the use of an image intensifier and a pituitary ronguer. The joint should be irrigated copiously to remove all loose intra-articular fragments. Inadvertent removal of a coronoid fragment should be avoided by noting fragment attachment to the anterior capsule. Fragments of bone in the coronoid fossa on the lateral radiograph are almost always from the coronoid, not the radial head. The status of the capitellum is evaluated for chondral injuries or osteochondral fractures. Associated fractures of the coronoid, olecranon, and proximal ulna are managed as indicated. Following fragment excision, ORIF, or radial head excision or replacement, the LCL complex and common extensor muscle origins should be carefully repaired back to the lateral condyle using nonabsorbable sutures through drill holes or with suture anchors. The fascial interval between the anconeus and ECU also should be closed to augment lateral stability of the elbow.

Following fragment excision, ORIF, or radial head excision or replacement and lateral soft-tissue closure, the elbow should be moved through an arc of flexion-extension while carefully evaluating for elbow stability in pronation, neutral, and supination. Pronation is generally beneficial if the lateral ligaments are still deficient, supination is beneficial if the medial ligaments are deficient, and neutral position is beneficial if both sides

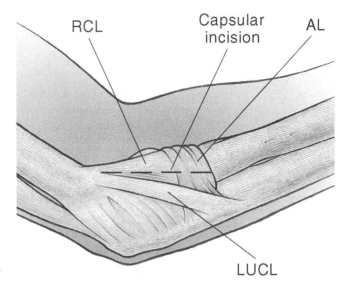

Figure 9 Ligament-sparing approach to the radial head. The RCL and annular ligament (AL) are incised obliquely at the midaxis of the radial head. The anterior portion of the RCL is elevated to allow exposure of the anterolateral aspect of the radial head, the area usually involved in displaced radial head fractures. This approach preserves the LUCL, an important varus and rotational stabilizer of the elbow.

have been damaged, either by the injury or the surgical approach. In patients who have an associated elbow dislocation, the MCL and flexor pronator origin should be repaired if the elbow subluxates in extension. The acceptable degrees of extension block required to prevent subluxation depend on a variety of factors but would tend to be between 30° and 60°.

Postoperative Management

The elbow that has undergone stable osseous and ligamentous repair should be splinted in extension and elevated; this will diminish swelling, protect the posterior wound, and decrease flexion contractures. In the setting of a more tenuous ligamentous repair or the presence of some residual instability at the end of the surgical procedure, the elbow should initially be splinted at 90° of flexion in the optimal position of forearm rotation to maintain stability.

Indomethacin, 75 mg daily for 3 weeks, should be considered in patients undergoing radial head surgery to control postoperative pain and swelling and to reduce the incidence of ossification. This medication should be avoided in patients with a history of peptic ulcer disease or known allergy. The efficacy of indomethacin in the prevention of heterotopic ossification around the elbow remains unproven.

For an isolated radial head fracture treated with an LUCL-sparing approach, active range of motion should be initiated on the day after surgery. A sling with the elbow maintained at 90° is used for comfort between exercises. A static progressive extension splint is fabri-

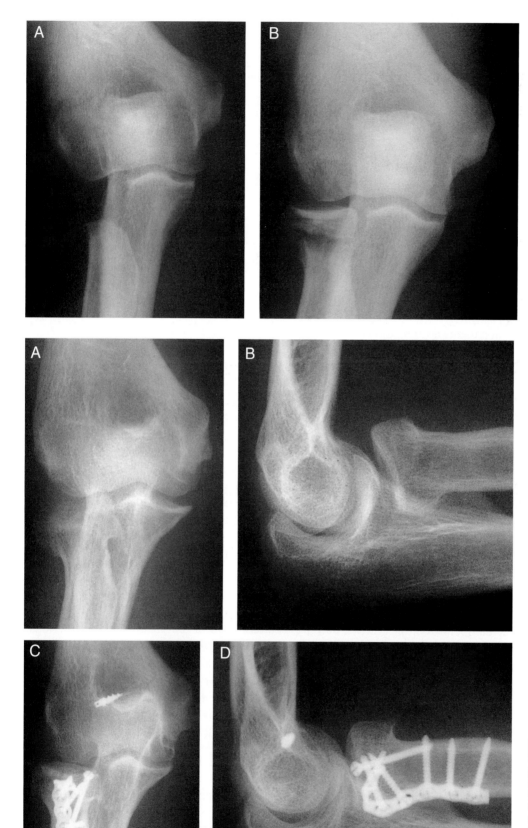

Figure 10 Nonunion of radial neck fracture. AP radiograph **(A)** demonstrating a nonunion of a radial neck fracture in a 52-year-old patient who fell while running 1 year earlier. The patient had persistent lateral elbow pain aggravated by resisted forearm rotation and a weak grip. Radiograph following arthroscopic radial head excision **(B)**. The patient had no pain and full motion 3 months postoperatively.

Figure 11 Malunion of radial neck fracture. AP **(A)** and lateral **(B)** radiographs of a 15-year-old girl who sustained a displaced fracture of the radial neck 18 months earlier, which was treated with closed reduction and casting. The patient had persistent lateral elbow pain and no supination. Radiographs following radial neck osteotomy demonstrate restoration of proximal radial anatomy **(C** and **D)**. The patient had no pain and 70° of supination 1 year postoperatively.

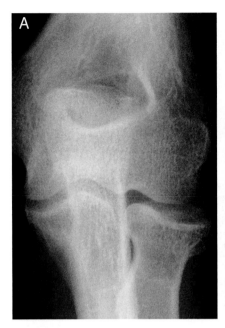
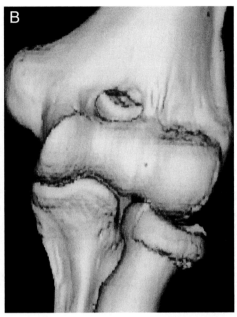
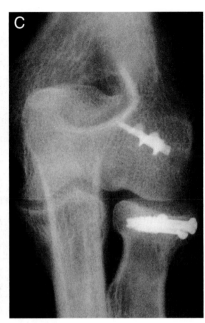

Figure 12 Malunion of radial head fracture. **A,** AP radiograph of a 21-year-old competitive swimmer who sustained a displaced fracture of the radial head 1 year earlier and was treated with early motion. She had persistent lateral elbow pain and clicking that prevented her return to athletics. **B,** CT scan demonstrates residual incongruity of the radial head. **C,** Radiograph following intra-articular radial head osteotomy demonstrates restoration of proximal radial anatomy. The patient had minimal pain and was able to return to swimming.

cated for nighttime use and continued for 12 weeks. Strengthening commences once fracture union is secure.

Patients with associated fractures and ligamentous injuries should commence active flexion and extension exercises within a safe arc 1 day postoperatively. A resting splint with the elbow maintained at 90° or a hinged brace is used for 3 to 6 weeks. Active forearm rotation is performed with the elbow at 90° of flexion to avoid stressing the medial and/or lateral ligamentous injuries or repairs. A static progressive night extension splinting program is initiated as ligamentous healing progresses and stability improves, usually at 6 weeks postoperatively. No passive stretching is permitted for 6 weeks postoperatively. Strengthening exercises are initiated once the fracture and ligament injuries have adequately healed, usually about 8 weeks postoperatively.

Complications

Osteonecrosis probably is common following ORIF of radial head fractures because the fragments typically have an absent or precarious blood supply. Fortunately, the patient is usually asymptomatic, the fragments usually heal uneventfully, and late collapse is uncommon.

Nonunion often is associated with osteonecrosis and seems to be more common in patients with displaced fractures involving the radial neck, particularly if the internal fixation is not secure. Revision ORIF with bone grafting or radial head excision or replacement may be used if the nonunion is symptomatic (Fig. 10).

Malunion is usually a consequence of inadequate fracture fixation or collapse resulting from osteonecrosis. Malunion may cause a restriction in forearm rotation, pain, or crepitus. Extra-articular (Fig. 11) or intra-articular osteotomy (Fig. 12) may be helpful in younger patients, whereas radial head excision or replacement may be considered in those who are older and have lower functional demands.

Osteoarthritis is seen as a consequence of articular cartilage damage from the initial injury, articular incongruity, or persistent instability. Pain and stiffness develop as the arthritis progresses. Radial head excision, either open or arthroscopic, can be helpful if the ulnohumeral joint is uninvolved.

Stiffness is a common sequela of radial head fractures and may be caused by capsular contracture or heterotopic ossification. If a capsular contracture is identified early, physical therapy combined with static progressive splinting using a flexion cuff and resting extension splint can be helpful. Turnbuckle splinting can be useful in patients who are not responsive to standard therapy. Open or arthroscopic capsular release restores a functional arc of motion in most patients.

Late axial or valgus instability is uncommon unless the radial head has been excised and not replaced. Salvage using radial head allografts has been reported; however, increasing experience and longer follow-up suggest a high incidence of complications such as nonunion, collapse, and resorption (Fig. 13). MCL or interosseous ligament reconstruction has not been reliable in restoring

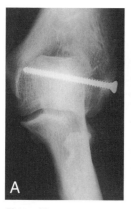
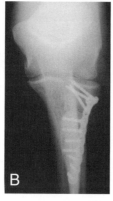
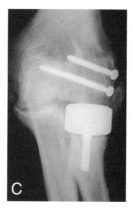
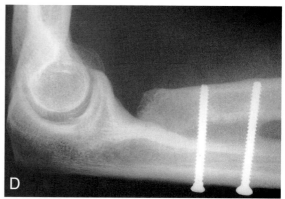

Figure 13 Essex-Lopresti allograft reconstruction. **A,** AP radiograph of a 36-year-old man who had a radial head excision for a comminuted radial head fracture 4 years earlier. He had persistent elbow and wrist pain that prevented his return to construction work. **B,** Radiograph following radial head replacement with a frozen allograft. Autogenous bone graft was used at the host-bone junctions. **C,** Unfortunately, the radial head went on to collapse and the allograft to a nonunion. **D,** One year following radioulnar fusion, the patient had no pain and had changed to a less physically challenging occupation.

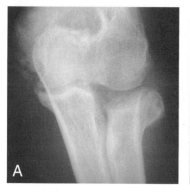
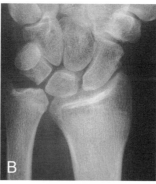
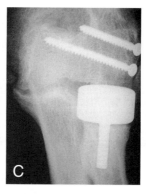
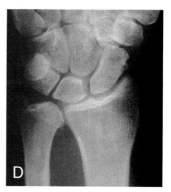

Figure 14 Essex-Lopresti prosthetic reconstruction. AP elbow radiograph **(A)** and posteroanterior wrist radiograph **(B)** of a 37-year-old man who had a radial head excision for a comminuted radial head fracture 3 years earlier. He had persistent severe elbow and wrist pain. Radiographs 2 years after metallic radial head replacement (Smith & Nephew Richards, Warsaw, IN) and an ulnar shortening osteotomy **(C** and **D)** are shown. He had a nonunion of the lateral epicondyle osteotomy used to provide exposure for the insertion of the monoblock radial head implant. The patient had mild discomfort and returned to work as a firefighter.

stability in the absence of a radial head replacement, probably because of attenuation of the soft-tissue repair. Metallic radial head arthroplasty may have a role to play in the salvage of these difficult clinical problems, provided that the capitellar cartilage is not excessively damaged and the proximal radius has not subluxated too far posteriorly to be realigned with the capitellum (Fig. 14).

Annotated Bibliography

Armstrong AD, Dunning CE, Faber KJ, Duck TR, Johnson JA, King GJ: Rehabilitation of the medial collateral ligament-deficient elbow: An in vitro biomechanical study. *J Hand Surg Am* 2000;25:1051-1057.

In a cadaveric study, muscle activity and forearm supination were demonstrated to improve the stability of the MCL-deficient elbow with the arm in the dependent position.

Beingessner DM, Bennett JD, King GJ: Intraarticular radial head osteotomy. *J Shoulder Elbow Surg* 1999;8:172-174.

A symptomatic malunited radial head fracture was successfully managed with an intra-articular radial head osteotomy.

Beredjiklian PK, Nalbantoglu U, Potter HG, Hotchkiss RN: Prosthetic radial head components and proximal radial morphology: A mismatch. *J Shoulder Elbow Surg* 1999;8:471-475.

The anatomic dimensions of the proximal radius obtained from the MRI scans of 46 patients were compared with those of a commercially available titanium implant. The metallic implant overestimated the dimensions of the radial neck and underestimated the thickness of the radial head, making it difficult to restore normal anatomy.

Boulas HJ, Morrey BF: Biomechanical evaluation of the elbow following radial head fracture: Comparison of open reduction and internal fixation vs excision, silastic replacement, and non-operative management. *Chir Main* 1998;17:314-320.

The authors reviewed 36 patients with fractures of the radial head treated with four different techniques. The best outcome was achieved with ORIF of displaced radial head fractures.

Cohen MS, Hastings H: Rotatory instability of the elbow: The anatomy and role of the lateral stabilizers. *J Bone Joint Surg Am* 1997;79:225-233.

In a series of cadaveric dissections, thick septae within the extensor muscle origins were thought to be important stabilizers against posterolateral rotatory instability of the elbow.

Diliberti T, Botte MJ, Abrams RA: Anatomical considerations regarding the posterior interosseous nerve during posterolateral approaches to the proximal part of the radius. *J Bone Joint Surg Am* 2000;82:809-813.

In a cadaveric study, the authors demonstrated that the lateral aspect of the proximal radius is best approached with the forearm maintained in supination to prevent injury to the posterior interosseous nerve. The safe zone was an average of 33 mm from the radial head in supination and 52 mm in pronation.

Dowdy PA, Bain GI, King GJ, Patterson SD: The midline posterior elbow incision: An anatomical appraisal. *J Bone Joint Surg Br* 1995;77:696-699.

In this study, the authors wanted to determine the relationship of the cutaneous nerves to the three usual skin incisions around the elbow. Eighteen cadaver arms were used in the study. It was found that the routine use of the posterior incision may reduce the incidence of symptomatic paresthesia and painful neuromas postoperatively.

Dunning CE, Zarzour ZD, Patterson SD, Johnson JA, King GJ: Muscle forces and pronation stabilize the lateral ligament deficient elbow. *Clin Orthop* 2001;388:118-124.

In a cadaveric study, muscle activity and forearm pronation were demonstrated to improve the stability of the LCL-deficient elbow with the arm in the dependent position.

Esser RD, Davis S, Taavao T: Fractures of the radial head treated by internal fixation: Late results in 26 cases. *J Orthop Trauma* 1995;9:318-323.

Twenty-six patients were assessed after ORIF of a displaced radial head fracture using the Mason classification and the Broberg and Morrey elbow score. Results were good or excellent in the majority of patients.

Frankle MA, Koval KJ, Sanders RW, Zuckerman JD: Radial head fractures associated with elbow dislocations treated by immediate stabilization and early motion. *J Shoulder Elbow Surg* 1999;8:355-360.

Twenty-one patients with radial head fractures and associated elbow dislocations were initially managed with closed reduction of the elbow. Four radial head fractures were treated nonsurgically, nine with open reduction, and eight with silicone radial head replacement. Six patients had persistent elbow instability requiring collateral ligament repair and/or use of an articulated external fixator. Initial radial head displacement predicted functional outcome.

Harrington IJ, Sekyi-Otu A, Barrington TW, Evans DC, Tuli V: The functional outcome with metallic radial head implants in the treatment of unstable elbow fractures: A long-term review. *J Trauma* 2001;50:46-52.

The authors report their experience with metallic radial head arthroplasty in 20 patients at an average follow-up of 12 years. The results were excellent or good in 16 and fair or poor in 4. The radial head prosthesis restored elbow stability when the fractured radial head occurred in combination with a dislocation of the elbow, rupture of the MCL, fracture of the coronoid, or fracture of the proximal ulna. Four patients underwent removal of the implant.

Hildebrand KA, Patterson SD, King GJ: Acute elbow dislocations: Simple and complex. *Orthop Clin North Am* 1999;30:63-79.

Up to 20% of dislocations of the elbow are associated with fractures. In this article, the authors discuss treatment principles of acute elbow dislocations and determine that simple dislocations have a better prognosis than do fracture-dislocations.

Hotchkiss RN: Displaced fractures of the radial head: Internal fixation or excision? *J Am Acad Orthop Surg* 1997;5:1-10.

In this article, the Hotchkiss modification of the Mason classification is discussed.

Ikeda M, Oka Y: Function after early radial head resection for fracture: A retrospective evaluation of 15 patients followed for 3-18 years. *Acta Orthop Scand* 2000;71:191-194.

The authors reviewed 15 patients treated with early radial head resection for a fracture of the radial head at an average 10-year follow-up. All patients had reduced elbow power, and only five patients were pain free.

Janssen RP, Vegter J: Resection of the radial head after Mason type-III fractures of the elbow: Follow-up at 16 to 30 years. *J Bone Joint Surg Br* 1998;80:231-233.

Twenty-one patients with a Mason type III radial head fracture treated by excision of the radial head were evaluated between 16 and 30 years follow-up. Only four patients had elbow pain. Of the 16 patients who had radiographic follow-up, 11 had mild degenerative arthritis of the elbow with joint space narrowing and osteophytes.

Jensen SL, Olsen BS, Sojbjerg JO: Elbow joint kinematics after excision of the radial head. *J Shoulder Elbow Surg* 1999;8:238-241.

In a cadaveric study, the authors demonstrated that even in the setting of intact collateral ligaments, the kinematics and stability of the elbow are altered by excision of the radial head.

King GJ, Zarzour ZD, Rath DA, Dunning CE, Patterson SD, Johnson JA: Metallic radial head arthroplasty improves valgus stability of the elbow. *Clin Orthop* 1999; 368:114-125.

In a cadaveric study, the authors demonstrated that silicone radial head arthroplasty did not improve the valgus stability of the MCL-deficient elbow. All three metallic radial head implants conferred stability similar to the native radial head.

King GJ, Zarzour ZD, Patterson SD, Johnson JA: An anthropometric study of the radial head: Implications in the design of a prosthesis. *J Arthroplasty* 2001;16:112-116.

The anthropometric features of 28 cadaveric proximal radii and 40 contralateral elbows of patients who had undergone radial head arthroplasties were measured. The native radial head was found to have an inconsistently elliptical shape, and the articular dish of the radial head was variably offset from the radial neck. The medullary canal of the radial neck correlated poorly with the diameter of the radial head, suggesting that a modular implant design is needed for radial head arthroplasty.

Morgan SJ, Groshen SL, Itamura JM, Shankwiler J, Brien WW, Kuschner SH: Reliability evaluation of classifying radial head fractures by the system of Mason. *Bull Hosp Jt Dis* 1997;56:95-98.

Twenty orthopaedic surgeons reviewed AP radiographs of 23 patients with an isolated radial head fracture and classified them according to the Mason classification. The intraobserver and interobserver reliability of this classification was fair to poor, indicating that the Mason classification based on plain radiographs is unreliable.

Moro JK, Werier J, MacDermid JC, Patterson SD, King GJ: Arthroplasty with a metal radial head for unreconstructible fractures of the radial head. *J Bone Joint Surg Am* 2001;83:1201-1211.

The authors report the functional outcome of 25 patients at an average follow-up of 3.5 years. The results were rated as 3 poor, 5 fair, and 17 good or excellent. The radial head prosthesis restored elbow stability when the fractured radial head occurred in combination with a dislocation of the elbow, rupture of the MCL, fracture of the coronoid, or fracture of the proximal ulna. There were mild residual deficits in strength and motion. No patients required removal of the implant.

Popovic N, Gillet P, Rodriguez A, Lemaire R: Fracture of the radial head with associated elbow dislocation: Results of treatment using a floating radial head prosthesis. *J Orthop Trauma* 2000;14:171-177.

Eleven patients with a comminuted radial head fracture and an associated elbow dislocation were evaluated following radial head replacement with a bipolar hemiarthroplasty. At an average follow-up of 32 months, eight patients had a good to excellent result, whereas three patients had a fair or poor result.

Sellman DC, Seitz WH, Postak PD, Greenwald AS: Reconstructive strategies for radioulnar dissociation: A biomechanical study. *J Orthop Trauma* 1995;9:516-522.

In a cadaveric study, the authors demonstrated that silicone radial head implants did not improve the axial stability of the interosseous ligament–deficient forearm. Metallic radial head implants restored stability similar to the intact radial head. Reconstruction of the interosseous ligament further increased stability.

Soyer AD, Nowotarski PJ, Kelso TB, Mighell MA: Optimal position for plate fixation of complex fractures of the proximal radius: A cadaver study. *J Orthop Trauma* 1998;12:291-293.

In a cadaveric study, the authors demonstrate that internal fixation of the proximal radius with a T-plate should be performed with the forearm in neutral rotation and the hardware placed laterally.

Szabo RM, Hotchkiss RN, Slater RR Jr: The use of frozen-allograft radial head replacement for treatment of established symptomatic proximal translation of the radius: Preliminary experience in five cases. *J Hand Surg Am* 1997;22:269-278.

A frozen-allograft radial head prosthesis was implanted in five patients who had disabling symptoms resulting from proximal translation following a radial head excision. Follow-up occurred at a mean time of 3 years (range, 1 to 7 years). All patients had pain relief and were satisfied with the outcome of the surgery.

Wallenbock E, Potsch F: Resection of the radial head: An alternative to use of a prosthesis? *J Trauma* 1997;43: 959-961.

This is a retrospective study of 23 patients who had a primary or secondary resection of the radial head 17 years prior to the review. The authors report 13 good, 5 satisfactory, and no poor results. Nine of their patients had some medial instability on stress testing. Six patients had proximal migration of the radius between 7 and 15 mm. The authors do not report if their patients had any osteoarthritis.

Classic Bibliography

Amis AA, Dowson D, Wright V: Elbow joint force predictions for some strenuous isometric actions. *J Biomech* 1980;13:765-775.

Davidson PA, Moseley JB, Tullos HS: Radial head fracture: A potentially complex injury. *Clin Orthop* 1993; 297:224-230.

Halls AA, Travill A: Transmission of pressures across the elbow joint. *Anat Rec* 1964;150:243-247.

Hotchkiss RN, Weiland AJ: Valgus stability of the elbow. *J Orthop Res* 1987;5:372-377.

Johnston GW: A follow-up of one hundred cases of fracture of the head of the radius with a review of the literature. *Ulster Med J* 1962;31:51-56.

Khalfayan EE, Culp RW, Alexander AH: Mason type II radial head fractures: Operative versus nonoperative treatment. *J Orthop Trauma* 1992;6:283-289.

King GJ, Evans DC, Kellam JF: Open reduction and internal fixation of radial head fractures. *J Orthop Trauma* 1991;5:21-28.

Knight DJ, Rymaszewski LA, Amis AA, Miller JH: Primary replacement of the fractured radial head with a metal prosthesis. *J Bone Joint Surg Br* 1993;75:572-576.

Mason ML: Some observations on fractures of the head of the radius with a review of one hundred cases. *Br J Surg* 1954;42:123-132.

Morrey BF, An KN: Articular and ligamentous contributions to the stability of the elbow joint. *Am J Sports Med* 1983;11:315-319.

Morrey BF, Tanaka S, An KN: Valgus stability of the elbow: A definition of primary and secondary constraints. *Clin Orthop* 1991;265:187-195.

Regan W, Morrey B: Fractures of the coronoid process of the ulna. *J Bone Joint Surg Am* 1989;71:1348-1354.

Stoffelen DV, Holdsworth BJ: Excision or Silastic replacement for comminuted radial head fractures: A long-term follow-up. *Acta Orthop Belg* 1994;60:402-407.

Chapter 34

Fractures of the Distal Humerus

David Ring, MD

Jesse B. Jupiter, MD

Introduction

Discussions of the treatment of fractures of the distal humerus continue to focus on four major issues: surgical exposures, fixation techniques for osteoporotic bone, fixation of fractures with small articular fragments, and management of the ulnar nerve. The availability of linked elbow prostheses has made it possible to treat fractures of the distal humerus with total elbow arthroplasty, but this is appropriate only for severe or irreparable fractures in older patients with limited functional demands. An understanding of the basic patterns of distal humeral fractures, methods of obtaining stable fixation, and potential complications as well as how to avoid them will help surgeons preserve the native elbow joint in young and active patients.

Evaluation

In a recent study of interobserver and intraobserver variation in the classification of fractures of the distal humerus based on radiographs, it was found that only very simple distinctions could be made reliably. Detailed distinctions, such as between the groups and subgroups of the Comprehensive Classification of Fractures (AO/ASIF), or the system of Mehne and Matta, were not consistently identifiable. This finding is not surprising given that radiographs are notoriously poor at demonstrating important injury characteristics. It has long been recognized that fracture classification can be difficult before surgical exposure; in fact, the system of Mehne and Matta, which distinguishes high and low T-shaped fractures, lateral and medial lambda-shaped fractures, and Y- and H-shaped fractures from among bicolumnar fractures, is based specifically on surgical exposure, not on radiographic appearance. The advent of high-quality CT scanning—three-dimensional (3-D) images in particular—has made it much easier to characterize the fracture and thereby plan surgical treatment (Fig. 1). The status of the articular surface of the distal humerus can be determined when the proximal ulna is subtracted from a 3-D scan.

No single classification system captures all factors important in the treatment of distal humeral fractures. Imaging studies should be used to define the size and fragmentation of the articular fragments before surgical treatment because they represent the most challenging aspect of treatment.

Two basic determinations must be made to plan the operation: (1) whether the fracture is best approached through a posterior approach (eg, olecranon osteotomy or triceps reflecting approach) or through a lateral approach, subluxating the ulnohumeral joint and (2) whether total elbow arthroplasty should be considered, in which case olecranon osteotomy should not be used.

Fractures with fragmentation of the anterior articular surface of the distal humerus are difficult to see and even more difficult to access through an olecranon osteotomy or triceps-elevating (Bryan-Morrey) exposure. This type of fragmentation is common among fractures of the lateral condyle and capitellum. A coronal shearing fracture, an apparent fracture of the capitellum that actually extends into the trochlea, is an example of this type of fracture. The orthopaedist should be aware that there is a spectrum of progressively complex lateral articular injuries, and that sometimes the posterior aspect of the lateral column is impacted or the posterior aspect of the trochlea is a separate fragment. A CT scan will usually define the extent of articular fragmentation. Fractures involving the lateral column and anterior articular surface of the distal humerus are best accessed through an extensile lateral exposure (Fig. 2).

The decision to use total elbow arthroplasty for treatment of a fracture of the distal humerus is usually based more on patient-related factors than on fracture-related factors. Most fractures of the distal humerus are complex fractures in osteoporotic, older individuals, and these factors alone do not merit total elbow arthroplasty. Many older patients remain healthy, active, and independent and are better treated by attempted osteosynthesis. However, frail elderly patients with very limited

A

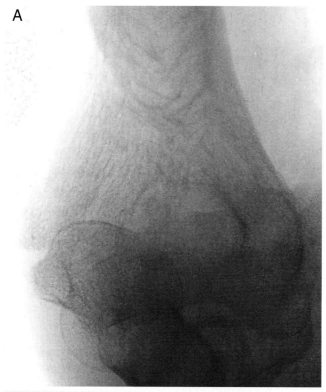

B

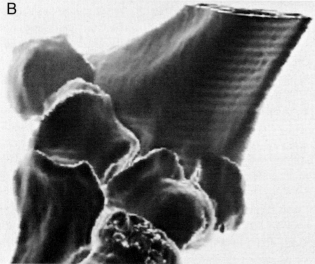

Figure 1 Standard radiographs are notoriously inadequate to determine fracture characteristics. **A,** This AP radiograph is difficult to interpret. **B,** A 3-D CT scan reveals very distal fracture lines with small articular fragments.

demands may be severely disabled by the need to protect an osteosynthesis or to wear a cast or splint. These patients may experience functional restoration and greater independence more quickly after total elbow arthroplasty because it can provide immediate stability without the need for protecting the limb. Many of these patients with the so-called "bag of bones" fracture would be treated nonsurgically in the past, but this nonsurgical treatment should be used only when there are extenuating contraindications to surgery.

In younger and more active patients, every attempt should be made to preserve the native elbow articulation because total elbow arthroplasty requires strict activity limitations and has a limited life span. Precise preoperative evaluation of the fracture with 3-D CT may help surgeons decide whether they have sufficient experience to attempt to repair the fracture or whether the patient should be referred to a surgeon with greater experience.

Surgical Treatment

Lateral Exposure

Complex fractures of the lateral column and anterior articular surface are best exposed through a lateral exposure. A lateral incision or a posterior incision with a lateral skin flap can be used. When the lateral epicondyle is fractured, mobilization of this fragment and the attached lateral collateral ligament will allow subluxation of the elbow, thereby improving exposure of and access to the articular surface of the distal humerus. Alternatively, the origin of the lateral collateral ligament can be mobilized either by sharp dissection or using an osteotomy of the lateral epicondyle. This type of extensive exposure is usually necessary for all but simple capitellar fractures. The articular fragments are realigned and provisionally fixed with smooth Kirschner wires (K-wires). The wires are then exchanged for Herbert screws (Zimmer, Warsaw, IN), mini-Acutrak screws (Acumed, Beaverton, OR), other screws that can be countersunk beneath the chondral surface, or absorbable PDS (polydioxanone) pins. Very small fragments can be secured with small, threaded K-wires countersunk beneath the articular surface. If the lateral epicondylar fragment is large or the posterior aspect of the lateral column has been disimpacted, one or two plates are used to repair the lateral column. If the lateral epicondylar fragment is small, it can be reattached with a figure-of-8 tension wire.

Posterior Exposures

Most fractures of the distal humerus are accessed through a posterior exposure. The optimal posterior exposure is debated. Most surgeons agree that an osteotomy of the olecranon provides the best exposure of the columns and articular surface of the distal humerus, but enthusiasm for this technique has been diminished by experience with hardware-related complications and healing problems at the osteotomy site. Exposures, such as the Bryan-Morrey approach, that elevate the insertion of the triceps from the proximal ulna as a continuous soft-tissue sleeve that is subsequently repaired represent a popular alternative. Problems with this exposure include occasional disruption of the triceps insertion, which is a very difficult problem to

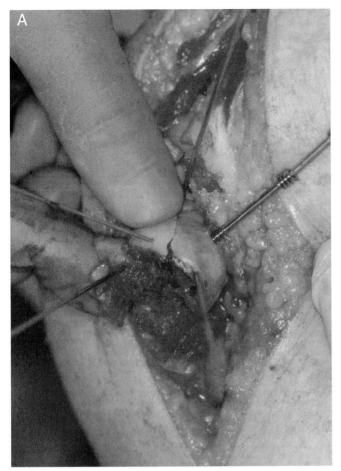 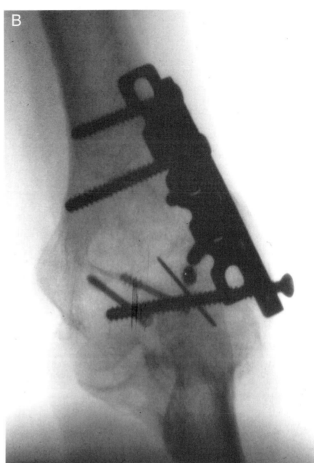

Figure 2 Fractures of the lateral column and anterior articular surface can be far more complex than they appear on radiographs. An extensile lateral exposure provides better exposure and access to these fragments than a posterior approach. **A,** Through a lateral skin incision the lateral epicondyle fragment has been mobilized distally, allowing subluxation of the elbow. The complex articular fragmentation has been reduced and provisionally secured with 0.062-in smooth K-wires. These wires are sequentially exchanged for Herbert screws. **B,** The lateral column was secured with two plates in orthogonal planes, in part to support the disimpacted posterior aspect of the lateral column. This AP radiograph shows that numerous implants were needed to repair the articular surface.

treat. In addition, the intact olecranon hinders access to the articular surface, with the result that a fracture line in the coronal plane (so-called multiplane fracture) could go unidentified or if identified would be difficult to reduce and repair. One advantage of leaving the olecranon intact is the ability to perform total elbow arthroplasty if indicated. Variations of triceps-elevating exposures include splitting the triceps in the midline and elevating the insertion medially and laterally, the so-called TRAP (triceps reflecting anconeus pedicle) approach in which the anconeus is elevated along with the triceps, or elevation from the lateral side (extended Kocher approach).

Another useful exposure that is becoming more popular is the bilaterotricipital exposure (Alonso-Llames approach). This exposure elevates the triceps from the intramuscular septum and the distal humerus both medially and laterally. The articular surface is exposed by incising the capsule on both sides, and the insertion of the triceps onto the olecranon is preserved. This exposure is adequate to treat extra-articular and many simple

articular fractures of the distal humerus, and it can provide sufficient exposure of more complex fractures to help decide whether internal fixation is feasible or total elbow arthroplasty should be used. If the surgeon decides to internally fix the fracture, an olecranon osteotomy or TRAP exposure can be created. If the surgeon decides to perform total elbow arthroplasty, the fragments can be excised and an arthroplasty placed without elevating the triceps insertion. Preserving the triceps insertion greatly facilitates rehabilitation and eliminates the risk of triceps detachment. One recent study recommends the Alonso-Llames approach based on measurements of greater extension strength at follow-up than with olecranon osteotomy or triceps-elevating exposures.

For posterior exposure of the distal humerus, it is useful to position the patient in the lateral decubitus position with the involved arm draped over a bolster. Some surgeons favor a supine position to facilitate hyperflexion in order to have a better view of the anterior articular surface. A sterile tourniquet is used. A straight posterior inci-

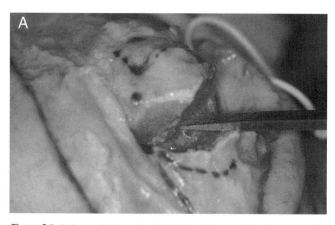
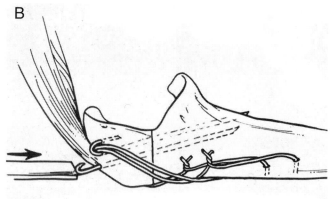

Figure 3 To limit complications associated with osteotomy of the olecranon, great care must be taken in the creation and repair of the osteotomy. **A,** A chevron-shaped osteotomy with cracking of the subchondral bone is easier to reposition and has greater inherent stability than a transverse osteotomy. **B,** The K-wires exit the anterior ulnar cortex distally and are bent 180° and impacted into the olecranon proximally to help prevent migration.

sion limits risk to cutaneous nerves. However, some surgeons favor curving the incision around the olecranon tip.

Ulnar nerve problems are extremely common. There is still some debate about how to handle the ulnar nerve. Most skilled elbow surgeons believe strongly that subcutaneous transposition of the nerve should be done routinely. Subcutaneous transposition limits the risk that the nerve will become bound up in scar tissue and fracture callus and prevents irritation by internal fixation devices; however, it is associated with a theoretical risk of injury caused by devascularization. Once the ulnar nerve is transposed, the groove below the medial epicondyle is available for the application of a contoured plate and screws.

Osteotomy
Careful attention to the details of creation and fixation of the olecranon osteotomy will greatly reduce the incidence of complications. A chevron-shaped osteotomy with the apex pointing distally facilitates anatomic repositioning, enhances stability, and provides a broader interface of cancellous bone to encourage healing. The osteotomy should be located at the depth of the semilunar notch, where there is little articular cartilage. This location is identified precisely because it can be seen after elevation of the anconeus muscle from its insertion on the olecranon. The osteotomy is initiated with a thin oscillating saw. The articular surface and subchondral bone are then cracked with a thin-bladed osteotome, resulting in a rough interdigitating surface, which further facilitates anatomic repositioning of the fragment (Fig. 3, *A*).

When exposure is complete, the fracture is carefully assessed, and the preoperative plan is modified according to the surgical findings. The order in which the various components of the injury are addressed may vary; articular reconstruction is typically done first, followed by fixation of each column to the humeral shaft.

Reduction and Fixation
Provisional reduction is obtained and held with smooth 0.045- or 0.062-in K-wires and, occasionally, bone clamps. If there is no articular comminution, then the trochlear spool is most stably reconstructed with an interfragmentary lag screw. In the face of comminution, the trochlear sulcus must carefully be reconstructed in both depth and width, and fixation should be achieved with a screw threaded into both medial and lateral fragments to maintain these relationships. All resulting gaps are filled with cancellous autograft from the iliac crest.

A fracture of the articular surface in the coronal plane is not uncommon. These fractures can be addressed with Herbert screws that recess beneath the articular cartilage.

Fixation of the articular fragments onto the osseous columns has historically been the weak point of internal fixation of distal humeral fractures. The keys to success include the use of well-contoured plates that are strong enough to resist bending or breakage before osseous union occurs and adequate fixation to the distal fragments, which is frequently the most difficult aspect of treating these fractures. The basic biomechanical concept of fixation in orthogonal planes has found particular favor in the treatment of fractures of the distal humerus; however, a recent biomechanical study demonstrated that parallel plates can provide equivalent fixation if they are thick enough. Some surgeons now favor this approach.

A number of authors recommend 3.5-mm reconstruction plates because they are stout enough to resist the deforming forces in this region and yet are easily contoured in three dimensions. This is particularly important in the distal humerus because the complex bony surfaces require equally complex and exacting contour of the plates. Some plating systems offer plates precontoured for application to the medial, lateral, and posterolateral columns.

The olecranon osteotomy is fixed with a tension band wire construct or plate. Some authors insert two parallel

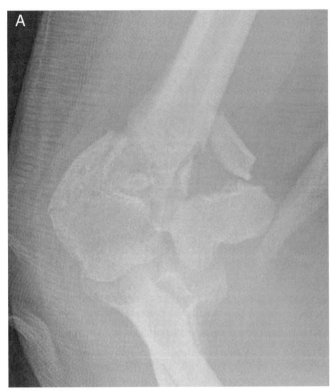

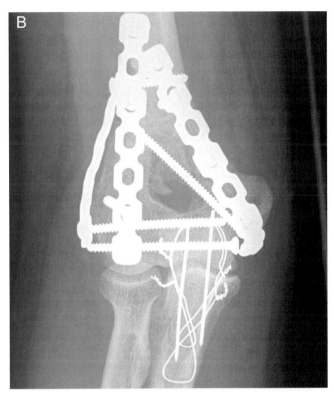

Figure 4 Fractures with very small articular fragments or poor quality bone may require modifications of standard plating techniques for adequate stability. A 38-year-old woman fell from a standing height and had a complex bicondylar fracture of the distal humerus with very small articular fragments. **A,** The AP radiograph obtained at the time of injury shows that the fracture is at the level of the olecranon fossa and has created very small articular fragments, particularly on the lateral side. **B,** On the medial side a plate was contoured to cradle the medial epicondyle. On the lateral side, two plates in orthogonal planes were used to better secure the lateral articular fragments.

0.045-in smooth K-wires aimed into the anterior cortex of the ulnar shaft at the junction with the coronoid process in an attempt to enhance fixation (Fig. 3, *B*). For the tension wire component, two 20- or 22-gauge wires are threaded through separate holes in the ulna and tightened on both sides of the osteotomy to ensure symmetric tensioning. The proximal tips of the K-wires are bent 180° and impacted into the olecranon beneath the triceps insertion. These technical aspects are important in limiting the prominence and potential for migration of the hardware.

Techniques for Use With Osteoporotic Bone

A large percentage of distal humeral fractures occur in elderly patients with osteoporosis. Some authors recommend using tension band wiring techniques to secure the medial and lateral columns when bone quality is poor. Several modifications of plate and screw fixation also are useful.

A plate applied to the posterior aspect of the lateral column can extend distally to the posterior border of the capitellum, increasing the number of screws in the distal fragment. A stable hold on the distal fragment is enhanced by directing the most distal screws proximally so that they converge on screws entering more proximally and engage the anterior cortex while avoiding the anterior surface of the capitellum. A second plate can be applied to

the lateral aspect of the lateral column. This double orthogonal plate fixation greatly enhances the security of fixation of small or osteopenic lateral fragments (Fig. 4).

On the medial side, when the plate is applied posteriorly, it can be contoured to wrap around the medial epicondyle. One or more additional screws can then be placed in the distal fragment, and a distal screw can be inserted in a directly superior direction. This screw is thereby directed perpendicular to the more proximal screws, creating a mechanical interlocking construct. The most distal screw can be a long screw directed up the medial column.

Another approach is to use plates placed directly medial and lateral (ie, parallel plating). With this approach, multiple screws engage the distal fragments and interdigitate with screws from the opposite plate (Fig. 5).

The fixation is tested through a full range of motion. Although in practice this is rarely necessary, loose screws can be reinforced with methylmethacrylate; care must be taken to avoid extravasation of the cement.

Total Elbow Arthroplasty

A recent report of the use of semiconstrained total elbow arthroplasty for the treatment of fractures of the distal humerus indicates that good results can be obtained. The average age of the patients was 72 years, and the

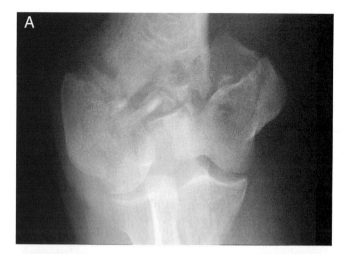

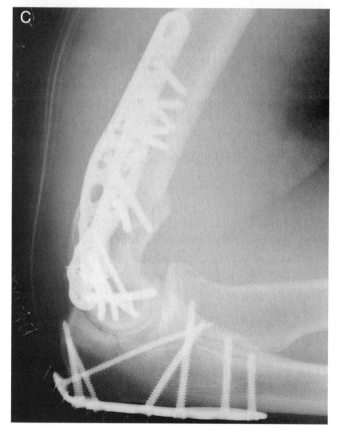

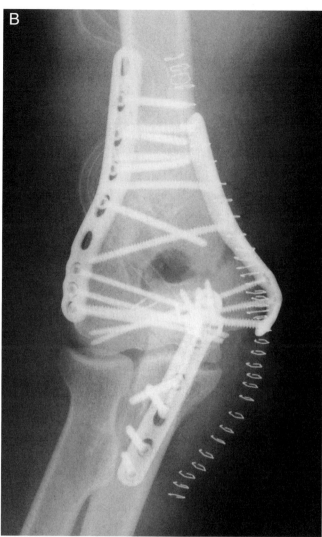

Figure 5 A, Distal humerus fracture with both intra-articular and supracondylar comminution. **B,** Parallel plate technique permits placement of six to seven long screws through the plates into the articular fragments, maximizing fixation of the distal segment and stability at the supracondylar level. **C,** The olecranon osteotomy can be fixed with a precontoured plate that is low profile and specifically designed as an alternative to tension band wires.

youngest patient was age 48 years. Ten of 21 fractures were in patients with rheumatoid arthritis, including the only two patients younger than age 60 years. The authors advise against using total elbow arthroplasty in younger patients. When total elbow arthroplasty is considered, an Alonso-Llames approach, which preserves the insertion of the triceps on the ulna, should be used (Fig. 6). When the decision is made to proceed with total elbow arthroplasty, the epicondylar fragments and the origins of the collateral ligaments are excised. This allows dislocation of the ulnohumeral joint and insertion of the prosthesis without disrupting the triceps mechanism.

Contaminated or Infected Fractures

Surgeons may be reluctant to apply plates and screws to infected fractures or fractures with extensive contamination or colonization related to a severe open wound. In this situation, the limb may be supported in a splint, cast, or external fixator while serial débridements, soft-tissue procedures, and parenteral antibiotics are used to eradicate the infection or colonization. An alternative during this period is to apply a thin wire (Ilizarov) external fixator that uses olive wires to secure and compress the articular fragments. This type of fixator allows functional elbow mobilization during the treatment of the wound,

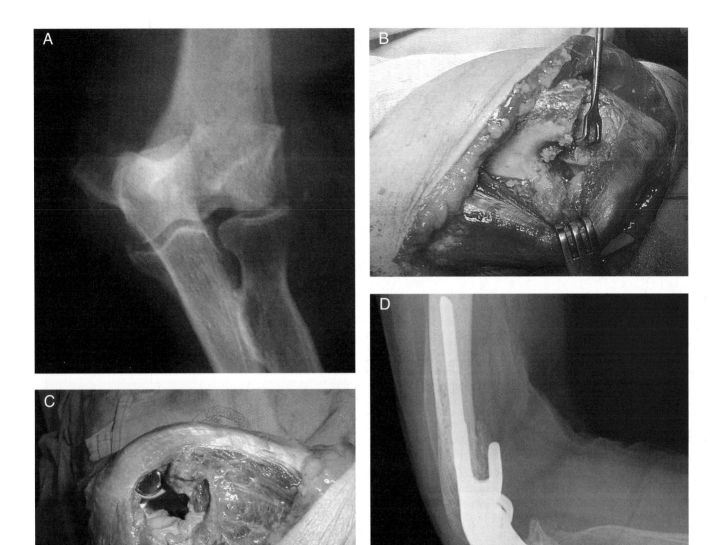

Figure 6 An 82-year-old woman who depended on a walker for ambulation and was becoming increasingly frail fell, fracturing her right distal humerus. Because the need to protect internal fixation would have confined her to a wheelchair until the fracture was healed, total elbow arthroplasty was performed. **A,** The initial AP radiograph shows a low extra-articular fracture. **B,** The bilaterotricipital, or Alonso-Llames, approach is useful when total elbow arthroplasty is considered because it allows total elbow arthoplasty **(C)** without detaching the triceps. **D,** Early lateral radiograph showing the implant. The patient started ambulating with her walker within a few days of surgery, regained full elbow mobility, and has not experienced any complications.

simplifies later treatment of the fracture, and in some cases provides definitive treatment.

Although hybrid external fixation of a comminuted fracture of the distal humerus caused by a low-velocity gunshot wound has been described (in analogy with a pilon fracture of the distal tibia), immediate internal fixation of such fractures is usually possible in the upper extremity.

Postoperative Care

Postoperative limb elevation for 24 to 36 hours and active digit motion are important to limit swelling. Early con-

trolled motion is key to the retention of elbow motion. When the fixation is secure and there are no soft-tissue concerns, active motion and functional use of the arm are started within 2 days. Gravity is used to facilitate elbow flexion by having the patient position the shoulder so that the limb is overhead. The forearm is supported by the uninjured arm as the patient brings the elbow into flexion. With the patient sitting upright, gravity is used to assist with extension. Muscle strengthening and endurance exercises are instituted by 8 to 12 weeks, when the surgeon is certain that osseous union has occurred. The use of patient-adjusted static progressive splints may help to improve motion for as long as 6 to 12 months postoperatively. Some surgeons use continuous passive motion in the early postoperative period.

Results and Complications

Although most patients experience satisfactory outcomes after surgical fixation of a fracture of the distal humerus, the need for a second procedure to address one or more complications is common. The results of treatment are closely tied to the occurrence of adverse events. Authors describing one recent series reported only 52% satisfactory results, ascribing most unsatisfactory results to complications of surgical treatment. Most of these complications relate to prominent or loose hardware and capsular contracture, but ulnar nerve dysfunction is also common. Nonunion and heterotopic bone blocking motion are uncommon severe complications. Subsequent surgeries to address these problems increase the rate of satisfactory results to approximately 75% to 80% in most series.

Complications can occur as a result of the surgical approach. After lateral collateral ligament detachment for a lateral exposure, poor healing of the ligament could lead to varus or posterolateral rotatory instability. Therefore, care must be taken to avoid varus gravitational stress in the early postoperative period.

Great care must be taken to minimize the prominence and potential for migration of the wires used for repair and olecranon osteotomy. The techniques outlined herein, including the use of two smaller-gauge tension wires, engaging the anterior ulnar cortex with the K-wires, and impacting the bent proximal ends of the K-wires into the olecranon beneath the triceps insertion, help to limit these problems.

Early active and gravity-assisted mobilization of the elbow within 1 or 2 days of surgery and the use of continuous passive motion or adjustable splints will help limit capsular contracture. The need for capsular contracture release is inevitable in some patients, but fortunately it is a fairly predictable method of restoring elbow mobility. It is probably wise to protect very complex fractures or tenuous fixation, particularly complex articular fractures in which nonunion might necessitate total elbow arthroplasty, and then perform secondary capsular release if needed once fracture healing is established.

Ulnar nerve dysfunction is very common after surgical treatment of a fracture of the distal humerus. One recent study recorded ulnar nerve dysfunction in 21 of 77 patients (27%) followed for longer than 1 year. The nerve can be irritated by implants or trapped in scar tissue. Irritation of the ulnar nerve can inhibit mobilization of the elbow and contribute to capsular contracture. Conversely, once the elbow becomes stiff, attempts to regain flexion

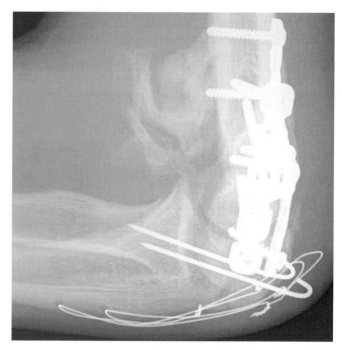

Figure 7 Heterotopic ossification that interferes with motion is uncommon after fracture of the distal humerus. This lateral radiograph demonstrates anterior heterotopic ossification that limited flexion to 100° after surgical fixation of a high-energy distal humeral fracture with extension deformity.

may irritate the ulnar nerve. Because the simple act of mobilizing and transposing the ulnar nerve can cause nerve dysfunction, presumably as a result of interrupting the vascular supply, the need for routine transposition still is debated. A number of authorities on elbow surgery advocate routine anterior subcutaneous transposition of the nerve because the prevalence of severe nerve dysfunction after routine mobilization seems far lower than that encountered in the reconstructive setting when the nerve has not been transposed. In spite of the traditional pessimism regarding the treatment of these often long-standing ulnar neuropathies, a recent study has demonstrated diminished pain and restoration of sensory and even motor function after release of the nerve.

Nonunion is usually the result of inadequate fixation. More specifically, nonunion occurs at the supracondylar level and is related to inadequate screw fixation of the plates to the distal fragments or lack of adequate contact between the fragments. Surgical reconstruction of an ununited distal humeral fracture is a demanding procedure that involves mobilization and possibly neurolysis of the ulnar nerve, resection of the nonunion site, anterior and posterior capsular release, and realignment and stabilization of the distal fragment, which is often small and osteoporotic. Using the techniques described earlier for fixation of osteoporotic bone and small articular fractures, including the use of a third plate when necessary, it is possible to gain stable fixation that allows immediate postoperative motion. Most nonunions are healed by this approach, with an average of 100° of ulnohumeral motion regained.

Semiconstrained total elbow arthroplasty has been used in the treatment of nonunited fractures of the distal humerus. Results have improved to the degree that this procedure can be considered an alternative for older patients with low functional demands.

Although one recent report cited heterotopic ossification in 49% of patients, only 6 of 77 patients (8%) had restriction of motion because of the heterotopic bone. This bone usually occurs anteriorly, under the brachialis, and can be resected if there is inadequate flexion (Fig. 7). Resection can be considered once the soft tissues are healed, edema has resolved, and the heterotopic bone begins to mature on radiographs. It is not necessary to wait longer than 6 months nor is it necessary for bone scan or alkaline phosphatase levels in the serum to normalize. The use of a single 700-cGy dose of radiation within the first few postoperative days may help prevent recurrence of the heterotopic bone. The use of nonsteroidal anti-inflammatory medications also has been suggested based on experience with total hip arthroplasty. There is no need for routine prophylaxis after surgical treatment of acute fractures, except perhaps in patients with closed head injuries.

Annotated Bibliography

Evaluation

Jacobson SR, Glisson RR, Urbaniak JR: Comparison of distal humerus fracture fixation: A biomechanical study. *J South Orthop Assoc* 1997;6:241-249.

A cadaveric biomechanical study of plate and screw fixation of fractures of the distal humerus confirmed that two reconstruction plates applied in orthogonal planes provide optimal fixation. The authors found no advantage to the addition of a third plate; however, the situations in which a third plate may be useful (poor bone quality, very small articular fragments) are difficult to simulate in the laboratory.

Wainwright AM, Williams JR, Carr AJ: Interobserver and intraobserver variation in classification systems for fractures of the distal humerus. *J Bone Joint Surg Br* 2000;82:636-642.

Study of the interobserver and intraobserver variation of radiographic classification of 33 fractures of the distal humerus showed that only very basic distinctions were reliable.

Surgical Treatment

Cobb TK, Morrey BF: Total elbow arthroplasty as primary treatment for distal humeral fractures in elderly patients. *J Bone Joint Surg Am* 1997;79:826-832.

Twenty-one fractures of the distal humerus in 20 patients (10 elbows with rheumatoid arthritis) were treated with semicon-

strained total elbow arthroplasty. The mean arc of ulnohumeral motion was 105°, and all of the patients had a good or excellent result. The authors caution that total elbow arthroplasty is not an alternative to osteosynthesis in younger patients.

Manueddu CA, Hoffmeyer P, Haluzicky M, Blanc Y, Borst F: Distal humeral fracture in adults: Functional evaluation and measurement of isometric strength. *Rev Chir Orthop Reparatrice Appar Mot* 1997;83:551-560.

Twenty-seven patients had surgical fixation of a fracture of the distal humerus through one of a variety of surgical exposures. Three fractures required a second operation. Seventy-three percent of patients were satisfied with the result. Based on a comparison of strength in the injured and uninjured arm, an approach accessing the distal humerus on either side of the triceps without elevating its insertion on the olecranon (the Alonso-Llames approach) was favored.

Morrey BF, Adams RA: Semiconstrained elbow replacement for distal humeral nonunion. *J Bone Joint Surg Br* 1995;77:67-72.

Semiconstrained elbow replacement produced satisfactory results in 36 patients studied. Repeated osteosynthesis has been shown to be ineffective in most patients.

Ochner RS, Bloom H, Palumbo RC, Coyle MP: Closed reduction of coronal fractures of the capitellum. *J Trauma* 1996;40:199-203.

Results of closed reduction and cast immobilization for capitellum fractures are given. The results reported are surprisingly good, although the authors are honest about the presence of cracking, locking, and pain in many of the patients.

O'Driscoll SW: The triceps-reflecting anconeus pedicle (TRAP) approach for distal humeral fractures and nonunions. *Orthop Clin North Am* 2000;31:91-101.

An alternative triceps elevating exposure that does not denervate the anconeus muscle and provides almost the same exposure as an olecranon osteotomy is described.

Patterson SD, Bain GI, Mehta JA: Surgical approaches to the elbow. *Clin Orthop* 2000;370:19-33.

This is an excellent review of useful approaches to the elbow and their historic development. The advantages of a bilaterotricipital approach (the Alonso-Llames approach; working on either side of the triceps without elevating its origin from the olecranon) over the triceps-elevating Bryan-Morrey exposure is discussed.

Pelto-Vasenius K, Hirvensalo E, Rokkanen P: Absorbable implants in the treatment of distal humeral fractures in adolescents and adults. *Acta Orthop Belg* 1996; 62(suppl 1):93-102.

Absorbable implants were used to repair 44 fractures of the distal humerus, half of them type B, or partial articular fractures, according to the Comprehensive Classification of Fractures. Eleven patients (25%) lost reduction, seven (16%) had infection, and four (9%) had a foreign body inflammatory response. Most of the poor results were in patients with type C or bicondylar, intra-articular fractures. There was a 25% rate of infection or noninfectious inflammatory response.

Pereles TR, Koval KJ, Gallagher M, Rosen H: Open reduction and internal fixation of the distal humerus: Functional outcome in the elderly. *J Trauma* 1997;43: 578-584.

Twelve patients older than age 60 years had surgical fixation of a fracture of the distal humerus with a plate and screws, with active mobilization initiated within a few days. There was no loss of fixation, and all of the fractures healed. The arc of ulnohumeral motion averaged 112°, and all patients had good or excellent results.

Petraco DM, Koval KJ, Kummer FJ, Zuckerman JD: Fixation stability of olecranon osteotomies. *Clin Orthop* 1996;333:181-185.

Biomechanical tests of three variations of olecranon osteotomy, transverse fixed with K-wires and tension wire, chevron fixed with screw and tension wire, and oblique fixed with screw and tension wire, could not demonstrate any advantages of one technique over another.

Poynton AR, Kelly IP, O'Rourke SK: Fractures of the capitellum: A comparison of two fixation methods. *Injury* 1998;29:341-343.

Twelve patients had surgical fixation of a fracture of the capitellum: six with K-wires, six with Herbert screws. Except for one pin tract infection, the groups were comparable.

Ring D, Jupiter JB, Toh S: Salvage of contaminated fractures of the distal humerus with thin wire external fixation. *Clin Orthop* 1999;359:203-208.

Five patients with infected or colonized fractures of the distal humerus were treated with thin wire external fixation. This fixation allowed immediate functional mobilization of the elbow. Subsequent procedures were frequently required, but the initial use of external fixation helped eradicate infection or colonization and improved the safety of subsequent surgeries.

Self J, Viegas SF, Buford WL Jr, Patterson RM: A comparison of double-plate fixation methods for complex distal humerus fractures. *J Shoulder Elbow Surg* 1995;4:10-16.

Patients treated with a modified method of fracture fixation of complex distal humerus fractures with medial and lateral plates and bolts exhibited increased strength and stability in early follow-up.

Skaggs DL, Hale JM, Buggay S, Kay RM: Use of a hybrid external fixator for a severely comminuted juxta-articular fracture of the distal humerus. *J Orthop Trauma* 1998;12:439-442.

An external fixator was used to secure a comminuted gunshot fracture of the distal humerus in a 14-year-old patient. Thin, Ilizarov-type wires were used to secure the articular fragments.

Voor MJ, Sugita S, Seligson D: Traditional versus alternative olecranon osteotomy: Historical review and biomechanical analysis of several techniques. *Am J Orthop* 1995;(suppl):17-26.

An argument in favor of extra-articular over intra-articular osteotomy of the olecranon is made using the technique of free-body analysis.

Results and Complications

Kinik H, Atalar H, Mergen E: Management of distal humerus fractures in adults. *Arch Orthop Trauma Surg* 1999;119:467-469.

Forty-six patients had surgical treatment of a fracture of the distal humerus using olecranon osteotomy, ulnar nerve transposition, fixation with two orthogonal plates, and early active mobilization. Two patients had nonunion or fixation failure, five had ulnar nerve dysfunction, and four had heterotopic bone blocking motion. Fourteen patients (30%) had an unsatisfactory range of motion. Patients often needed a second surgery to address ulnar nerve dysfunction, hardware problems, or stiffness to achieve a satisfactory result.

Kundel K, Braun W, Wieberneit J, Ruter A: Intraarticular distal humerus fractures: Factors affecting functional outcome. *Clin Orthop* 1996;332:200-208.

Ninety-nine fractures, 77 with follow-up of 1 year or longer, were reviewed. The percentage of satisfactory results (52%) was lower than in prior series. Diminished outcome was related to ulnar neuropathy, heterotopic ossification, and capsular contracture. The authors concluded that healing of the distal humerus in good alignment does not, in itself, ensure a good result.

McKee MD, Jupiter JB, Bosse G, Goodman L: Outcome of ulnar neurolysis during post-traumatic reconstruction of the elbow. *J Bone Joint Surg Br* 1998;80:100-105.

Long-term follow-up of patients with posttraumatic ulnar neuropathy treated with ulnar nerve neurolysis and transposition documented substantial improvement in most patients. Improvements in pain and sensation were accompanied by motor return in many cases.

Classic Bibliography

Ackerman G, Jupiter JB: Non-union of fractures of the distal end of the humerus. *J Bone Joint Surg Am* 1988; 70:75-83.

Figgie MP, Inglis AE, Mow CS, Figgie HE: Salvage of non-union of supracondylar fracture of the humerus by total elbow arthroplasty. *J Bone Joint Surg Am* 1989; 71:1058-1065.

Helfet DL, Hotchkiss RN: Internal fixation of the distal humerus: A biomechanical comparison of methods. *J Orthop Trauma* 1990;4:260-264.

John H, Rosso R, Neff U, Bodoky A, Regazzoni P, Harder F: Operative treatment of distal humeral fractures in the elderly. *J Bone Joint Surg Br* 1994;76:793-796.

Jupiter JB: Complex fractures of the distal part of the humerus and associated complications. *J Bone Joint Surg Am* 1994;76:1252-1264.

Jupiter JB, Goodman LJ: The management of complex distal humerus nonunion in the elderly by elbow capsulectomy, triple plating, and ulnar nerve neurolysis. *J Shoulder Elbow Surg* 1992;1:37-46.

Jupiter JB, Neff U, Holzach P, Allgower M: Intercondylar fractures of the humerus: An operative approach. *J Bone Joint Surg Am* 1985;67:226-239.

McKee M, Jupiter J, Toh CL, Wilson L, Colton C, Karras KK: Reconstruction after malunion and nonunion of intra-articular fractures of the distal humerus: Methods and results in 13 adults. *J Bone Joint Surg Br* 1994; 76:614-621.

Schemitsch EH, Tencer AF, Henley MB: Biomechanical evaluation of methods of internal fixation of the distal humerus. *J Orthop Trauma* 1994;8:468-475.

Södergård J, Sandelin J, Böstman O: Mechanical failures of internal fixation in T and Y fractures of the distal humerus. *J Trauma* 1992;33:687-690.

Chapter 35

Proximal Ulnar Fractures and Fracture-Dislocations

David Ring, MD

Jesse B. Jupiter, MD

Introduction

Proximal ulnar fractures include isolated olecranon or coronoid fractures, Monteggia fractures, and complex fracture-dislocations. Complex, multifragmented fractures of the proximal ulna are usually associated with instability of the radioulnar and/or ulnohumeral articulations. Anteriorly directed fractures include the classic anterior Monteggia fracture (which does not involve the ulnohumeral joint) and the anterior (transolecranon) fracture-dislocation of the elbow. Posteriorly directed fractures, all considered to be posterior Monteggia fractures, are characterized by an apex posterior fracture of the ulna. These include a spectrum of injuries with the fracture variously located in the diaphysis or the metaphysis, or directly involving the ulnohumeral joint. Although each pattern is associated with distinct pathoanatomy, pitfalls, and prognosis, the key to successful management of all fractures of the proximal ulna is secure restoration of anatomic alignment with a plate and screws.

Classification

Olecranon Fractures

In the Mayo classification of olecranon fractures, three factors are identified as having a direct influence on treatment: fracture displacement, comminution, and ulnohumeral instability (Table 1). Type I fractures that are nondisplaced or minimally displaced are classified as either noncomminuted (type IA) or comminuted (type IB) and are treated nonsurgically. Type II fractures are characterized by displacement of the proximal fragment without elbow instability; they require surgical treatment. Type IIA fractures, which are noncomminuted, are treated with tension band wire fixation. When the fracture is oblique, an ancillary interfragmentary compression screw can be added. Type IIB fractures are comminuted and require plate fixation. Type III fractures are characterized by instability of the ulnohumeral joint. In fact, type III fractures can be so complex that they are com-

TABLE 1	Mayo Classification of Olecranon Fractures
I Nondisplaced or minimally displaced
IA Noncomminuted
IB Comminuted
II Displacement of proximal fragment without elbow instability
IIA Noncomminuted
IIB Comminuted
III Displacement of proximal fragment with instability of the ulnohumeral joint

monly recognized as one of the various types of complex fracture-dislocations of the elbow. These fractures, which include anterior (transolecranon) fracture-dislocations of the elbow and posterior Monteggia pattern injuries, are generally distinguished by anterior or posterior displacement of the forearm with respect to the trochlea of the distal humerus. Anterior (transolecranon) fracture-dislocations are often associated with open wounds, which occasionally require modification of the surgical approach or the consideration of soft-tissue flaps.

Coronoid Fractures

Coronoid fractures can occur as isolated injuries or in association with fractures of the olecranon or radial head and dislocations or subluxations of the elbow. These fractures are discussed in chapter 36.

Monteggia Fracture-Dislocations

Fractures of the proximal ulna with dislocation of the proximal radioulnar joint are called Monteggia fracture-dislocations. The most commonly used classification of these injuries is based on the direction of dislocation of the radial head: type I, anterior; type II, posterior; type

III, lateral; type IV, any direction, associated with a diaphyseal fracture of the radius. Anterior and lateral Monteggia fractures can be associated with injury to the posterior interosseous nerve. Fracture-dislocations can injure the ulnar nerve; high-energy injuries can be associated with compartment syndrome.

Evaluation

Radiographs should be evaluated for displacement of the fracture fragments, fracture of the radial head, fracture of the coronoid process, alignment of the radial head with the capitellum, and alignment of the trochlea with the coronoid. Approximately two thirds of posterior olecranon fracture-dislocations and posterior Monteggia fractures with fracture of the ulna at the metaphyseal or diaphyseal level have associated fractures of the radial head. Most posterior olecranon fracture-dislocations and about half of anterior fracture-dislocations of the olecranon have an associated fracture of the coronoid process.

Fragmentation of the coronoid process and the character of the radial head fracture may be best assessed using CT. Three-dimensional views are particularly useful.

Treatment

Type I Fractures

Stable, minimally displaced fractures can be treated with a brief period of immobilization (2 to 4 weeks) in a splint followed by active mobilization. Minimally displaced fractures are uncommon, and in practice, fractures of the olecranon therefore rarely are treated nonsurgically. Moreover, the notorious propensity of the elbow for stiffness and the relative simplicity and safety of surgical treatment lead most patients and surgeons to prefer internal fixation and immediate active functional mobilization.

Type IIA Fractures

Simple transverse fractures are well treated with tension band wire fixation. The use of two figure-of-8 tension wires makes it possible to use smaller, 22-gauge wires that may limit hardware prominence. Kirschner wires (K-wires, 0.045-in) have been found to be more than adequate to avoid hardware prominence and migration. The K-wires are drilled obliquely into the anterior ulnar cortex distal to the coronoid process and then retracted about 1 cm for later impaction. The two figure-of-8 tension wires are twisted on both the ulnar and radial limbs until all of the slack of the wires is taken up. Alternatively, the tension wires can be tied with a Harris wire-tier on the lateral side to maximize tension and minimize prominence. The K-wires are then trimmed and bent 180° at the proximal end. This bent end is then impacted into the olecranon to pre-

vent migration. The triceps tendon, which can be split slightly to permit deep impaction, is then sutured over the K-wires.

For simple oblique fractures, placement of an interfragmentary compression screw between the proximal and distal fragments will greatly enhance the security of the fixation. This screw is neutralized by the tension band wire technique.

Type IIB Fractures

With comminuted fractures, tension band techniques are less effective and the fixation device, which will experience larger loads, should be stronger. In this situation, a plate provides more secure fixation, and narrowing of the trochlear notch can be avoided. The plate must be contoured to wrap around the proximal aspect of the olecranon; precontoured plates are available for this purpose. This contour allows for a greater number of screws in the proximal fragment. The most proximal screw is oriented orthogonally to more distal screws, which may enhance fixation. If the olecranon fragment is small, osteopenic, or fragmented, figure-of-8 tension wires engaging the triceps insertion will greatly enhance the security of fixation and should be strongly considered in many cases. Distally, the plate will extend onto the apex of the ulnar diaphysis. Although this might seem to be a cause for concern, a plate in this position will provide strong fixation provided the bone quality is good and the screws are well placed.

Treatment of olecranon fractures with excision of the proximal fragments and advancement of the triceps insertion may be appropriate in infirm older patients; this method is used infrequently. Even comminuted fractures can be effectively treated with open reduction and internal fixation.

Type III Fractures and Other Complex Fractures of the Proximal Ulna

These injuries, best thought of as complex fracture-dislocations of the elbow, are characterized by several different injury patterns. The most important distinction is between injuries that involve primarily the radioulnar articulation and those that involve primarily the ulnohumeral articulation. One of the unique aspects of the posterior Monteggia fracture-dislocation is its involvement of both articulations. The key to effective treatment of complex fractures of the proximal ulna is stable, anatomic realignment including restoration of the contour and dimensions of the trochlear notch. Realignment of the ulna restores the radioulnar relationship. This relationship is usually stable even though the annular ligament is torn by virtue of the intact interosseous ligament. Realignment of the trochlear notch is essential to ensure ulnohumeral stability. Stable fixa-

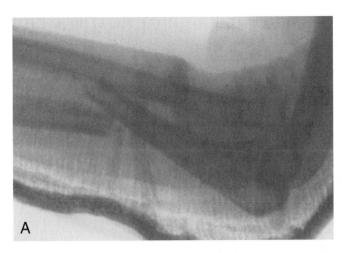
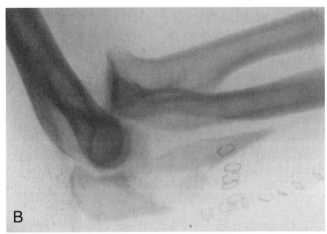

Figure 1 A, In the classic anterior Monteggia fracture, there is an apex anterior fracture of the ulnar diaphysis with anterior dislocation of the radial head from the proximal radioulnar joint. **B,** Although the anterior (transolecranon) fracture-dislocation of the elbow features anterior dislocation of the radial head with respect to the capitellum, the radioulnar relationship is relatively spared. The entire forearm dislocates anteriorly and the ulnohumeral dislocation is disrupted, often with the creation of a large coronoid fracture and extensive fragmentation of the trochlear notch.

tion of the coronoid is required to restore the function of the medial collateral ligament. Whenever the radial head is exposed or the ulnohumeral joint is unstable, the lateral collateral ligament should be carefully and securely repaired, including reattaching its origin to the lateral epicondyle using either suture anchors or drill holes through bone.

The goal in treatment of complex fractures of the proximal ulna is to restore the relationship between the olecranon and coronoid articular facets without narrowing or widening the trochlear notch. Comminution usually involves the region between these two important structures and is best accomplished using the trochlea of the distal humerus as a template. If healing occurs, the trochlear notch will function well.

Anterior (Transolecranon) Fracture-Dislocations of the Elbow
Anterior dislocation of the ulnohumeral joint with a fracture of the olecranon often involves separation of the coronoid as a single large fragment. In addition, the fragmentation may extend distally into the ulnar diaphysis. Because this injury features anterior dislocation of the radial head in relation to the capitellum, it has been considered as a Monteggia fracture or equivalent (Fig. 1). However, this injury is actually quite distinct in that the radioulnar relationship is maintained and the entire forearm dislocates anteriorly. The anterior (transolecranon) fracture-dislocation of the elbow is primarily an injury of and a threat to the function of the ulnohumeral, rather than the radioulnar, articulation. Although in both injuries optimal treatment consists of stable, anatomic realignment of the proximal ulna, the anatomy, treatment considerations, and prognosis are substantially different.

Monteggia Fractures
Monteggia injuries are very common in children. Anterior fracture-dislocations are common; on occasion the radial diaphysis is fractured as well. Anterior and anterolateral dislocations of the radial head are similar except that lateral displacement may be more likely to injure the posterior interosseous nerve. One injury unique to the immature skeleton consists of a buckle fracture of the proximal ulnar metaphysis with lateral subluxation of the radiocapitellar joint. Apex posterior fractures of the ulna with posterior displacement of the radial head (the posterior Monteggia lesion) are extremely rare in children.

In adult patients, posterior displacement of the radial head predominates. The majority of these posterior fractures occur in older patients, most of them women. The association of the posterior injury pattern with osteoporosis has been reported, including a recent study detailing an association with chronic steroid use. Anterior and anterolateral displacement are less common and seem to be associated with high-energy injuries and complex upper extremity trauma. According to a recent study of adult Monteggia injuries at Massachusetts General Hospital, five of eight patients had either a Gustilo and Anderson type 3 open wound (two with brachial artery injuries) or a major ipsilateral skeletal injury such as an ulnohumeral dislocation or an ipsilateral humerus fracture.

Posterior Monteggia Fractures
Posterior Monteggia fractures are defined as the combination of an apex posterior fracture of the proximal ulna and posterior dislocation of the radial head. There is a spectrum of injuries with similar features that vary according to

the associated capsuloligamentous damage, fracture and dislocation of the radial head, and the morphology of the fracture, which often involves a triangular or quadrangular fragment of the ulna that includes the anterior ulnar cortex and sometimes the coronoid process.

Some authors have suggested that Monteggia injuries are most precisely defined as fractures of the forearm associated with dislocation of the proximal radioulnar joint. This definition might exclude many type A fractures in which the radioulnar relationship appears to be relatively preserved; however, given the common anatomic features and management issues of apex posterior fractures of the proximal ulna, they are probably best considered as a group.

Posterior Monteggia fractures involve both the elbow and the forearm joints directly. In particular, the stability of the ulnohumeral articulation can be compromised by fracture of the radial head; injury to the lateral collateral ligament complex as the radial head dislocates posteriorly; apex posterior alignment of the proximal ulna contributing to posterior subluxation of the radial head and diminished effective height of the coronoid; and sometimes fracture of the coronoid process. One of the most difficult aspects of the management of these injuries is that the potential for ulnohumeral instability is often not recognized and the surgeon may not be prepared to deal with it when it is encountered.

Fractures of the Coronoid

Fractures of the coronoid associated with complex fractures of the proximal ulna usually involve 50% to 100% of the height of the coronoid. An earlier report noted poor results in treating these large coronoid fractures, but none of the patients studied had undergone surgical fixation. If the coronoid fragments are large and non-comminuted, the prognosis is good if accurate alignment and secure fixation are achieved (Fig. 3). Large fractures of the coronoid are associated with more limited injury to the capsuloligamentous stabilizers of the elbow. The anterior capsule and the insertion of the medial collateral ligament remain attached to the coronoid. Therefore, realignment of the coronoid restores the trochlear notch and the anterior buttress and also restores the capsuloligamentous stabilizers. Of course, the coronoid may be comminuted, and if so can be difficult to treat.

One distinction between anterior (transolecranon) and posterior (posterior Monteggia) olecranon fracture-dislocations is that the lateral collateral ligament is spared in anterior fractures but is probably torn in the majority of posterior fractures. The injury to the lateral collateral ligament (among the other factors mentioned above) creates the potential for posterolateral rotatory instability of the elbow. In contrast, ulnohumeral insta-

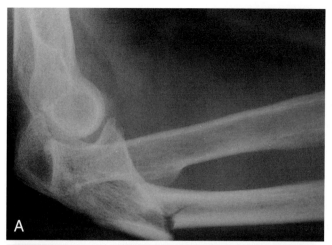
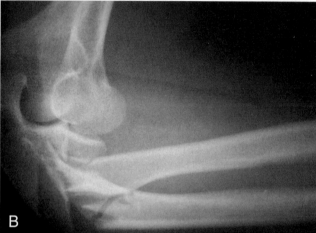
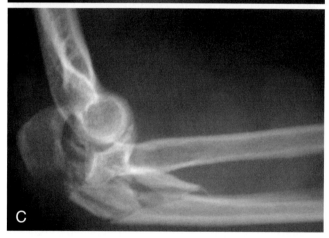

Figure 2 Radiographs showing posterior Monteggia fractures. These fractures occur in a spectrum with the ulnar fracture occurring at the diaphysis **(A)** or the metaphysis **(B)**, or involving the ulnohumeral articulation itself **(C)**.

the location of the ulnar fracture (Fig. 2). These have been subclassified as type A when the fracture is at the level of the trochlear notch (involving the olecranon and often the coronoid processes); type B, in the metaphysis just distal to the trochlear notch; and type C, in the diaphysis. Type D fractures are multifragmented and involve more than one region. These fractures are inherently unstable by virtue of

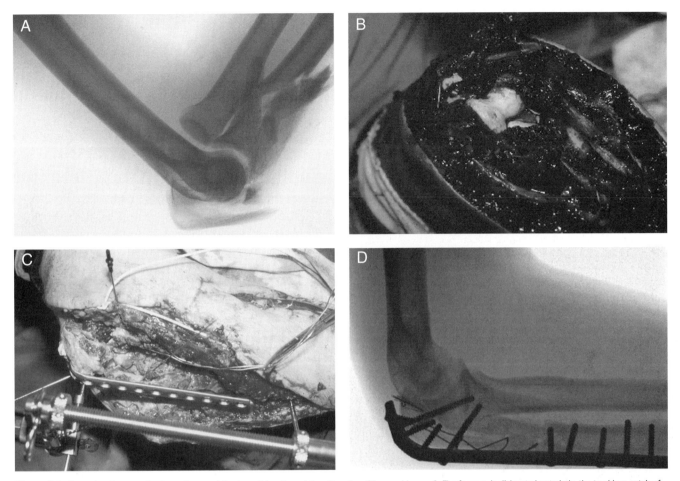

Figure 3 Radiographs of an anterior (transolecranon) fracture-dislocation of the elbow in a 21-year-old man. **A,** The forearm is dislocated anteriorly, the trochlear notch of the ulna is extensively fragmented, and the coronoid is separated as a single large fragment. **B,** Surgical exposure shows that the distal humerus is protruding through the proximal ulna. Muscle and periosteal attachments are preserved. **C,** A Mast small distractor is used to facilitate manipulative reduction. A stout, smooth K-wire holds the olecranon aligned. **D,** Plate and screw fixation supplemented by a tension wire has restored anatomic alignment of the ulna. Near full elbow motion was restored.

bility is rare after surgical fixation of an anterior (transolecranon) fracture-dislocation.

The fracture of the olecranon provides access to the coronoid process through the ulnohumeral articulation. The coronoid fragment can be realigned and provisionally stabilized by transfixing it either to the distal ulnar fragment or to the distal humerus using K-wires. The latter option proves useful as fragmentation of the ulna often extends into the diaphysis. In addition, or as an alternative, a skeletal distractor or external fixator can be used to realign the ulna. The olecranon fragment is first brought into anatomic alignment (for 90° of elbow flexion) and secured to the trochlea using a 5/64-in K-wire. Distraction can then be applied between this wire and a Schantz screw placed in the ulnar diaphysis. This distraction often pulls the coronoid into anatomic alignment as it realigns the elbow, and it helps maintain alignment while the plate and screws are applied (Fig. 4).

If adequate alignment of the coronoid is still not accomplished, a final option is manipulation of the coro-

noid through either a lateral or a medial exposure. The lateral exposure is useful in the treatment of posterior Monteggia fractures because exposure of the radial head is frequently necessary. Elevation of the radial wrist extensors and brachialis from the anterior humerus and development of a distal interval in the common extensor musculature provides access to the coronoid.

A medial exposure may be required because many coronoid fractures are more medially based. Medial exposure is obtained after isolating and protecting the ulnar nerve. The flexor pronator muscles can be elevated off the ulna, split longitudinally, or reflected off the medial epicondyle and proximal ulna. Fixation of the coronoid is accomplished with screws entering through the plate or adjacent to it and providing interfragmentary compression where appropriate. Supplementation with an anterior or anteromedial plate may be necessary.

Using these techniques, very little muscle or periosteum need be elevated from the bone. If precontoured plates are not available, a long plate is contoured to the

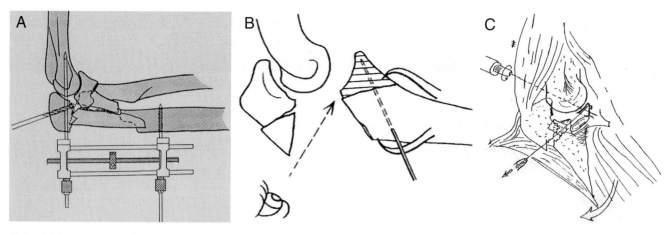

Figure 4 Schematic representation of various methods for realigning the coronoid process in a complex fracture of the proximal ulna. **A,** Distractor as described by Mast. *(Reproduced with permission from Mast J, Jakob R, Ganz R: Planning and Reduction Technique in Fracture Surgery. Heidelberg, Germany, Springer-Verlag, 1989, p 195.)* **B,** Depiction of the ulnohumeral joint; access is provided by the fracture of the olecranon. *(Reproduced with permission from Heim U: Combined fractures of the radius and the ulna at the elbow level in the adult: Analysis of 120 cases after more than 1 year. Rev Chir Orthop Reparatrice Appar Mot 1998;84:142-153.)* **C,** Provisional reduction is secured using a smooth K-wire passed through the distal humerus. *(Reproduced with permission from Hastings H II, Engles DR: Fixation of complex elbow fractures: Part II. Proximal ulna and radius fractures. Hand Clin 1997;13:721-735.)*

dorsal surface of the proximal ulna and around the olecranon process. Plates placed on the medial or lateral aspect of the ulna are not as effective biomechanically as those placed posteriorly. The triceps insertion does not need to be elevated. The proximal contour of the plate allows for a greater number of screws in the metaphyseal olecranon fragment. The most proximal screw can be a very long screw oriented longitudinally down the shaft of the ulna or into the anterior cortex and orthogonally to more distal screws. Distal to the fracture, the plate is applied directly to the apex of the ulnar diaphysis, which becomes triangular distal to the coronoid. The flexor and extensor carpi ulnaris muscles are separated to allow the plate to rest directly on the bone, but they are not otherwise elevated from the bone.

Fractures of the Radial Head

Once the ulnar fracture is secured, the stability of the elbow and forearm should be evaluated. Most anterior (transolecranon) fractures and many posterior fractures will be stable at this point. The radial head is commonly fractured in posterior Monteggia injuries, and this must be addressed if there is either a block to forearm rotation or instability of the ulnohumeral articulation.

When repair or replacement of the radial head is indicated, a lateral skin flap should be elevated and a second muscular interval created. Simultaneous exposure of the proximal radius and ulna via elevation of the intervening anconeus, extensor carpi ulnaris, and supinator muscles may increase the risk of radioulnar synostosis. The lateral collateral ligament is often injured, usually via avulsion from the lateral epicondyle, and can be used to improve exposure of the radial head. Although excision without replacement of the radial head has been adequate in many cases, the potential for ulnohumeral instability merits prosthetic replacement for most fractures not amenable to surgical fixation.

Postoperative Management

In most cases, treatment according to these guidelines will be sufficiently secure and reliable to allow functional mobilization and active, gravity-assisted elbow range-of-motion exercises within a few days. Prophylaxis against heterotopic ossification is not administered routinely, but it is considered in patients with injury to the central nervous system and patients in whom repeat elbow surgery has been performed in the early postinjury period. Once early fracture healing has been established (around 6 weeks), patients can use turnbuckle splints or the equivalent to improve motion.

Complications

A number of complications are associated with the treatment of complex fractures of the proximal ulna. These include inadequate or loose fixation leading to malalignment or nonunion of the ulna; instability of the ulnohumeral joint; and loss of motion, which can be caused by heterotopic ossification.

Tension band wires and long screws are often inadequate in the treatment of fracture-dislocations of the olecranon and proximal ulna, even when the fracture appears relatively simple. In addition, plates placed on the medial or lateral surface of the ulna seem more likely to loosen than plates placed on the posterior or dorsal surface, probably because they allow fewer screws to be placed in the proximal fragment; also, the forces exerted by the triceps and brachialis create adverse mechanics. The treatment of malalignment and nonunion consists of realignment of the ulna, débridement of fibrous and synovial tissue and sclerotic bone, and stable fixation with a contoured dorsally applied plate (Fig. 5).

Ulnohumeral instability after failed treatment of a proximal ulnar fracture is treated by realigning the ulna, repairing or reconstructing the coronoid, replacing the radial head with a prosthesis, repairing the lateral collateral ligament complex, and protecting the entire construct with hinged external fixation for 4 to 6 weeks (Fig. 6). Reconstruction of the coronoid can be performed using a fragment of the radial head or a portion of the olecranon tip when necessary.

Posttraumatic contractures are common after these injuries. The contracted capsule and heterotopic bone

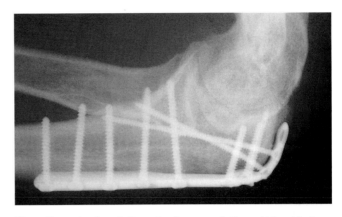

Figure 5 Lateral radiograph 10 months after open reduction and internal fixation and bone grafting with revision plating for an olecranon nonunion. The use of a congruent olecranon plate, which is available in different configurations, permits maximization of fixation in the proximal olecranon fragment. In these patients, five screws are placed in the proximal fragment in different planes, with interdigitation of those screws. Two of them can be used as compression screws across the nonunion as well.

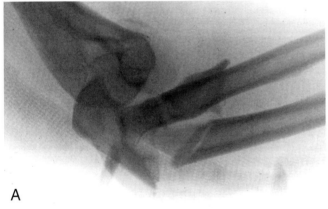

A

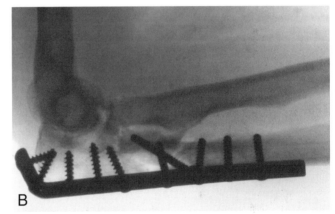

B

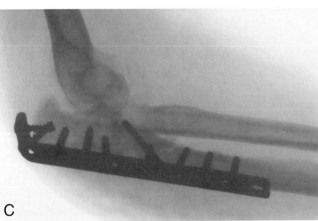

C

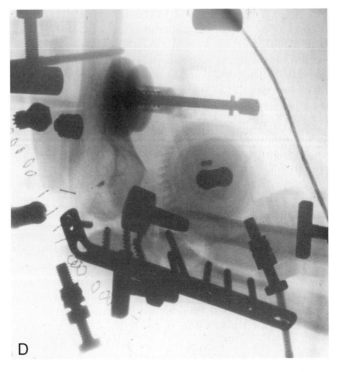

D

Figure 6 Radiographs from a 75-year-old woman with ulnohumeral instability after surgical fixation of a posterior Monteggia fracture. **A,** Lateral radiograph at the time of injury demonstrates a complex fracture of the proximal ulna involving the trochlear notch. There is a large coronoid fragment and a fracture of the radial head. The ulnohumeral joint is located, but disrupted. **B,** Initial surgical radiograph shows ulnar fixation, but the coronoid is not reduced anatomically. The radial head fracture has not been addressed. **C,** The ulnohumeral joint dislocated. **D,** Reconstructive treatment consisting of reconstruction of the coronoid process using a fragment of the radial head, prosthetic replacement of the radial head, reattachment of the lateral collateral ligament complex, and temporary hinged external fixation, restoring stability to the joint.

are excised, taking care to protect the ulnar and radial nerves. If the medial and lateral collateral ligaments are ossified, they may fracture as the elbow is mobilized. The resulting instability may necessitate temporary hinged external fixation. Prophylactic radiation may help limit the potential for heterotopic bone to reform and may make it safer to intervene early. Nonsteroidal anti-inflammatory medication has proved useful in the management of heterotopic bone around the hip, but it has been less well studied in the elbow.

Annotated Bibliography

Classification

Givon U, Pritsch M, Leby O, Yosepovich A, Amit Y, Horoszowski H: Monteggia and equivalent lesions: A study of 41 cases. *Clin Orthop* 1997;337:208-215.

Pediatric and adult injuries of various types, including "Monteggia equivalent" injuries are combined in this article. The majority of the "type 1 equivalent" injuries were probably misidentified posterior Monteggia fractures.

Haddad ES, Manktelow AR, Sarkar JS: The posterior Monteggia: A pathological lesion? *Injury* 1996;27: 101-102.

Five of six patients with posterior Monteggia fractures were receiving chronic corticosteroid treatment. The authors cite previous studies suggesting that the posterior Monteggia fracture may represent an alternative injury resulting from the same mechanism as posterior dislocation. The authors agree that the posterior Monteggia lesion may be associated with osteoporotic bone.

Hastings H, Engles DR: Fixation of complex elbow fractures: Part II. Proximal ulna and radius fractures. *Hand Clin* 1997;13:721-735.

This article offers organized thinking about simple and complex fractures of the proximal ulna. Several useful technical tips are described.

Heim U: Combined fractures of the radius and the ulna at the elbow level in the adult: Analysis of 120 cases after more than 1 year. *Rev Chir Orthop Reparatrice Appar Mot* 1998;84:142-153.

One hundred twenty combined fractures of the proximal radius and ulna registered in the AO Documentation Center in Davos, Switzerland, were reviewed and subclassfied as involving the coronoid and radial head (CR—25 cases); olecranon and radial head (OR—22 cases); coronoid, olecranon, and radial head (COR—41 cases); or metaphyseal ulna and radial head (MR—32 cases). Many of the 95 OR, COR, and MR fractures could be considered posterior Monteggia injuries or posterior Monteggia-type fracture-dislocations of the elbow. Good results were obtained in OR fractures with stable fixation of the olecranon and resection of the radial

head. Good results were rare among COR fractures, particularly when the radial head was resected. One third of MR cases had nonunion of the ulna—this was more common after radial head resection.

Reynders P, Groote W, Rondia J, Govaerts K, Stoffelen D, Broos PL: Monteggia lesions in adults: A multicenter BOTA study. *Acta Orthop Belg* 1996;62(suppl 1):78-83.

This multicenter review of 67 patients illustrates the challenges and inconsistencies in classification and management. Pitfalls in management included unstable fixation of the ulna, the use of postoperative cast immobilization, and exposure of the radius and the ulna simultaneously (the Boyd exposure). Only 54% of patients had satisfactory results because of complications such as healing problems, radioulnar synostosis, and persistent dislocation of the radial head.

Ring D, Jupiter JB, Sanders RW, Mast J, Simpson NS: Trans-olecranon fracture-dislocation of the elbow. *J Orthop Trauma* 1997;11:545-550.

Seventeen patients with an anterior (transolecranon) fracture-dislocation of the elbow—13 identified from a study of "Monteggia" injuries at Massachusetts General Hospital—were reviewed. Despite the complexity of the fractures—including a large fracture of the coronoid in eight patients and fragmentation extending into the diaphysis in six patients—union and good functional results were predictable. This injury disrupts the ulnotrochlear and not the radioulnar joint. The capsuloligamentous structures are relatively spared so that restoration of the normal contour and dimensions of the trochlear notch restores stability.

Ring D, Jupiter JB, Simpson NS: Monteggia fractures in adults. *J Bone Joint Surg Am* 1998;80:1733-1744.

Overall, 40 of 48 adult patients with Monteggia fractures obtained good or excellent function according to the rating of Broberg and Morrey. Twenty-six patients had fracture of the coronoid—all as a single large fragment (Regan and Morrey type III). Patients with Bado type I injuries were younger (average age of 26 years), more often male (71%), and were often injured in very high-energy accidents, and ipsilateral fractures and neurovascular injuries were common. However, 13 of 26 patients (50%) with a posterior Monteggia fracture associated with fracture of the radial head either required a second surgical procedure within the first 4 months of the injury or had an unsatisfactory final result.

Ring D, Jupiter JB, Waters PM: Monteggia fractures in children and adults. *J Am Acad Orthop Surg* 1998;6: 215-224.

The similarities and distinctions between pediatric and adult Monteggia injuries are described. The key to the treatment of all such injuries is secure, anatomic realignment of the ulna.

Treatment

Tapasvi S, Diggikar MS, Joshi AP: External fixation for open proximal ulnar fractures. *Injury* 1999;30:115-120.

This article reports the use of external fixation in the treatment of 21 patients with open proximal ulnar fractures. Eighteen were type 2 and three were type 3A according to the classification of Gustilo and Anderson. All of the fractures healed and the functional results were reported as good or excellent in all patients. Despite these apparently good results, the role of external fixation is unclear given the safety of plate and screw fixation for open fractures of the upper extremity. The authors cite an advantage for plastic surgical procedures, but external devices usually hinder such procedures. Furthermore, 12 patients required skin grafts, one a rotational flap, and one a pedicle flap—far more soft-tissue work than is usually required for type 2 wounds.

Complications

Biyani A, Olscamp AJ, Ebraheim NA: Complications in the management of complex Monteggia-equivalent fractures in adults. *Am J Orthop* 2000;29:115-118.

This article reports loosening of fixation or failure to heal in five patients with complex fractures of the proximal ulna. All five "Monteggia equivalent"cases appear to be posterior Monteggia fractures, but were not identified as such. Surgeons should be aware that fracture of the radial head is very common among posterior Monteggia injuries and does not merit separate classification.

Cobb TK, Morrey BF: Use of distraction arthroplasty in unstable fracture dislocations of the elbow. *Clin Orthop* 1995;312:201-210.

A small group of patients is reviewed and the principles of reconstruction outlined in this article. Some of these patients had complex fractures of the proximal ulna. Although the results are not predictably excellent, these patients had severe problems, and their conditions usually improved substantially.

Gallay SH, McKee MD: Operative treatment of nonunions about the elbow. *Clin Orthop* 2000;370: 87-101.

This study of ununited fractures about the elbow presents an extensive discussion of the decision-making and treatment options for olecranon nonunions, but it provides limited information about nonunion after more complex fractures of the proximal ulna.

Ring D, Jupiter JB: Reconstruction of posttraumatic elbow instability. *Clin Orthop* 2000;370:44-56.

Complex fractures of the proximal ulna can be associated with ulnohumeral instability. This article discusses the management of these problems in detail. The osseous and articular contributions to stability must be restored and the ligaments repaired or reconstructed. In many cases, temporary hinged external fixation is helpful to protect these repaired structures.

Classic Bibliography

Danziger MB, Healy WL: Operative treatment of olecranon nonunion. *J Orthop Trauma* 1992;6:290-293.

Jupiter JB, Leibovic SJ, Ribbans W, Wilk RM: The posterior Monteggia lesion. *J Orthop Trauma* 1991;5: 395-402.

Papagelopoulos PJ, Morrey BF: Treatment of nonunion of olecranon fractures. *J Bone Joint Surg Br* 1994;76: 627-635.

Chapter 36

Coronoid Fractures

Shawn W. O'Driscoll, PhD, MD

Introduction

Coronoid fractures are most commonly seen in association with radial head fractures as part of the "terrible triad" (coronoid fracture, radial head fracture, and elbow dislocation). They are seen less commonly as isolated fractures or as part of complex olecranon fracture-dislocations. Coronoid fractures are caused by axial loading with or without varus or valgus or by rotational torques applied to the elbow. The injury pattern is determined by the position of the elbow at the time of injury and the loading pattern across the elbow. Until recently, a clear understanding of these fractures has been lacking, and thus little has been written regarding their management. However, most elbow surgeons would currently agree with a recent study of 120 fracture-dislocations of the elbow in which the coronoid was identified as the key component in these injuries.

Classification

Coronoid fractures have been classified into three types according to the height of the fragment involved. However, clinical experience has revealed fracture patterns that are not classifiable by this system, suggesting that a more appropriate classification system might be based on anatomic location of the primary fracture as follows: tip, anteromedial facet, and base (body). Subtyping within each category is based on the severity (amount of coronoid loss) of the fracture. This classification system accounts for comminution, elbow stability, and associated injuries and provides guidelines for surgical approach and treatment.

Evaluation

A coronoid fracture should be suspected with all elbow dislocations, especially if the radial head is fractured. A common mistake is to misidentify a coronoid fragment as a radial head fragment; it is helpful to know that a dislocated elbow with a radial head fracture usually has an associated coronoid fracture. Clinical examination should include evaluation for tenderness or bruising at the origin of the collateral ligament complexes and common flexor and extensor origins, especially on the lateral side, where avulsion may not be obvious without an index of suspicion.

Plain AP and lateral radiographs are sometimes adequate, but oblique views can be helpful. Lateral (sagittal) tomograms or CT scans are highly useful in identifying the location of the fracture and the severity of comminution. It is useful to remember that the coronoid fragment is bigger than it appears on the radiograph because of the cartilage cap on the fragment. Stress radiographs permit accurate determination of the instability patterns and therefore which constraints have been disrupted. Lateral collateral ligament (LCL) injuries may be missed unless stress radiographs are taken.

Examination under anesthesia including stress radiographs is an important part of the assessment of any elbow fracture-dislocation with the potential for instability. This includes evaluation for varus, valgus, and posterolateral rotatory instability. Varus posteromedial rotatory instability has only recently been recognized. A corollary of posterolateral rotatory instability, it occurs during axial loading of the elbow during flexion. The combination of varus and internal rotation moments during axial loading of the flexed elbow produces a fracture of the anteromedial coronoid and disruption (usually avulsion) of the LCL (Fig. 1). The coronoid fracture may be large and comminuted, or it may be small and involve only the segment between the tip and sublime tubercle, which is the attachment site of the anterior bundle of the medial collateral ligament (MCL). This injury, which is discussed later, is significant in that it results in ulno-humeral joint incongruity, which can lead to premature posttraumatic arthritis.

Coronoid Tip Fractures

These coronal plane fractures rarely involve more than one third to one half of the coronoid tip and do not extend medially past the sublime tubercle. They usually occur as a result of a posterolateral rotatory elbow subluxation or dis-

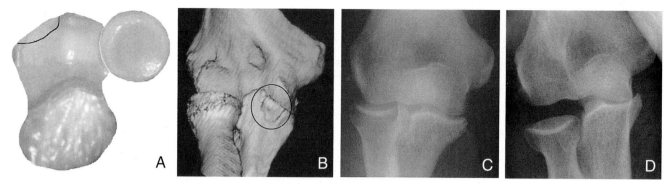

Figure 1 Location of the anteromedial coronoid fracture fragment. **A,** A schematic illustration. **B,** A three-dimensional CT reconstruction. (Fracture fragment indicated in figure B by the small circle). AP radiographs with (**C**) and without (**D**) varus posteromedial rotatory stress applied; C appears to be an almost normal radiograph, whereas D reveals significant varus instability and apparent narrowing of the medial ulnohumeral joint. The displacement and mechanism of injury are as described and illustrated in Figure 2. *(Reproduced with permission from the Mayo Foundation, Rochester, MN.)*

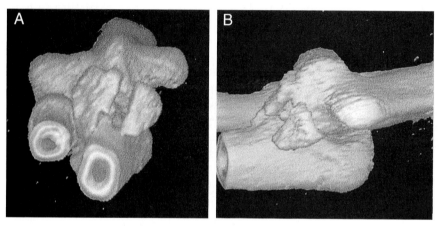

Figure 2 Mechanism of injury for anteromedial coronoid fractures. **A,** An anteromedial subtype 3 coronoid fracture, with involvement of not just the anteromedial fragment but the tip and the sublime tubercle as well. **B,** Varus posteromedial displacement is seen. (Courtesy of Mark Cohen, MD.)

location. The effect of this injury on elbow stability is proportionate to the amount of coronoid lost or fractured. One study found that if the radial head is fractured, fixation of tip fractures involving as little as one sixth of the coronoid is required to maintain elbow stability. Another study noted that elbow dislocation after radial head excision only occurred when the coronoid was also fractured. If treatment of a radial head fracture includes surgical repair, these coronoid tip fractures can be fixed adequately through the lateral exposure with transosseous sutures, fine threaded Kirschner wires (K-wires), or a combination of the two. Occasionally, larger fragments can be fixed with screws. This is performed through the lateral exposure used for treating the radial head fracture. The LCL is virtually always disrupted when a dislocation has occurred, and it should be repaired if surgical treatment is being undertaken. If the elbow has not apparently dislocated and is stable, these fractures can be treated nonsurgically. The authors of a study reporting on two patients with minimally displaced coronoid tip fractures that progressed to nonunion and resulted in contractures suggested that displacement and hypertrophy of the coronoid fragment were responsible. Caution is required when treating isolated coronoid fractures (ie, those with no apparent radial head

fracture or elbow dislocation), as they appear benign but usually are fracture-subluxations with avulsion of the LCL.

Anteromedial Coronoid Fractures

Anteromedial fractures have not been addressed in the literature. The initial fracture (subtype 1) is located anteromedially, between the tip of the coronoid and the sublime tubercle, in an oblique plane between the coronal and sagittal planes (Fig. 1). Medially, the fracture line usually exits the cortex in the anterior half of the sublime tubercle (ie, in the anterior portion of the anterior bundle of the MCL). Laterally, the fracture exits just medial to the tip of the coronoid. Comminution can extend to the tip (subtype 2), the sublime tubercle (subtype 3), or the body of the coronoid, depending on the energy of the injury.

The mechanism of injury is varus posteromedial rotation that occurs with axial loading. Flexion and abduction torque at the shoulder that occurs during elbow flexion under axial load causes the elbow to go into varus (disrupting the LCL) and the medial trochlea to ride up onto the anteromedial coronoid, which is fractured off by a shearing mechanism (Fig. 2).

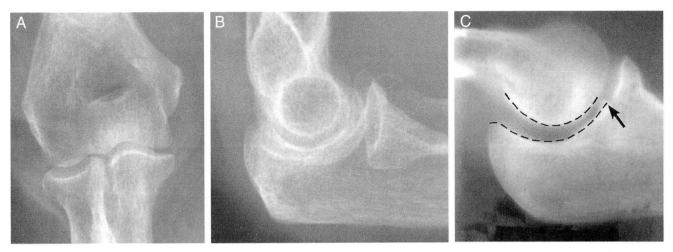

Figure 3 AP **(A)** and lateral **(B)** radiographs of an anteromedial subtype 2 coronoid fracture, showing anatomic joint alignment and no apparent significant displacement. **C,** Lateral trispiral tomogram (taken through the medial portion of the ulnohumeral articulation with slight gravitational varus stress on the elbow) shows an anteromedial subtype 2 fracture (involving the anteromedial coronoid and the tip) with joint incongruity caused by varus posteromedial rotatory subluxation. The medial trochlea has displaced anteriorly and distally along with the anteromedial coronoid fragment, which it displaced and with which it remains congruent. This results in point contact between the medial trochlea and the coronoid at the fracture site (arrow), which over the course of a few months leads to medial trochlear erosion. The incongruity is indicated by the ulnohumeral joint being widened posteriorly and converging anteriorly (indicated by converging dotted lines). *(Reproduced with permission from the Mayo Foundation, Rochester, MN.)*

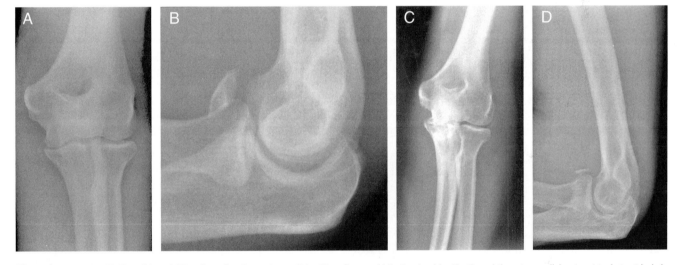

Figure 4 Preoperative AP **(A)** and lateral **(B)** radiographs of an anteromedial subtype 2 coronoid fracture involving the tip and the anteromedial segment to, but not including, the sublime tubercle. AP **(C)** and lateral **(D)** radiographs taken 1 year after reduction and transosseous suture fixation of the fragments, showing medial ulnohumeral collapse and early arthritis. *(Reproduced with permission from the Mayo Foundation, Rochester, MN.)*

Associated injuries include disruptions of the collateral ligaments and occasionally a fracture of the radial head. It is safe to assume with an anteromedial coronoid fracture that the LCL has been disrupted. The LCL is usually avulsed beneath the common extensor tendon origin; this condition may be missed unless stress radiographs are obtained or the tendon is opened to explore the ligament. Although an isolated anteromedial coronoid fracture may appear benign, it is usually a fracture-subluxation with avulsion of the LCL, and the elbow will tend to articulate incongruently under axial load or gravitational varus stress (Fig. 3). Such incongruity can lead to rapid onset of arthritis (Fig. 4). The authors of a recent biomechanical study found that a loss of up to 40% of the coronoid did not change the resistance of the elbow to direct posterior subluxation; however, they did not evaluate stability with coupled motions in posterolateral or varus posteromedial rotation.

Although the optimal treatment of anteromedial coronoid fractures has yet to be identified, protection against gravitational varus stress is critical. Many of these injuries require some form of surgical treatment, possibly anatomic reduction and either rigid internal fixation or protection with an external fixator. In addi-

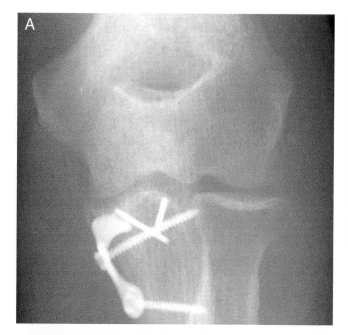

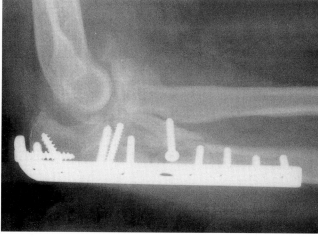

Figure 6 Radiograph of a patient with a comminuted olecranon coronoid fracture-dislocation. The anteromedial coronoid fragment remained displaced despite attempts to lag the coronoid fragments in place. This resulted in joint incongruity and early posttraumatic arthritis, subsequently requiring a total elbow arthroplasty.

Basal Coronoid Fractures

Basal fractures involve the body of the coronoid rather than just the tip or the anteromedial facet. On the medial side, the fracture emerges in or below the insertion of the MCL on the sublime tubercle. Though elbow congruity and stability may be severely disrupted, the extent of soft-tissue disruption is often less than that seen with tip fractures. However, the authors of one study found that results after treatment of transolecranon fractures involving both the radial head and the coronoid were rarely good, with arthritis developing in 36 of 41 patients. These fractures are usually quite comminuted, but the coronoid fragment may be large if it is part of an olecranon fracture-dislocation. The authors of another study reported good results in eight patients with transolecranon fractures following fixation of a large coronoid fragment. Comminution of the trochlear notch did not preclude a good result provided that stable, anatomic fixation of the coronoid was achieved.

Basal coronoid fractures not involving the olecranon are reduced and held with fine wires or screws and neutralized with a plate placed on the anteromedial surface of the ulna. Elevation of a depressed medial or central fragment of the coronoid may be necessary. The elbow also can be neutralized with a hinged external fixator, which is necessary if stable anatomic reduction cannot not be attained. Any ligamentous disruption (usually the LCL complex or annular ligament) is repaired. Transolecranon fracture-dislocations (basal subtype 2 fractures) are managed by attempting a reduction of the coronoid fragment through the olecranon fracture. A posterior precontoured plate is used for these fractures. Sometimes it is possible to lag the coronoid fragments, but comminution may make this impossible. Obtaining adequate reduc-

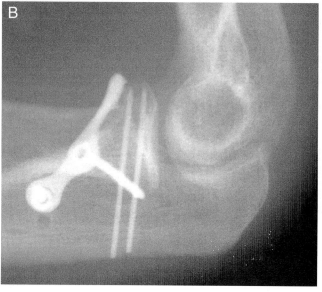

Figure 5 AP (A) and lateral (B) radiographs of an anteromedial coronoid fracture fixed with a congruent plate and two fine threaded K-wires. *(Reproduced with permission from the Mayo Foundation, Rochester, MN.)*

tion, the LCL must be repaired if a hinged fixator is not used. The surgical exposure can be directly anterior or medial. Medial access to the fracture is possible by reflecting a portion of the common flexor-pronator origin from the epicondyle and ulna after transposing the ulnar nerve. One technique for anatomic reduction involves placing threaded 0.062 K-wires through the ulna into the anteromedial fracture fragments and using a precontoured buttress plate (Fig. 5). The anteromedial facet of the coronoid (between the tip and sublime tubercle) is the critical fragment to be buttressed if there is comminution.

tion and stability of the anteromedial coronoid fragment is critical. Failure to do so will likely result in joint incongruity and early posttraumatic arthritis (Fig. 6).

Postoperative Management

Postoperative management consists of splinting of the elbow in extension for about 36 hours, followed by early motion. If the posterior tension band has been restored and is secure, full active motion is permitted. A hinged brace offers some protection, but only when the elbow is relatively extended. When the security of fixation is in question, motion is limited to an arc from 30° to 110° for the first 3 to 6 weeks. Stiffness is likely to result if the elbow is immobilized postoperatively, so motion should be started in almost all cases. A hinged external fixator is used to protect the elbow when fracture displacement or joint subluxation is a concern. If a choice is required between stability and mobility, stability should be chosen. A stiff but congruent elbow is easier to correct than one that has been chronically incongruent because of the cartilage erosion that occurs in the latter. Gravitational varus stress in the postoperative period is probably the major factor causing displacement of the coronoid. This can be avoided by neutralizing the elbow with a hinged external fixator. If no fixator is used, the patient must be instructed regarding the importance of not positioning the forearm in the horizontal or inclined plane. In other words, the elbow should always be positioned such that the forearm is in the vertical plane when it is moved.

Annotated Bibliography

Ameur NE, Rebouh M, Oberlin C: Anterior transbrachial approach of the coronoid apophysis. *Chir Main* 1999;18:220-225.

The authors propose a midline anterior incision retracting the biceps tendon laterally and splitting the brachialis muscle longitudinally, allowing direct access to the fracture.

Bousselmame N, Boussouga M, Bouabid S, Galuia F, Taobane H, Moulay I: Fractures of the coronoid process. *Chir Main* 2000;19:286-293.

The authors report that an anteroposterior screw worked well for fixing small coronoid fragments when no comminution was present.

Closkey RF, Goode JR, Kirschenbaum D, Cody RP: The role of the coronoid process in elbow stability: A biomechanical analysis of axial loading. *J Bone Joint Surg Am* 2000;82:1749-1753.

The authors found that a loss of up to 40% of the coronoid did not change the resistance of the elbow to direct posterior subluxation. However, they did not evaluate stability with coupled motions in posterolateral or varus posteromedial rotation. Isolated coronoid fractures involving this much of the coronoid are usually anteromedial fracture-subluxations, which are potentially serious injuries. An isolated coronoid fracture (ie, a coronoid fracture without a radial head fracture or apparent dislocation) is highly likely to be an anteromedial fracture-subluxation with LCL injury and the potential for joint incongruity.

Heckman JD (ed): *Fractures in Adults*. Philadelphia, PA, Lippincott-Raven, 1996, pp 980-981.

A general review and approach to coronoid fractures is given in the context of elbow injuries in general.

Liu SH, Henry M, Bowen R: Complications of type I coronoid fractures in competitive athletes: Report of two cases and review of the literature. *J Shoulder Elbow Surg* 1996;5:223-227.

Two cases of minimally displaced coronoid tip fractures that progressed to nonunion resulted in contractures. Displacement and hypertrophy of the coronoid fragment were thought to be responsible.

O'Driscoll S: Olecranon and coronoid fractures, in Norris TR (ed): *Orthopaedic Knowledge Update: Shoulder and Elbow*. Rosemont, IL, American Academy of Ortho-paedic Surgeons, 1997, pp 405-413.

The state of understanding and treatment of coronoid fractures is reviewed. A comparison with current knowledge reveals a significant advance in 5 years.

Ring D, Jupiter JB, Sanders RW, Mast J, Simpson NS: Transolecranon fracture-dislocation of the elbow. *J Orthop Trauma* 1997;11:545-550.

Eight patients with transolecranon fractures also underwent fixation of a large coronoid fragment. Comminution of the trochlear notch did not preclude a good result provided that stable, anatomic fixation of the large coronoid fragment was achieved.

Classic Bibliography

Amis AA, Miller JH: The mechanisms of elbow fractures: An investigation using impact tests in vitro. *Injury* 1995;26:163-168.

Cage DJ, Abrams RA, Callahan JJ, Botte MJ: Soft tissue attachments of the ulnar coronoid process. *Clin Orthop* 1995;320:154-158.

Copf F, Holz U, Schauwecker HH: Biomechanical problems in elbow joint dislocations with coronoid and capitulum radii fractures. *Langenbecks Arch Chir* 1980;350: 249-254.

Josefsson PO, Gentz CF, Johnell O, Wendeberg B: Dislocations of the elbow and intraarticular fractures. *Clin Orthop* 1989;126-130.

O'Driscoll SW: Classification and spectrum of elbow instability: Recurrent instability, in Morrey BF (ed): *The Elbow and Its Disorders*. Philadelphia, PA, WB Saunders, 1993, pp 453-463.

O'Driscoll SW: Elbow instability. *Hand Clin* 1994;10: 405-415.

Regan W, Morrey B: Fractures of the coronoid process of the ulna. *J Bone Joint Surg Am* 1989;71:1348-1354.

Section 7

Miscellaneous Shoulder Topics

Section Editor:
Robert D. Leffert, MD

Chapter 37

Brachial Plexus Injuries in the Adult

Robert D. Leffert, MD

Introduction

Brachial plexus injuries occur in a wide variety of situations, but they are not commonly seen in most orthopaedic practices. Moreover, because treatment is constantly evolving and requires a team of health care providers working together, treatment of these injuries can be difficult and time-consuming. This chapter reviews both the basic aspects of brachial plexus injuries as well as more recent developments.

Although most injuries to the brachial plexus are caused by traction to the nerves, which occurs in high-velocity situations such as motorcycle accidents and automobile crashes, they also may occur during falls and in industrial accidents involving machines. Unfortunately, some injuries are iatrogenic, resulting from surgery, invasive radiologic studies, or radiation therapy for neoplasms.

The mechanism of traction injury is a good model with which to advance the understanding of these injuries. When a force is applied to increase the distance between the head and the shoulder, forcibly depressing the shoulder girdle, or causing longitudinal traction on the arm, the ability of the surrounding soft tissues to protect the underlying nerves from traction-elongation may be exceeded, and a variety of neuropathologic conditions can occur. These conditions can range from a relatively benign neurapraxia, which has an excellent prognosis, to neurotmesis, or actual tearing of the nerves. Tearing can occur either within the nerve substance or from the nerve's origin at the spinal cord. In the latter situation, the outlook for functional recovery is generally extremely poor, although there has been some interesting work on reimplantation of avulsed spinal nerves. For some of the lesions along the continuity of the nerve, there is the possibility of restoring function by means of grafting or providing axons from other sources. Furthermore, in situations where neural reconstruction fails or is not applicable, peripheral reconstruction using techniques adapted from the treatment of polio can be used with benefit.

The biomechanical considerations of traction injuries must include the magnitude of the force applied to the tissues, the position of the head and arm at the moment of impact, and the integrity or lack thereof of the skeletal framework. These considerations will determine not only the severity of nerve injury, but also its distribution within the brachial plexus. For example, patients who sustain widely displaced fractures of the clavicle or actual lateral dislocation of the scapula on the thorax are liable to have severe traction injuries that may not only render the limb permanently paralyzed but also cause significant vascular complications that can be life-threatening.

Anatomy

In the anatomy of the idealized and most common form of the brachial plexus, the C5 through T1 anterior primary rami exit their neural foramina to form the three trunks that are arranged within the supraclavicular fossa. In addition, in 65% of plexus dissections, C4 contributes to the upper trunk to form a prefixed plexus; in significantly fewer bodies, T2 joins the lower trunk to constitute a postfixed plexus. When applied to either a diagnostic or a surgical situation, the placement of C4 and T2 assume significant importance. The divisions of the plexus are located behind the clavicle, and the cords and the axillary artery originate beneath the coracoid process. Unfortunately, variations in the form of the plexus are common and have been both an impediment to understanding its anatomy and a historic source of debate. Since the application of microsurgical techniques to the repair of the nerves, several studies have been done on the intraneural topography. However, even these are limited because of the variations that occur within the general population.

The muscles supplied by the root collaterals of the brachial plexus that are susceptible to both manual muscle testing and electromyographic study are the rhomboids and the serratus anterior. In traction lesions, the ability to differentiate root avulsions from distal ruptures is of prime importance because the latter are practically irreparable. Electrodiagnostic or clinical evidence of denervation of these muscles provides strong presumptive evidence that the nerve root under consideration has been avulsed.

The clavicle usually is thought of as a simple mechanical strut for the shoulder girdle; it also serves to protect the brachial plexus from excessive traction as long as it is intact. Rarely will lesions occur acutely beneath the clavicle as a result of impingement or laceration by fracture fragments. However, extension of a supraclavicular lesion beneath the clavicle may involve the distal parts of the plexus. With direct injury to the clavicle and subsequent malunion or nonunion of fractures, compression lesions of the underlying plexus can occur over time.

Injuries that appear to be confined to the infraclavicular portions of the plexus usually are caused by fractures or fracture-dislocations of the glenohumeral joint and humerus. They are not ordinarily traction lesions but instead are caused by local compression, and their prognosis for recovery without surgery generally is good. If the fracture fragments are sharp, there may be actual laceration of the neural elements (neurotmesis); fortunately, this is not common. In some infraclavicular paralyses specific to the axillary nerve, local traction caused by excessive distraction of the humerus occasionally may result in neurotmesis.

Supraclavicular Injuries

Clinical Examination

As previously described, most high-velocity brachial plexus injuries result from traction and produce a variety of distributions and degrees of pathology. The required determination is between a distal lesion and an avulsion of the nerve root from the spinal cord. The patient may have sustained other injuries, including head injury, which may compromise the examiner's ability to recognize the presence of the plexus injury or to define its specifics. Additional life-threatening conditions may occupy the attention of the trauma surgeons until the patient's condition has stabilized. Many of these nerve injuries are first encountered by physicians and surgeons who may be expert at saving the patient's life but who lack familiarity with the evaluation of the nerve injury, resulting in a wait-and-see approach that can prejudice functional recovery of the limb. The nature of the injury must be quickly defined so that treatment can begin. Alternatively, the patient may be referred to a center where he or she can be started on a rehabilitative program that may involve either direct repair or peripheral reconstruction of the nerves. Although there is little indication for an emergency cervical myelogram, and electrodiagnostic studies are of little use before 3 weeks

postinjury, the evaluation should be completed and the treatment algorithm well defined within 3 months.

The patient with an acute supraclavicular injury of the brachial plexus can have a variety of neurologic deficits. It therefore is imperative to urgently document the precise extent of the loss to provide a basis for determining whether the injury is improving, static, or actually getting worse. It would be most unlikely for a traction injury that is incomplete initially to worsen unless there is an accompanying vascular injury that produces further compression on the already injured nerves. Such situations are more likely, for example, when there has been an iatrogenic brachial plexus injury as a result of a subclavian vein puncture. However, a poorly documented initial evaluation places the subsequent treating surgeon and the patient at a significant disadvantage.

Certain aspects of an adequate orthopaedic examination of an injured patient are especially important for examination of a patient with a brachial plexus injury. The face must be carefully examined for the presence of Horner's syndrome, which consists of ptosis of the eyelid, an abnormally small pupil, enophthalmos, and absence of sweating on the ipsilateral side of the face. The presence of Horner's syndrome usually indicates that the first thoracic nerve root has been avulsed from the spinal cord. It generally is considered a poor prognostic sign if the patient also has an anesthetic, flail limb. Horner's syndrome may, however, be seen in a small group of patients whose lesions are confined to the lower trunk of the brachial plexus. They generally lack finger flexion and intrinsic function in the hand as well as sensibility in the little finger and the medial side of the forearm. Such patients are unusual, both in the adult population and in the pediatric population with birth paralysis referred to as Klumpke's paralysis.

After a gentle evaluation of the integrity and range of motion of the cervical spine, attention is turned to the area of the supraclavicular fossa and the clavicle. In an acute injury, if there is swelling above the clavicle or other evidence of hematoma, the physician can assume there is a supraclavicular traction injury. However, if a Tinel's sign can be elicited by percussion over the brachial plexus in this area, then at least one nerve root has not been avulsed from the spinal cord. In the chronic situation, when swelling has gone down, the area of the plexus may feel indurated, which indicates the presence of scarring. Tinel's sign should be sought in this situation as well, with the same rationale as in the acute situation.

The skeletal components of the shoulder girdle should then be assessed for their integrity, stability, and range of motion. A displaced fracture of the clavicle predisposes the patient to increased severity of a traction lesion of the plexus. A dislocated shoulder may be the cause of the injury to the plexus, which may not be supraclavicular at all but infraclavicular. This situation is described further in the next section. The skeletal integrity of the remainder of the limb should be rapidly but carefully determined.

Attention should then be directed to careful manual muscle testing, first of the unaffected side, and then of the injured limb. Performing an identical examination on both sides, starting with the unaffected side, ensures that the patient understands what is expected and gives the examiner a baseline to compare with what is normal for that patient. Although pain or the presence of open wounds may condition the responses, it usually is possible to obtain an accurate picture of muscle strength. The examination should begin with the scapular muscles, including the trapezius, serratus anterior, and rhomboids, and then proceed to the deltoid and rotator cuff as well as the latissimus and the pectoralis major. Both the clavicular portions of the latter, innervated by C5 and C6, and the sternocostal portion, supplied by the rest of the plexus, must be palpated as strength is assessed because this palpation often will provide important information regarding the distribution of the lesion. If the patient is hesitant or cannot move the limb, having the patient cough vigorously while the examiner palpates both muscles may test the latissimus. The contraction of the latissimus, if it occurs, is involuntary with cough.

Elbow extension and flexion are then tested, remembering that even in the absence of biceps and brachialis, strong elbow flexion may be possible with an intact brachioradialis. In a C5-C6 lesion, however, elbow flexion will be lost because of the common innervation that all of these muscles share.

The examination of wrist extension can be particularly deceptive because even with complete loss of the C5-C6 innervated radial wrist extensors, the patient may retain reasonably strong wrist extension if the extensor carpi ulnaris and the finger extensors are spared. The effect of these muscles can be ruled out by having the patient make a fist and then attempt to extend the wrist against resistance.

The remainder of the manual muscle test is conducted in standard fashion. Although there are numerous systems for recording motor power, the one that is most preferred is that of the British Medical Research Council, which rates a normal muscle as 5 and one that is completely paralyzed as 0. It is imperative not only to perform a careful manual muscle test, but also to record the results in detail. Visible atrophy of muscle takes several months to occur, but if it is completely absent in a limb that is alleged to be completely paralyzed, the physician must look for another reason for the patient's loss of function.

The sensory evaluation of a patient with a posttraumatic brachial plexopathy need not be time-consuming to be complete. For most patients, simple testing with light touch and pinprick will suffice. Only in chronic situations with minimal positive physical findings will further investigations of sensibility be applicable. Here, too, the skin should be evaluated for the presence or absence of normal sweating. Sensory deficits should be carefully recorded and compared with known patterns of peripheral nerve and dermatomal distribution. A patient with complete loss of brachial plexus function will retain sensibility in the axilla and the upper medial aspect of the arm because these areas are supplied by the T2 spinal nerve. Although avulsion injuries usually do not produce long tract signs, spasticity may develop in the lower extremities if scarring encroaches on these tracts with the passage of time.

Finally, the vascular status of the limb must be assessed in terms of peripheral pulses and the possibility of a compartment syndrome. Unfortunately, these additional lesions may complicate diagnosis and in some cases, if not promptly recognized, can result in complete functional loss of the limb.

Clinical examination of the patient with an anesthetic, flail limb will take the least amount of time. However, the ultimate total evaluation and establishment of a prognosis will prove to be the most difficult. These are the most severe of the traction injuries, and the combination of Horner's syndrome and a totally paralyzed and insensate upper extremity virtually ensures that normal function will not be regained under any circumstances. It is in treating these patients, however, that the most progress has been made in the last half of the 20th century, before which most of these patients were advised to have the limb amputated. The general adoption of microsurgical techniques has changed this situation, and new developments continue to evolve.

The prognosis for spontaneous recovery is considerably better for patients with incomplete lesions, particularly lesions of the upper trunk. Some of these patients may recover completely. For patients with other lesions, the possibilities range from complete loss of limb function to a return to normal function.

The time required for neurologic recovery may be lengthy. During that time, stiffness and edema of the limb must be prevented or aggressively treated so that the recovery of neural function does not translate into functional recovery.

Common Patterns of Neurologic Loss

A C5-C6 lesion, or upper trunk lesion, causes loss of shoulder abduction and lateral rotation as well as elbow flexion. There is also weakness of wrist extension because of the deficit of the radial wrist extensors. The sensory deficit extends from the lateral aspect of the arm, the radial side of the forearm, to include the thumb and index finger. The C5, C6, and C7 lesion adds additional paralysis of the wrist and finger extensors as well as loss of triceps function to the above pattern.

Loss of function of the entire plexus produces an anesthetic, flail arm and hand and usually is accompanied by Horner's syndrome. In the uncommon C8 and T1 pattern, the patient loses finger flexion as well as intrinsic function in the hand, although the sensory deficit usually is restricted to the little finger and the medial side of the forearm. The prognosis for each category worsens with the extent of the lesion; an anesthetic, flail arm rarely recovers unless the condition is caused by an infraclavicular lesion.

Infraclavicular Injuries

These injuries are identified largely by the history of the injury and its mechanism. They are distinct from the traction injuries described in the previous sections in that they are the result of a local injury to the infraclavicular portions of the brachial plexus resulting from fractures and fracture-dislocations in the region of the shoulder joint. Excluded from this category are injuries that result from displaced fractures of the clavicle and traction injuries that extend from above the clavicle. Unless there are obvious indications of supraclavicular injury, such as the presence of Horner's syndrome or the finding of a large swelling in the supraclavicular fossa, the patient with a fracture or fracture-dislocation of the proximal humerus can be presumed to have an infraclavicular injury until proven otherwise. If, however, sharp and oblique fracture fragments are seen on the radiographs, the prognosis for these lesions is worse than for other infraclavicular injuries.

In 1965, records from the Royal National Orthopaedic Hospital in London were retrospectively reviewed and it was determined that the isolated axillary nerve lesion that accompanied closed shoulder dislocation had a poor prognosis. The problem with this conclusion was the bias of the sampled patient population; these patients were documented because they had clinically recognizable and persistent axillary nerve lesions and were culled from a nerve injury center. Subsequent experience has clearly demonstrated that many patients with shoulder dislocations have some element of axillary nerve injury that is not detected in the emergency department evaluation. Most of these patients will recover even if they do have significant axillary nerve lesions at initial examination. However, if there is neither clinical nor electrodiagnostic evidence of recovery by 3 months following injury, the axillary nerve should be surgically explored. If it is technically possible to graft the nerve, there is a reasonable chance of functional recovery. Unfortunately, some of these lesions simply are not repairable.

Although the prognosis for neurologic recovery of infraclavicular lesions is good, it is vital to maintain the range of motion of the joints because if the nerves recover but the joints are stiff, function will be severely compromised. In addition, the problem of edema is a very real one that is much easier to prevent than to treat. The outlook for functional recovery for all muscles proximal to the intrinsics of the hand is good, but the period of recovery may be as long as 3 years from the time of injury.

Mechanisms of Injury

Burners and Stingers

Burners and stingers are closed injuries to the brachial plexus that usually occur during contact sports, most often football. After collision with another player, the patient suddenly has acute pain and numbness in the affected extremity accompanied by a variable degree of weakness. Although these injuries are common, the etiology remains somewhat unclear and is probably multifactorial. Most burners and stingers are due to traction induced in the classic mode, by forcing the head and shoulder apart. Some probably are caused by acute pressure of the edge of the shoulder pad on the brachial plexus when the player is struck from the side. Most of these injuries are essentially benign and the player recovers completely, sometimes even immediately. However, the physician must entertain the possible diagnosis of a cervical disk herniation in patients in whom the symptoms persist. In addition, repeated episodes may cause cervical stenosis. From a practical point of view, a player with persistent symptoms or neurologic deficit should be excluded from further competition until the nature of the problem is clearly defined and all of the symptoms have resolved completely.

Open Injuries

Open injuries can be produced by a variety of objects and mechanisms. The simplest of these injuries is a sharp wound such as might be caused by a knife or a shard of glass. In this situation, with a defined deficit, it can safely be assumed that the lesion is a neurotmesis and that the nerves have been transected sharply. Although the technical problems involved in such repairs may be increased by the more urgent accompanying vascular lesion, there is no reason to delay their repair. Repair of both the upper and the intermediate trunks may lead to functional recovery, although it is unusual to observe a complete recovery. Nevertheless, a sharp cut usually makes the identification of the extent of the injury easier, and the gap that is produced usually does not require the interposition of a graft.

Although microsurgical repair of injured peripheral

nerves has advanced, unfortunately high-velocity military firearms have become more generally available and have infiltrated civilian criminal life. Until recently, it was possible to confidently separate civilian from military wounds and opine that many gunshot wounds would produce incomplete lesions that would improve with time. However, today's high-velocity bullets cause considerably more damage because of the shock waves they generate in the tissues. The consequent pathology results in more extensive nerve lesions than might otherwise be expected, thus decreasing the possibility of functional recovery.

The incidence of chainsaw injuries has diminished as a result of new safety features on chainsaws and better public education regarding their use. Nevertheless, when such injuries do occur, particularly at the root of the neck, they can threaten both life and limb. Rarely can the emergency surgeon be concerned with identifying and attempting to repair the individual nerves beyond indicating, on a simple map in the operative note, the location of any nerves that are found. Before attempting secondary nerve repair, the secondary surgeon should do ancillary diagnostic testing, as for a traction lesion, because the injury caused by a chainsaw involves not only laceration but also traction that may result in root avulsions. The secondary surgeon usually will encounter a field of massive scarring where little will be recognizable initially. The use of a Doppler probe has been found to be helpful in such situations.

Postanesthetic Paralysis

Postanesthetic paralysis results from injury to the brachial plexus of a patient undergoing surgery under either general or regional anesthesia. In the case of general anesthesia, the mechanism of injury usually is traction induced by the patient's position on the operating table. This type of injury must be differentiated from that caused during surgical manipulation because these are two distinct entities with differing prognoses and implications. The increasing use of regional anesthesia by means of brachial plexus block both for the procedure and for postoperative pain management brings with it the possibility of injury to the brachial plexus.

The surgical patient under general anesthesia must be safeguarded by periodic intraoperative observation to avoid hyperabduction of the arm beyond 90° or excessive lateral flexion of the neck because these are common mechanisms by which intraoperative brachial plexus injuries are incurred. Fortunately, the ultimate prognosis for these injuries is good, although if they are degenerative in nature, recovery time may be lengthy.

The injuries to the brachial plexus that sometimes are seen after cardiac surgery usually involve the lower trunk of the brachial plexus and are caused by a differ-

ent mechanism. Wide retraction of the split sternum can cause the nerves to be compressed between the retropulsed clavicle and the first rib. These injuries may have permanent aftereffects expressed as paralysis of the intrinsic muscles of the hand. The complication usually can be avoided by a lower placement of the rib-spreader.

Significant injuries properly attributable to regional block are unusual, but transient paralysis of the ipsilateral diaphragm is almost guaranteed and usually has little clinical significance. The occasional nerve injury can result from contaminated solutions or rough probing in the attempt to elicit multiple paresthesias. Direct injection into the nerves should be avoided.

Radiation Injuries

Since the refinement of therapeutic radiation techniques, radiation injuries have become significantly less common. The extensive skin changes and fibrosis that in the past were almost expected in the patient who received radiation therapy for breast cancer are no longer seen. Although radiation injuries are less common and less severe, the nature of the pathology, when it occurs, remains the same and results from fibrosis of the blood vessels supplying the nerves. Peripheral nerves formerly were considered to be highly resistant to the effects of ionizing radiation, but further consideration has clearly demonstrated that this is untrue. However, the process takes considerably longer than previously believed. The initial clinical manifestations may be faint paresthesias in the limb, with onset as long as 5 to 10 years after the radiation treatment. These paresthesias may then progress relentlessly to loss of function. Although some authors have reported benefits from various surgical maneuvers, including attempts at neovascularization, these injuries remain problematic.

Ancillary Diagnostic Studies in the Evaluation of Closed Injuries

Radiographic Studies

Appropriate plain radiographic studies must be obtained for the patient with a brachial plexus injury, as well as adequate cervical spine and shoulder girdle radiographs. Obvious pathologic conditions of the cervical spine may accompany a brachial plexus injury. In addition, displaced fractures of the cervical transverse processes usually, but not invariably, indicate avulsion of the nerve root at that level. A pronounced cervical scoliosis usually indicates extensive cervical root avulsions. The integrity of the clavicle and the skeletal components of the shoulder girdle must be established. Markedly comminuted fractures of the scapula often are associated with brachial plexus injury and sometimes with vascular injury as well. If the glenohumeral joint is dislocated or there is a proximal humeral fracture, then the possibility of infraclavicular injury must be considered.

Chest radiographs must be examined not only for the possibility of intrathoracic pathology but also to rule out paralysis of the ipsilateral diaphragm. Because the phrenic nerve shares some of its origin with the brachial plexus, diaphragmatic paralysis usually indicates high root avulsion.

If clinical examination determines the possibility of a vascular lesion, appropriate contrast vascular studies should be ordered. These studies are indicated particularly in a patient with a widely displaced fracture of the clavicle and so-called scapulothoracic dissociation, with its possibility of serious hemorrhage to the point of exsanguination.

Although some authors advocate MRI for demonstration of root avulsions, MRI scans usually lack sufficient resolution to provide as much information about the integrity or lack thereof of the cervical roots as does CT myelography. However, one group of authors demonstrated that MRI can provide additional information that can be used to establish the level of the lesion and also may provide information about injury to the plexus outside the spinal canal.

In patients with anesthetic, flail limbs who are thought to have sustained major root avulsions, myelography is indicated, but not until about 1 month following the injury. Studies done immediately after an injury have shown contrast material actually running out of the spinal column, through the torn meninges, and into the axilla. When a nerve root is avulsed, the meninges almost always are torn away with the neural elements; after a few weeks, these tissues will become scarred and form pouches, or pseudomeningoceles. Contrast material will collect in these pouches, which therefore can be revealed by myelography. Although it is possible to find intact nerve filaments within a pseudomeningocele, it is very unusual, so a positive finding on myelography usually is consistent with root avulsion.

Electrodiagnostic Studies

Wallerian degeneration and its electromyographic manifestations do not become apparent until about 3 weeks after an injury that causes either axonotmesis or neurotmesis, the two categories of degenerative nerve lesion. Therefore, unless there is some reason to believe that the patient had a preexisting nerve lesion, there is no indication for obtaining these tests sooner. The surgeon must, however, indicate precisely what information is needed from the electromyogram. Written requests to sample the serratus anterior and rhomboids as well as the weak or paralyzed muscles of the limb will ensure that the desired

information will not be overlooked. Fibrillation potentials in a totally paralyzed muscle do not come as a surprise. But it is vital that not only the limb and girdle muscles be sampled with needle electrodes, but that the cervical paravertebral muscles be carefully examined as well. The cervical paravertebral muscles are arranged segmentally and are supplied by the posterior primary rami of the same nerve roots that give off the anterior primary rami to the brachial plexus. If they are denervated, this is good evidence of root avulsion. Examination of the neck muscles is technically the most difficult part of the examination and also the most painful for the patient.

The anatomic configuration explains the usefulness of conduction velocity determinations in the peripheral nerves of the patient who has sustained a traction injury of the brachial plexus. Anything that interrupts continuity of the cell body and the axon will result in a loss of conduction in the peripheral nerve. This situation pertains to attempts to measure motor conduction velocity in patients with a ruptured nerve root or a nerve with a more distal injury. However, because the dorsal root ganglion is outside the spinal cord, if the nerve root is avulsed proximal to it, there will be no loss of continuity between that nerve cell body and its axon. Therefore, despite the fact that the cutaneous distribution of the nerve root will be anesthetic, the velocity of conduction of the sensory components of a nerve derived from a root that has been avulsed from the cord will be normal or only slightly reduced. Motor conduction in this situation will be lost in both nerve root avulsion and distal rupture.

Histamine testing of axon reflexes, which involved injection of small amounts of histamine into anesthetic areas of skin to observe the wheal and flare phenomenon, was one of the standard modes of evaluation used before the refinement of electrodiagnostic and radiographic techniques. Unfortunately, it was difficult to use for viewing the fingers, particularly for evaluation of the C7 root distribution. Moreover, there was always a risk of provoking a generalized histamine reaction in susceptible patients. There is little or no indication for the use of this test today.

Surgical Treatment

Neurologic Reconstruction

As previously indicated, the diagnostic evaluation of a patient with a brachial plexus injury should be completed before 3 months postinjury. Decisions about surgical intervention on the nerves depend on this assessment, which results in a presumptive diagnosis of both the location of the nerve injury and its degree of severity. An open injury caused by a sharp, penetrating instrument with corresponding loss of motor and sensory function will most likely be a neurotmesis. If there is no accompanying vascular or intrathoracic lesion, then as soon as the general condition of the patient permits, either a primary or an early secondary surgical exploration is indicated. The likelihood of such a lesion producing a gap that will require a nerve graft is small; nevertheless, the patient should be draped for surgery in a way that allows access to potential donor sites such as the sural nerves in the legs.

Low-velocity gunshot wounds historically have been considered to have a tendency to improve with time, so that there is usually considerably less urgency in their surgical exploration. If the neurologic deficit is partial, the patient may be observed for 2 or 3 months to determine whether there is any evidence of nerve regeneration and reinnervation. The use of neurolysis in this situation usually is not of benefit because it will not encourage the nerves to grow faster than they would have without surgery. However, if nerve regeneration, as demonstrated by an advancing Tinel's sign, interval manual muscle testing, and appropriate electrodiagnostic studies, does not appear to be occurring, then the plexus should be explored with a view toward verifying the nerve lesion and reconstructing it if possible. In this situation, the use of intraoperative electrodiagnostic monitoring with nerve stimulation and determination of somatosensory-evoked potentials is now considered essential.

As in the peripheral nervous system in general, the benefits of the use of neurolysis in the brachial plexus remain to be proved by rigorous evaluation and standards. Although neurolysis has been used in many patients with great ultimate enthusiasm when the patient has recovered, many of those patients would have gone on to recover without surgery. Therefore, the surgeon must carefully consider this possibility when contemplating a neurolysis for a plexus lesion. This decision can be difficult if there is inadequate documentation of the initial nerve deficit or its subsequent course. However, when it is clearly established that regeneration has ceased well within the window in which such recovery can be reasonably expected, neurolysis is indicated. There has been some enthusiasm for its use in cases of radiation fibrosis of the brachial plexus following therapeutic radiation. Because of the difficulty of the dissection and the basically ischemic nature of the pathology, the possibility of actually increasing the deficit is a very real one. There are some reports of attempts to bring fresh blood supply to the fibrotic plexus by means of either free or pedicled omental grafts, but these must be interpreted with caution.

The greatest surgical progress has been made in treating the patient with an anesthetic, flail arm caused by a traction injury. Although efforts at surgical reconstruction in these cases date to the beginning of the 20th cen-

tury, by the 1930s, enthusiasm for this surgery had waned to the point of extinction. Thereafter, either nothing was done surgically, or, upon confirmation of a total lesion, a decision was made whether to amputate the arm above the elbow and fuse the shoulder so that a functional prosthesis could be fitted. After the early 1960s, microsurgical techniques were adapted not only to repairing transected nerves but also to using grafts to overcome the larger gaps caused by traction injuries. These techniques provided hope for recovery of some degree of function in the arms of patients with complete lesions. Although the clinical symptoms may be severe (ie, the anesthetic, flail arm), even severe traction injuries usually do not result in complete avulsion of the nerve roots at the spinal cord level. More often there will be a mixture of root avulsions and distal ruptures in the trunks or related structures. The former usually affects the outflow of C8 and T1, a level at which there still is no possibility of functional recovery.

Repair of the avulsed spinal nerve root has been attempted by many. One author, who reported on a long series of animal experiments with replantation of roots, has applied these techniques to humans with some evidence of functional success. However, this surgery has not reached the status of general inclusion in the treatment of brachial plexus injuries.

The use of nerve transfer techniques to provide a source of axons in cases of root avulsion or irreparable proximal lesions has had some useful results. Donor sites have included the cervical plexus, collateral branches of the ipsilateral brachial plexus, phrenic nerve, spinal accessory nerve, and intercostal nerves; cross-body transfers of the contralateral C7 root also have been performed. Many of these procedures have resulted in voluntary control of previously paralyzed muscles. However, it also is important to evaluate these procedures critically in terms of their day-to-day usefulness to the patients.

Free muscle transfers also may have a role in functional reconstruction when more conventional procedures are not feasible. In several patients who had free gracilis transfers to the paralyzed elbow, that elbow functioned voluntarily by reinnervation through intercostal nerves.

Whether or not vascularization can improve the surgical outcome of nerve transfers and grafts continues to be the subject of debate. Combinations of aggressive plexus and peripheral reconstruction have produced results that bear review.

Peripheral Reconstruction of the Limb

Patients with permanent residuals of injury to the brachial plexus, either because spontaneous recovery is unsuccessful or because surgery could not be performed or failed, may realize significant benefit from peripheral reconstruction procedures. These techniques have been adapted from their use in poliomyelitis and peripheral nerve injuries. However, patients with poliomyelitis do not lack sensibility, so their functional benefits from the same level of motor improvement will be greater than those in the corresponding patient with a brachial plexus paralysis.

Numerous innovative procedures have been designed for the restoration of shoulder control. The most commonly used procedure involves transposition of the insertion of the trapezius muscle to the humerus. In satisfied patients who have had this surgery, shoulder abduction improved an average of 63° and shoulder flexion an average of 60°. Although there have been enthusiasts for this procedure as well as similar reports of good results, consideration of the complex kinesiology of the shoulder indicates it is somewhat naive to assume that anything resembling normal shoulder function can be attained by these means. Furthermore, disturbance of the trapezius, either because its innervation has been partially used as a source of axons for reinnervation more distally, or because it has been used as a tendon transfer, seriously compromises the possibility of its function as the prime mover of a fused shoulder.

A detailed consideration of birth paralyses of the brachial plexus is beyond the scope of this chapter. However, this subject is well covered in the literature.

A complete lesion of the upper trunk deprives the patient of the use of both the deltoid and lateral rotators of the humerus. Any elevation of the limb that remains is attributable to a combination of trapezius and serratus function, so these two muscles must be essentially intact for a shoulder fusion to be indicated. Previously, prolonged postoperative immobilization in a shoulder spica cast was required; however, the use of rigid compression plating has obviated the need for this cast, making the postoperative period considerably more comfortable. Excessive abduction in the scapular plane should be avoided because this invariably will lead to chronic fatigue and discomfort about the shoulder girdle. The most common position for shoulder fusion is 20° of abduction, 30° of forward flexion, and 30° of medial rotation. In most cases, this position will provide the patient with a strong and functional, albeit somewhat limited, range of motion.

A variety of tendon transfers are available for patients with incomplete paralysis of the deltoid and rotator cuff. These can provide surprisingly good function.

Flexion of the elbow can be partially restored by one of several well-documented surgical procedures involving tendon transfer. The oldest of these involves proximal transfer of the flexor-pronator muscles from the medial epicondyle to the shaft of the humerus. Its effec-

tiveness can be augmented if there is good abduction and forward flexion of the humerus, which will eliminate some of the effects of gravity at the elbow. However, this transfer does not provide really strong elbow flexion. Transfer of the sternocostal portion of the pectoralis major produces much stronger flexion, although it does require a stable and controlled shoulder. The sacrifice of an intact triceps for a flexor transfer generally is a bad bargain unless there is no alternative. Results of latissimus dorsi transfer leave much to be desired because the muscle shares the same innervation as the elbow flexors and generally is not strong enough for transfer in lesions of the upper trunk.

When considering paralytic problems about the forearm and hand, most of the same principles applicable to peripheral nerve deficits in general may be used. However, it is good to remember that the sensory picture may differ.

Pain Management

In almost all instances of total brachial plexus paralysis, and to a lesser degree in those injuries that are less severe, neurogenic pain is a factor. It can be quite distressing to the patient and can frustrate attempts at rehabilitation. The pain is not usually the same as that of phantom limb, but it is associated with sensory deprivation and most often with root avulsions. It is not alleviated by sympathetic blockade or surgical sympathectomy because if the T1 root has been avulsed, the patient has in effect already had a sympathectomy at a more proximal level, that of the spinal cord. Treating the pain with increasing doses of narcotics usually is ineffective. Several drugs provide some relief, including gabapentin and carbamazepine. Both of these drugs should be carefully titrated, beginning with small doses and gradually increasing them. Both the dosage schedules and the potential complications should be reviewed thoroughly before they are prescribed. Only about one third of patients with severe pain due to brachial plexus injury will obtain significant relief from these drugs.

Other modalities of treatment, including the transcutaneous nerve simulator, may provide some benefit, but the problem in their evaluation is control of the many variables in both the degree of injury and the overall treatment programs instituted for the patients. Nevertheless, there is virtually no downside to using the transcutaneous nerve simulator. The roster of discarded neurosurgical procedures both on the central nervous system and peripherally is quite long. However, the dorsal root entry zone procedure appears to be the most effective and long-lasting in its results. In addition, there is some evidence that reconstruction of the nerves has a positive benefit for pain caused by deafferentation. It cannot be too strongly stated that amputation of the limb is not indicated as a treatment for the pain of brachial plexus injury.

Amputation

Since the advent of increased neural reconstruction of the traumatized brachial plexus over the past 40 years, there has been a significant shift away from amputation, which was formerly the major option for a patient with an anesthetic, flail arm. Considering the options available to treat brachial plexus injuries, there are very limited indications for amputation of the limb. As previously noted, pain is not one of them. However, amputation may be necessary either to save a life or to improve quality of life. For example, advising amputation of the insensate paralyzed arm of a patient who repeatedly sustains non-healing burns or ulcerations with infection would be reasonable. Amputation may be an option for the patient who has a totally useless arm and has undergone a series of unsuccessful attempts at surgical reconstruction.

For an amputation to result in the successful fitting of a prosthesis for function, it must be done in a timely manner. A patient who is fitted for a prosthesis more than 18 months after injury is unlikely to use the device because by that time, the patient is likely to have learned to function with one hand. From a technical point of view, if proprioception is preserved in the elbow, even with imperfect cutaneous sensibility, the ultimate function will be significantly enhanced by retention of the elbow joint. Otherwise, a midhumeral level amputation is optimal. In most cases, because the glenohumeral joint will be flail, the activation of the prosthesis will require a shoulder fusion, which can be done at the same time as the amputation. Although it would be tempting to try to fit the patient in such a situation with a myoelectric prosthesis, these devices generally are very expensive and of little use for the patient with a brachial plexus injury.

Annotated Bibliography

Carlstedt TP: Spinal nerve root injuries in brachial plexus lesions: Basic science and clinical application of new surgical strategies. *Microsurgery* 1995;16:13-16.

In this article, the author details pioneering application of laboratory experiments to the clinical situation. Further developments bear watching.

Carlstedt T, Grane P, Hallin RG, Noren G: Return of function after spinal cord implantation of avulsed spinal nerve roots. *Lancet* 1995;346:1323-1325.

Pioneering applications of laboratory experiments to the clinical situation are detailed in this article.

Carvalho GA, Nikkhah G, Matthies C, Penkert G, Samii M: Diagnosis of root avulsions in traumatic brachial plexus injuries: Value of computerized tomography myelography and magnetic resonance imaging. *J Neurosurg* 1997;86:69-76.

This prospective study compares the accuracy of CT myelography and MRI in diagnosing root avulsion and demonstrates the superiority of CT myelography.

Gilbert A (ed): *Brachial Plexus Injuries*. London, UK, Martin Dunitz, 2001.

This is a collection of articles on various aspects of diagnosis and treatment of brachial plexus injuries by 39 different authors. The emphasis is on surgery, and approximately one third of the volume is devoted to obstetric palsy.

Gilbert A, Berger A: General concept and conclusions regarding treatment of traumatic brachial plexus birth injury lesions. *Orthopade* 1997;26:729-730.

The authors discuss their experience in treatment of birth injuries.

Gu YD, Ma MK: Use of the phrenic nerve for brachial plexus reconstruction. *Clin Orthop* 1996;323:119-121.

The authors describe a clinical series of 180 patients who sustained brachial plexus injuries and had phrenic nerve transfer for restoration of elbow flexion. The results are extraordinary.

Ochiai N, Nagano A, Sugioka H, Hara T: Nerve grafting in brachial plexus injuries: Results of free grafts in 90 patients. *J Bone Joint Surg Br* 1996;78:754-758.

The authors assessed the results of free nerve grafts in 90 patients with brachial plexus injuries and found that flexor and extensor muscles in the elbow and shoulder girdle had relatively good results, but results in the flexor and extensor muscles of the forearm and the intrinsic hand muscles were extremely poor.

Spinner RJ, Kline DG: Surgery for peripheral nerve and brachial plexus injuries or other nerve lesions. *Muscle Nerve* 2000;23:680-695.

This is an algorithm for the integration of electrodiagnostic techniques into the evaluation of plexus injuries.

Classic Bibliography

Barnes R: Traction injuries to the brachial plexus in adults. *J Bone Joint Surg Br* 1949;31:10.

Birch R, Dunkerton M, Bonney G, Jamieson AM: Experience with the free vascularized ulnar nerve graft in repair of supraclavicular lesions of the brachial plexus. *Clin Orthop* 1988;237:96-104.

Bonney: Prognosis in traction lesions of the brachial plexus. *J Bone Joint Surg Br* 1959;41:4.

Carlstedt T: Experimental studies on surgical treatment of avulsed spinal nerve roots in brachial plexus injury. *J Hand Surg Br* 1991;16:477-482.

Chuang DCC, Yeh MC, Wei FC: Intercostal nerve transfer of the musculocutaneous nerve in avulsed brachial plexus injuries: Evaluation of 66 patients. *J Hand Surg Am* 1992;17:822-828.

Codman EA: *The Shoulder*. Brooklyn, NY, G. Miller, 1934.

Friedman AH, Nashold BS Jr, Bronec PR: Dorsal root entry zone lesions for the treatment of brachial plexus avulsion injuries: A follow-up study. *Neurosurgery* 1988; 22:369-373.

Friedman AH, Nunley JA II, Goldner RD, et al: Nerve transposition for the restoration of elbow flexion following brachial plexus avulsion injuries. *J Neurosurg* 1990;72:59-64.

Gilbert A, Tassin: Obstetrical palsy: A clinical, pathologic, and surgical review, in Terzis E (ed): *Microreconstruction of Nerve Injuries*. Philadelphia, PA, WB Saunders, 1987.

Kerr AT: The brachial plexus of nerves in man: The variation in its formation and its branches. *Am J Anat* 1918;23:285.

Leffert RD: *Brachial Plexus Injuries*. New York, NY, Churchill Livingstone, 1985.

Leffert RD: Clinical diagnosis, testing, and electromyographic study in brachial plexus traction injuries. *Clin Orthop* 1988;237:24-31.

Leffert RD, Pess GM: Tendon transfers for brachial plexus injury. *Hand Clin* 1988;4:273-288.

Leffert RD, Seddon HJ: Infraclavicular brachial plexus injuries. *J Bone Joint Surg Br* 1965;47:9.

LeQuang C: Postirradiation lesions of the brachial plexus: Results of surgical treatment. *Hand Clin* 1989; 5:23-32.

Merle M, Dautel G: Vascularized nerve grafts. *Hand Surg* 1991;16:483-488.

Millesi H: Brachial plexus injuries: Management and results. *Clin Plast Surg* 1984;11:115-120.

Millesi H: Surgical treatment of brachial plexus injuries. *J Hand Surg* 1977;2:367.

Nagano A, Tsuyama N, Ochiai, et al: Direct nerve crossing with the intercostal nerve to treat avulsion injuries to the brachial plexus. *J Hand Surg Am* 1989;14:980-985.

Narakas AO, Hentz VR: Neurotization in brachial plexus injuries: Indication and results. *Clin Orthop* 1988; 237:43-56.

Nashold BS Jr, Ostdahl RH: Dorsal root entry zone lesion for pain relief. *J Neurosurg* 1979;51:59.

Rowe CR: Re-evaluation of the position of the arm in arthrodesis of the shoulder in the adult. *J Bone Joint Surg Am* 1974;56:913.

Seddon HJ: Reconstructive surgery of the upper extremity, in *Poliomyelitis, Second International Poliomyelitis Congress*. Philadelphia, PA, Lippincott, 1952.

Sedel L: Repair of severe traction lesions of the brachial plexus. *Clin Orthop* 1988;237:62-66.

Sedel L: Results of surgical repair of brachial plexus injuries. *J Bone Joint Surg Br* 1982;64-54.

Yeoman PM: Cervical myelography in traction injuries of the brachial plexus. *J Bone Joint Surg Br* 1968;SO:25.

Yeoman PM, Seddon HJ: Brachial plexus injuries: Treatment of the flail arm. *J Bone Joint Surg Br* 1961;43:3.

Chapter 38

Thoracic Outlet Syndrome

Robert D. Leffert, MD

Introduction

In the course of their practice, orthopaedic surgeons will see patients who present with paresthesias and numbness in the upper limb. Usually, these symptoms are determined to be a result of either cervical radiculopathy or peripheral nerve compression. Occasionally, however, these patients are found to have neurovascular compression within the thoracic outlet, or thoracic outlet syndrome (TOS).

TOS is not a single entity, and it produces a wide range of symptoms. Therefore, diagnosis can be difficult, and the disorder remains extremely controversial. To better understand and manage TOS, it is helpful to review the anatomy and pathology of the syndrome as well as the history of its treatment.

Anatomy

The area of the thoracic outlet extends from the supraclavicular fossa to the axilla, between the clavicle and the first rib. Within it, the cervical nerve roots become the trunks of the brachial plexus as they pass through a triangle formed by the anterior scalene muscle medially and the middle scalene muscle laterally. The first rib is the base of this triangle, and the suprapleural membrane separates the apex of the lung from the first rib.

The apex of the axilla anterolaterally is formed by the clavicle, subclavius muscle, the upper border of the scapula and subscapularis muscle dorsally, and the anterolateral border of the first rib medially. The cords of the brachial plexus and axillary vessels then pass beneath the coracoid process.

The first rib is divided into three parts. The first segment extends from the head to the neck. The second segment is oriented almost perpendicular to the first segment and serves as the attachment for the middle scalene, the first digitation of the serratus anterior, and the muscles of the first intercostal space. The third, or vascular segment, contains the scalene tubercle, which is the attachment of the anterior scalene muscle, the costoclav-icular ligaments, and the attachment of the subclavius muscle. The subclavian vein normally is found between the subclavius and costoclavicular ligaments and the anterior scalene. The subclavian artery is located posterior to the anterior scalene and, next to it, the lower trunk of the brachial plexus crosses the first rib. Unfortunately, variations in this arrangement are not rare and may constitute a significant puzzle for the surgeon.

History

In 1947, studies focused on the arterial manifestations of TOS, originally referred to as scalenus anticus syndrome. Diagnosis was made in nonemergent situations by performing Adson's test, in which the patient's arm is placed in a dependent position and the patient is asked to rotate the neck to the affected side and hyperextend the neck. The patient takes a deep breath while the examiner palpates the pulse at the wrist. If the pulse disappears, a positive diagnosis is made. Unfortunately, this test is not particularly reliable because in many normal women the pulse can be obliterated by placing the arm in various positions. The surgical procedure designed to relieve the problem, anterior scalenotomy, resulted in many therapeutic failures.

Wright's test, which involves elevation and external rotation of the arm in various positions, also was developed in the 1940s. This clinical test has been considerably more reliable if the patient does not know what to expect or what constitutes a positive sign. Bracing the patient's shoulders back or forcefully depressing the shoulder girdles also usually will elicit symptoms in patients with a compromised thoracic outlet. Fatigue of the elevated arm with repetitive flexion and extension of the fingers, described by Roos in the 1960s, is another positive sign; this has also proved to be a useful clinical test.

For a time, clinicians believed that the presence of extra or cervical ribs was indicative of TOS. However, it was soon apparent that compression within the thoracic

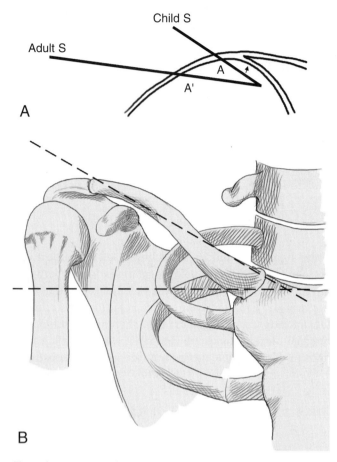

Figure 1 A, This hypothetical drawing from Todd's 1912 article illustrates the descent of the shoulder (S) in growth from infancy to adulthood. The clavicle (the darker black line) is represented as if its inner extremity were fixed, as was thought possible at the beginning of Todd's research. The arrowhead represents the site of pressure on the nerve by the first rib. A and A' = corresponding points of the nerve in childhood and adulthood. **B,** This diagram shows the clavicular angle. This is the angle that the clavicle makes with the horizontal. The clavicular angle appears exaggerated in the drawing because the angle actually is measured in an oblique manner and is greater than the true vertical elevation of the bone.

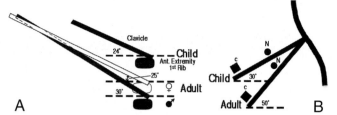

Figure 2 These two diagrams from Todd's 1912 article show the clavicular angle in the child and the adult and also the descent of the anterior end of the first rib. The clavicular angles shown are averages. **A,** This figure is intended to show that as the shoulder sinks, it tends to stretch the lowest trunk of the brachial plexus over the first rib. The rib itself also tilts downward and thus in the normal subject nullifies the tendency to stretching of the nerve by allowing it to travel to its distribution with a less marked upward curve. This compensation is normally less marked in women. **B,** This diagram represents how the descent of the first rib with growth compensates for the stretching effect of the descent of the shoulder on the nerve. The curved black line represents the vertebral column. The straight black line represents the first rib in childhood and in adult age. The costal angles are given in degrees. C, the black square, represents the position of the inner end of the clavicle in infancy and adulthood. The black circle N is the crossing of the first rib by the lower trunk of the brachial plexus.

outlet sometimes occurred when no extra ribs were present, and that some patients with extra ribs had no symptoms. For example, extra ribs were found in a small percentage of the population who had undergone chest radiographs for other reasons.

Compression within the thoracic outlet, particularly by the first rib on the lower trunk of the brachial plexus, can be caused by changes in the patient's posture that could be influenced by development and sexual differences in body habitus (Figs. 1 and 2). In Todd's classic article, the intent was to show how the descent of the shoulder would tend to stretch the nerve over the first rib, were it not that the influence of the descent of the first rib compensates for the descent of the shoulder. Unfortunately, despite the fact that Todd's article was written in English, it was largely neglected by most thoracic outlet surgeons because it appeared in a German medical journal. Over the years, the emphasis began to

shift, and it became apparent that other structures within the thoracic outlet, either singly or in combination, could be compressed. Furthermore, it became apparent that anything that altered the alignment of the shoulder girdle or the competence of the scapular suspensor muscles, particularly the trapezius, could induce neurovascular compression. Both whiplash injuries and pathologies of the glenohumeral joint, particularly instability, were recognized as contributing factors.

In an attempt to make order out of the apparent chaos, some writers, mostly neurologists, noted that the diagnosis was true neurogenic TOS only if the nerves were compressed. However, they also noted that TOS could have a vascular component. Patients without verifiable neurogenic or neurovascular TOS who had the presumptive diagnosis of TOS were considered to have "disputed-type" TOS, a term implying skepticism. Unfortunately, this attitude still persists in some quarters.

In a renewed attempt to find a more definitive test for TOS, various ancillary diagnostic tests were championed as being diagnostic of the syndrome. These included electrodiagnostic, vascular, and radiographic studies.

Clinical Presentation

TOS is most prevalent among women of childbearing age. In most series, women outnumber men by about 3.5:1. In addition, obesity and very large breasts are factors that can contribute to the genesis of compression. If the symptoms and signs result from neural compression, the patient may experience painful paresthesias in the upper limb that are positionally induced and often nocturnal. There may be hand weakness or atrophy in the distribution of the ulnar nerve, occasionally in the thenar muscles. In addition, there may be weakness of the deep flexors of the little and ring fingers and sensory loss over the medial side of the hand and forearm. Some patients may have neck or chest pain, and when the latter is present, it may be misdiagnosed as cardiac disease. In the most extreme cases, arterial compression can result in gangrene of the limb; in less severe situations, it can result in symptoms of arterial insufficiency. Venous compression can develop acutely as a result of thrombosis of the subclavian vein, resulting in a swollen and cyanotic limb. This manifestation has been called "effort thrombosis" or Paget-Schroetter syndrome. When compression is intermittent, the swelling may come and go with activity. Some patients may have headaches or central nervous system disturbances resulting from abnormalities in their cerebral circulation, induced by TOS.

Physical Examination

In all cases it is necessary, after taking a careful history, to perform a complete examination of the cervical spine, shoulder girdles, and upper extremities, including neurologic testing. Of the various provocative maneuvers, which have been described briefly, the most useful is Wright's test, which is done by abducting the arm to shoulder height and then externally rotating the limb fully while palpating the pulses at the wrist. The physician must determine the degree of stability of the glenohumeral joint prior to doing this test to avoid misdiagnosing patients with dead-arm syndrome. Some patients may have both TOS and dead-arm syndrome concurrently, and each condition must be considered and treated to achieve a satisfactory therapeutic result. Also, with the arm in the abducted position, the status of the ulnar nerve must be verified to assure that a subluxating ulnar nerve is not made symptomatic by flexing the elbow. The patient with significant neurovascular compression usually will experience tingling at the same time the pulses at the wrist are obliterated. The diagnosis can be further strengthened by auscultation over the proximal axillary artery for the presence of a bruit. There may be significant color change in the limb as it is elevated.

The overhead exercise test of Roos is usually positive in patients with significant compression, but Adson's test usually has a low yield. In the clinical evaluation of TOS, at least one and preferably two of the provocative maneuvers should reproduce the symptoms.

As in any clinical evaluation, differential diagnosis is mandatory. For TOS, the following entities must be ruled out: (1) cervical radiculopathy, (2) carpal tunnel syndrome, (3) supraclavicular fossa pathology, (4) lung tumors, (5) brachial neuritis, (6) complex regional pain syndrome, and (7) psychiatric disorders.

It is helpful to remember that double crush syndrome may occur with both carpal tunnel syndrome and ulnar

neuropathy, but it occurs less often with cervical radiculopathy. The upper type of TOS, in which compression takes place in the interscalene interval, is difficult to differentiate from the effects of cervical radiculopathy. It is clear, therefore, that a careful neurologic evaluation is mandatory. Particular attention should be paid to the sensory examination of the medial forearm, which is supplied by the first thoracic nerve rather than the ulnar and which serves to differentiate the two sites, even with the same pattern of motor deficit.

Ancillary Diagnostic Studies

Radiographs of the cervical spine and chest are obtained in all patients; the purpose of the latter is to detect apical lung tumors. Significant cervical spine pathology is not common in the affected age group, but when present, it must not be ignored. Cervical ribs or overly long transverse processes at C7 that can be the attachment of congenital bands are found occasionally; these can cause compression if the posture of the shoulder girdle is altered. The effectiveness of both CT scans and MRI studies in the diagnosis of TOS has been reported recently, but the efficacy of these modalities remains to be substantiated. Similarly, experience with the combination of neurography and MRI is limited.

Noninvasive vascular studies using Doppler ultrasonography or digital plethysmography have been used to identify arterial compression, but these tests, like the provocative maneuvers, frequently give false-positive results. Nevertheless, in patients in whom intrinsic vascular disorders are suspected, such testing can be of value. Although arteriography still is done in some centers as a result of this presumptive diagnosis, it usually is not necessary unless there is strong suspicion of the presence of an aneurysm of the subclavian artery. Such aneurysms have been reported in patients with large cervical ribs or other bony abnormalities that might be expected to produce arterial compression. According to one study, a woman in her 20s presented with distal arterial insufficiency in the forearm that was believed to be caused by local thrombosis but actually was the result of embolization from a subclavian-axillary aneurysm at the junction of a large cervical rib fused to the first rib, where the constriction took place. The patient required a vein graft after resection of the aneurysm and of the cervical and first ribs; results were satisfactory following surgery.

Occlusion of the subclavian vein within the thoracic outlet may occur suddenly following intensive exercise of the upper limbs, hence the name "effort thrombosis." Effort thrombosis is characterized by dramatic and painful swelling of the arm and hand accompanied by cyanosis. In addition, swelling and pain in the pectoral region occurs, caused by collateral blood flow around the thrombosed venous segment. The condition constitutes an emergency that is best managed by interventional radiology using either urokinase or streptokinase to lyse the clot. The pretreatment venogram may depict significant external compression. Following a period of anticoagulation therapy, usually 3 or 4 months, an elective resection of the first rib will significantly diminish the possibility of another thrombosis. Recently, some authors have advocated immediate surgical decompression without the intervening period of anticoagulation therapy.

The most controversial ancillary diagnostic studies are those that involve electrodiagnosis. The best correlation between the results of testing and those of the clinical neurologic examination occurs in patients in whom the compression is largely on the lower trunk of the brachial plexus. However, the deficits in those patients are usually discernible by means of careful clinical neurologic examination alone. Moreover, such cases, which can be comfortably designated as true neurogenic TOS, are not common; many more patients with significant, genuine, and verifiable symptoms caused by thoracic outlet compression will have normal electrodiagnostic studies. Initial reports of the ability to diagnose this condition by the relatively crude measurement of the velocity of ulnar nerve conduction through the thoracic outlet have not stood the test of time. Enthusiastic reports of the efficacy of somatosensory evoked potentials and other late responses also have been controversial. More recently there has been support for the determination of the sensory nerve action potential of the medial cutaneous nerve of the forearm as a more reliable diagnostic tool. Nevertheless, there is no electrodiagnostic standard for the diagnosis of TOS, and the diagnosis remains a clinical one. This finding does not mean that electrodiagnostic studies should not be obtained in the evaluation of such patients because more peripheral sites of compression or double crush syndromes may thus be identified.

Conservative Therapy

Unless an acute neurovascular compression with potentially irreversible clinical consequences is found, most patients with TOS are treated conservatively after diagnostic evaluation. Patients who are overweight are urged to reduce their weight and begin a general exercise program in addition to specific exercises for the shoulder girdles. Unfortunately, there is a tendency to treat all patients with TOS with the same exercises, many of which actually provoke symptoms and should not be done. These exercises, which include cervical traction and significant shoulder stretching exercises as well as those that involve sharply bracing the shoulders back or repetitively exercising the arms overhead, persist in the liter-

ature and in the protocols of many physical therapy departments. In the vast majority of patients, these exercises will prove to be provocative and intolerable.

Each patient must be evaluated individually with reference to specific postural abnormalities, and a gentle and progressive program of strengthening exercises for the shoulder girdle musculature should be begun. As the patient progresses in the ability to tolerate the exercises, additional exercises can be added. It is important for the surgeon to be in communication with both the patient and the therapist to enable midcourse therapy corrections when necessary. Favorable results are unlikely to be perceived in less than 2 or 3 months. If there is significant compression, conservative management will not succeed, but about 80% of patients can be treated conservatively.

In women with very large or pendulous breasts and slumping posture, the combined effect is to increase pressure on the structures within the thoracic outlet. In some patients, the condition can be significantly helped by proper breast support, and those who do not respond to this simple measure may benefit from reduction mammoplasty. Because patients who are significantly emotionally depressed often have slumping posture, treatment of any underlying depression is an important part of treating patients with TOS. In addition, patients who undergo surgery for TOS without preoperative attention to clinical depression have a poor prognosis for relief of their symptoms.

Indications for Surgery

TOS clearly is a complicated condition that requires attention to the individual issues of each patient. A carefully supervised exercise and postural program over a 3- or 4-month period will be unsuccessful in some patients. In a recently published article on a series of patients treated with transaxillary first rib resection, the average time between the initial consultation and the surgical procedure was 11 months.

TOS associated with intractable pain is very difficult to treat, and it is often problematic to determine when or if a particular patient should have surgery. Significant neurologic deficits in the hand of a TOS patient with moderate to severe intrinsic atrophy or weakness are an indication that surgery should be performed sooner rather than later, but the likelihood of complete recovery of motor function following decompression is not good.

Impending vascular catastrophe, either arterial or venous, or the presence of an aneurysm requires the aid of a vascular surgeon. Fortunately, patients with these conditions usually do not present to the orthopaedic surgeon primarily. Nevertheless, they do constitute an urgent indication for surgical intervention.

Surgical Procedures

Although it is beyond the scope of this chapter to describe in detail the technique of the various surgical procedures used in the treatment of TOS, it is of value to discuss the advantages and disadvantages of each. For many years the most popular surgical procedure, which was also the easiest technically, was to release the anterior scalene muscle from the first rib through a supraclavicular incision. Even this seemingly simple operation had reported complications of death from hemorrhage, and over time it was realized that symptoms recurred in patients who appeared to have benefited initially. Therefore, this approach has largely been abandoned, although some surgeons still use the supraclavicular approach to resect the anterior scalene muscle and even the first rib. Resection of the first rib by the transaxillary route is the procedure of choice for most primary patients. This technically demanding procedure requires a commitment to anatomic study and should be learned with the assistance of a more experienced surgeon.

Because of the narrow configuration of the thoracic outlet encountered from below with the axillary approach, anesthesia must achieve adequate muscular relaxation. This is best induced by the newer short-acting muscle relaxants. An adequate number of surgical assistants will facilitate the ease of performance of the surgery as well as its safety. The use of slings to suspend the arm should be avoided because of the possibility of a traction injury to the brachial plexus.

Resection of the clavicle to treat TOS was advocated by some, but this indication is extremely rare because the clavicle is an important factor in maintaining the position of the shoulder girdle and the patency of the outlet. Even in situations where the clavicle must be divided for vascular access, provision for osteosynthesis should be made at the end of the procedure. Significant soft-tissue stripping of the bone will encourage nonunion and should be avoided.

The posterior approach to the thoracic outlet for resection of the first rib gives excellent access to the posterior third and the neural structures. This approach uses essentially the same incision as is used for high thoracoplasty, which means that it must traverse the trapezius and rhomboid muscles. Because the health and strength of these muscles is of primary importance for suspension of the scapula, this approach is best avoided except in unusual circumstances. These circumstances might include revision surgery or surgery in patients who are extremely obese or muscular and for whom other anatomic approaches might be problematic.

The release of the pectoralis minor muscle for treatment of TOS is of historic interest, but it probably has no place in the modern armamentarium. It would be extremely unusual for the area beneath the coracoid process to be the primary or sole locus of compression-causing symptoms of neurovascular compromise.

Results of Surgery

The patient populations that could be described as having good, fair, and poor results are almost impossible to compare because of the many factors that influence this disorder. Several large series have indicated approximately 75% of the surgically treated patients as having good and excellent results, with 15% having had fair results. The latter were patients who required occasional nonnarcotic analgesics. About 10% of patients either are unimproved or claim the condition was made worse by the surgery.

Complications

Noncommunicating pneumothorax may occur during the course of resection of the first rib or even with scalenectomy because of the proximity of the very thin apical pleura to the rib. As long as this is noticed during surgery, it should not be a significant problem because noncommunicating pneumothorax usually can be managed either by means of aspiration at the end of the procedure or by the use of a chest tube for 24 hours postoperatively.

Because the intercostal brachial nerve, which is about the diameter of a digital nerve, is in the middle of the surgical field when the transaxillary approach is used, it is at risk. By means of gentle retraction and partial neurolysis, it usually can be spared. Nevertheless, some patients will have transient numbness along the posterior aspect of the arm postoperatively. In a very small percentage of patients, this may be manifest as dysesthesia and can be extremely unpleasant.

Winging of the scapula will result from injury to the long thoracic nerve and will cause significant weakness of the shoulder girdle in forward elevation of the arm. Scapular winging is a significant complication if it does occur and can usually be avoided by knowledge of the path of the nerve, particularly on the chest wall.

The danger of hemorrhage should any of the large vessels be breached during the decompression of the thoracic outlet is a very major potential complication for which the surgeon should be adequately prepared in terms of available assistance and transfusion if necessary.

Finally, injury to the lower trunk of the brachial plexus may occur if its position is not verified and kept under surveillance at all times during the procedure. Unfortunately, such injuries usually result in permanent loss of function of the muscles that these nerves supply.

Annotated Bibliography

Azakie A, McElhinney DB, Thompson RW, Raven RB, Messina LM, Stoney RJ: Surgical management of subclavian-vein effort thrombosis as a result of thoracic outlet compression. *J Vasc Surg* 1998;28:777-786.

This is a very well-documented and illustrated study of 33 patients who underwent surgical decompression of primary subclavian vein thromboses with early surgical decompression following thrombolysis. More than 90% of patients had complete relief of their symptoms and durable vein patency on positional venography.

Edwards DP, Mulkern E, Raja AN, Barker P: Transaxillary first rib excision for thoracic outlet syndrome. *J Roy Coll Surg Edinb* 1999;44:362-365.

This is a retrospective study of 52 first rib resections with good documentation.

Hood DB, Kuehne J, Yellin AE, Weaver FA: Vascular complications of thoracic outlet syndrome. *Am Surg* 1997;63:913-917.

This is a retrospective review of 17 patients with TOS and vascular complications. Ten patients presented with acute axillosubclavian vein thrombosis and three had acute symptoms of upper extremity emboli. Three presented with chronic arm claudication. Their management is discussed in detail.

Leffert RD, Perlmutter GS: Thoracic outlet syndrome: Results of 282 transaxillary first rib resections. *Clin Orthop* 1999;368:66-79.

This article details the authors' 21 years of experience with the Roos transaxillary approach for the treatment of TOS. Many of the patients had been misdiagnosed as having other peripheral nerve compressions, and many of them also had workers' compensation claims. The results are generally favorable, and serious complications were few and of minor character.

McCarthy MJ, Varty K, London NJ, Bell PR: Experience of supraclavicular exploration and decompression for treatment of thoracic outlet syndrome. *Ann Vasc Surg* 1999;13:268-274.

The authors of this study of 31 patients who underwent 37 thoracic outlet decompressions by the supraclavicular approach, using anterior scalenectomy and removal of fibrous bands or cervical ribs, conclude that supraclavicular scalenectomy and cervical rib excision with selective first rib excision is a safe and effective procedure for most patients with TOS.

Toso C, Robert J, Berney T, Pugin F, Spiliopoulos A: Thoracic outlet syndrome: Influence of personal history and surgical technique on long-term results. *Eur J Cardiothorac Surg* 1999;16:44-47.

The conclusion of this study is that surgical decompression is more successful when TOS is traumatic or subacute. The transaxillary approach was preferred.

Wilbourn AJ: Thoracic outlet syndromes. *Neurol Clin* 1999;17:477-497.

This review discusses the three types of TOS in which neurologic symptoms are believed to be caused by compromise of the brachial plexus fibers.

Classic Bibliography

Clagett OT: Presidential address: Research and prosearch. *J Thorac Cardiovasc Surg* 1962;44:153-166.

Kunkel JM, Machleder HI: Treatment of Paget-Schroetter syndrome: A staged, multidisciplinary approach. *Arch Surg* 1989;124:1153-1158.

Leffert RD, Gumley G: The relationship between dead arm syndrome and thoracic outlet syndrome. *Clin Orthop* 1987;223:20-31.

Machleder HI: Evaluation of a new treatment strategy for Paget-Schroetter syndrome: Spontaneous thrombosis of the axillary-subclavian vein. *J Vasc Surg* 1993;17:305-317.

Roos DB: Transaxillary approach for first rib resection to relieve thoracic outlet syndrome. *Ann Surg* 1966;163:354-358.

Sanders RJ, Pearce WH: The treatment of thoracic outlet syndrome: A comparison of different operations. *J Vasc Surg* 1989;10:626-634.

Todd TW: The descent of the shoulder after birth. *Anatomischer Anzeiger Centralblatt für die gesamte wissenschaftliche Anatomie* 1912;41:385-397.

Urschel HC Jr, Razzuk MA, Wood RE, Parekh M, Paulson DL: Objective diagnosis (ulnar nerve conduction velocity) and current therapy of the thoracic outlet syndrome. *Ann Thorac Surg* 1971;12:608-620.

Wilbourn AJ: The thoracic outlet syndrome is overdiagnosed. *Arch Neurol* 1990;47:328-330.

Wilbourn AJ, Lederman RJ: Letter: Evidence for conduction delay in thoracic-outlet syndrome is challenged. *N Engl J Med* 1984;310:1052-1053.

Wright IS: The neurovascular syndrome produced by hyperabduction of the arms: The immediate changes produced in 150 normal controls and the effects on some persons of prolonged hyperabduction of the arms, as in sleeping, and in certain occupations. *Am Heart J* 1945;29:1-19.

Chapter 39

Accelerated Postoperative Shoulder Rehabilitation

W. Ben Kibler, MD

J.B. McMullen, MS, ATC

Introduction

Advances in the treatment of shoulder injuries have led to improvements in the restoration of shoulder function after those injuries. More anatomic and physiologic surgical techniques have led to less perioperative morbidity and more secure tissue repairs, thereby allowing earlier application of rehabilitation protocols that emphasize physiologic and biomechanical restoration of the entire kinetic chain. This improvement is reflected in anecdotal reports of earlier return to functional status.

The evolution of this type of accelerated application of rehabilitation and return to functional status is similar to that of accelerated knee rehabilitation, and it relies on the same principles. They are: (1) proper preoperative preparation; (2) anatomic surgical restoration; (3) assurance of biomechanically appropriate motion at surgery; (4) early assisted or active assisted motion; (5) closed-chain axial loading rehabilitation protocols; (6) functional joint positions during rehabilitation; and (7) physiologic progressions as improved functions are acquired. These principles may be applied to shoulder rehabilitation with modifications as required by the anatomic differences between the knee and the shoulder.

Principles That Aid Accelerated Shoulder Rehabilitation

Evaluation of Related Deficits

Many shoulder injuries occur through microtrauma-based overload and may be associated with local or distant deficits in flexibility, strength, strength balance, and mechanics. Examples include glenohumeral internal or external rotation deficits, scapular dyskinesis, acromioclavicular joint arthrosis, low back and hip inflexibility, thoracic kyphosis, poor lifting or carrying technique, and alterations in throwing or serving mechanics. These deficits are in addition to the anatomic lesions and resulting swelling and pain. The preoperative physical examination must establish the presence or absence of all of these possible problems, and preoperative preparation must minimize these problems, all of which may have deleterious physiologic or biomechanical consequences in the postoperative phase of treatment.

Leg and Trunk Control

Deficits in flexibility, especially on the contralateral side, must be identified, and proper stretching exercises must be instituted preoperatively. Hip and trunk extension strength is important for the development of core strength, or the strength of the musculature around the hips, trunk, and spine, which is critical in controlling posture, generating and transferring force, and increasing the activation of extremity muscles. These exercises include ipsilateral leg/trunk extensions and contralateral leg/trunk diagonal patterns (Fig. 1) that improve rotational control. They may be done with a stable base or on an unstable base, such as a trampoline or wobble board, which increases proprioceptive input. Other exercises include lunges and step-ups/step-downs. These exercises may be executed with or without scapular involvement.

Scapular Control

The scapula frequently is involved with shoulder injuries. Scapular dyskinesis, or alterations in position or motion of the scapula, is caused by weakness or inhibition of the periscapular muscles, especially the lower trapezius and serratus anterior, and/or overactivity of the upper trapezius. This dyskinesis results in lack of control of scapular retraction, contributing to internal shoulder impingement; lack of control of acromial elevation with excessive shoulder "shrugging," contributing to external shoulder impingement; and lack of a stable base of muscle origin, contributing to rotator cuff weakness. Lower trapezius and serratus anterior strengthening in the injured athlete by means of isolated exercises is difficult in the early rehabilitation phases because of neurologic inhibition of the acti-

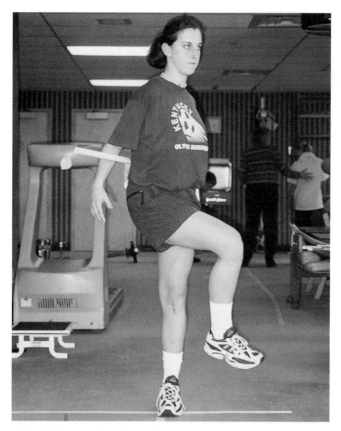

Figure 1 Diagonal patterns for rotational control over one leg.

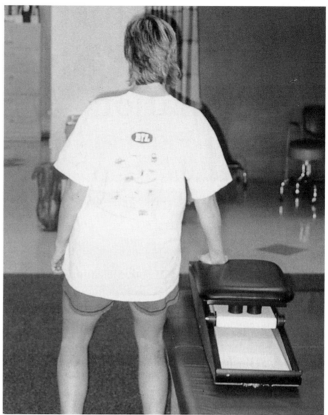

Figure 2 Low row exercise is effective for stabilization of the lower scapular border.

vation of these muscles. Their activation can be facilitated by proximal muscle activation. Diagonally directed hip/trunk extension and scapular retraction and protraction, ipsilateral trunk extension/scapular retraction/arm extensions (low row exercises; Fig. 2), and trunk extension/bilateral scapular pinches are good exercises that accomplish scapular control without creating shear stresses on the injured shoulder joint. The low row exercises also are effective in reducing upper trapezius hyperactivity, reducing the "shrugging."

Shoulder Flexibility

Scapular protraction and retraction and glenohumeral internal and external rotation frequently are compromised by inflexibility in association with shoulder injuries. Either as a cause or a result of loss of retraction control, all of the structures that attach to the coracoid may be contracted. This contraction results in point tenderness to palpation over the coracoid and along the pectoralis minor and short head of the biceps. There is frequently a feeling of stiffness and/or tightness in this area when the scapula is actively or passively retracted toward the midline. These structures may be stretched by the "open book" stretch by placing the patient supine with a rolled up towel between the scapulae, followed

by massage. If paresthesias due to thoracic outlet syndrome are reported, this maneuver should not be continued. Placing the arms at the patient's sides decreases the possibility of producing paresthesias. Limitation of glenohumeral rotation is almost universal in association with shoulder injuries. True estimation of internal rotation deficit should be done by goniometric assessment. Spinal-level estimation has 7° of freedom in the test and does not correlate with the biomechanically important glenohumeral internal rotation. Internal/external rotation stretching should be done by applying a rotational stress to the arm as the scapula is stabilized (Fig. 3).

Shoulder Strength

Shoulder muscles should be strengthened as much as is anatomically possible. If the rotator cuff is not involved in the injury, closed-chain exercises for rotator cuff strengthening (discussed later) will not place shear stress on the joint. Rotator cuff strength frequently improves as scapular control is gained as a result of the more stable base of muscle origin.

Early Postoperative Motion

Early joint motion under controlled circumstances is encouraged in many accelerated shoulder rehabilitation

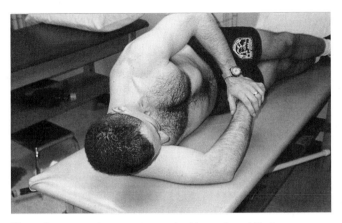

Figure 3 Stretching of the posterior capsule with scapular stabilization.

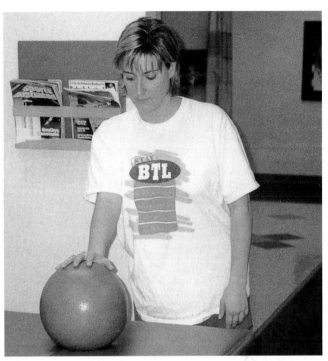

Figure 4 Closed-chain axial loading for motion. The patient can be moved to any position around the ball that is safe and comfortable, and rotational movement can be started.

protocols. This motion may prevent restricted range of motion, decrease pain, and allow the shoulder joint to be moved to biomechanically optimal positions to reproduce normal physiologic muscle activations and proprioception. However, unlike the knee, which has relatively few degrees of freedom, the shoulder has many degrees of freedom and can assume many passive positions, so care must be taken in positioning the arm in relation to the body and loading the arm so that excessive shear is avoided.

Continuous Passive Motion

Continuous passive motion (CPM) has been advocated as a means of obtaining range of motion following all types of shoulder surgery. Its most common use is following capsular release for postoperative adhesions or adhesive capsulitis. The major impediment to widespread use of CPM is the inability to control the mechanical axis of the glenohumeral joint and to limit movement of the joint to a specifically desired plane. Rotation is the most commonly restricted movement, but this is the hardest to control and to reproduce reliably using the machines currently available. Better-designed machines may eventually produce the desired effect of early specific motion with protection of the repair.

Closed-Chain Axial Loading for Motion

Early motion with protection of the surgical repair can be instituted by closed-chain stabilization of the hand on an object (table, wall, or ball), moving the body to a position that is protective, and then instituting motion (Fig. 4). No shear is placed on the repair, and no open-chain loading is applied. Increased motion can be achieved by active-assisted wand exercises in single planes of motion, by advancing the placement of the hand on the wall, or by increasing the distance of the arm away from the body as healing progresses.

Early Achievement of 90° of Abduction

Many athletic and industrial activities in the shoulder occur around 90° of abduction. This position is optimum for most muscle geometry and activation, reproduces proprioception, and allows optimal rotation. Surgical repairs for instability and labral injuries should be assessed intraoperatively to make sure this position can be achieved without undue stress on the repair. Early closed-chain motion and active-assisted motion with a wand can then be started. Many protocols try to achieve 90° of abduction by 3 to 5 weeks. When this position is achieved, scapular and arm strengthening can be started with low shear stresses on the joint.

Closed-Chain Axial Loading for Strengthening

Closed-chain rehabilitation protocols link the trunk to the scapula and the scapula to the arm. This allows strengthening of the scapular and arm musculature as a unit.

Scapular Control

The earliest and safest exercises are the scapular clock exercises (Fig. 5) with the hand placed at various positions depending on the state of healing. The scapula is moved in elevation (12 o'clock) to depression (6 o'clock) and in protraction (3 o'clock) to retraction (9 o'clock). The patient stands during the exercises to allow trunk

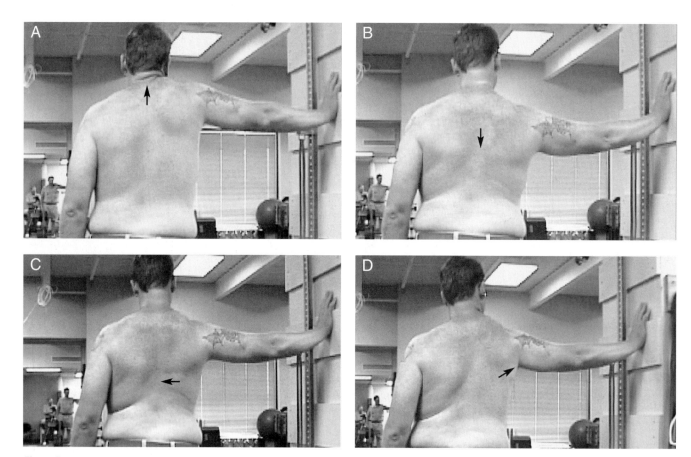

Figure 5 Scapular clock exercises. The scapula is moved between elevation/depression (12 o'clock/6 o'clock) (**A** and **B**) and retraction/protraction (3 o'clock/9 o'clock) (**C** and **D**).

extension to facilitate the activity of the scapular stabilizers. These exercises decrease deltoid activation, thereby eliminating upward shear, and activate the rotator cuff to control concavity/compression. Another safe scapular activation is the low row for control of the lower scapula (Fig. 2). Progressions for scapular and arm strengthening can be accomplished by incorporating the arm into the trunk/scapula exercises. These exercises are called "dumps" (Fig. 6) because the patients appear to be dumping material out of cans. Extra resistance can be created by moving the arm away from the body, by increasing the load, and by increasing the distance moved. Sport- or activity-specific positions and motions can be simulated. Other progressions include push-ups on the wall or floor; push-ups plus, with thoracic elevation; press-ups; and arm hugs.

Rotator Cuff Activation

The rotator cuff has two main roles in shoulder function— increasing capsular stiffness by increasing ligamentous stiffness and maintaining concavity/compression of the glenohumeral joint. Rotator cuff activation is coupled with and follows scapular stabilization so that the muscles

are physiologically activated off a stabilized base and are mechanically placed in an optimum length-tension arrangement. Rotator cuff activation is seldom isolated to one muscle but is integrated within its component parts. Closed-chain axial loading exercises are efficient in reproducing these patterns. Early loading can occur through weight shifts on a table or ball with the arm at low elevations (Fig. 4). Advanced integration of rotator cuff activation with the trunk and scapula can be accomplished by rotator cuff clock exercises, wall washes (Fig. 7), punches, and proprioceptive exercises with oscillating blades. These exercises can be made sport- or activity-specific by varying the position of the arm and trunk. Internal and external rotation strengthening can be done by using rubber resistance tubing with trunk extension and 90° arm abduction (Fig. 8). Isolated rotator cuff exercises may be used if strength deficits persist, but these should be instituted only after scapular control is gained.

Aquatic Therapy

Aquatic therapy has been shown to be beneficial in achieving early improvements in range of motion, decreasing pain on glenohumeral joint mobilization, and

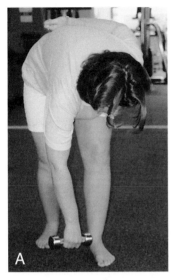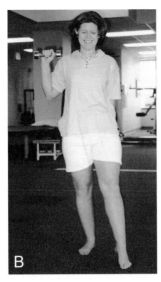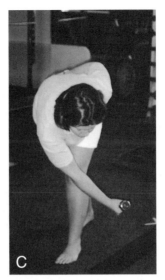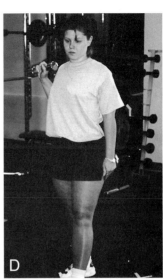

Figure 6 Shoulder dumps may be done ipsilaterally (**A** and **B**) or diagonally (**C** and **D**).

allowing safe levels of activation of the rotator cuff and synergistic muscles. Muscle activation intensity during arm elevation in water is significantly less than activation intensity on dry land. The activation intensities are similar to the levels reported for closed-chain rotator cuff clock exercises. These exercises can be used at the same early stage as the scapular control and clock exercises and have similar margins of safety in terms of controlled motion and muscle activation.

Power Development

Power is required for throwing in sports and dynamic work in activities of daily living. Power is generated through the entire kinetic chain. Plyometric, or stretch/shortening, exercises are the best way to develop power. Plyometrics can be instituted in uninjured areas early in rehabilitation but must be deferred to later stages in injured areas because of the large ranges of required motions and large forces developed.

Lunges, vertical jumps, depth jumps, and slides are lower extremity plyometric exercises. Trunk and upper extremity plyometric exercises include rotation diagonals, medicine ball rotations, and dumbbell rotations.

Special Concerns in Accelerated Shoulder Rehabilitation

Pain

Pain is a powerful inhibitor of muscle activation. This principle is especially important when dealing with shoulder rehabilitation because of the large contribution of coordinated muscle activation to joint motion, position, stability, and function. Accelerated programs may create pain if not monitored properly for arm position, joint load, joint shear, or muscle tension. The visual analog scale is used to objectively measure pain levels. Pain should be kept below 4 (out of a maximum of 10) during the rehabilitation exercises. Instead of pushing through the pain with the exercise, the reasons for the pain should be evaluated, and joint position, arm position, body position, or muscle load should be altered to keep pain in the 0 to 4 range. This allows minimal pain-based muscle inhibition and deters the patient from assuming pain avoidance postures or motions, which include excessive shoulder shrugging, hitching of the shoulder with motion, or avoidance of certain ranges of motions.

Use of Exercise Machines

Exercise machines are a traditional modality in classic rehabilitation. They are relatively inexpensive and readily available, and exercise protocols for their use have been established. However, several features of exercise machines limit their use in accelerated rehabilitation, especially in the early stages. First, their load application is usually at the distal end in an open-chain fashion and creates joint shear. Second, they functionally isolate single muscles or specific groups of related muscles, using activation patterns that are not integrated. Third, they usually emphasize activation of the anterior muscles around the shoulder and deemphasize the important posterior shoulder and scapular muscles. If exercise machines are used, they are most effective in the later stages for extra strengthening and acquisition of plyometric power development. If the load is applied in the right direction along the arm, muscle activation and joint loading can achieve closed-chain characteristics.

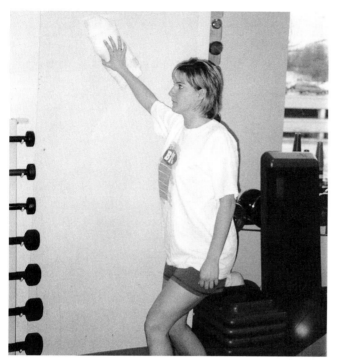

Figure 7 Wall wash. The arm is moved along a smooth surface at comfortable elevations. Trunk and leg movement provide increased stabilization and muscle activation.

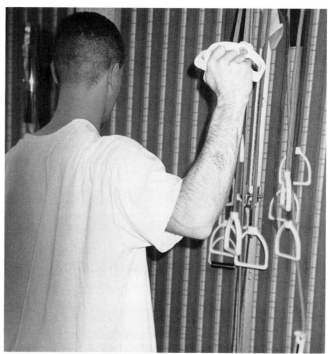

Figure 8 Internal/external rotator cuff strengthening should be done at arm elevations around 90°.

Progressions

Because accelerated rehabilitation focuses on functional return of the shoulder as part of a kinetic chain, there is less emphasis on specific timing or stages and more emphasis on acquisition of key functions in the kinetic chain. These functions may be used as markers for progressions in the rehabilitation protocol. These points include normal pelvis control over the planted leg, hip and trunk extension, control of scapular retraction, glenohumeral range of motion, and coupled scapulohumeral motion in normal patterns. As each functional marker is achieved, more advanced exercises may be used.

Substitute patterns can be seen in some patients if these functional markers are not achieved. These patterns include lumbar lordosis with pelvic tilt, shoulder shrugging with thoracic kyphosis, upward scapular rotation, and scapular retraction instead of shoulder rotation. These patterns must be corrected to allow kinetic chain function, or substitute patterns will be present and will decrease the ability to achieve normal functional return of the entire kinetic chain.

Accelerated rehabilitation is accelerated only in relation to protocols that wait to begin rehabilitation until shoulder healing is complete. Normal physiologic timing of healing of shoulder repairs must be respected, but many of the facets of accelerated rehabilitation—leg/ trunk control, scapular control, and range of motion in safe planes—can be instituted in the acute repair stage of

the postoperative period, from 1 to 3 weeks after surgery. Closed-chain placement protects the arm and shoulder from shear and tensile loads, and its use allows the initiation of scapular and glenohumeral rehabilitation— flexibility exercises, scapular clocks, low rows, and axial loading—during the 3- to 6-week stage of tissue remodeling. Power development and other strenuous exercises require normal healing and should be delayed until the patient demonstrates healed tissue.

Summary

Accelerated shoulder rehabilitation along physiologic and biomechanical principles appears to be safe and produces no excessive shear on the repair. Attention must be paid to the details of joint position, arm and body motion, and muscle activation to allow successful progressions. These protocols are still evolving, but they appear to be efficacious in allowing the early, safe return to athletic and activity function, with outcomes similar to those of accelerated knee rehabilitation.

Annotated Bibliography

Burkhart SS, Morgan CD, Kibler WB: Shoulder injuries in overhead athletes: The "dead arm" revisited. *Clin Sports Med* 2000;19:125-158.

This is a good review of shoulder mechanics and injury and provides an overview of physical findings associated with shoulder injury.

Happee R, Van der Helm FC: The control of shoulder muscles during goal directed movements: An inverse dynamic analysis. *J Biomech* 1995;28:1179-1191.

This detailed article demonstrates through inverse dynamics how humeral motion is linked with scapular motion to achieve shoulder function.

Kelly BT, Roskin LA, Kirkendall DT, Speer KP: Shoulder muscle activation during aquatic and dry land exercises in nonimpaired subjects. *J Orthop Sports Phys Ther* 2000;30:204-210.

This is a good overview of the effect the aquatic environment has on muscle activation to decrease strain and shear.

Kibler WB: The role of the scapula in athletic shoulder function. *Am J Sports Med* 1998;26:325-337.

The author provides an update on scapular function and dysfunction and methods of examination and rehabilitation.

Kibler WB, Livingston BP: Closed chain rehabilitation for the upper and lower extremities. *J Am Acad Orthop Surg* 2001;9:412-421.

This is a review of the biomechanical basis of closed-chain rehabilitation and exercise protocols for clinical application.

Lephart SM, Henry TJ: The physiologic basis for open and closed chain rehabilitation for the upper extremity. *J Sports Rehab* 1996;5:71-87.

This is a good review of the physiologic basis for different types of exercises, the role of proprioceptive feedback, and exercises for clinical application.

Classic Bibliography

Dillman CJ, Murray TA, Hintermeister RA: Biomechanical differences of open and closed chain exercises with respect to the shoulder. *J Sports Rehab* 1994;3:228-238.

Chapter 40

CPT® and ICD-9-CM Coding for the Shoulder Surgeon

Richard J. Friedman, MD, FRCSC

Introduction

Every patient encounter, whether it is an office visit or a surgical procedure, must be documented by the physician in a medical record. The medical record contains the evaluation and treatment plan, as well as additional information that can be communicated to other physicians. Insurance carriers use the medical record to provide accurate and timely claims. The medical record also is used as a resource for utilization and quality control, research, and education. In addition, it is considered a legal document that verifies that care was provided. Thus, the importance of a thorough, accurate, and properly coded medical record cannot be overemphasized.

CPT

Each service or procedure performed by a physician is identified by a five-digit Current Procedural Terminology (CPT®) code, which accurately identifies and simplifies reporting of the service. CPT is a systematic listing and coding of procedures and services developed and published by the American Medical Association (AMA) and has become the universal language that all physicians use to bill for their services; it is used by the government and insurance carriers for subsequent reimbursement of physician services. Each year CPT is updated, published in book and electronic formats in November, and in effect on January 1 of the following year. All changes are listed in Appendix B of CPT. All orthopaedic surgeons and their office staff should review these changes and implement them beginning January 1. Although insurance carriers often lag behind the annual changes, it is critical that the surgeon and staff are up to date.

ICD-9

Each diagnosis is identified by a three- to five-digit numeric or V code from the International Classification of Diseases, Ninth Revision, Clinical Modification (ICD-9-CM or ICD-9). ICD-9 is a system developed by the World Health Organization that classifies diagnoses into numeric codes that range from 001.0 to 999.9 and is divided into 17 classifications, including musculoskeletal diseases, diseases defined by body systems, congenital anomalies, symptoms, signs and ill-defined conditions, and injuries. The V codes range from V01.0 to V82.9 and describe the circumstances of a patient visit unrelated to injury or disease. V codes are used for preventive medicine visits, physical examinations, postoperative follow-up examinations outside the global service period, and physical therapy.

CMS

The Centers for Medicare and Medicaid (CMS), formerly the Health Care Financing Administration (HCFA), is the government agency responsible for establishing reimbursement policies for Medicare and Medicaid; CMS establishes reimbursement policies that often are followed by private insurance carriers. In 1998, HCFA reported a loss of $23 billion as a result of fraud and abuse. Of this loss, 42% has been attributed to upcoding or miscoding of evaluation and management (E/M) services. In addition, CMS is directed by Congress and the Office of the Inspector General to limit expenses and reduce costs. Therefore, CMS makes changes in reimbursement in the context of budget neutrality, so that when funds are allocated for a new CPT code, reimbursement is reduced elsewhere to pay for the new code. For example, if a new CPT code is created for revision total shoulder arthroplasty (TSA), CMS would most likely pay for this by decreasing the amount reimbursed for all primary TSAs. If most orthopaedic surgeons do not perform revision TSAs, this type of change would penalize the majority while benefiting only a small number of surgeons. Therefore, any request for a new code must be considered very carefully for its full impact on all orthopaedic surgeons.

AAOS Role in Coding

The American Academy of Orthopaedic Surgeons' (AAOS) CPT and ICD-9 Coding Committee was established to ensure that Academy members are kept informed about current issues regarding CPT and ICD-9 coding. The Committee also represents orthopaedic interests in coding-related issues on a national level. Four members of AAOS Coding Committee sit on the AMA CPT Advisory Committee. The AMA's 11-member CPT Editorial Committee, which is composed of physicians and other members of the health care industry and government, revises the CPT annually. An orthopaedic surgeon has served on the CPT Editorial Committee at various times in the past.

New Code Development

Numerous orthopaedic procedures, shoulder procedures in particular, have not been assigned a CPT code; however, a limited number of new codes are introduced annually. Any individual–be it a physician, nurse, or industry representative–can request creation of a new code. Physicians, however, generally are more successful in soliciting the AMA CPT Editorial Committee for new codes.

The most appropriate course of action for a physician who wishes to propose a new CPT code for a shoulder procedure is to submit the request, in writing, to the American Shoulder and Elbow Surgeons (ASES) CPT Committee. This committee can assist the physician in gathering the necessary information required by the AMA to support and justify the request. A number of factors must be analyzed when a new code is considered so that the new code will benefit most orthopaedic surgeons and not inadvertently penalize them. If the ASES CPT Committee believes that the request has merit, it will be submitted for review to the AAOS Coding Committee. From there, it is forwarded to the AMA Department of Coding, at which point the official process begins–a process that generally takes 2 years.

Coding Tips

CPT coding must be a collaborative effort between the physician and the office staff. A physician must be involved because he or she is the only one who really knows and understands the service that was provided. CPT coding is not always uniequivocal; often, there may

be several correct ways to code a procedure. Thus, an informed surgeon should always code the procedure rather than relying on a lay individual. Therefore, the surgeon must learn and use the CPT language because it is not always intuitive or identical to the clinical terms that often are used. For example, when a surgeon applies a plate to a humeral fracture, correct CPT terminology would be open treatment of a humerus fracture, not open reduction and internal fixation as one would intuitively think. Using the correct terminology results in improved and timely reimbursement.

Proper Use of CPT Codes

It is important to note that the government and insurance carriers consider the use of any CPT code that describes a surgical procedure to be for major surgery, even if the patient has not had surgery. For example, a patient is referred to an orthopaedic surgeon's office for consultation. Following examination, the surgeon determines that the patient has a nondisplaced ulnar nightstick fracture with minimal tenderness and elects to treat the fracture with a compression bandage. The proper way to code the encounter is to assign the appropriate E/M code, add the appropriate modifier (in this case, modifier –57), and the CPT code for closed treatment of an ulnar shaft fracture, without manipulation, (25530). Modifier –57 is used when an E/M service results in the initial decision to perform surgery within 24 hours, and closed treatment of a fracture without manipulation is considered surgery. (Further explanations of modifiers and E/M services appear later in this chapter.) Alternatively, the surgeon could choose to bill the E/M code initially but not the procedure code, then subsequently charge for follow-up visits, because there is no 90-day global period as there is for a procedure code.

One easy way to begin consistently coding is to ensure that CPT and ICD-9 codes are added to the patient's operative note. Each operative note should contain all of the information necessary for the insurance carrier to process the claim and reimburse the surgeon in a timely fashion. The diagnosis and any relevant comorbidities, such as obesity, diabetes, and smoking, should be listed in the operative note, using exact ICD-9 language. The CPT code should be listed after the procedure, using exact CPT language from the book, and any appropriate modifier(s) should be included. To facilitate this practice, a CPT book should be present in every operating room and at every dictating station in the operating room suite. The first paragraph of the operative note should outline the indications for the procedure and explain explicitly the reasons and justification for using any modifiers, followed by the description of the procedure itself.

The medical record must support the CPT and ICD-9 codes used, and the appropriate diagnosis code must match the procedure performed. For example, if a TSA (CPT code 23472) was performed for arthritis of the shoulder joint, ICD-9 code 715.91 (Osteoarthrosis and allied disorders) is an appropriate diagnostic code; however, subacromial impingement (ICD-9 code 726.2, Peripheral esthesopathies and allied syndromes), would not be appropriate. To help orthopaedic surgeons and their office staff code correctly, the AAOS has both text and electronic resources to help cross-reference CPT and ICD-9 codes.

Proper Billing Procedures

The federal government considers billing a procedure as "insurance only" to be fraud and abuse; therefore, "insurance only" billing is never allowed for Medicare or Medicaid billing. Other insurance carriers have followed suit. This is based on the premise that if the physician is willing to give the patient a discount, then he or she must offer the insurance carrier the same discount. For example, if the physician sees his or her partner's relative and submits a bill to the insurance carrier, the physician is required to collect any outstanding part of the bill that the insurance carrier does not cover. If asked, the physician must provide proof to the insurance carrier that a reasonable effort was made to collect. According to Medicare, a reasonable effort means that three bills were sent to the patient. The government does not require a physician to pursue the outstanding amount beyond this.

Handling Denials

Once a surgeon submits a claim, the insurance carrier responds with an explanation of benefits that details what the surgeon was paid and/or what or why part or all of the payment was denied. The orthopaedic surgeon should review every denial or reduced reimbursement personally in a timely fashion and should appeal any incorrect reimbursement as quickly as possible.

Generally, a denial occurs for one of three reasons: the surgeon made an error in coding, the insurance company made an error in coding, or the insurance company simply refused to pay. Whatever the reason, the denial must be dealt with expeditiously so that the surgeon can be reimbursed; in these instances, the surgeon's input can be invaluable, as well as greatly appreciated by the office staff. Clearly, the more input the surgeon has from the outset, the higher the likelihood that a claim will be paid in a timely fashion. Therefore, the importance of submitting the initial claim correctly cannot be overemphasized; resubmissions and appeals are costly and time consuming.

Resubmission of a denied claim should be accompa-nied by any requested supporting documentation and then sent directly to the insurance company's medical director. The medical director is a physician who usually is more willing to consider an orthopaedic surgeon's explanation of a claim rather than that of the office staff's. If appealing to the medical director fails, a formal appeal should be filed with the insurance carrier. Although the formal appeals process is often protracted, tedious, and time consuming, it is important that the appeal is pursued to the very end. Most appeals can be won with perseverance.

Precertification

Precertification and preauthorization from the insurance carrier are often required before a patient can undergo surgery. Precertification permits the surgeon to perform the procedure and obtain a precertification number. Preauthorization gives the surgeon approval for the codes he or she will use and the amount of reimbursement. Therefore, the surgeon must provide the insurance carrier with the CPT code(s) that likely will be used to describe the surgical procedure(s) being performed. The surgeon should try to be as inclusive as possible when deciding beforehand what procedures may be performed. It is certainly easier to ask for more and use less, rather than the reverse. To facilitate this process and other insurance carrier issues, a list of contact names at the physician's 10 most commonly used insurance carriers should be easily available for the office staff's use.

Consultations

Any time a surgeon sees a patient at the request of another physician, the service can be billed as a consultation. Whether the consulting physician assumes further care of the patient or treats the patient is irrelevant to the use of consultation codes. A consultation performed in the surgeon's office or emergency department is billed as an outpatient consultation, and an E/M code in the 9924X series is used. This includes a patient sent to the surgeon's office by an emergency department physician. Any follow-up visit of an outpatient consultation is billed subsequently as an established patient visit, and E/M codes in the 9921X series are used. If the orthopaedic surgeon sees a patient who has been admitted to the hospital, E/M codes in the 9925X series are used. Subsequent visits are billed as an inpatient consultation follow-up visit using E/M codes in the 9926X series.

Three conditions must be met to qualify as a consultation. First, the consultation must meet appropriate E/M documentation guidelines for the level of service billed. Second, the request for the consultation should be documented by the requesting physician in the patient's medical record, although it is not necessary for the consulting physician to document the request. Third, the findings of the consultation must be communicated in writing to the requesting physician. The last two requirements can be met easily if the consulting physician sends a letter to the requesting physician that documents both the request for the consultation and the findings. It also fosters good communication among physicians, which helps with patient care and future referrals.

A confirmatory consultation, or second opinion, can be requested by any individual, such as a health care professional, lawyer, insurance carrier, or patient. The consulting physician must document that the visit is for a second opinion and note any other physicians who have treated the patient and other treatments that have been rendered. In these cases, E/M codes in the 9927X series are used.

If a patient with a hip fracture is referred to an orthopaedic surgeon by an emergency department physician, the consulting physician can bill for an outpatient consultation if the patient is evaluated in the emergency department, a history and physical examination are performed, and the patient is hospitalized for surgery. In this instance, a modifier –57 should be added to the E/M code (9927X series) if surgery will be performed within 24 hours. Alternatively, the consulting physician may recommend that the patient be admitted to the consulting physician's service to be seen the next morning. At that time, the consulting physician obtains a history and examines the patient. Billing in this instance would be for an initial hospital visit using E/M codes in the 9922X series (initial hospital care), not the outpatient or inpatient consultation codes.

Compliance

The federal government has made compliance to and enforcement of proper coding and billing procedures a priority. The Federal Bureau of Investigation and the Departments of Justice and Health and Human Services are involved in the investigation and prosecution of suspected fraud and abuse. A distinction between fraud and abuse is whether the physician knew, or should have known, what was being done wrong.

Random audits are conducted but these are not common and generally simply ask for documentation, usually of an E/M visit. This type of audit generally is not as involved as one conducted in response to a report of sus-

pected abuse. A lawsuit can be initiated by anyone who suspects fraud and abuse can file a lawsuit–be it an accountant or disgruntled former employee. A so-called whistle-blower can receive 15% to 30% of any monies the government recovers as a result of the information provided. With the latter type of audit, the government is not required to examine all the records in question. Rather, a small sampling can be thoroughly reviewed, and the findings extrapolated to the whole practice. The total number of violations is thus an estimated number based on the extrapolation, and there is a $10,000 fine for each infraction. In addition, the government can share the information with other insurance carriers, who then have the authority to conduct their own audit of the practice and impose fines for violations found.

Therefore, every physician, whether a solo practitioner or part of a large multiple specialty group, should have a compliance program in place for the physician and office staff, as well as adequate documentation of each patient visit. Internal and possibly external audits should be part of any compliance program. Educating physicians and staff must be ongoing and documented. As part of a compliance program and to help prepare for any type of audit, every physician must know his or her own profile and how it compares to local, regional, and national norms. The profile can be obtained relatively easily from the state Medicare carrier.

Coding for Arthroscopic Procedures

As technology improves, new techniques are developed to help physicians treat their patients. New procedures may be developed or new methods of performing an established procedure may become popular before scientific evidence of safety and efficacy is available. When safety and efficacy data to support a new procedure or technique have been published in peer-reviewed journals, the procedure or technique may become established or the standard of care. However, the development of a CPT code often lags behind technologic advances and perhaps, for numerous reasons, may never be created. As a result, coding for the procedure often is confusing and frustrating for both the office staff and the orthopaedic surgeon.

CPT codes do not yet exist for numerous arthroscopic shoulder procedures. Historically, orthopaedic surgeons have used the CPT code corresponding to the open procedure for an arthroscopic procedure. For example, a Bankart procedure done arthroscopically would be coded the same way as an open Bankart repair, using CPT code 23455 (Capsulorrhaphy, anterior; with labral repair [eg, Bankart procedure]).

This is not the correct way to code arthroscopic procedures. Conflicting advice was given in the past on the best way to code arthroscopic procedures. In 1999, the AMA and HCFA explicitly stated that under no circumstances should CPT codes for open procedures be used for arthroscopic procedures. This proclamation is not specific to orthopaedic surgery but rather covers all endoscopic procedures. If a code does not exist for the arthroscopic procedure, CPT code 29999 (Unlisted procedure, shoulder arthroscopy), is to be used.

CMS now considers the use of open codes for arthroscopic procedures to constitute fraud and abuse. To illustrate how seriously CMS considers the problem, various insurance carriers have hired "bounty hunters" to review 5 years of records to uncover instances in which open codes may have been used for arthroscopic procedures. Although physicians cannot change what they have done in the past, they can clearly document through their compliance program that once they became aware of this clarification, they stopped using codes for open procedures for arthroscopic procedures and began using the unlisted arthroscopy code.

Coding for Unlisted Procedures

Historically, insurance carriers have refused to pay for unlisted CPT codes. However, they have begun to realize that many established procedures have no corresponding CPT codes and that they must reimburse physicians fairly and equitably for the their work. Each practice must have a plan for reporting unlisted arthroscopic procedures and justification for the fee requested. The commitment for reimbursement for these unlisted procedure codes should be obtained from the insurance carrier before the surgery is performed electively. Leverage is always greater when negotiations with the insurance carrier occur prior to surgery. It may be difficult at first, but once a process is developed to report unlisted procedures, it can be applied to the 10 most common unlisted procedures with the practice's 10 most used insurance carriers. Insurance carriers are as interested in saving time and money as physicians, and if the physician and carrier can agree ahead of time how these unlisted arthroscopic procedures will be handled, the physician will find the increased reimbursement and decreased payment time worth the effort.

Specific steps should be taken for reporting unlisted procedures to insurance carriers. First, the CPT book should be consulted to determine whether a code exists for the procedure performed. If no code exists for an arthroscopic procedure, such as an arthroscopic rotator cuff repair, the unlisted procedure, CPT code 29999, should be used.

A cover letter, which can be modified depending on the procedure, should then be developed to attach to the operative report. In the letter, an existing CPT code that is similar to what was done arthroscopically should be identified and listed. This code, called a comparison code, must be a fair comparison to the unlisted procedure or the insurance carrier will reject the claim. The comparison code should involve the same body part and the same or similar approach and/or procedure; for example, for the arthroscopic rotator cuff repair, the comparison code would be 23412 (Repair of ruptured musculotendinous cuff, rotator cuff; chronic).

Next, two or three aspects of the procedure performed that make it more or less difficult (or the same level of difficulty) than the existing comparison procedure should be listed. Based on this, a percent of difficulty should be assigned to the unlisted code. In other words, was the procedure performed more difficult (eg, 120%, or 1.2), less difficult (eg, 80%, or 0.8), or the same level of difficulty (100%, or 1) compared to the comparison code?

The relative value units, or reimbursement fee, assigned to the comparison code should be checked and communicated to the insurance carrier with a notation that the fee should be adjusted according to the percent of difficulty (up, down, or unchanged) calculated. An explanation of the fee adjustment should be provided as well. Procedures that are normally included in the global service data list should not be unbundled.

For example, an arthroscopic rotator cuff repair with three suture anchors involves less dissection compared to the open procedure, but arthroscopically placing the suture anchors and tying the knots may be more difficult. Therefore, the level of difficulty may be considered the same whether an open or arthroscopic procedure was performed (100%). In this case, the cover letter should be as simple and brief as possible and should include the fee for the comparison code ($XXX). The payor also should be informed that the procedures have similar levels of difficulty, require no adjustment to the fee, and the arthroscopic procedure should be paid at the same rate as the comparison code ($XXX × 1).

The comparison code for an arthroscopic thermal capsulorrhaphy of the anterior and inferior capsule would be CPT code 23466 (Capsulorrhaphy, glenohumeral joint, any type multidirectional instability). In most instances, the level of difficulty of an arthroscopic procedure is less than what it would be if an open procedure were performed; therefore, the fee charged would be the reimbursement fee for CPT code 23466 multiplied by the reduced level of difficulty.

Any payment requests for an unlisted procedure should be reasonable and honest. If the orthopaedic surgeon is uncertain of how the process works, he or she should speak to colleagues who have a similar practice profile or contact his or her specialty society or the AAOS CPT and ICD Coding Committee. After the first time, the process becomes much easier. The time invested initially to develop comparisons for the most common unlisted procedures and the busiest insurance carriers will save the office staff and the physician a great deal of work and provide timely reimbursement.

Modifiers

A modifier is defined in the AMA's *Current Procedural Terminology CPT 2002* as follows: "A modifier provides the means by which the reporting physician can indicate that a service or procedure that has been performed has been altered by some specific circumstance but not changed in its definition or code." Although most modifiers will not increase the amount of reimbursement, they will help prevent delays in processing a claim and payment. An example would be a patient who fell 2 months after undergoing a total hip arthroplasty and sustained a Colles' fracture that was reduced with closed treatment and application of a cast. Because the Colles' fracture was sustained during the 90-day global service period, any claim submitted for the Colles' fracture would be rejected automatically unless modifier –79 (unrelated procedure or service by the same physician during the postoperative period) was attached to the CPT code. This modifier indicates that the closed treatment to reduce the fracture during the 90-day postoperative period was an unrelated procedure to the total hip arthroplasty.

Modifiers usually are expressed as a hyphenated two-digit number added to the E/M or CPT code. Alternatively, the modifier can be included as a five-digit number (099XX) that is listed in addition to the E/M or CPT code used. Most insurance carriers will honor the modifiers listed in CPT. However, with certain modifiers, such as –22 (unusual procedural services), insurance carriers will always delay the claim awaiting an internal review. To minimize the delay, the operative note should be attached to the claim when submitted and a written request should be made that the claim be sent straight to adjudication.

Although all of the modifiers are described fully in CPT, some of the more common ones used by orthopaedic surgeons are emphasized here. E/M modifiers include –21, –24, –25, and –26.

Modifier –24 is used for an unrelated E/M service provided by the same physician during a postoperative period. For example, if the orthopaedic surgeon treats a patient for a sprained wrist 2 months after a total knee arthroplasty, modifier –24 should be appended to the code for the appropriate level of E/M service provided.

A different ICD-9 code from that used for the original procedure must be used as well.

Modifier –25 is for a significant, separately identifiable E/M service provided by the same physician on the same day of the procedure or other service. For example, an orthopaedic surgeon who examines a new patient in the office, diagnoses the patient's condition as subacromial impingement, and injects the subacromial space at that time can use CPT code 20610 (Arthrocentesis, aspiration and/or injection; major joint or bursa) for the injection and append modifier –25 to the code for the appropriate level of E/M service. Modifiers –24 and –25 prevent claims from being rejected, eliminating the need for resubmission and allowing timely reimbursement for services provided.

Modifier –26 (professional component) can be appended to the CPT code if the orthopaedist reads radiographs that he or she ordered but that were neither taken in the surgeon's office nor read by a radiologist. However, the orthopaedist must generate and sign a report that this was done and place it in the patient's medical record. An orthopaedic surgeon who reviews radiographs that were previously read by a radiologist cannot bill for reading the radiographs. However, the content of the office notes and the fact that the orthopaedist reviewed the radiographs should be considered when determining the level of E/M service to bill.

Altered service modifiers include –22 (unusual procedural services) and –52 (reduced services). Modifier –22 is one of the most commonly used, and potentially abused, modifiers that exist. An unmodified CPT code generally covers an easy to difficult range of cases. However, when the service provided is greater than that usually required for the listed procedure, modifier –22 can be added to the CPT code. Use of this modifier, however, requires documentation of the unusual conditions or events requiring increased work and time (for example, for a procedure for which a CPT code does not exist, such as revision rotator cuff repair). Documentation must include the key words "altered surgical field." It is best to ask for approval of this modifier during the precertification as well as asking that the claim be sent straight to adjudication. Modifier –52 (reduced services) is used when the service performed was clearly reduced compared to the standard procedure. For example, if a surgeon performed a revision total hip arthroplasty, both components, but only replaced the acetabular liner (because of polyethylene wear) and the femoral head with one with a longer neck (because of recurrent dislocations), the surgeon should use CPT code 27134 (Revision of total hip arthroplasty; both components, with or without autograft or allograft). However, modifier –52 should be added to the CPT code to demonstrate that this was clearly reduced services compared to a standard revision total hip arthroplasty.

The global service period covers the 24 hours before the procedure and the first 90 days (in most cases) after the procedure. During this period, the work value assigned is 10% for the preoperative work, 69% for the surgical portion, and 21% for the postoperative care. If one physician performs the surgical procedure and another provides the preoperative and/or postoperative care, then the physician who performed the surgery adds modifier –54 (surgical care only) to the CPT code. The physician who provided the postoperative care adds modifier –55 (postoperative management only) to the CPT code. This situation may occur if the surgeon who performed the procedure went out of town and his or her partner assumed the follow-up care for the complete global service period. A physician who provides preoperative care but does not perform the surgical procedure should add modifier –56 (preoperative management only) to the CPT code. This situation may occur if a physician admits a patient while on call and performs the initial work-up but not the surgery. These modifiers allow physicians with different roles in patient care to bill the same CPT code and receive reimbursement for that portion of the work they performed. Alternatively, if a physician provides only postoperative care for a patient and the surgeon did not use these modifiers, then an appropriate level E/M code may be used.

Regional or general anesthesia provided by the surgeon should be documented by adding modifier –47 (anesthesia by surgeon) to the CPT code, and the surgeon also should bill for the anesthetic procedure provided. However, Medicare does not pay for this modifier. Note also that this modifier cannot be used for conscious sedation provided by the surgeon during a procedure such as closed treatment of a fracture with manipulation or for local or hematoma block anesthesia.

Bilateral procedures performed during the same surgical session should be identified with modifier –50 (bilateral procedure). For multiple procedures performed at the same session by the same provider, the primary procedure, which is the one with the highest reimbursement, is listed first. Modifier –51 (multiple procedures) is then applied to each additional procedure. Most insurance carriers discount all subsequent procedures after the primary surgery by a previously agreed upon percentage. However, if the physician has the opportunity to negotiate contract rates with an insurance carrier, it may be worthwhile to point out that because the global service concept allows 69% for the surgery, with bilateral or multiple procedures the physician should receive 69% for subsequent procedures, not 50%. Modifier –51 applies only to multiple procedures other than E/M services.

To avoid rejected claims, resubmissions, and payment delays, modifiers must be used when performing any procedure on a patient during the global postoperative period. If the same surgeon repeats the initial procedure, modifier –76 (repeat procedure by same physician) should be added to the CPT code. If another surgeon repeats the original procedure, then modifier –77 (repeat procedure by another physician) should be used. During the postoperative period, if the patient requires another procedure that is related to the initial surgery, modifier –78 (return to the operating room for a related procedure during the postoperative period) should be added to the CPT code. In the event that, during the postoperative period, a physician performs another procedure or service that is unrelated to the original procedure, modifier –79 (unrelated procedure or service by the same physician during the postoperative period) is used.

Although the global service period includes the 24 hours prior to the procedure, if an E/M service is provided that results in the initial decision to perform the surgery, modifier –57 (decision for surgery) is added to the code for the appropriate level of E/M service. For example, if a physician admits a patient to the hospital in the evening with a displaced four-part proximal humeral fracture, performs the initial evaluation, and decides to perform a hemiarthroplasty the following morning, he or she would bill E/M code 99222–57 for the preoperative evaluation and CPT code 23616 (Open treatment of proximal humeral (surgical or anatomical neck) fracture, with or without internal or external fixation, with or without repair of tuberosity(s); with proximal humeral prosthetic replacement) for the surgical procedure. This will not increase reimbursement; however, the E/M code will not be rejected as being part of the global service period, and the physician will receive timely reimbursement without the difficulties and the added work of having to resubmit a rejected claim.

Modifier –59 (distinct procedural service) is used to unbundle procedures that may appear to the insurance carrier as bundled procedures and addresses computer coding edits. In other words, the physician may need to indicate that a procedure or service was distinct or independent from other services performed on the same day. Modifier –59 is used to identify procedures or services that are not normally reported together but are appropriate under the circumstances. As defined in the AMA's *Current Procedural Terminology CPT 2002*, "this may represent a different session or patient en-counter, different procedure or surgery, different site or organ system, separate incision/excision, separate lesion, or separate injury not ordinarily encountered or performed on the same day by the same physician." The reimbursement for modifier –59 is the same as for modifier –51.

Modifier –59 would be used with arthroscopic procedures in which different procedures are performed at different anatomic sites within the same joint at the same time through different incisions. An example would be a physician who performs an arthroscopic subacromial decompression in the subacromial space as well as an extensive dĕbridement of the glenohumeral joint for tears of the biceps tendon, anterior and posterior labrum, and undersurface partial rotator cuff tears. The first procedure would be billed using CPT code 29826 (Arthroscopy, shoulder, surgical; decompression of subacromial space with partial acromioplasty, with or without coracoacromial release). The second procedure would be coded as 29823 (Arthroscopy, shoulder, surgical; dĕbridement, extensive), and modifier –59 would be appended to this code. Billing in this manner will allow reimbursement for the second procedure. If modifier –51 (multiple procedures) was used, the claim would be rejected.

E/M Guidelines

New E/M guidelines were established in 1995 and 1997, and at the time of publication of this text, physicians could select which set of guidelines they would use based on which was more beneficial. In general, the 1997 guidelines are more favorable for orthopaedic surgeons. However, in December 2000, CMS (formerly HCFA) published a revised draft of new guidelines, but then stopped all work on new guidelines in July 2001. Physicians can determine the status of any new guidelines by logging onto the CMS website for E/M guidelines at http://www.cms.hhs.gov.

Vignettes

This section presents several vignettes depicting the types of patient encounters for which an orthopaedic surgeon may have to submit a claim. Following the description of the encounter, diagnosis, and treatment, possible CPT codes for billing are suggested.

E/M Vignette

A 55-year-old woman who has not been a patient for 4 years comes to the orthopaedic surgeon's office for evaluation of shoulder pain. After the patient has been examined and radiographs obtained, the physician determines that she has acute subacromial impingement and gives the patient a subacromial injection with cortisone and lidocaine.

CPT codes: E/M code 99203–25 (Office or other outpatient visit for the evaluation and management of a new patient, requiring a detailed history, detailed examination, and medical decision making of low complexity) and CPT procedure code 20610.
Alternate codes: 99203, 99025, and 20610

Surgery Vignette

A right-handed 46-year-old tennis player has pain in her right shoulder and is unable to hit a serve or overhead shot. The orthopaedic surgeon diagnoses impingement and, after nonsurgical treatment fails, performs a diagnostic shoulder joint arthroscopy, diagnostic subacromial arthroscopy, subacromial bursectomy, arthroscopic subacromial decompression with excision of an acromioclavicular joint spur, and coracoacromial ligament release.
CPT code: 29826

Surgery Vignette

A right-handed 66-year-old retired painter has pain in his right shoulder and weakness with elevation. The orthopaedic surgeon diagnoses impingement with a rotator cuff tear and, after nonsurgical treatment fails, performs a shoulder joint arthroscopy with extensive dĕbridement of a torn labrum, partial biceps tear, and partial undersurface rotator cuff tear, an arthroscopic subacromial decompression, and open rotator cuff repair.
CPT codes: 29826, 29823–59, and 23412–59

Surgery Vignette

A right-handed 63-year-old retired electrician has pain in his right shoulder and weakness with elevation. The orthopaedic surgeon diagnoses impingement with a rotator cuff tear and, after nonsurgical treatment fails, performs a shoulder joint arthroscopy with extensive dĕbridement of a torn labrum, partial biceps tear, and partial undersurface rotator cuff tear, an arthroscopic subacromial decompression, and an arthroscopic rotator cuff repair.
CPT codes: 29826, 29823–59 and 29999–59

Surgery Vignette

A right-handed 72-year-old man with rheumatoid arthritis who had a total shoulder arthroplasty 17 years ago now has pain, and radiographs show loosening of both components. At surgery, all loose components are removed and a cemented revision total shoulder arthroplasty is performed.
CPT codes: 23331, 23472–59
Alternate code: 23472–22

Bibliography

Websites and Electronic Format

American Academy of Orthopaedic Surgeons Website: http://www.aaos.org

The Centers for Medicare & Medicaid Services (CMS) Website: http://www.cms.hhs.gov

CodeX, Rosemont, IL, American Academy of Orthopaedic Surgeons, 2002.

Print Format

AAOS Guide to CPT Coding for Orthopaedic Surgery 2000, Rosemont, IL, American Academy of Orthopaedic Surgeons, 2000.

Gallagher PE, Smith SL (eds): *Medicare RBRVS: The Physician's Guide.* Chicago, IL, American Medical Association, 2000.

Complete Global Service Data for Orthopaedic Surgery, 2002, Rosemont, IL, American Academy of Orthopaedic Surgeons, 2002.

CPT/ICD-9 Cross-Reference for Orthopaedic Surgery, 2002, Rosemont, IL, American Academy of Orthopaedic Surgeons, 2002.

Current Procedural Terminology CPT 2002, Chicago, IL, AMA Press, 2002.

Physician ICD-9-CM, Volumes 1 & 2, Salt Lake City, UT, Medicode, 2001.

Chapter 41

Outcomes Analysis in the Shoulder and Elbow

Robin R. Richards, MD, FRCSC

Introduction

The assessment of outcomes following treatment is an important component of clinical care. All stakeholders in the health care system—patients, third-party payers, physicians, hospital administrators, and government officials—need to know whether health care interventions are effective, the degree to which they affect the health of patients, and, in relative terms, the cost-effectiveness of treatment. The concepts of quality assurance and continuous improvement demand that measurements be available to use as yardsticks against which to assess the outcomes of treatment. Over the past two decades there has been an explosion of interest in the assessment of general health outcomes and of outcomes in the shoulder and elbow. This chapter details the history of shoulder and elbow outcomes assessment, describes the methodology used to assess outcomes measures, provides a critical analysis of the outcomes measures currently available, and makes some recommendations regarding the use of outcomes measures in clinical practice.

History

Codman is credited with introducing the concept of outcomes assessment in the early 1900s. He espoused the concept of the "end result idea," wherein the clinician would critically evaluate the results of treating even routine problems to identify and understand treatment failures so that the care of future patients could be improved. Until recently, outcomes of shoulder and elbow reconstruction usually were assessed in terms of treatment efficacy, defined by observer-based measures such as range of motion, stability, and deformity, together with radiographic assessment of fracture union or prosthetic alignment. Such observer-based assessments of effectiveness have several disadvantages, however. They ignore the consumer of the product and do not address the larger concept of patient health or the effect of the shoulder or elbow disorder on the general well-being of the patient. Also, because the observer-based measures are specific to the shoulder and elbow, their use makes it impossible to compare the efficacy of these interventions with those of health care interventions in other fields of medicine, for which a common measurement instrument would be needed. For these reasons, patient-based outcomes assessment tools, which are widely accepted for the assessment of general health, are valuable. In recent years, general health outcomes measures have been used to determine the effect of shoulder and elbow conditions on patient well-being, and patient-based outcomes instruments have been developed for the shoulder, the elbow, and the upper extremity as a whole.

Development of Outcomes Measures

Outcomes are best viewed through a disablement paradigm. Disablement is a global term that reflects all of the diverse consequences that disease, injury, or congenital abnormalities may have on human function. Pathologic conditions may lead to impairment, which is an anatomic or physiologic loss of structure or function that may be the direct or secondary result of pathology. Outcomes measures are developed through a process involving (1) identification of a specific patient population, (2) generation of items (questions), (3) item (question) reduction, (4) pretesting of the outcomes instrument, and (5) determination of the measurement properties of the instrument (validity, reliability, and responsiveness).

Types of Outcomes Measures

The decision about which measure to use should be based on many factors, including the population being studied, the purpose of the assessment (routine assessment versus clinical research), the training required, the time required for administration and scoring, and the availability of normative data. Generic health, joint-specific, limb-specific, and disease-specific instruments

TABLE 1	Instruments for Assessment of Outcomes in the Shoulder and Elbow

Generic Health
Arthritis Impact Measurement Scale
Duke Health Profile
Index of Well-Being
Short Form-12 (SF-12)
Short Form-36 (SF-36)
Sickness Impact Profile
Nottingham Health Index

Joint-Specific
Shoulder
American Shoulder and Elbow Surgeons (ASES) Standardized Assessment
Constant Score
L'Insalata Shoulder Rating Questionnaire
Neer Rating Sheet
Shoulder-Arm Disability Questionnaire
Shoulder Disability Questionnaire
Shoulder Pain and Disability Index (SPADI)
Shoulder Pain Score
Shoulder Rating Questionnaire
Shoulder Rating Scale
Shoulder Severity Index (SSI)
Simple Shoulder Test (SST)
Subjective Shoulder Rating Scale
UCLA End-Result Score
University of Pennsylvania Shoulder Score
Wheelchair User's Shoulder Pain Index

Elbow
ASES Standardized Assessment
Broberg and Morrey
Ewald et al
Hospital for Special Surgery
Mayo Elbow Performance Index
Pritchard

Limb-Specific
Disabilities of the Arm, Shoulder and Hand (DASH)
Modified American Shoulder and Elbow Surgeons (M-ASES)
Musculoskeletal Functional Assessment
Toronto Extremity Salvage Score
Upper Extremity Function Scale

Disease-Specific
AC Separation Scoring System
Rowe's Rating for Bankart Repair
Western Ontario Shoulder Instability Index (WOSI)
Western Ontario Osteoarthritis Score

are available for outcomes assessment in the shoulder and elbow (Table 1).

Generic Health Instruments

In the past, the function of the shoulder and elbow traditionally has been assessed using measures that reflect the local impact of a disorder rather than the impact of that disorder on the ability of the patient to function in daily life. Generic health instruments provide information that is comparable across different patient groups regarding the impact of the condition of interest and any coexisting conditions on general health. The Short Form-36 (SF-36) is a commonly used generic health status instrument that has been found to be a reliable and valid measure of the health of patients with musculoskeletal conditions (Fig. 1). The SF-36 has eight indices of health: physical function (PF), social function (SF), role function relating to physical limitations (RP), role function relating to emotional limitations (RE), mental health (MH), vitality and energy (VE), bodily pain (BP), and general health (GH). In addition, two summary scores can be calculated: the Physical Health Component Summary Score (PCS) and the Mental Health Component Summary Score (MCS).

Joint-Specific Outcomes Instruments

Joint-specific health instruments have been found to be more responsive than generic health status instruments in assessing conditions of the upper extremity (Fig. 2). The greater responsiveness is probably the result of including specific items that are relevant to the patient group being studied. The disadvantages of joint-specific instruments are the need for numerous scales and the inability to compare outcomes across various conditions, populations, or interventions. Studies of joint-specific instruments have demonstrated lower correlations with generic measures of health than with each other. Joint-specific instruments tend to be less powerful in their ability to discriminate between levels of overall health, a role better fulfilled by generic health measures such as the SF-36.

Limb-Specific Outcomes Instruments

Limb-specific outcomes instruments are based on the supposition that the upper extremity functions as a kinematic chain. According to this model, the shoulder, elbow, forearm, and wrist position the hand for grasping and for manipulation of the environment. Studies of limb-specific instruments have shown close correlation with joint-specific and disease-specific measures, although limb-specific instruments tend to have a lower degree of responsiveness. Nevertheless, a limb-specific instrument may be appropriate when the diagnosis is less certain or when more than one part of the extremity is affected. For

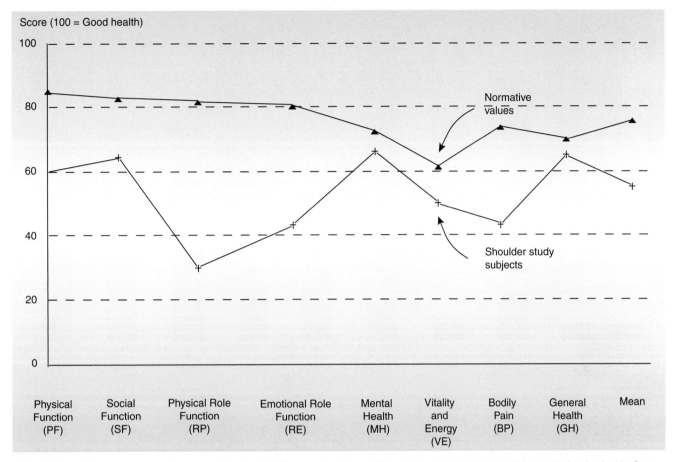

Figure 1 Graph of the mean scores on the acute version of the SF-36 for normal subjects and the mean scores for patients with problems related to the shoulder. Some of the dimensions (physical function, physical role function, emotional role function) assessed on the SF-36 are sensitive to the impact of the problems related to the shoulder. *(Reproduced with permission from Beaton DE, Richards RR: Measuring function of the shoulder: A cross-sectional comparison of five questionnaires. J Bone Joint Surg Am 1996;78:882-890.)*

example, it would be appropriate to measure the effect of a condition involving the shoulder, elbow, wrist, and hand on the patient's ability to use a telephone.

The Disabilities of the Arm, Shoulder and Hand (DASH) questionnaire focuses on functional limitations, symptoms, and psychosocial problems. Patient-completed limb-specific functional questionnaires such as the DASH questionnaire have been developed with careful attention to psychometric principles of instrument design. Whole-limb questionnaires can be used to assess functional outcomes after the treatment of specific joint disorders in the upper extremities. The use of outcomes measures designed to assess the function of the entire limb may help to determine the relative impact of disorders affecting various anatomic sites in the upper extremities.

It may be appropriate to use a combination of joint-specific, limb-specific, disease-specific, and generic health status instruments for detailed research studies. However, for most clinicians, the use of a generic and either a joint-specific or a limb-specific outcomes instrument would be sufficient for routine assessment and follow-up.

Disease-Specific Outcomes Instruments

Disease-specific outcomes measures are designed to assess specific conditions in individual joints. An example of a disease-specific outcomes measure is the Western Ontario Shoulder Instability Index (WOSI). Disease-specific outcomes measures generally are very responsive to small changes in the condition for which they were designed. The disadvantage of these measures is their limited usefulness in comparing outcomes across different disorders, anatomic sites, and populations and the need for a plethora of outcomes measures to assess all conditions affecting the shoulder and elbow.

Application of Outcomes Measures

The lack of a widely accepted outcomes measure can lead to confusion when attempting to determine the severity of an impairment. Patient-completed functional questionnaires have been developed and tested by psychometric and clinimetric methods. When an observer questions a patient with regard to function and then records the response, the possibility of observer bias is

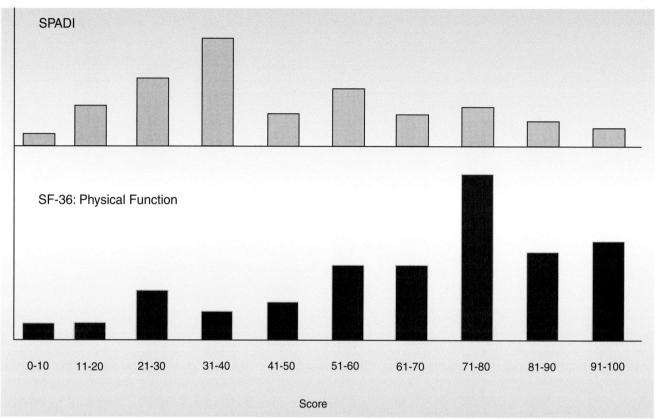

Figure 2 Graph comparing the responses obtained from a joint-specific outcomes instrument, the SPADI, and a generic health status instrument, the SF-36. The SF-36 depicts a healthier state than the joint-specific instrument. Both questionnaires were administered at the same time to the same sample of subjects who had pain in the shoulder. The bars represent the percentage of the sample in each score range. *(Reproduced with permission from Beaton DE, Richards RR: Measuring function of the shoulder: A cross-sectional comparison of five questionnaires.* J Bone Joint Surg Am *1996;78:882-890.)*

introduced. Patient-completed questionnaires can be completed by telephone or mail, do not require a physical examination, and can be used to derive raw scores rather than categorical rankings.

Administration

The response methodology for outcomes instruments can include yes or no answers, Likert scales, or visual analog scales. Visual analog scales take longer to score than other response methodologies if the value of the patient's response must be determined manually. Yes or no answers limit the number of possible responses and may also limit the responsiveness of the instrument. Many contemporary outcomes instruments use Likert scales, although the ideal number of response options for a Likert scale has not been determined.

Assessment of Pain

Some investigators question whether both pain and function scores should be combined in a total score. Because pain affects function to a variable extent, some believe that it should not be included to generate a score of functional limitations. This issue can be ad-

dressed by scoring and reporting pain and functional limitations separately. Because a clinical result is important to the clinician, the outcomes of therapies designed for the treatment of the shoulder and elbow should ideally be described on the basis of three measures: a separate patient-derived assessment of function, an assessment of pain, and a clinical examination.

Categorical Rankings Versus Aggregate Scores

A review of the literature reveals at least 14 different definitions for categorical rankings (excellent, good, fair, poor) that have been used to describe outcomes after elbow surgery. Clinicians may mistakenly assume that the categorical rankings used in independently designed scoring systems describe similar levels of impairment. This lack of standard definitions for categorical rankings hinders accurate communication among investigators and is an impediment to the objective comparison of the results of different studies. For example, the developers of different elbow scoring systems have assigned different weights to each domain and different ranges of values to each categorical ranking (Table 2). The outcomes measures currently in general use for the elbow are based on

TABLE 2 | Distribution and Weighting of Domains in Five Elbow Scoring Systems

Instrument	Score (*Points*)						
	Pain	Motion	Strength	Stability	Function	Deformity	Total
Hospital for Special Surgery	30	28	10	0	20	12	100
Ewald et al	50	10	0	0	30	10	100
Pritchard	50	25	25	0	0	0	100
Broberg and Morrey	40	25	10	10	15	0	100
Mayo Elbow Performance Index	45	20	0	10	25	0	100

(Reproduced with permission from Turchin DC, Beaton DE, Richards RR: Validity of observer-based aggregate scoring systems as descriptors of elbow pain, function, and disability. J Bone Joint Surg Am 1998;80:154-162.)

assessment domains such as range of motion, pain, and ability to perform daily activities, which are scored separately. Scores are then aggregated and assigned categorical rankings that range from excellent to poor. The same patient could therefore have different raw scores and different or similar categorical rankings based on which scoring system is used.

Scoring systems based on categorical rankings compartmentalize results into several categories or domains that clinicians use in decision making. Such scoring systems may be more appealing to clinicians than other outcomes measures such as patient-completed functional questionnaires. However, the admixture of clinical and functional criteria can create a confusing array of variables, and questioning of a patient by an observer introduces the possibility of observer bias during the collection and interpretation of data. Objective analysis of five commonly used elbow scoring systems demonstrated that the systems differed remarkably with regard to the aspects of elbow function that they were designed to assess (Table 3).

The wide variability among the systems limits the interchangeability of the scoring systems. When categorical rankings are ignored and raw aggregate scores are used, there is a surprising trend toward agreement among different elbow scoring systems. The same phenomenon probably applies to shoulder outcomes instruments, although shoulder instruments have not been subjected to the same degree of scrutiny in this regard. The differences among scoring systems are so pervasive that categorical rankings cannot be relied on to provide meaningful comparisons either with the same cohort of patients or between cohorts. The results of studies based on categorical rankings of different scoring systems cannot be compared or combined.

An ideal instrument for the assessment of a joint would measure pain, function, and disability simultaneously and accurately. Observer-based aggregate scoring systems seem to be reliable for the assessment of the clinical aspects of impairment of the elbow. Unfortunately, the variable admixture of clinical and functional criteria and the use of variably defined categorical rankings impair their validity. Patient-completed functional questionnaires can be valid and reliable instruments for the assessment of the shoulder and elbow and are not limited by observer bias.

Assessing Outcomes Measures

A wide variety of outcomes measures are available. Because most clinicians will use an outcomes measure both as an initial assessment tool and as a method of determining a patient's progress over time, the initial selection of an appropriate outcomes measure is important. The measurement properties of different instruments should be assessed to be certain of the accurate appraisal of outcomes. Outcomes measurements may have varying strengths depending on the population being assessed or the reason for their use. The selection of an outcomes measure must be context-specific and should be based on evidence that the instrument has the necessary measurement properties in the population being sampled for a study or assessment. The quality of an outcomes measure can be assessed objectively, and, given the plethora of outcomes measures that have been developed, it is advisable to use an outcomes measure for which there are data on its measurement properties. The measurement properties of an outcomes measure that are important to clinicians are validity, reliability, and responsiveness.

TABLE 3 | Distribution of Categorical Ranking in Five Elbow Scoring Systems

Instrument	Distribution of Categorical Rankings (%)				
	Failed	Poor	Fair	Good	Excellent
The Hospital for Special Surgery	25	16	28	21	11
Ewald et al	NA*	42	33	13	12
Pritchard	NA	14	NA	41	45
Broberg and Morrey	NA	26	39	16	18
Mayo Elbow Performance Index	NA	21	21	38	20

*NA = not applicable

(Reproduced with permission from Turchin DC, Beaton DE, Richards RR: Validity of observer-based aggregate scoring systems as descriptors of elbow pain, function, and disability. J Bone Joint Surg Am 1998;80:154-162.)

Validity

Conceptually, an instrument is considered valid if it measures what it is supposed to measure. Different terms are used to describe different facets of validity. Face validity, in which the items (questions) chosen appear to make sense to the subject using the instrument, is the simplest but weakest form of validity. Content validity is satisfied when it is proved that the scale measures all important aspects of the condition to be examined. Construct validity is the degree to which an outcomes measure can be shown to be associated with other measures that have a specific relationship with the system being measured. Testing of construct validity builds confidence in an outcomes measure. Comparison of the data generated by the outcomes measure with patient- and physician-derived assessments of the severity of the impairment, the level of pain, the ability to perform normal activities of daily living, and the responses on other contemporary patient-completed questionnaires can be used to test construct validity. Convergent validity determines whether an outcomes measure correlates with similar scales or dimensions of a scale. Divergent validity demonstrates lack of correlation between dissimilar scales or dimensions of a scale. Discriminant validity is the ability of an outcomes measure to discriminate across the levels of severity for a patient population.

A variety of statistical measures are used in determining validity, including the Pearson product-moment correlation coefficient. A detailed discussion of the methodology of determining validity is beyond the scope of this chapter.

Reliability

Reliability is the degree to which repeated administration of a measurement tool on stable subjects will yield the same results. Shoulder and elbow outcomes instruments should be sufficiently reliable that the score derived from the use of the outcomes measure is the same when the questionnaire is completed on different occasions, providing that there has been no change in the patient's clinical condition for the problem being measured. Reliability is determined by statistical techniques such as the one-way, random effects intraclass correlation coefficient; the two-way analysis of variance to determine the intraclass correlation coefficient; and Spearman rank correlation coefficients (Fig. 3). Clinicians also can assess the percentage of subjects having identical scores and the number of patients whose responses have moved from one category to another between testing.

Responsiveness

Responsiveness is the ability of an instrument to detect true changes in patient status beyond random variability. Some authors believe that responsiveness is the most important property of health status evaluation instruments. Knowing the responsiveness of an instrument helps the investigator select appropriate outcomes measures and estimate the sample size required to assure adequate statistical power. Responsiveness is assessed by defining a cohort of patients whose health condition probably has changed between testing. For instance, patients with advanced rotator cuff disease or glenohumeral osteoarthritis could be compared before and after rotator cuff repair or total shoulder arthroplasty.

To determine responsiveness, the difference between the preoperative and postoperative scores (change score) is determined. A statistical measure called the

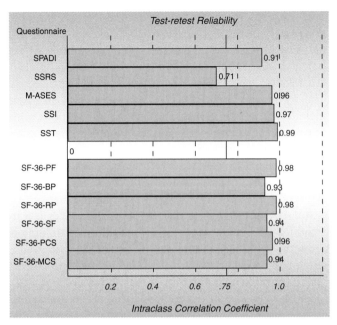

Figure 3 Graph comparing the reliability of five different joint-specific shoulder questionnaires and the SF-36. All of the outcomes measures meet the acceptable level (0.75 intraclass correlation coefficient), with the exception of the Subjective Shoulder Rating Scale (SSRS). *(Reproduced with permission from Beaton D, Richards RR: Assessing the reliability and responsiveness of 5 shoulder questionnaires.* J Shoulder Elbow Surg *1998;7:565-572.)*

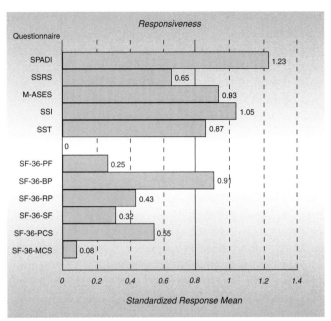

Figure 4 Standardized response means of five different joint-specific shoulder outcomes instruments and the SF-36 in patients who stated that they had improved between testings. The vertical line is the lower limit of what is considered by Cohen to indicate a "large" response. As a general rule, the joint-specific questionnaires are more responsive than the SF-36. *(Reproduced with permission from Beaton D, Richards RR: Assessing the reliability and responsiveness of 5 shoulder questionnaires.* J Shoulder Elbow Surg *1998;7:565-572.)*

standardized response mean (mean change score divided by the standard deviation of the change scores) can be used to assess the relative responsiveness of questionnaires. The standardized response mean transforms the change score into a standard unit of measure allowing comparison among different instruments. The standardized response mean has been used frequently to assess the relative responsiveness of various health status instruments for assessment of the impact of musculoskeletal conditions (Fig. 4). A higher standardized response mean indicates greater sensitivity to clinical change. Cohen's standard has been used by investigators in this field to compare the responsiveness of outcomes measures.

A number of other indices have been used to assess the relative responsiveness of self-administered questionnaires. Other statistical measures include the effect size (mean change score divided by the standard deviation of the initial scores), relative efficiency (squared ratio of *t* statistic), Guyatt's responsiveness statistic (clinically important difference divided by variability in stable subjects), and correlation with external criteria. The magnitude of a responsiveness statistic can vary depending on the time that has elapsed (3-month scores are likely to be lower than 6-month scores) or the type of procedure that was performed (different treatments have different effects). Differences in responsiveness statistics should not be considered by themselves to

indicate the quality of a particular instrument because such statistics must be reviewed in the context of the patient group being tested.

Specific Outcomes Instruments

Generic Outcomes Instruments

As described earlier, the SF-36 measures eight health concepts: physical functioning (10 items), social functioning (two items), role limitations due to physical problems (four items), role limitations due to emotional problems (three items), mental health (five items), energy and fatigue (four items), bodily pain (two items), and general health perception (five items). A number of studies have assessed the reliability, validity, and responsiveness of the SF-36 for upper extremity conditions. Concern has been expressed that the SF-36 physical functioning dimension lacks upper limb content. The SF-12, an abbreviated version of the SF-36, has been developed, although its measurement properties have not been as well defined for musculoskeletal disorders.

Joint-Specific Instruments for the Shoulder

The measurement properties of several outcomes measures designed specifically for the shoulder have been described (Tables 2 and 3). The American Shoulder and Elbow Surgeons (ASES) Standardized Assessment

Form Shoulder Score Index was developed in 1994. The instrument consists of a patient self-assessment section and a clinician assessment section. An advantage of the activities of daily living section and the pain scale is ease of administration. The patient self-assessment section of the ASES form can be completed independently of an examiner or by telephone interview.

The Shoulder Pain and Disability Index (SPADI) was introduced in 1991. This outcomes instrument uses a 100-point system, incorporating visual analog scales for all items. The Simple Shoulder Test (SST) developed at the University of Washington consists of 12 functional items and does not directly assess pain, range of motion, or strength. Two of the questions relate to pain, seven to function, and three to range of motion. The response to each item requires either a yes or a no. The dichotomous scale of the SST provides excellent reliability but may constrain its use as an evaluative instrument.

The University of California, Los Angeles (UCLA) End-Result Score was first used in 1986. It is a 35-point scale including 10 points for pain, 10 points for function, five points for active forward elevation, five points for strength and forward elevation, and five points for patient satisfaction. The data are reported in terms of categorical rankings. The scale has been criticized because it uses descriptive items for pain and function. Furthermore, the inclusion of patient satisfaction makes it difficult to use the scale before treatment. When using the scale, it is best to report numeric results and avoid use of the categorical rankings.

The University of Pennsylvania Shoulder Score uses two 100% scoring systems based on patient self-assessment and objective measures of range of motion and strength. There are three pain scales, a patient satisfaction scale, and a self-assessment of function.

The Constant Score is a 100-point scoring system in which 35 points are derived from the patient's reported pain and function and the remaining 65 points are allocated for assessment of range of motion and strength. Age- and gender-matched normative data are available for the Constant Score. The Constant Score has been criticized for having only one pain scale and for including a nonstandardized strength test as part of the instrument. Because a large portion of the Constant Score is derived from objective measures, patients who are unable to return to the clinic will be lost to follow-up, which may lead to incomplete data collection.

Joint-Specific Outcomes Measures for the Elbow

Several elbow scoring systems are in general use (Tables 2 and 3), none of which assesses function exclusively. The systems assess pain, function, range of motion, stability, deformity, and strength to varying degrees. Most

outcomes studies performed using these systems report the results in terms of categorical rankings, which immensely impairs the usefulness of these systems. Much better comparative information would be available if the results were reported in terms of aggregate scores. The recently described ASES Elbow Evaluation Form includes patient and physician assessment sections, with the patient evaluation section containing visual analog scales for pain and a series of questions relating to function of the extremity.

The system of the Hospital for Special Surgery has a simple format. The cost of administering the instrument is low because the only necessary equipment is a 5-lb weight, a 2-lb weight, and a goniometer. Little training is required by the examiner, and the use of the system in a clinic is practical. Stability of the elbow is not included in the testing. The scaling is ordinal and is done easily.

The Ewald system has a clear format. The associated costs are low because only a goniometer is needed. Little training is required to administer the system, which can be used in a clinic, but it is difficult to assess valgus and varus deformity in patients who have flexion contractures. Neither strength nor stability is included in the Ewald scale, and motion is assessed only in terms of flexion and extension. The scaling is ordinal, pain is weighted heavily, and motion is weighted lightly.

The Pritchard system can be confusing, particularly with regard to scoring of range of motion. Several weights are required to administer the system, although little training is needed and the system is suitable for use in a clinic. The system does not assess function, deformity, or stability. Pain is weighted heavily, and the score is ordinal.

The system of Broberg and Morrey has a clear format, and the cost of the necessary equipment is low. Little training is required to administer the system, and it is suitable for use in a clinic. Deformity is not included in the content, the scaling is ordinal and done easily, and the weighting of the domains seems reasonable.

The Mayo Elbow Performance Index has a clear format. The associated costs are low because only a goniometer is required. Little training is needed, and the system is suitable for use in a clinic. Neither strength nor deformity is included in the content of the scale, and motion is assessed only in terms of flexion and extension. The scaling is ordinal, and function and motion are weighted less heavily than pain.

Limb-Specific Outcomes Instruments

The DASH questionnaire was developed as an instrument that would measure the impact on function of a wide variety of musculoskeletal conditions affecting the upper limbs. The multidisciplinary group that developed the DASH designed the instrument to quantify disability (predominately physical function) and symptoms in individuals with upper limb disorders. The DASH is a 30-item questionnaire with two optional modules to measure the impact of a disorder when playing a musical instrument or sport or when working. Respondents circle one of five responses, and the score is transformed to a 0 to 100 scale. A higher score indicates greater disability. Normative data are currently being gathered for the DASH. The 30-item questionnaire includes 21 physical function items, six symptom items, and three social/role function items; the sports and performing arts modules have four items. The development and recommended use of the DASH is outlined in a detailed user's manual.

Another limb-specific instrument is the modified version of the ASES Standardized Shoulder Assessment Form (M-ASES) developed by Beaton and Richards. These authors added five questions to the original joint-specific questionnaire to assess patients with any type of upper extremity diagnosis, rather than only shoulder-related conditions. Studies have shown this limb-specific questionnaire to be valid, reliable, and responsive.

Future Developments

Standardization of outcomes assessment has been called for by various authors because it would facilitate communication among investigators, clinicians, health care administrators, and the general public. Comparison and pooling of data across studies and the conduct of multicenter trials would be encouraged by the standardization of outcomes assessment. Much work remains to be done in determining the most appropriate outcomes measures for various purposes. More comparative studies are needed to be able to recommend one instrument over another. For instance, in a study of outcomes after surgical treatment for recurrent posterior shoulder instability, a disease-specific measure for shoulder instability was found to be the most responsive, followed by a joint-specific measure and a limb-specific measure (DASH), although the differences were not statistically significant. However, the DASH was easier to score than the other two measures and would allow for comparison between studies if it were widely used. The SF-36 was not responsive to change in this patient population. Further work is needed to complete investigation of the measurement properties of a number of outcomes instruments in specific patient populations.

Summary

Ideally, an outcomes instrument measures phenomena that are directly relevant to a patient and provides a comprehensive assessment of the impact of a condition on a patient's daily life. Although subjective complaints may be difficult to quantify, pain and disability may be the most valid outcomes measures because they are directly relevant to patients. Self-administered questionnaires, which are not subject to observer bias, have been shown to be more responsive than traditional physical measures such as range of motion, strength, dexterity, and sensation. Comparisons between studies based on different scoring systems are generally not valid, and the categorical rankings of different systems are not interchangeable. When categorical rankings are used, the data should also be reported in terms of aggregate scores. In general, both generic and joint-specific measures of health status should be used when assessing function of the shoulder and elbow. The role of limb-specific and disease-specific instruments is evolving at this time. The use of patient-completed functional questionnaires should allow and possibly encourage the comparison of results from different studies.

Annotated Bibliography

Beaton DE, Richards RR: Measuring function of the shoulder: A cross-sectional comparison of five questionnaires. *J Bone Joint Surg Am* 1996;78:882-890.

This study reports on a prospective comparison of the validity of five questionnaires used in the assessment of shoulder function. The questionnaires (SPADI, SST, Subjective Shoulder Rating Scale, M-ASES Shoulder Patient Self-Evaluation Form, and the Shoulder Severity Index) performed similarly in describing function of the shoulder and in discriminating between levels of severity. The shoulder questionnaires performed differently than the SF-36, confirming the need to use both disease-specific and generic health status measures to assess the shoulder.

Beaton D, Richards RR: Assessing the reliability and responsiveness of 5 shoulder questionnaires. *J Shoulder Elbow Surg* 1998;7:565-572.

This study reports on a prospective comparison of five different shoulder questionnaires and the SF-36 in a sample of patients with shoulder pain. All the shoulder questionnaires had acceptable reliability ratings and measured responsiveness more effectively than did the SF-36. Both types of questionnaires should be used in outcomes evaluations.

Chipchase LS, O'Connor DA, Costi JJ, Krishnan J: Shoulder impingement syndrome: Preoperative health status. *J Shoulder Elbow Surg* 2000;9:12-15.

Eighty-one patients with chronic shoulder impingement syndrome resistant to conservative treatment completed a generic (SF-36) and a shoulder-specific (SST) questionnaire. The patient scores were found to be significantly lower in all health dimensions of the SF-36 than those of the normal population. The results of the SST demonstrated that the patients were functionally very limited, particularly in being unable to work full time at their usual job and being unable to lift a weight over their head.

Conboy VB, Morris RW, Kiss J, Carr AJ: An evaluation of the Constant-Murley shoulder assessment. *J Bone Joint Surg Br* 1996;78:229-232.

The authors analyzed the Constant-Murley (1987) assessment for 25 patients with shoulder pathology. The instrument was easy to use but imprecise in repeated measurements. There was a ceiling effect (most scores at the maximum) in patients with shoulder instability, suggesting that this instrument may not measure disability accurately in these patients.

Gartsman GM, Brinker MR, Khan M, Karahan M: Self-assessment of general health status in patients with five common shoulder conditions. *J Shoulder Elbow Surg* 1998;7:228-237.

Before undergoing treatment, 544 patients with five common shoulder conditions completed the SF-36 health survey. Comparison with published data demonstrated that the severity of the shoulder conditions was comparable in rank to that of five major medical conditions: hypertension, congestive heart failure, acute myocardial infarction, diabetes mellitus, and clinical depression.

King GJ, Richards RR, Zuckerman JD, et al: A standardized method for assessment of elbow function: Research Committee, American Shoulder and Elbow Surgeons. *J Shoulder Elbow Surg* 1999;8:351-354.

This report concerns the adoption of a standardized method of assessment for the elbow. The method consists of a patient evaluation section containing visual analog scales for pain and a series of questions relating to function of the extremity. The responses are scored on a four-point ordinal scale. The physician assessment section includes motion, stability, strength, and physical findings. The authors suggest that the adoption of a standardized method of outcomes assessment would stimulate multicenter studies and improve communication among professionals who assess and treat patients with elbow disorders.

Kirkley A, Griffin S, McLintock H, Ng L: The development and evaluation of a disease-specific quality of life measurement tool for shoulder instability: The Western Ontario Shoulder Instability Index (WOSI). *Am J Sports Med* 1998;26:764-772.

The authors developed a disease-specific quality of life measurement tool for patients with shoulder instability. The steps included identification of a specific patient population, item generation, item reduction, and pretesting. The final instrument had 21 items and was tested for validity, reliability, and responsiveness. The responsiveness of the instrument compared favorably with that of five other shoulder outcomes instruments, a general health outcomes measure, and measurement of range of motion. The authors suggest that their instrument be used as a primary outcomes measure in patients with shoulder instability.

L'Insalata JC, Warren RF, Cohen SB, Altchek DW, Peterson MG: A self-administered questionnaire for assessment of symptoms and function of the shoulder. *J Bone Joint Surg Am* 1997;79:738-748.

The authors developed a self-administered questionnaire to assess symptom severity and function of the shoulder. Their instrument has separate domains including global assessment, pain, daily activities, recreational and athletic activities, work, satisfaction, and areas for improvement. Each domain is graded separately and weighted to arrive at the total score. The self-administered shoulder questionnaire was found to be valid, reliable, and responsive to clinical change.

McKee MD, Yoo DJ: The effect of surgery for rotator cuff disease on general health status: Results of a prospective trial. *J Bone Joint Surg Am* 2000;82:970-979.

The general health status of 71 patients who underwent open acromioplasty and subacromial bursectomy was assessed preoperatively and postoperatively. The preoperative SF-36 scores were significantly below normative data for the domains of physical function ($P = 0.02$), role function-physical ($P = 0.001$), and pain ($P = 0.003$). Postoperatively, the scores for pain ($P = 0.0001$), role function-physical ($P = 0.06$), and vitality ($P = 0.01$) improved. The authors concluded that surgery for chronic rotator cuff disease reliably and significantly improved general health status.

Turchin DC, Beaton DE, Richards RR: Validity of observer-based aggregate scoring systems as descriptors of elbow pain, function, and disability. *J Bone Joint Surg Am* 1998;80:154-162.

Five different elbow-scoring systems were used to evaluate the same group of patients. There was a remarkable lack of concordance with regard to the aspects of elbow function that were discussed. Only slight to moderate correlation between the systems was observed when the systems were compared on the basis of categorical rankings. Good correlation was observed when the systems were compared based on raw scores. Comparisons between studies based on different scoring systems are not valid, and the categorical rankings of different systems are not interchangeable.

Classic Bibliography

Broberg MA, Morrey BF: Results of delayed excision of the radial head after fracture. *J Bone Joint Surg Am* 1986;68:669-674.

Codman EA: *The Shoulder, Rupture of the Supraspinatus Tendon and Other Lesions In or About the Subacromial Bursa*. Boston, MA, Thomas Todd, 1934.

Ellman H, Hanker G, Bayer M: Repair of the rotator cuff: End-result study of factors influencing reconstruction. *J Bone Joint Surg Am* 1986;68:1136-1144.

Ewald FC, Scheinberg RD, Poss R, Thomas WH, Scott RD, Sledge CB: Capitellocondylar total elbow arthroplasty. *J Bone Joint Surg Am* 1980;62:1259-1263.

Pritchard RW: Total elbow arthroplasty, in *Joint Replacement in the Upper Limb*. London, England, Mechanical Engineering Publications, 1977, p 67.

Chapter 42

Regional Anesthesia for Shoulder Surgery

Alan Buschman, MD

Jeffrey L. Swisher, MD

Introduction

Regional anesthetic blockade is a technique in which major nerve roots, trunks, or branches are blocked by the well-placed injection of local anesthetics. Because major peripheral nerves are easy to access, many orthopaedic procedures are particularly well suited for regional block, either alone or in combination with general anesthesia. Surgery on the shoulder and the upper arm represents an excellent opportunity to take advantage of the benefits of regional anesthesia.

Although regional anesthesia has been used for more than 100 years, training in its use has been lacking in many US anesthesia programs. This issue has been addressed extensively in the literature. A recent survey found that although 97.8% of US anesthesiologists use some regional anesthetic techniques in their practice, relatively few use peripheral nerve blocks. Of the anesthesiologists surveyed, 59.7% performed fewer than five nerve blocks per month, demonstrating the need for increased exposure to peripheral nerve blocks.

This chapter focuses on the rationale for the use of regional blockade for shoulder and upper arm surgery. Traditional blocks are described, as well as what is new and emerging in this field. The goal is to familiarize the orthopaedic surgeon with techniques believed to offer major advantages over a general anesthetic from the standpoint of surgical stability, postoperative recovery, and pain relief.

Benefits and Reliability of Regional Anesthesia

The benefits of regional anesthesia can be both direct and indirect. They include improved surgical and perioperative outcome and cost efficiencies. Improved outcomes are due primarily to superior postoperative pain relief and decreased reliance on postoperative narcotics, decreased time of hospital stay, and more rapid and effective postoperative physical therapy. Cost efficien- cies may result from shorter surgical times because an efficiently delivered regional anesthetic decreases both induction time (time before the patient is ready for surgery) and emergence time (time before the patient is ready to leave the operating room). In addition, time in the postanesthesia care unit and total hospitalization time are decreased because of the patient's greatly diminished postoperative pain and increased level of alertness. Finally, regional anesthesia requires a coordinated care plan from the surgeon, anesthesiologist, and the operating room nursing staff, which results in a better informed and educated patient and higher hospital satisfaction scores.

A primary concern of many orthopaedic surgeons is that administration of regional anesthetics takes extra time and, therefore, delays surgery, but the opposite is in fact the case. In a supportive operating room environment, manned by experienced individuals, regional anesthesia causes minimal to no delays in surgical start times. In many circumstances, total surgery time actually is reduced because less time is required for emergence from anesthesia. When a block provides the only anesthetic, the patient can be moved immediately to the recovery room after application of dressings. When a combination of regional and general anesthesia is used, the emergence time is shorter because only a minimal amount of general anesthetic is needed to keep the patient asleep; the analgesic requirements are met by the block. The patient emerges quickly, and analgesia continues into the postoperative period. Factors that facilitate support of regional anesthesia vary from institution to institution and may include a preoperative block room, which is a separate room in which blocks are initiated before the patient enters the operating room; extra help in the operating room; experienced anesthesia technicians; and preoperative patient education.

Numerous studies have assessed the success rate of regional anesthetics. Experienced practitioners report interscalene block success rates, ie, adequate intraopera-

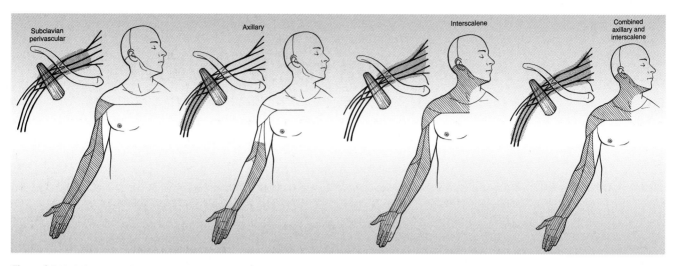

Figure 1 Typical distribution of local anesthetic solution and sensory patterns after injection at various points. *(Reproduced with permission from Urmey WF: Upper extremity blocks, in Brown DL (ed):* Regional Anesthesia and Analgesia. *Philadelphia, PA, WB Saunders, 1996, pp 254-278.)*

TABLE 1	Recommendations for Major Nerve Blocks and Maximum Local Anesthetic Doses in 70-kg Adult			
Local Anesthetic	Dose (mL)	Maximum Dose, (mg) Without Epinephrine	Maximum Dose, (mg) With Epinephrine	Duration of Analgesia (h)
Ester-linked				
Cloroprocaine 2%	40 to 50	800	1,000	1.5 to 3
Amide-linked				
Prilocaine 1.5%	40 to 55	500	600	1.5 to 3
Lidocaine 1.5%	40 to 55	400	500	2 to 4
Mepivicaine 1.5%	40 to 55	400	500	3 to 5
Bupivicaine 0.5%	40 to 50	175	225	9 to 11
Ropivicaine 0.5%	40 to 50	225	225	9 to 11
Levobupivicaine 0.5%	40 to 50	300		9 to 11*

*Data at present indicate duration similar to bupivicaine

tive or postoperative analgesia, ranging from 95% to 98%. To achieve these success rates, a thorough understanding of surface and deep anatomy, nerve physiology, and local anesthetic pharmacology, as well as regional anesthesia technique, is needed. Success also depends on preoperative preparation of the patient by the surgeon, including a discussion regarding anesthesia techniques, possible complications or side effects, and postoperative pain management.

Choice of Regional Block

In general, the type of surgical procedure should determine the choice of block (Fig. 1). Surgery of the shoulder or elbow requires that local anesthetic be injected more proximally in the brachial plexus, ie, by an interscalene, supraclavicular, subclavian perivascular, or coracoid approach. Although elbow surgeries can be performed successfully with an axillary block, an interscalene block is preferable when possible. For surgical procedures on the forearm and hand, the local anesthetic is injected more distally in the brachial plexus, ie, an axillary, forearm, wrist, or Bier block. After the point of injection is chosen, the choice of local anesthetic and its volume and concentration are critical for block success (Table 1).

Before the selection of a regional anesthetic, a full

review of the patient's history and physical examination is required to ascertain whether the patient is an appropriate candidate. An allergy to a particular local anesthetic agent should be investigated. Most reported allergies to local anesthetics are actually reactions either to epinephrine or to a preservative in the multiuse local anesthetic preparations. When patients report having experienced palpitations and tachycardia after the use of local agents during a dental procedure, the actual cause often is the rapid uptake of epinephrine caused by the extremely high concentration of epinephrine (1:10,000) in the agents used for dental anesthesia. In these patients, any type of agent is acceptable. If a patient reports that a rash or swelling developed following local anesthesia, then a reaction to the preservative or local anesthetic agent should be investigated. A list of contraindications to regional anesthesia is provided in Table 2.

The block most commonly used at this time for shoulder surgery is the interscalene brachial plexus block. The techniques, complications, and choice of local anesthetics described in this chapter are important guidelines for interscalene blocks as well as many other nerve blocks.

Interscalene Brachial Plexus Block

The interscalene block is indicated for surgery of the upper extremity and shoulder. It can be used for hand surgery, although it usually requires supplemental ulnar nerve blockade because incomplete blockade of the C8 and T1 roots (medial cord of the plexus) is common. Compared with the classically described supraclavicular block, the interscalene approach is farther from the subclavian artery and the cupola of the lung, reducing the risk of subclavian injury or pneumothorax. However, because of the close proximity of the carotid and vertebral arteries as well as the epidural and subarachnoid spaces, hematoma formation or central neuraxial blockade is a risk. Moreover, the presence of the stellate ganglion, the phrenic nerve, and the recurrent laryngeal nerve in the same anatomic area as the brachial plexus usually leads to a temporary Horner's syndrome, hoarseness, and ipsilateral diaphragm paralysis (Fig. 2).

Administration

Two people are preferred to administer an interscalene block. This two-person technique leaves the anesthesiologist free to use two hands: one hand to locate the interscalene groove, and the other hand to control/stabilize the block needle (Fig. 2). The anesthesiologist stands either at the patient's head or on the side receiving the block. The head should be turned toward the contralateral shoulder with the neck in neutral or a slightly extended position. The assistant helps with injection of the local anesthetic and feels for motor responses. If the patient is placed in a

TABLE 2	Contraindications to Regional Anesthesia

Allergy to local anesthetic agent

Deep sedation prior to block placement

General anesthesia prior to block placement

Uncooperative patient due to age, language, mental status

Patient refusal

Local infection, active septicemia

Local neoplasm

Abnormal anatomy

Neurologic deficit

Coagulopathy

Warfarin, heparin, antiplatelet agents

Severe respiratory compromise

Vocal cord lesions on contralateral side

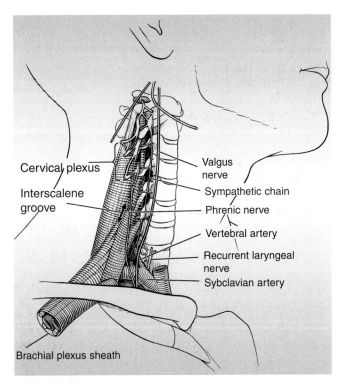

Figure 2 Elongated brachial plexus and surrounding structures. *(Reproduced with permission from Urmey WF: Upper extremity blocks, in Brown DL (ed): Regional Anesthesia and Analgesia. Philadelphia, PA, WB Saunders, 1996, pp 254-278.)*

slightly reverse Trendelenburg position, the external jugular vein will be less distended. Having the patient elevate the head against slight resistance helps to identify the lateral border of the sternocleidomastoid muscle. Posterior to the lateral border of this muscle, the interscalene groove is formed by the anterior and medial scalene mus-

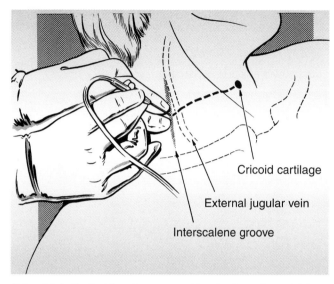

Figure 3 Palpating the interscalene groove and inserting the needle to administer an interscalene block. *(Reproduced with permission from Bridenbaugh LD: The upper extremity: Somatic blockade, in Cousins MJ, Bridenbaugh PO (eds): Neural Blockade in Clinical Anesthesia. Philadelphia, PA, Lippincott, 1988, pp 387-416.)*

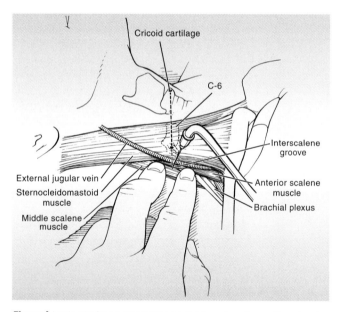

Figure 4 Landmarks for needle placement into interscalene groove. *(Reproduced with permission from Urmey WF: Upper extremity blocks, in Brown DL (ed): Regional Anesthesia and Analgesia. Philadelphia, PA, WB Saunders, 1996, pp 254-278.)*

cles. The anesthesiologist can determine that this is the correct groove by tracing it to the clavicle; the interscalene groove runs to the middle third (Fig. 3). Sandwiched between the interscalene muscles and the prevertebral fascia are the roots and the trunks of the brachial plexus. The superior portion of the interscalene groove will be palpable at the level of C6. This spot can be identified at the same coronal plane as the cricoid cartilage. A small skin wheal is raised at this level, between the two scalene

muscles, and a short-beveled 4-cm × 22-gauge needle or a 22-gauge nerve stimulator needle is inserted perpendicular to the skin (Fig. 4).

The needle should be inserted in a direction that avoids unintentional entry into the epidural or spinal space: medial, 45° caudal, and at a slight dorsal angle. In a thin patient, the nerves of the plexus are located within several millimeters of the skin at this level, so the needle should be advanced slowly, millimeter by millimeter (Fig. 5).

Proper placement of the needle is confirmed by the patient report of a paresthesia in the shoulder, arm, or hand. A paresthesia occurs when the tip of the needle physically stimulates the nerve bundle. A paresthesia may be elicited by contacting nerve fibers at the proximal end in the root or the trunk or more distally in the terminal branches. Paresthesias are extremely reliable indicators of end point in the location of specific nerves. To avoid damaging the nerve, a specifically designed short-beveled needle always should be used for nerve blocks. There is controversy, however, over the safety of this method because it is possible for the needle tip to enter the nerve bundle and cause damage to individual fascicles. The literature is not definitive on this matter, and many authors advocate this use of paresthesias as the safest and most reliable way to obtain peripheral nerve blockade.

The use of a peripheral nerve stimulator is another method by which proper placement can be determined. Required equipment includes a constant current generator (nerve stimulator) and an insulated needle. The principle is that of an electric circuit. A positive reference electrode is applied to the patient, and the stimulating electrode is attached to an insulated needle. The needle is insulated so that current is delivered only at the tip of the needle rather than along its length. These needles are available in a variety of gauges and lengths. Typically, the shorter needles are 20 to 24 gauge, whereas the longer needles are 18 to 20 gauge. For an interscalene block, a 22-gauge, 50-mm needle is most appropriate. The nerve stimulator is set at 2 mA, and the amperage is slowly decreased so that a motor response from the deltoid, upper arm, or forearm is elicited at 0.5 mA or less. The assistant should palpate the arm to differentiate between localized neck and scapular contractions and arm movement from deltoid, biceps, triceps, or brachioradialis contractions. Too-anterior needle placement causes diaphragmatic contraction (phrenic nerve), and too-posterior placement yields trapezius motion (spinal accessory nerve). A blind or deep injection should not be made, because such injections increase the risk of central neuraxial blockade and/or intravascular injection. If paresthesia is encountered during placement of the needle, the anesthesiologist can either switch to a paresthesia technique or redirect the needle and continue using the nerve stimulator technique.

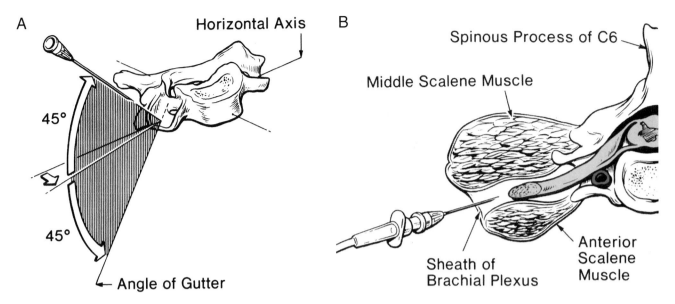

Figure 5 Needle direction for interscalene block in relation to spine **(A)** from anterolateral view and **(B)** from above. *(Reproduced with permission from Bridenbaugh LD: The upper extremity: Somatic blockade, in Cousins MJ, Bridenbaugh PO (eds): Neural Blockade in Clinical Anesthesia. Philadelphia, PA, Lippincott, 1988, pp 387-416.)*

After confirmation of an upper arm motor response at less than 0.5 mA, the syringe is aspirated to test for intravascular or subarachnoid injection. The next step is to test for intraneural needle placement by injecting 1 mL of local anesthetic. An intraneural injection will produce lancinating pain; the needle should be withdrawn slightly. This is followed by administration of anesthetic in 5-mL increments until 40 to 50 mL has been injected (Table 1).

Volume of Anesthetic

Whether using a paresthesia technique or a nerve stimulator, the response during the placement of the needle will be from a small portion of a nerve plexus. To anesthetize the entirety of the plexus requires the appropriate volume of local anesthetic to spread evenly around the plexus. A number of authors have advocated using lower volumes of anesthetic and directing the flow of the local anesthetic during injection with either digital pressure for interscalene block or even a tourniquet for axillary block. Several investigators have attempted to determine whether this is a successful strategy. Most have failed to demonstrate an increase in the extent or the quality of block. It is also possible that excessive pressure applied to the neck in the vicinity of the interscalene groove will result in bradycardia or even asystole as a result of pressure on the carotid sinus. Thus, using a larger volume of anesthetic is the preferred method to improve the rate of successful blocks and increase duration of postoperative pain relief.

Precautionary Measures

Care should be taken to avoid systemic toxicity by using the following precautionary measures: careful aspiration for blood, incremental injection of local anesthetic, and addition of a small amount of epinephrine (eg, 1:200,000 or 1:400,000 concentration). Epinephrine serves three important functions. First, it can be used as an indicator of intravascular injection. Even with frequent aspiration, intravascular injection is still possible. By adding 2.5 to 5 mg/mL epinephrine to the local anesthetic, intravascular injection will result in immediate tachycardia and hypertension. As little as 1 mL (2.5 mg of epinephrine) injected into the vascular system can show a response. If aspiration for blood is negative but an increase in heart rate is noted, the injection is stopped immediately. Stopping the injection can avert a massive local anesthetic toxic reaction. A second reason for epinephrine is to achieve local vasoconstriction, which decreases the rate of systemic absorption and increases block duration by up to 50%. The final advantage of epinephrine is that it increases the amount of anesthetic required to reach toxicity (Table 1). When systemic absorption is slowed, peak blood levels are lowered, thereby enhancing patient safety.

Whenever large volumes of local anesthetic are used, it is important to consider patient weight. Toxic doses are calculated for adults weighing 70 kg; smaller doses should be used for children and small adults under 70 kg.

Complications and Side Effects

Local anesthetic toxicity from unintended intravascular injection (either arterial or venous) or toxicity from sys-

TABLE 3 | Complications of Regional Anesthesia

Complication	Pathophysiologic Effect
Common to all Types of Regional Anesthesia	
Intravascular injection	CNS and cardiovascular compromise
Local anesthetic overdose	CNS and cardiovascular compromise
Nerve trauma, hematoma	Motor and sensory deficit
Particular to Interscalene Brachial Plexus	
Phrenic nerve block	Decreased ventilatory capacity, dyspnea
Laryngeal nerve block	Ipsilateral vocal cord palsy, hoarseness
Stellate ganglion block	Horner's syndrome
Pneumothorax	Dyspnea, hypoxemia
Spinal or epidural injection	Spinal anesthetic, respiratory compromise, bradycardia, hypotension
Sitting position hypotension	Hypotension and bradycardia

temic absorption after block placement is a risk common to all regional anesthetics. Some authors advocate performing blocks with a nerve stimulator while the patient is under general anesthesia and deeply sedated. However, a conscious patient is the best defense against both intraneural or intravascular injection. Historically, most of the case reports involving nerve injuries have been for patients who have been deeply sedated or receiving general anesthesia. Local anesthetic toxicity initially manifests itself as central nervous system (CNS) impairment and, subsequently, cardiovascular toxicity. The initial CNS symptoms are sensory changes, which include lightheadedness, dizziness, difficulty focusing, mental confusion, tinnitus, circumoral numbness, shivering, muscle twitching, and tremors. At higher blood levels, generalized tonic-clonic convulsions occur.

The cardiovascular system is more resistant than the CNS to the effects of local anesthetic drugs. For this reason, higher blood levels are required for cardiovascular responses. Initially, the anesthesiologist should see increased sympathetic tone from the excitatory CNS phase, which causes hypertension and tachycardia. As local anesthetic blood levels increase, myocardial and vascular depression are displayed as conduction changes, decreased cardiac output, vasodilation, and hypotension. If blood levels continue to increase, bradycardia, ventricular arrhythmias, and ultimately cardiovascular collapse occur.

Interscalene blocks have also been shown to cause ipsilateral phrenic nerve blockade, which results in transient unilateral diaphragmatic paralysis. This effect is seen in nearly 100% of patients, and the rate is not diminished with lower injectant volumes, lower local anesthetic concentrations, or addition of digital pressure to prevent upward spread. Pulmonary functional residual capacity is reduced an average of 35%. Generally, this reduction in functional residual capacity has little clinical relevance; however, the condition of patients who have preexisting pulmonary disease with diminished pulmonary reserves may become worse. If a general anesthetic with positive pressure ventilation is used, this effect may not be seen until the postoperative period, when the patient is extubated and breathing spontaneously. Inappropriate patient selection can lead to intraoperative hypoxemia or postoperative respiratory insufficiency with the need for postoperative mechanical ventilation.

Patient positioning is important. The sitting or beach chair position is associated with bradycardia and hypotension in approximately 20% of patients with shoulder problems who are given regional anesthesia. As noted previously, Horner's syndrome is an almost universal complication associated with interscalene blocks, as is recurrent laryngeal nerve block and subsequent hoarseness. The application of a neural block at the neck carries with it the risk of pneumothorax, vertebral artery injection, spinal or epidural anesthesia, and airway compromise from hematoma formation or bilateral recurrent nerve blockade. Complications such as intraneural injection, hematoma formation, and local anesthetic allergic reaction should be considered because they are common to all types of regional anesthesia (Table 3).

Intraoperative Neurologic Complications

Fortunately, neurologic complications after shoulder surgery are rare. However, there is an intrinsic risk resulting from patient positioning, surgical approach, retraction, infection, hematoma, and direct neurologic injury, with the rate of complications varying with the procedure. For total shoulder arthroplasty, the brachial plexus injury rate is approximately 2.8%.

Patients undergoing open shoulder procedures should have an appropriate preoperative review of the risks for axillary or musculocutaneous neurapraxias. Anesthesiologists also should review the risks of nerve injury due to regional anesthesia.

When surgical neurologic injury is suspected, a systematic evaluation of the patient is essential, as well as a thorough review of the techniques used during both the administration of anesthetic and the surgical procedure. It is often helpful to order a prompt neurologic consultation. Electromyography and nerve conduction studies often can locate the injury to a central plexus or a more peripheral site, but these studies may not show definitive results until 3 weeks after surgery.

Although idiopathic brachial plexitis (IBP) is not a complication of interscalene block, it is a neurologic disease of the shoulder and may be included in the differential diagnosis for postoperative neurologic dysfunction. IBP also has been called brachial plexus neuropathy, multiple neuritis, acute brachial radiculitis, localized nontraumatic neuropathy, neuralgic amyotrophy, and paralytic brachial neuritis. The annual incidence of IBP has been reported to be 1.64 per 100,000 people. It is characterized by brachial pain, followed by patchy atrophy of the shoulder girdle and arm muscles. Many cases reported in the literature are described as occurring spontaneously and not necessarily associated with surgery. Those that are associated with surgery have mostly been reported following general anesthesia rather than regional anesthesia and after procedures as diverse as hysterectomies and appendectomies. Following surgery, the patient appears to recover all or most neurologic function, then rapid functional deterioration develops.

Patients with IBP often have severe pain similar to that of reflex sympathetic dystrophy, followed by the onset of motor deficits. Electromyographic studies may reveal an asymmetric involvement of the brachial plexus, and 30% of patients may also have involvement on the contralateral side. Aside from obvious etiologies such as direct nerve trauma, little has been proven to implicate interscalene blocks. To evaluate a suspected case of IBP, electromyography and nerve conduction studies are helpful.

Determination of Block Success

One of the finer points in providing skillful regional anesthesia is the ability to determine quickly whether a given block will be successful for the indicated surgery. In most cases, within a minute or two after injection of the faster-acting local anesthetics (eg, lidocaine, mepivacaine), loss of pinprick or temperature sensation or the inability of the patient to raise his or her arm should indicate a successful block. The loss of temperature sensation is an early indication of a successful block, and once enough time has elapsed the deep sensory and motor blocks will appear. If a surgical procedure is to be performed under light sedation, a rapid-acting local anesthetic is advised. The longer-acting local anesthetics can require 30 minutes or more to take full effect. These longer-acting agents often are used for postoperative pain management; if they are used for intraoperative anesthesia, heavy sedation or a general anesthetic will be required to start an operation expeditiously.

Combined Regional and General Anesthesia

For many orthopaedic procedures such as arthroscopies, it is possible and even desirable to provide minimal sedation in addition to the regional anesthetic block. For major surgery of the shoulder, such as a total arthroplasty or repair of a humeral fracture, combining the block with a light general anesthetic may be preferred. Regional anesthesia is combined with general anesthesia for major shoulder surgery for a number of reasons: (1) Often, the patient's head must be immobilized for a prolonged period. This immobilization can lead to patient restlessness and fatigue. (2) Use of the long-acting anesthetic 0.5% bupivacaine with either 1:200,000 or 1:400,000 epinephrine provides postoperative pain relief for a minimum of 10 hours, but at the expense of a slower onset time. The addition of a general anesthetic allows the surgeon to begin operating immediately and gives patients long-lasting postoperative pain relief, no intraoperative recall, and rapid awakening at the end of surgery. (3) If management of the patient's airway is an issue, the anesthesiologist may choose to intubate the patient with a laryngeal mask airway or an endotracheal tube. Although it is possible to convert a patient who has been sedated to general anesthesia after surgery has begun, the confined space of the shoulder drapes makes this quite difficult. (4) Newer general anesthetics such as propofol and the shorter-offset inhalational agents do not cause prolonged postoperative sedation and produce minimal nausea. Therefore, the addition of a general anesthetic has little to no effect on the benefits of the regional anesthetic such as prolonged pain relief, diminished incidence of urinary retention and nausea, and shorter hospitalization time.

Postoperative Brachial Plexus Blocks: Infusions and Adjuvants

There has been much interest in ongoing postoperative brachial plexus blockade through the use of local anesthetic infusions or local anesthetic mixed with a variety of helper medications called adjuvants. Primary among the reasons for this interest is the desire to extend pain relief further into the postoperative period in order to provide patient comfort and, potentially, to avoid other complications associated with prolonged pain. Reasons for postoperative infusions include to provide extremity sympathectomy for replant surgery, to ameliorate high narcotic requirements, to prevent reflex sympathetic dystrophy, and to increase postoperative range of motion and enhance physical therapy.

The addition of companion drugs, or adjuvants, to local anesthetics is an area of active research and debate. The purpose of adjuvants is threefold: (1) to improve analgesia, (2) to prolong anesthetic duration, and (3) to improve the safety of the local anesthetic administration either by reducing the effective dose or by limiting the systemic absorption.

The history of adjuvant usage can be traced to the beginning of the use of local anesthetics in the late 19th century. The first clinically used local anesthetic, cocaine, although effective, proved difficult to use because of its systemic toxicity. Braun conceived of using extracts of the adrenal glands, adrenaline, to provide vasoconstriction and, therefore, decreased systemic absorption. Along with newer and safer synthetic local anesthetics such as procaine, the use of adrenaline provided not only safer anesthesia but also greater duration of anesthetic blockade.

With the discovery of the endorphins and their endogenous receptors in the CNS, significant changes occurred in the use of adjuvants for local anesthetics. In 1979, Wang demonstrated that small doses of morphine given by spinal injection provided prolonged and effective analgesia. Subsequently, it has become routine anesthetic practice to add opiates such as morphine and opioids such as fentanyl or sufentanil to local anesthetics to both enhance and prolong the analgesia of central neuraxial blockade. In addition to opiates, several other classes of agents have been tried in this manner, such as α-2 agonists (clonidine, dexmetatomidine), acetylcholinesterase inhibitors (neostigmine), and N-methyl-D-asparate antagonists (ketamine). Most of these have met with variable success, typically because of an undesirable side effect profile.

The success of central neuraxial adjuvants has led to their use in the peripheral nervous system as well. However, aside from the addition of epinephrine to local anesthetics to serve as a test marker for intravascular injection or as a means of limiting intravascular spread, the results obtained have been less promising. Although there are opiate receptors in the periphery, it is less clear that their function is to mediate analgesia; hence, addition of opiates and opioids to local anesthetic solutions in peripheral blocks has not yielded results comparable to those obtained when they are used in central blockades. The use of clonidine for this purpose is slightly more encouraging. Several articles document increased duration of analgesia with the addition of clonidine; however, side effects such as sedation limit the beneficial effect.

Summary

Appropriately administered regional anesthesia can offer patients the latest in medical technology with minimal risk of complications. Rapid detection of toxic local anesthetic reactions from either intravascular injection or excessive dosages is of prime importance. At a minimum, the basic guidelines for the safe application of regional anesthesia include a thorough knowledge of local anesthetic pharmacology, modest premedication with benzodiazepines, the addition of epinephrine, proper monitoring, and incremental injections. Cardiovascular monitoring should start at the very beginning of regional anesthesia,

that is, during the application of a block, and continue well after maximum blood levels are achieved. Resuscitation drugs and equipment should be readily available to treat hypotension, cardiac conduction changes, ventricular fibrillation, or arrest. If seizures or cardiovascular collapse occur, the ability to intubate and ventilate the patient should be immediately available. Any physician who administers regional anesthesia should be familiar with these resuscitative measures because toxicity signs and symptoms can progress in a matter of minutes from minor tinnitus to ventricular arrest.

Regional anesthesia for shoulder surgery has become a mainstay for both surgeons and anesthesiologists. On the horizon are faster- and longer-acting local anesthetics, improved postoperative infusion techniques, and new adjuvants. As perioperative pain management improves, patients show faster postoperative recovery and improved surgical outcome.

Annotated Bibliography

Benefits and Reliability of Regional Anesthesia

D'Alession JG, Rosenblum M, Shea KP: A retrospective comparison of interscalene block and general anesthesia for ambulatory surgery shoulder arthroscopy. *Reg Anesth* 1995;20:62-68.

Patients having shoulder procedures in an ambulatory surgery unit were given either an interscalene block or a general anesthetic. Results showed that patients who received an interscalene block had a decrease in intraoperative time (53 ± 12 versus 62 ± 13 min, $P ± 0.0001$), postanesthesia care unit time (72 ± 24 minutes versus 102 ± 40 minutes, $P = 0.0001$), and unplanned postoperative admissions (0 versus 13, $P = 0.004$).

Ritchie ED, Tong D, Chung T, et al: Suprascapular nerve block for postoperative pain relief in arthroscopic shoulder surgery: A new modality? *Anesth Analg* 1997;84:1306-1312.

Patients undergoing arthroscopic shoulder surgery were given a suprascapular nerve block with 10 mL of 0.5% bupivicaine with 1:200,000 epinephrine. A suprascapular nerve block will anesthetize 70% of the sensory area to the shoulder. Postoperative nausea, pain, and hospital discharge times were reduced.

Silverstein WB, Moin US, Brown AR: Interscalene block with a nerve stimulator: A deltoid response is a satisfactory endpoint for a successful block. *Reg Anesth Pain Med* 2000;25:356-359.

A nerve stimulator was used to guide interscalene blocks in 160 patients. The first motor twitch encountered and subsequent success rates were noted. Sixty-one patients had a biceps response, 54 had a deltoid response, and 45 had a deltoid-biceps combination of motor responses. Only one block, in the deltoid group, failed in the study. A motor response of the shoulder or arm was found to be indicative of a successful block. The overall success rate was greater than 99%. Deltoid innervation

(C5-6) is a more proximal component of the brachial plexus, and the search for more distal paresthesias or motor responses is not necessary and might lead to a higher nerve injury rate.

Interscalene Brachial Plexus Block

Fibuch EE, Mertz J, Geller B: Postoperative onset of idiopathic brachial neuritis. *Anesthesiology* 1996;84:455-458.

A case of idiopathic brachial neuritis (IBN) is reported in an otherwise healthy 44-year-old woman who underwent a diagnostic hysteroscopy, dilation, and curettage. Onset was noted 12 hours postoperatively, and follow-up examinations at 4 weeks and 8 weeks confirmed the diagnosis. The authors hypothesize that the etiology for this case of IBN included autoimmune response after general anesthesia, surgical stress, and the activation of a dormant virus, or spontaneous occurrence. Full resolution of symptoms took 11 months.

Liguori GA, Kahn RL, et al: The use of metoprolol and glycopyrrolate to prevent hypotension/bradycardic events during shoulder arthroscopy in the sitting position under interscalene block. *Anesth Analg* 1998;87:1320-1325.

One hundred fifty patients were anesthetized with interscalene blocks for arthroscopy in the beach chair position. Prospective prophylaxis with metoprolol, glycopyrrolate, or placebo was used to evaluate intraoperative hypotension and bradycardia. Hypotension and bradycardia were seen in 28% of the placebo group, 5% of the metoprolol group, and 22% of the glycopyrrolate group. This reaction may be exacerbated by the increased cardiac contractility from the beta-2 agonism of the epinephrine in the local anesthetic solution and is likely related to the Bezold-Jarisch reflex. Beta blockade therefore decreases the intraoperative incidence of bradycardia and hypotension. Intraoperative hypotension should be treated with fluid loading and vasoconstrictors.

Lynch NM, Cofield RH, Silbert PL: Neurological complications after total shoulder arthroplasty. *J Shoulder Elbow Surg* 1996;5:53-61.

In a study of 417 total shoulder arthroplasties from 1975 to 1989, there were 18 cases of neurologic deficits (in 17 patients) after surgery. Surgical approach can affect the incidence of injury. Patients taking methotrexate had a 57% incidence of neurologic injury.

Pessannante AN: Spinal anesthesia and permanent neurological deficit after interscalene block. *Anesth Analg* 1996;82:873-874.

An interscalene block was placed after the induction of general anesthesia using a nerve stimulator technique. The patient received both an intrathecal and brachial root intraneural injection of local anesthetic. Interscalene blocks should not be placed in overly sedated or anesthetized patients.

Walton JS, Folk JW, Friedman RJ: Complete brachial plexus palsy after total shoulder arthroplasty done with interscalene block. *Reg Anesth* 2000;25:318-321.

A 36-year-old man with juvenile rheumatoid arthritis received an interscalene block with 0.5% bupivicaine and 1:200,000 epinephrine. The patient had a total shoulder arthroplasty, and 24 hours after surgery motor function was absent in the axillary, radial, musculocutaneous, and median nerves. All neurologic deficits had resolved 26 weeks postoperatively. An algorithm for postoperative evaluation and treatment of brachial plexus palsy is presented. The authors suggest that preoperative methotrexate may increase the risk of brachial plexus palsy.

Postoperative Brachial Plexus Blocks: Infusion and Adjuvants

Azad SC, Beyer A, Romer AW, et al: Continuous axillary brachial plexus analgesia with low dose morphine in patients with complex pain syndromes. *Eur J Anesthesiol* 2000;17:185-188.

In this prospective study, nine patients with complex pain syndromes of the arm were treated with morphine at a dosage of 0.16 mg/h (3.84 mg/day) through a continuous axillary brachial plexus catheter. Previously, these patients had taken tramadol orally with poor pain relief. With the morphine treatment, all patients reported improvement of pain while at rest or during physical therapy. No major opioid side effects occurred, and the authors reported that this would be beneficial therapy for patients with regional pain syndrome.

Muittari P, Kirvela O: The safety and efficacy of intrabursal oxycodone and bupivacaine in analgesia after shoulder surgery. *Reg Anesth Pain Med* 1998;23:474-478.

The subacromial bursa was injected with 10 mL of either bupivicaine or oxycodone plus bupivicaine. There was no difference in postoperative relief.

Murphy DB, McCartney CJ, Chan VW: Novel adjuvants for brachial plexus block: A systematic review. *Anesth Analg* 2000;90:1122-1128.

This is an excellent review of adjuvants including opioids, tramadol, clonidine, and neostigmine. Twenty-four studies are summarized. Although an ideal study with clonidine was not found, it is suggested that only clonidine provided significant additional analgesia when the dose was limited to 150 mg. Bradycardia, hypotension, and sedation should be monitored postoperatively.

Summary

Brown DL (ed): *Regional Anesthesia and Analgesia.* Philadelphia, PA, WB Saunders, 1996.

This is a complete text for review of all aspects of regional anesthesia including techniques, local anesthetic drug profiles, complications, risks and benefits, and equipment for injection, monitoring, and resuscitation.

Classic Bibliography

Arnason BG, Ashury AK: Idiopathic polyneuritis after surgery. *Arch Neurol* 1968;8:500-507.

Bazin JE, Massoni C, Bruelle P, et al: The addition of opioids to local anesthetics in brachial plexus block: The comparative effects of morphine, buprenorphine and sufentanil. *Anesthesiology* 1977;52:858-862.

Braun H: ueber den Einfluss der Vitalitat der Gewebe auf die ortlichen und allgemeinen Giftwirkungen local-anasthesirender Mittel und uber die Bedeutung des Adrenalins fur die Localanasthesie. *Arch Klin Chir* 1903;69:541.

Brown AR, Weiss R, Greenberg C, et al: Interscalene block for shoulder arthroscopy: Comparison with general anesthesia. *Arthroscopy* 1993;9:295-300.

Cousins MJ, Bridenbough: *Neural Blockade in Clinical Anesthesia.* Philadelphia, PA, Lippincott, 1988.

Eddie RR, Deutsch S: Cardiac arrest after interscalene brachial plexus block. *Anesth Analg* 1977;56:446-447.

Malamut RI, Marques W, England JD, et al: Postsurgical idiopathic brachial neuritis. *Muscle Nerve* 1994;17:320-324.

Moote C: Abstract: Random double blind comparison of intra-articular bupivacaine and placebo for analgesia after outpatient shoulder arthroscopy. *Anesthesiology* 1994;81:A49.

Stein C: Peripheral mechanisms of opioid analgesia. *Anesth Analg* 1993;76:182-191.

Tsairis P, Dyck PJ, Mulder DW: Natural history of brachial plexus neuropathy. *Arch Neurol* 1972;27:109-117.

Wang JK, Naus LA, Thomas JE: Pain relief by intrathecally applied morphine in man. *Anesthesiology* 1979;50:149-151.

Chapter 43

Clinical Guidelines for Shoulder Pain

Edward Baldwin Self, Jr, MD

Introduction

There is justification for the prevalence of clinical guidelines in medicine today. However, many guidelines are developed by parties outside the medical profession, including government agencies (Centers for Medicare and Medicaid Services), big businesses, and third-party payers (insurance companies), whose goals may be different from the goals of the medical profession. The motivation for many guidelines may be to control costs, rather than to improve quality of care. Too often, these guidelines lack appropriate input from physicians and are not based on scientific methodology. When clinical guidelines have been properly developed with physician input, however, their application can lead to higher quality and more efficient patient care.

A common misconception is that a guideline represents a rigid pathway or standard of care. This is not so. A guideline is not intended to embrace all appropriate methods of treatment, nor does it exclude other appropriate methods of treatment. A guideline is simply a guide, similar to the center line in a highway. It is designed to guide physicians through a sequence or series of diagnostic and treatment decisions toward a care standard or practice pattern that is intended to result in an improved outcome.

A guideline seeks to change particular patterns of practice. From a position on the right side of the tail of the bell-shaped curve representing all practice patterns (Fig. 1, *A*), a shift of the pattern of care to the left (Fig. 1, *B*) will result in both an improved quality of care and an increased number of providers dispensing that care. Thus, both a higher quality of care and a narrower, more efficient pattern of practice are achieved.

Development of Clinical Guidelines

As leading experts in musculoskeletal health care, the American Academy of Orthopaedic Surgeons (AAOS) has affirmed that clinical guidelines should be developed by physicians, with the goal of achieving quality patient care. Guideline development is based on state-of-the-art scientific methodology, through the careful identification, evaluation, and synthesis of the best available scientific evidence, including both current literature and expert consensus opinion. A collaborative approach that uses the expertise of practitioners in both orthopaedic and nonorthopaedic medical specialties reduces bias and increases the validity of the final guideline.

The shoulder pain guidelines developed by the AAOS in conjunction with the American Shoulder and Elbow Surgeons (ASES) were initiated by physicians. They have arisen from recognized medical care issues, including marked geographic variation in practice patterns, the demand for consistent and high-quality patient care, and the desire to control the spiraling costs of medical care. These guidelines seek to improve practice patterns, improve quality of patient care, and improve the cost-effectiveness of care.

Evidence Analysis Workgroups

The AAOS has directed its members, in conjunction with the musculoskeletal specialty societies, to assume a leadership role in guideline development. They are to generate evidence-based guidelines that are founded on the best scientific evidence and expert consensus opinion available.

This guideline development process is a challenging one and involves a significant learning curve regarding the extensive subject of scientific methodology. For this reason, the ASES Evidence Analysis Workgroup functions as a permanent subcommittee of the AAOS Guidelines Committee.

Evidence Analysis Workgroups have been established for eight orthopaedic subspecialties (hand, shoulder and elbow, spine, knee, hip, foot and ankle, pediatrics, and sports medicine). Members of each workgroup collaborate with other appropriate medical specialties and third parties.

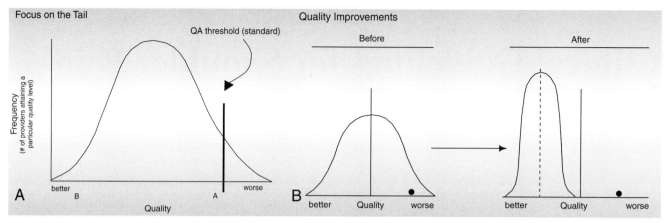

Figure 1 A, This graph represents the frequency of practice patterns of all qualities of care. **B,** This graph represents the effect of improved practice patterns (improved care quality).

Established in 1996, the ASES Workgroup first developed expertise in evidence analysis and scientific methodology. They subsequently have used their expertise to serve as a resource to both the AAOS and the ASES in three distinct areas: (1) guideline development, (2) assessment and critique of guidelines developed by external organizations and agencies, and (3) identification and prioritization of future research needs.

The AAOS Clinical Guideline on Shoulder Pain

The Revised Phase I Shoulder Pain Guideline consists of two elements: The Support Document and the Treatment Algorithm. Both appear at the end of this chapter. This guideline is designed to assist the initial treating physician during the first 4 to 6 weeks of treatment of a new patient with shoulder pain.

The Support Document is a summary text of the guideline. It consists of three sections: overview (including the goals, scope and organization, methodology, literature review, and bibliography), definition of terms relating to the six differential diagnoses of shoulder pain, and recommendations for future research.

The Treatment Algorithm (or flowchart) provides for assessment of information through a comprehensive patient assessment, including history, physical examination, and imaging evaluation (if indicated). It guides the physician through four critical exclusionary diagnoses (including tumor, infection, acute fracture or dislocation, and noncervical referred pain), concluding with the determination of a differential diagnosis. After assessment of the differential diagnosis, the user is then guided through initial treatment and subsequent modifications of treatment. Should further treatment be indicated subsequent to the initial treatment period of 6 to 8 weeks (due to unsatisfactory or incomplete outcome), referral to a shoulder specialist is advised.

The Phase I Shoulder Pain Guideline has been approved by the AAOS Guidelines Committee, the Council on Research, and the Board of Directors.

Guideline Development and Practice

Understanding the science of guideline development allows orthopaedic surgeons in the AAOS and ASES to become actively involved in the guideline evolution process, thereby participating in and reaffirming medical leadership in the establishment of health care policy. This scientifically based process allows physicians to impact the important issues of maximizing quality of care, refining practice patterns, and containing costs. Through this process and by better defining the indications for specialty care, orthopaedists may help to preserve patients' access to such care.

The ASES Evidence Analysis Task Force serves as an important resource to members of both the ASES and the AAOS. This task force creates and maintains protocols for guideline development and revision but also can assess guidelines developed by other organizations and agencies. By this process, future research needs within the AAOS and ASES also can be identified and prioritized.

In view of the importance of informed consent and recent increased involvement by the patient in treatment options and decision making, a well-designed guideline can be used for patient education. It can provide patients with a better understanding of available options (both surgical and nonsurgical) prior to treatment, which should enhance the patients' understanding of both treatment options and possible outcomes.

Guidelines, outcomes, and practice patterns are closely interrelated. Practice guidelines developed using scientific methodology, when combined with analysis of treatment outcomes, promote the evolution and the definition of best practice patterns. Best practice patterns, when followed, result in improved outcomes (Fig. 1, *B*).

The Future

Guideline use and development will improve if certain conditions are met. First, guidelines need to be distributed to and understood by physicians. Internal distribution can occur through the appropriate specialty societies. External dissemination can occur from a listing with the National Guideline Clearinghouse (www.guideline.gov/index.asp), as well as through endorsement by external organizations.

Second, a standard procedure for guideline development, revision, and evaluation needs to be established. This procedure will permit proper evaluation and critique of both guidelines developed by AAOS and those submitted by external organizations.

Finally, the underlying scientific methodology, which determines the strength of a guideline, needs to be further refined. Future research necessary to support guideline recommendations currently based on consensus needs to be identified and carried out.

Summary

The Phase I Shoulder Pain Guideline should be used by initial treating physicians for new patients with shoulder pain. Through the use of such guidelines, physicians have the opportunity to better impact important health care issues, including quality of care, practice patterns, and cost. Finally, the close interrelationship among guidelines, best practice patterns, and outcomes must be understood. Through this process, physicians can refine the need and indications for specialty care and thus help to maintain patients' access to it.

Annotated Bibliography

Barratt A, Irwig L, Glasziou P, et al: Users' guides to the medical literature. XVII: How to use guidelines and recommendations about screening: Evidence-Based Medicine Working Group. *JAMA* 1999;281:2029-2034.

This guide reviews how a physician should assess guidelines on screening, pointing out the importance of weighing the benefits and harms of screening, as well as the values placed on these benefits and harms by different individuals.

Benson K, Hartz AJ: A comparison of observational studies and randomized, controlled trials. *N Engl J Med* 2000;342:1878-1886.

This comparison of treatments is based on observational studies versus those based on randomized, controlled trials documents no significant difference in treatment results between the two groups.

Daum WJ, Brinker MR, Nash DB: Quality and outcome determination in health care and orthopaedics: Evolution and current structure. *J Am Acad Orthop Surg* 2000;8:133-139.

This article is a discussion of the evolution of health care to its current state including the adoption of current industrial economic principles characterized by three elements: the use of practice standards (guidelines), the implementation of continuous quality improvement techniques, and the use of outcome studies.

Drummond MF, Richardson WS, O'Brien BJ, Levine M, Heyland D: Users' guides to the medical literature: XIII. How to use an article on economic analysis of clinical practice. A: Are the results valid?: Evidence-Based Medicine Working Group. *JAMA* 1997;277:1552-1557.

When making recommendations for treatment of large patient groups, physicians must consider not only benefits and risks of treatment, but also whether or not the benefits are worth the resources consumed. Physicians must become knowledgeable regarding economic analyses to be able to make informed resource allocation decisions. This guide assists the physician in this complex area of guideline development and analysis, specifically addressing how to evaluate the validity of the different study methods.

Griffen FD, Fischer JE: Practice guidelines and liability implications. *Bull Am Coll Surg* 1997;82:29-33.

This is a forthright discussion regarding guidelines, including what they are, why they are written, who writes them, and who reads and uses them. The authors are not enamored of practice guidelines, but they emphasize that if guidelines are deemed essential, they must be written with the goal of quality patient care advocacy in mind.

Guyatt GH, Naylor CD, Juniper E, Heyland DK, Jaeschke R, Cook DJ: Users' guides to the medical literature. XII: How to use articles about health-related quality of life: Evidence-Based Medicine Working Group. *JAMA* 1997;277:1232-1237.

Physicians treat patients to prevent future morbidity, to increase longevity, and to make patients feel better. This guide offers advice to the physician regarding measurement of such important issues as the patient experience, including functional, emotional, and social issues.

Jadad AR, Gagliardi A: Rating health information on the Internet: Navigating to knowledge or to Babel? *JAMA* 1998;279:611-614.

With the development of the Internet, information of unprecedented magnitude is available. To obtain both useful and valid information that is credible and applicable requires an understanding of the sources of information as well as how to assess its reliability. This article identifies instruments used to rate various Web sites that provide health information and also rates 47 different rating instruments used to evaluate these Web sites.

National Guidelines Clearinghouse. Available at: http://www.guideline.gov/index.asp.

Developed by the Agency for Health Care Policy and Research in partnership with the American Medical Association and the American Association of Health Plans, the NGC is designed to promote quality health care by making available the latest clinical practice guidelines that are based on scientific evidence, at one location on the Web. This site seeks to enhance health care quality by promoting the dissemination, implementation, and use of clinical practice guidelines based on scientific evidence.

Naylor CD, Guyatt GH: Users' guides to the medical literature. XI: How to use an article about a clinical utilization review: Evidence-Based Medicine Working Group. *JAMA* 1996;275:1435-1439.

Many factors, including quality concerns, patient preference, and cost containment help to determine what treatment physicians provide and how their outcomes are assessed. This guide helps the physician to determine which treatment may be proper for which patient, and how to properly assess a Utilization Review or Clinical Audit.

Stroup DF, Berlin JA, Morton SC, et al: Meta-analysis of observational studies in epidemiology: A proposal for reporting: Meta-analysis of Observational Studies in Epidemiology (MOOSE) group. *JAMA* 2000;283:2008-2012.

Most orthopaedic guidelines are based on observational studies, rather than random, controlled studies with meta-analysis. This article examines the reporting of meta-analysis of observational studies, demonstrating how the proper use of meta-analysis can improve the quality of the observational study itself.

Swiontkowski MF, Buckwalter JA, Keller RB, Haralson R: The outcomes movement in orthopaedic surgery: Where we are and where we should go. *J Bone Joint Surg Am* 1999;81:732-740.

This is a history of the AAOS effort in outcomes study from 1991 to the present.

Classic Bibliography

Amadio PC: Outcome measurements. *J Bone Joint Surg Am* 1993;75:1583-1584.

Eddy DM: Clinical Decision Making: From theory to practice: Anatomy of a decision. *JAMA* 1990;263:441-443.

Eddy DM: Clinical decision making: From theory to practice. Guidelines for policy statements: The explicit approach. *JAMA* 1990;263:2239-2243.

Eddy DM: Clinical decision making: From theory to practice. Principles for making difficult decisions in difficult times. *JAMA* 1994;271:1792-1798.

Eddy DM: Clinical decision making: From theory to practice. The challenge. *JAMA* 1990;263:287-290.

Eddy DM: Comparing benefits and harms: The balance sheet. *JAMA* 1990;263:2493,2498,2501.

Guyatt GH, Rennie D: Users' guides to the medical literature. *JAMA* 1993;270:2096-2097.

Guyatt GH, Sackett DL, Cook DJ: Users' guides to the medical literature: II. How to use an article about therapy or prevention: A. Are the results of the study valid?: Evidence-based Medicine Working Group *JAMA* 1993;270:2598-2601.

Guyatt GH, Sackett DL, Cook DJ: Users' guides to the medical literature: II. How to use an article about therapy or prevention: B. What were the results and will they help me in caring for my patients?: Evidence-based Medicine Working Group. *JAMA* 1994;271:59-63.

Guyatt GH, Sackett DL, Sinclair JC, Hayward R, Cook DJ, Cook RJ: Users' guides to the medical literature: IX. A method for grading health care recommendations: Evidence-Based Medicine Working Group. *JAMA* 1995;274:1800-1804.

Hayward RS, Wilson MC, Tunis SR, Bass EB, Guyatt G: Users' guides to the medical literature: VIII. How to use clinical practice guidelines: A. Are the recommendations valid?: The Evidence-Based Medicine Working Group. *JAMA* 1995;274:570-574.

Jaeschke R, Guyatt G, Sackett DL: Users' guides to the medical literature: III. How to use an article about a diagnostic test: A. Are the results of the study valid?: The Evidence-Based Medicine Working Group. *JAMA* 1994;271:389-391.

Jaeschke R, Guyatt GH, Sackett DL: Users' guides to the medical literature: III. How to use an article about a diagnostic test: B. What are the results and will they help me in caring for my patients?: The Evidence-Based Medicine Working Group. *JAMA* 1994;271:703-707.

Laupacis A, Wells G, Richardson WS, Tugwell P: Users' guides to the medical literature: V. How to use an article about prognosis: Evidence-Based Medicine Working Group. *JAMA* 1994;272:234-237.

Levine M, Walter S, Lee H, Haines T, Holbrook A, Moyer V: Users' guides to the medical literature: IV. How to use an article about harm: Evidence-Based Medicine Working Group. *JAMA* 1994;271:1615-1619.

Lohr KN, Field MJ: A provisional instrument for assessing clinical practice guidelines, in Field MJ, Lohr KN (eds): *Guidelines for Clinical Practice: From Development to Use*. Washington, DC, National Academy Press, 1992; pp 346-409.

Oxman AD, Cook DJ, Guyatt GH: Users' guides to the medical literature: VI. How to use an overview: The Evidence-Based Medicine Working Group. *JAMA* 1994; 272:1367-1371.

Oxman AD, Sackett DL, Guyatt GH: Users' guides to the medical literature: I. How to get started: The Evidence-Based Medicine Working Group. *JAMA* 1993; 270:2093-2095.

Schoenbaum SC, Sundwall DN (eds): *Using Clinical Practice Guidelines to Evaluate Quality of Care*. Rockville, MD, US Dept of Health and Human Services, Public Health Service Agency for Health Care Policy and Research, 1995, vol 1 and 2, AHCPR publication 95-0045.

Schon DA (ed): *The Reflective Practitioner: How Professionals Think in Action*. New York, NY, Basic Books, 1983, pp 241-253.

Wilson MC, Hayward RS, Tunis SR, Bass EB, Guyatt G: Users' guides to the medical literature: VIII. How to use clinical practice guidelines: B. What are the recommendations and will they help you in caring for your patients?: The Evidence-Based Medicine Working Group. *JAMA* 1995;274:1630-1632.

Universe Of Adult Patients With Localized Shoulder Pain Symptoms — Phase I Guideline

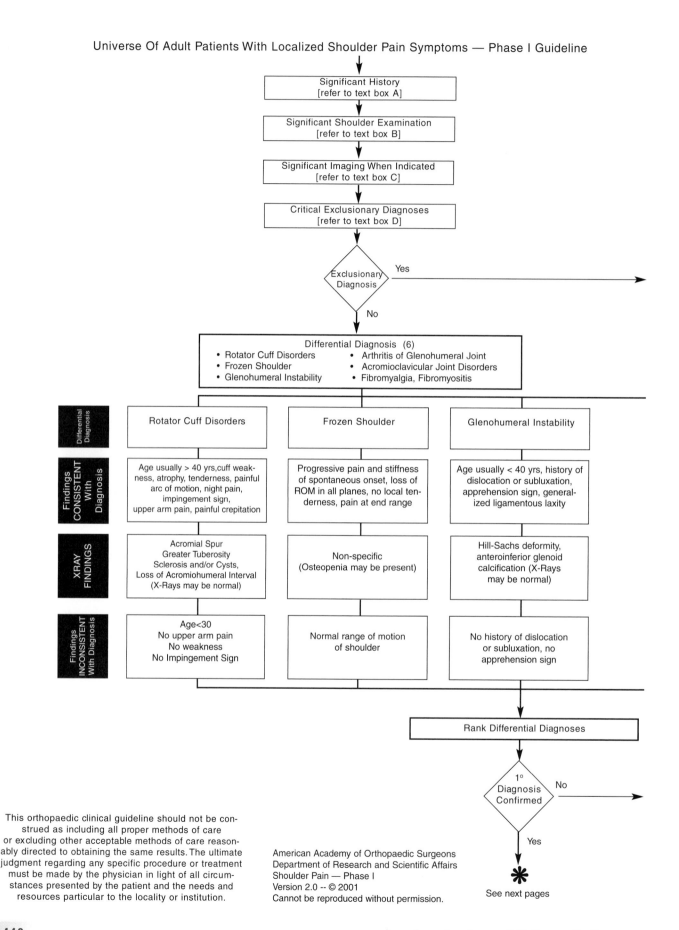

American Academy of Orthopaedic Surgeons
Department of Research and Scientific Affairs
Shoulder Pain — Phase I
Version 2.0 -- © 2001
Cannot be reproduced without permission.

American Academy of Orthopaedic Surgeons

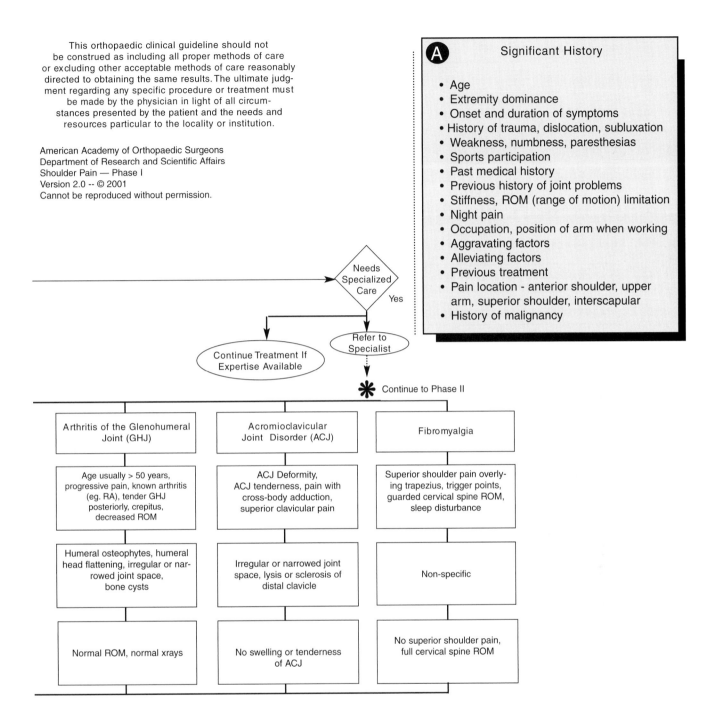

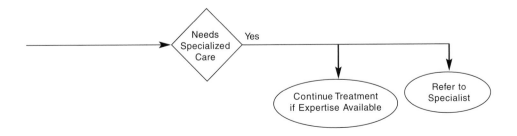

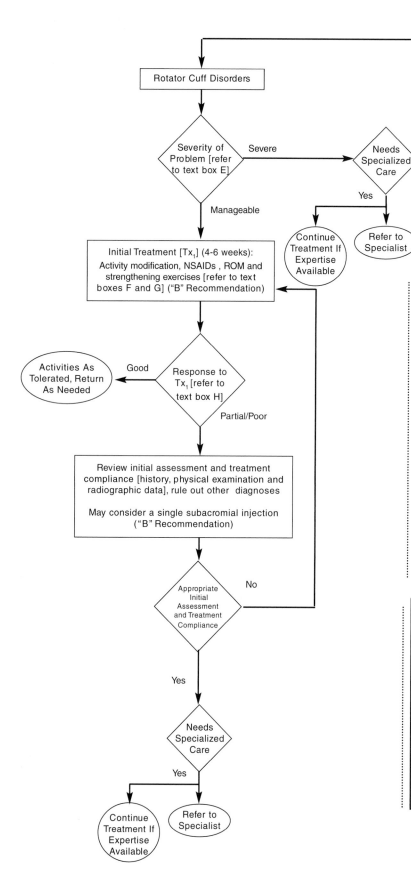

This orthopaedic clinical guideline should not be construed as including all proper methods of care or excluding other acceptable methods of care reasonably directed to obtaining the same results. The ultimate judgment regarding any specific procedure or treatment must be made by the physician in light of all circumstances presented by the patient and the needs and resources particular to the locality or institution.

American Academy of Orthopaedic Surgeons
Department of Research and Scientific Affairs
Shoulder Pain — Phase I
Version 2.0 -- © 2001
Cannot be reproduced without permission.

B Significant Shoulder Examination

- Observation (swelling, atrophy, deformity)
- Tenderness localized to bursa, acromioclavicular joint, glenohumeral joint
- Range of motion (active and passive) in planes of elevation, external rotation, internal rotation, cross body adduction
- Provocative tests for impingement, instability
- Motor and sensory upper extremity assessment
- Non-contributory cervical spine examination
- NB: examination should be bilateral, and each side compared for symmetry
- Distal Upper Extremity Exam

C Initial Imaging

- True AP in 0° external rotation
- Lateral in scapular plane
- Axillary view

When imaging studies are indicated during the initial evaluation and treatment of a patient with shoulder pain, appropriate plain "x-rays" should be obtained. More sophisticated imaging studies (such as shoulder MRI, ultrasound, or arthrography) are not indicated.

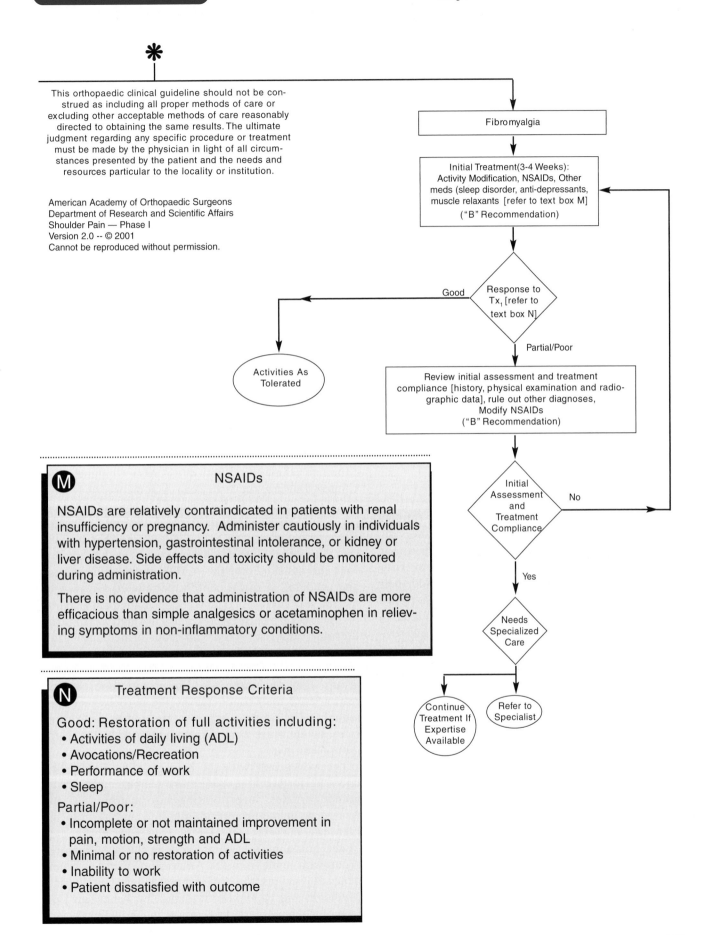

This orthopaedic clinical guideline should not be construed as including all proper methods of care or excluding other acceptable methods of care reasonably directed to obtaining the same results. The ultimate judgment regarding any specific procedure or treatment must be made by the physician in light of all circumstances presented by the patient and the needs and resources particular to the locality or institution.

American Academy of Orthopaedic Surgeons
Department of Research and Scientific Affairs
Shoulder Pain — Phase I
Version 2.0 -- © 2001
Cannot be reproduced without permission.

Fibromyalgia

Initial Treatment(3-4 Weeks):
Activity Modification, NSAIDs, Other meds (sleep disorder, anti-depressants, muscle relaxants [refer to text box M]
("B" Recommendation)

Response to Tx₁ [refer to text box N]

Good

Activities As Tolerated

Partial/Poor

Review initial assessment and treatment compliance [history, physical examination and radiographic data], rule out other diagnoses, Modify NSAIDs
("B" Recommendation)

Initial Assessment and Treatment Compliance

No

Yes

Needs Specialized Care

Continue Treatment If Expertise Available

Refer to Specialist

Ⓜ   NSAIDs

NSAIDs are relatively contraindicated in patients with renal insufficiency or pregnancy. Administer cautiously in individuals with hypertension, gastrointestinal intolerance, or kidney or liver disease. Side effects and toxicity should be monitored during administration.

There is no evidence that administration of NSAIDs are more efficacious than simple analgesics or acetaminophen in relieving symptoms in non-inflammatory conditions.

Ⓝ   Treatment Response Criteria

Good: Restoration of full activities including:
• Activities of daily living (ADL)
• Avocations/Recreation
• Performance of work
• Sleep

Partial/Poor:
• Incomplete or not maintained improvement in pain, motion, strength and ADL
• Minimal or no restoration of activities
• Inability to work
• Patient dissatisfied with outcome

AAOS Clinical Guideline on Shoulder Pain: Support Document

Overview

Goals and Rationale

This clinical guideline has been created to improve patient care by outlining the appropriate information gathering and decision making processes involved in managing shoulder pain in adults. Musculoskeletal care is provided in many different settings by many different providers. This guideline has been created as an educational tool to guide qualified physicians through a series of diagnostic and treatment decisions in an effort to improve the quality and efficiency of care.

This guideline should not be construed as including all proper methods of care or excluding methods of care reasonably directed to obtaining the same results. The ultimate judgment regarding any specific procedure or treatment must be made by the treating physician after a full assessment of all circumstances presented by a patient, including the needs and resources of a particular locality or institution.

Scope and Organization

This document addresses the diagnosis and treatment of localized shoulder pain in skeletally mature individuals, not arising from acute trauma, infection or tumor. Shoulder pain is frequently associated with overuse, especially in athletes and adult patients. Shoulder pain is also many times attributable to complex syndromes, as opposed to a single injury or condition. The increasing elderly population and a more generally active society is responsible for a significant increase in the number of people suffering from localized shoulder pain.

This guideline is intended to address issues faced by first contact physicians only, and provide information through the patient's first 6 to 8 weeks of treatment. This guideline does not address all possible conditions associated with localized shoulder pain, only those that account for the majority of initial visits to a physician. The guideline addresses the following conditions: rotator cuff disorders, frozen shoulder, glenohumeral instability, arthritis of the glenohumeral joint, acromioclavicular joint disorders, and fibromyalgia. The guideline provides the user with information used during the initial assessment of the patient, through several critical exclusionary diagnosis and then on to the determination of a differential diagnosis. Once a differential diagnosis is reached, the user continues on to a flow chart

specific to that diagnosis. Each diagnosis-specific flow chart guides the user through the initial treatment and possible modified treatment. The flow charts end where referral to a musculoskeletal specialist is recommended.

Methodology

Panel

Original authors: Freddie Fu, MD, Chairman, Answorth Allen, MD, Clifford Colwell, MD, Evan Flatow, MD, Keith Watson, MD, John Brems, MD, W. Benjamin Kibler, MD, Jeffrey Saal, MD. Phase I revision panel: Edward Self, MD, Chairman, John Brems, MD, Jeffrey Abrams, MD, Frank Cordasco, MD, Keith Watson, MD, Kenneth Butters, MD.

Process Overview

The guideline was originally developed by a multi-professional panel led by the American Academy of Orthopaedic Surgeons Task Force on Clinical Algorithms in cooperation with the AAOS Committee on Clinical Policies, the American Association of Neurological Surgeons, the American College of Physical Medicine and Rehabilitation, the American College of Rheumatology, as well as individuals in other medical specialties including family practice. The workgroup, with the assistance of the AAOS and various private and academic medical centers, completed a review of the relevant literature. The workgroup then participated in a series of meetings in which information from the literature was extracted and transformed into draft "decision trees." Information from the literature was supplemented by the consensus opinion of the workgroup when necessary. Multiple iterations of written review were then conducted by the participating individuals. Modifications, when supported by references from the literature were then incorporated by the workgroup chairman.

The workgroup, with the help of Value Health Sciences, performed a new literature search, reviewed and graded articles, incorporating information into the revised guideline as appropriate. Information from the literature was supplemented by consensus. The update of the guideline was completed by the AAOS workgroup with input from the American College of Emergency Physicians, the American Academy of Physical Medicine and Rehabilitation, and the American College of Rheumatology. In addition, individual physicians practicing in family medicine, emergency medicine, physical medicine and rehabilitation, rheumatology, and shoulder surgery were asked to participate in a field test of the revised guideline and to submit comments. The workgroup members and specialty society representatives completed an objective evaluation of the 1996 guideline. These evaluations assisted the workgroup in focusing on areas of the guideline that needed expansion or revision.

The revised guideline was reviewed and approved by various groups within the AAOS including the Evidence Analysis Work Group, Guidelines Committee, Council on Research, Board of Councilors, and Board of Directors.

In developing and revising this guideline the original task force and the workgroup made every effort to be consistent with the American Medical Association's (AMA) Attribute of Practice Parameters. In brief, the guideline was developed by a physician's organization with scientific and clinical expertise and it is based on a reliable methodology that integrates science and consensus. It is comprehensive and specific, is based on current information, and will be widely disseminated.

Evaluation of Existing Guidelines

A search of MEDLINE, the National Guidelines Clearinghouse and the AMA's Clinical Practice Guidelines Directory (1999) was performed. Only one relevant guideline was located. The Washington State Medical Society published medical treatment guidelines for use in workers' compensation situations. One guideline "Criteria for Shoulder Surgery" was reviewed by the workgroup.

Literature Review

A search of MEDLINE was performed in order to update the literature used to develop the original guideline. English language journals were searched from 1988 to 2000, human studies of adults over 19 years of age were included. Of the abstracts generated by the search 140 articles were graded by the workgroup and included in the bibliography.

Weighing the Evidence

All literature sited in the bibliography were reviewed and evaluated for quality according to the following categories:

Type I: Meta-analysis of multiple, well-designed controlled studies; or high-power randomized, controlled clinical trial.

Type II: Well-designed experimental study; or low-power randomized, controlled clinical trial.

Type III: Well-designed, nonexperimental studies such as nonrandomized, controlled single-group, pre-

post, cohort, time, or matched case-control series.

Type IV: Well-designed, nonexperimental studies, such as comparative and correlational descriptive and case studies.

Type V: Case reports and clinical examples.

Consensus/Opinion as it is Used in Bibliography

Articles representing expert consensus and not meeting the rigid I to V measurement are noted to represent consensus/opinion.

Consensus Development

The workgroup participated in a series of conference calls and meetings in which information from the literature search was extracted and incorporated into the original algorithm. Information from the literature was supplemented by the consensus opinion of the workgroup when necessary. Multiple iterations of the guideline were then completed and reviewed by workgroup members, ASES leadership, and a multidisciplinary group of physicians selected by workgroup members. Modifications (when supported by references from the literature) were then incorporated by the workgroup chairman.

Strength of Recommendation

The strength of the guideline recommendations for or against an intervention was graded as follows:

A   Type I evidence or consistent findings from multiple studies of types II, III, or IV

B   Types II, III, or IV evidence and findings are generally consistent

C   Types II, III, or IV evidence, but findings are inconsistent

D   Little or no systematic empirical evidence

Revision Plans

The guideline will be reviewed in 2005.

Definition of Terms

Musculoskeletal Specialist: Any licensed medical doctor who has completed a resident training program focused on the management of musculoskeletal conditions, including but not limited to orthopaedists, physiatrists and rheumatologists.

Differential Diagnoses

Rotator Cuff Disorders

Definition of the Problem

Rotator cuff disorders represent that spectrum of pathology (acute and chronic), which result in dysfunction of the rotator cuff. The acute manifestation (any age), may be represented by a painful condition or occasionally by a functional impairment, or both, representing the variances between soft tissue inflammation (minimal structural involvement) and irritation to the extreme of complete cuff avulsion (marked structural involvement). The chronic manifestation (more common over 40 years of age) is often associated with a gradual increase in symptoms, especially in the face of repetitive activity at or above shoulder level. A precise precipitating event is identified by patients in only about one half of the cases. Rotator cuff disease is a quite common cause of shoulder pain in patients over 40, and therefore a high index of suspicion will lead to appropriate evaluation.

Recommendations

The focus of initial evaluation should be determination of the structural integrity of the rotator cuff. Marked inability to raise the arm is an ominous sign and would lead to a high level of concern. However, many patients (even those with substantial structural deficits), will often demonstrate surprisingly good active range of motion. Closer examination is often needed to accurately assess rotator cuff function. Guarding (due to pain) may exaggerate the assessment of rotator cuff injury. Plain radiographs, while helpful in advanced stages, are often unrevealing (but are important to rule out reactive calcific tendinitis which can mimic an acute and severe rotator cuff process), and yet may reveal signs of chronic impingement—subacromial spurring, excrescences at the greater tuberosity. Strength testing of the rotator cuff, testing in active abduction and resisted external rotation (elbow flexed and at the side), will be helpful in assessing single tendon tears from larger tears. However, in the presence of guarding (due to pain), it may be necessary to block the pain (with an injection of local anesthetic into the subacromial space), in order to get a valid test of rotator cuff function.

Differential diagnosis would include calcific tendinitis, cervical radiculitis and viral plexopathy (Parsonage Turner syndrome). When clinical evaluation indicates rotator cuff integrity, treatment should employ (1) avoidance of irritating activity; (2) anti-inflammatory medications if tolerated; (3) exercises to recover and maintain passive range of motion; (4) exercises to strengthen the rotator cuff once acute symptoms are abated ("B" recommendation). If there is minimal or only partial response to the above treatment regimen over several weeks, consideration should then be given to a subacromial injection including a mixture of local anesthetic and a short-acting corticosteroid preparation ("B" recommendation). The above regimen should then be reinstated.

Clinical Outcomes

The majority of patients presenting with rotator cuff disorders will respond favorably to the above program within several weeks. For those who do not respond, attention should be directed toward further accuracy of diagnosis and the possibility of such structural compromise that more specialized care is indicated.

Alternative Approaches

In the severely debilitated and fragile patient who cannot tolerate, nor participate, in the above regimen, it may be necessary to utilize alternative measures for pain control (such as TNS unit, analgesics, topicals, etc), and increased activity modification.

Frozen Shoulder

Definition of the Problem

Frozen shoulder (adhesive capsulitis) is a condition of uncertain etiology characterized by significant restriction of both active and passive shoulder motion that occurs in the absence of another known intrinsic shoulder disorder.

Recommendations

The initial goal in the treatment of patients with idiopathic frozen shoulder or adhesive capsulitis is to provide pain relief. Nonsteroidal anti-inflammatory medications and analgesics are useful for this purpose. Analgesic medications used prior to the therapy will facilitate the performance of these exercises ("B" recommendation). Patients with adhesive capsulitis or idiopathic frozen shoulder should be placed on a physician directed exercise program with the goal of maintaining and regaining range of motion. This program should initially focus on stretching; after motion is regained, strengthening should be instituted ("B" recommendation). Patients who do not respond to this initial treatment over an 8-week period may be referred to an appropriate specialist, as indicated ("B" recommendation). Patients with diabetes and hypothyroidism may require a more prolonged treatment program.

Expected Clinical Results

This program will generally result in improvement in shoulder function and decrease in shoulder pain over time.

Alternative Approaches

No treatment is an alternative approach. There has been some evidence to suggest that at 18 months following the onset of adhesive capsulitis, many patients improve without treatment. However, there can be significant residual impairment even after this amount of time has elapsed.

Glenohumeral Instability

Definition of the Problem

Glenohumeral instability is a common etiology of shoulder pain in the young active patient. Glenohumeral instability occurs when excessive glenohumeral translation produces pain, apprehension, or dysfunction. Pain can be episodic, intermittent, or prolonged. "Apprehension" indicates that the patient avoids positioning the arm in such a way that may reproduce a pain or a fear of dislocation. "Dysfunction" indicates the inability of playing a sport, vocational limitations, or even interference with activities of daily living. Although apprehension and dysfunction may result in the avoidance of pain, they may also result in more restrictive impairment.

Recommendations

Patients with shoulder-related pain are commonly evaluated by family physicians, emergency room staff, rheumatologists, therapists, and orthopaedists. Once exclusionary diagnoses are eliminated (including fracture, tumor, infection, and pain radiating from another area) the shoulder can be further examined as a source of pain.

Evaluation

The first-contact physician should begin the evaluation with an appropriate history. Certain generalizations can be made, but exceptions are not uncommon. Patients are often less than 40 years old and often have had a prior injury. This may include a traumatic dislocation or subluxation. Some patients describe a subjective event that has caused the arm to suddenly "fall asleep," usually not associated with objective neurologic findings—often described as dead arm syndrome (pain induced subjective paresis). Pain can be associated with arm positioning, sporting, or exertional activities, and may be related to overuse. Some patients will describe a painful click that can be reproduced with certain arm movements.

The physical examination is used to reproduce the provocative actions. Certain patients may be able to demonstrate the position that creates pain or apprehension. Patients with apprehension may be unwilling to place the arm in a provocative position. In this instance, if the physician places the arm in the provocative position, the patient will often make a facial grimace or a verbal warning ("apprehension") to avoid this position. Translation testing can be performed in a relaxed patient by centering the humeral head on the glenoid and shifting the head in various directions (anterior, inferior, posterior) to see if it can sublux onto or over the edge. This should be compared to the contralateral extremity to identify discrepancies. Other joints can be

briefly examined to determine a baseline laxity for an individual.

Radiographs can be helpful to identify glenohumeral instability. The initial imaging series (see text box C) may identify changes along the glenoid rim or an impression defect on the humeral head that may result due to instability.

There are several types (categories) of instability a patient may present with. For the purposes of a screening examination to provide initial treatment, the categories include anterior instability, posterior instability, multidirectional instability, and voluntary or habitual instability.

Anterior Instability Anterior is the most common form of glenohumeral instability. This may be the most dramatic form when a patient has presented to an emergency room with the humeral head locked in an anteriorly displaced position in front of the glenoid. When an acute anterior dislocation is reduced, the arm should be placed in a simple sling and the patient should be referred to a specialist. Patients who did not require a reduction, do not demonstrate apprehension, and have minimal pain may proceed to an exercise approach to strengthen the rotators and scapular stabilizers ("B" recommendation). Poor response to this exercise program should result in referral to a specialist.

Should this patient subsequently present with continued symptoms of recurrent anterior glenohumeral instability, symptoms may include pain ('apprehension') when the arm is placed in the provocative "cocked" or throwing position.

Posterior Instability Patients are not always aware of posterior instability but can describe pain associated with activities. Some individuals can demonstrate the subluxation and/or the reduction which was once asymptomatic but now problematic. The provocative position of forward flexion and internal rotation may result in apprehension or pain. The humeral head can be displaced posterior to the glenoid in an acute posterior dislocation. Careful review of x-rays, particularly an axillary and trauma views, should avoid missing this diagnosis. Posterior dislocation should be referred to the specialist for reduction.

Multidirectional Instability Multidirectional instability of the glenohumeral joint occurs when the humeral head subluxates symptomatically in more than one direction (including inferiorly). It is associated with increased translation posterior, anterior, or inferior (creating a 'sulcus sign'). Many of these patients have an atraumatic onset, perform repetitive movements, and demonstrate a similar laxity in the nonpainful extremity. Certain sporting activities such as swimming, gymnastics, and overhead throwing, may produce pain to the predisposed lax shoulder. Activity reduction, temporary sling use for support, and early rotator cuff strengthening may reduce discomfort. If muscular re-education can maintain stability, a long-term approach towards exercises should follow ("B" recommendation). If the response is poor, referral to a specialist is recommended.

Voluntary, Habitual Instability Certain patients voluntarily subluxate or dislocate their shoulder. These patients have minimal pain and may have different motives for seeking medical aid, for example, medications, attention, etc. These patients must be educated to avoid abnormal shoulder posturing. Patients may need additional consultation for behavior modification/psychologic evaluation if condition becomes disabling. The major difference between a habitual subluxater and one who reluctantly demonstrates their abnormal subluxation is the motivation of the patient. There are individuals who have the ability to subluxate their shoulders, but once it becomes painful, wish it to stop. If they are unable to stop subluxating, and seek medical attention, they are not included in this habitual category. Early specialist referral may be warranted.

Other Diagnoses
There may be some overlap with other diagnoses for shoulder pain. Rotator cuff tears may result from a shoulder dislocation, especially in middle-age or older age groups. Patients may demonstrate symptoms of pain, weakness, and dysfunction as a result of a traumatic dislocation due to persisting rotator cuff pathology. In this case, symptoms from both impingement and instability may be evident on physical examination. Further imaging and referral to a specialist is suggested.

Certain patients with a long-standing history of instability may develop joint pain from arthritis. A small percentage of patients with a history of glenohumeral instability may have pain at rest, nighttime pain, and limits to terminal motion. Radiographs may not be diagnostic if early in the disease pattern. Further studies may or may not be of help. Gently stretching programs, nonsteroidal anti-inflammatory medication, heat and/or ice is the initial approach ("B" recommendation). If unsuccessful, consultation with a specialist is recommended.

Expected Clinical Results
Results depend on the type of instability and the age of the patient. Patients with joint laxity and subluxation have a greater chance of success with a nonoperative approach and exercise program, than the young athlete with an acute traumatic injury.

Alternative Approaches
Upon early consultation with a specialist, the patient

may be allowed to complete the season possibly with bracing.

Arthritis of the Glenohumeral Joint

Definition of the Problem
Multiple causes of glenohumeral arthritis exist and attempts should be made to secure a specific cause, for example, cuff arthropathy, arthritis of dislocation, avascular necrosis, part of a systematic disease (rheumatoid arthritis or ankylosing spondylitis), and osteoarthritis.

The shoulder stiffness from arthritis should be separated from that of frozen shoulder by history and physical examination as well as radiographs, and evaluation of the contralateral shoulder. Definition of the problem using evaluation instruments such as SF36 and SST are especially important.

Patients with arthritis of the glenohumeral joint generally are over 50 years of age with progressive pain, crepitus, and decreased range of motion. Radiographs may document head flattening, irregular or narrowed joint space, and bone cysts.

Recommendations
Initial treatment includes activity modification, NSAIDs and physical therapy to maintain motion and strength, but not to aggravate the problem ("B" recommendation). When considering long-term NSAIDs, appropriate lab tests and involvement of the primary care physician for overall medical treatment is indicated. Intra-articular corticosteroid injections are not recommended. No recommendation is made for glucosamine/chondroitin sulfate at this time. On follow-up examination, other diagnoses are again ruled out, compliance reviewed, and the NSAID perhaps changed ("B" recommendation). Specialist referral is indicated if the patient is not improved or with progressive loss of motion.

Shoulder replacement may be indicated in advanced cases of painful glenohumeral arthritis with failed conservative management. Age, activity level, bone, muscles, and tendon quality, and type of arthritis are all factors in deciding whether humeral head alone or the humerus plus glenoid are replaced. Open débridement of the arthritic shoulder is not thought to be helpful.

Expected Clinical Results
Control of pain, maintenance of limited shoulder function and delay in the need for shoulder joint replacement are all expected results of initial treatment.

Alternative Approaches
Intra-articular corticosteroid injections are not recommended. No recommendation is made for glucosamine/chondroitin sulfate or vicsosupplementation.

Acromioclavicular Joint Disorder

Definition of the Problem

Pain or injury involving the acromioclavicular (AC) joint or lateral clavicular region. Although the majority of problems related to this anatomic area are traumatic in origin, some painful conditions may be related to atraumatic diseases.

The skeletally mature patient who presents with an injury to the AC joint (superior shoulder pain) may be seen in an emergency room setting or in a practitioner's office. The individual may be seen by a wide variety of physicians including, family physician, internists, neurologists or orthopaedists. The first contact physician should begin the evaluation with a history and physical examination. Because the majority of injuries to the AC joint are traumatic, radiographic assessment of the shoulder girdle should be considered. What is more controversial is the question of whether weighted radiographic views are necessary or valuable in the diagnosis and treatment of injuries to the AC joint. The weight of the evidence (consensus) suggests such weighted radiographs are not necessary in initial evaluation except as specified below. Critical diagnoses are excluded including fractures or dislocation of the glenohumeral joint, vascular or neurologic injuries and gross deformities of the AC joint region which suggest a high grade injury.

Recommendations

Isolated Osteoarthritis of the AC Joint This clinical condition often manifests itself as a part of the impingement syndrome and rotator cuff disease. Isolated arthritis of this joint is commonly seen as a late sequelae of type II AC joint injuries many years in the past. Patients have difficulty rolling on to their affected shoulder while sleeping and have difficulty reaching across their chest such as is required to cleanse their opposite axilla. Radiographs will demonstrate sclerosis of the lateral aspect of the acromion and hypertrophic spurs on the superior and inferior aspects of both the acromial and clavicular sides of the joint. Treatment should consist of NSAIDs and activity modification specifically diminishing repetitive activities ("B" recommendation). Perpetuation of symptoms should result in referral to a specialist for consideration of injection therapy of other surgical alternatives.

Osteolysis of the Clavicle Osteolysis is a relatively uncommon condition associated with the distal clavicle. Although it is seen in female, it is distinctly more common in males and most often associated with weight lifting activities. In fact it carries the eponym "weight lifter's shoulder." Pain is of insidious onset, and typical of most AC joint pathology, patients complain of pain when rolling onto the affected shoulder while sleeping

or when reaching across their body to reach their opposite axilla. Overhead lifting activities also provoke pain. There is tenderness to direct palpation over the joint and swelling is occasionally discernable. Radiographs are characteristic and usually diagnostic with resorption of the lateral clavicle, widening of the joint space and a tapered appearance of the lateral clavicle. This is a self-limiting condition and rarely if ever requires surgical treatment. Cessation of offending activities, NSAIDs and patient education provide adequate treatment ("B" recommendation). Rarely intra-articular steroids may provide benefit. If symptoms persist beyond three months, referral to the specialist is indicated.

Expected Clinical Results

Many patients who rest the affected arm for two to three weeks and are dedicated to a rehabilitation program which emphasizes recovery of shoulder range of motion and strength can anticipate near full painless function of the limb. Occasionally type II injuries may have residual pain with activity but only very few AC joint injuries find need for surgical intervention. For painful osteoarthritis of the AC joint unresponsive to medical management, surgical excision of the lateral clavicle may be indicated.

Alternative Approaches

Some physicians may recommend earlier arthroscopic management of AC joint injuries. Joint débridement, lateral clavicle excision and open reduction of the chronic AC joint separation remain alternate treatment options. However the long history of satisfactory outcomes from a nonsurgical approach to treatment of AC injuries suggests that the vast majority of these conditions can be successfully treated by the first contact physician.

Fibromyalgia

Definition of the Problem

Fibromyalgia is characterized by the diffuse musculoskeletal pain, often presenting in the shoulder girdle. The definition from a multicenter criteria committee includes widespread pain of at least 3 months duration, including areas about the shoulder, for example, trapezius at the midpoint of upper border and supraspinatus at origins above the scapular spine near the medial border. Multiple trigger points are also present usually with guarded cervical spine motion and fatigue with sleep disturbances. These trigger points are often over the trapezius muscle and near ligament or muscular attachments to the bone. Induration may be present, localized to the tender areas. Muscle strength studies have not shown weakness to conform to the patient's perceived fatigue. Laboratory and radiographic testing are characteristically negative. The cause of fibromyalgia is unknown, but may be related to chronic muscular tension or sleep disturbance, causing chemical abnormalities. Fibromyalgia patients may have clinical depression and may require mental health consultation.

Recommendations

The focus of initial treatment should be on the sleep disturbance with bedtime low-dose tricyclic antidepressants. Suspension of caffeine use has been suggested ("B" recommendation). In addition, activity modification (aerobic exercise) and NSAIDs are advised ("B" recommendation). A follow-up visit at 4 weeks to allow patient reassessment, review the diagnosis, and evaluate patient compliance is necessary. Appropriate specialist care may then be indicated.

Expected Clinical Results

The discomfort associated with fibromyalgia is generally chronic, with waxing and waning symptoms which may be affected by mood changes. Some improvement is expected following explanation of the problem to the patient, and initial treatment.

Alternative Approaches

Naturopathic medicines, DMSO, massage, or chiropractic care may be chosen by the patient for this disease which is often poorly understood by the treating physician.

Rehabilitation

Aerobic exercise may be considered. Ultrasound, electrical stimulation and other modalities are commonly used by therapists but have not been proven to be beneficial.

Future Research Recommendations

The Revision Panel for the Clinical Guideline on Shoulder Pain believes that additional outcome studies, which assess outcomes resulting from the use of specific guidelines are necessary and beneficial. The further refinement and defining of "best practice patterns"—improving the evidence upon which guideline recommendations are based—may then serve as an improved model for further guideline revision and improvement.

The Revision Panel recommends the following three additional studies be designed and initiated at this time, to be designed utilizing best scientific methodology: (1) Indications and Efficacy for Shoulder Rehabilitation (Rotator Cuff and Scapular Stabilizer Strengthening with Restoration of Range of Motion) as Initial Treatment of Shoulder Impingement Syndrome; (2) Indications and Efficacy for Steroid Injection to Treat Patients Presenting with Shoulder Pain; (3) Evaluation and Critique of the AAOS Clinical Guideline of Shoulder Pain—Methods of Dissemination, Application, and Efficacy.

The Revision Panel recommends that the AAOS develop a clinical guideline on acute shoulder injury to address issues related to acute shoulder trauma.

References

Rotator Cuff Disorders

1. Bigliani LU; Cordasco FA; McIlveen S; et al. Operative repair of massive rotator cuff tears: Long-term results. *J Shoulder Elbow Surg* 1992 May/June; 1(3): 120-130. (IV).

2. Bigliani LU; Norris TR; Fischer J; et al. The relationship between the unfused acromial epiphysis and subacromial impingement lesions. *Orthop Trans* 1983; 7(1): 138. (V)

3. Bigliani LU; D'Alessandro DF; Duralde XA; McIlveen SJ. Anterior acromioplasty for subacromial impingement in patients younger than 40 years of age. *Clin Orthop* 1989 Sep;(246):111-6. (IV)

4. Cofield RH. Rotator cuff disease of the shoulder. *J Bone Joint Surg [Am]* 1985 Jul;67(6):974-9. (Consensus/ opinion)

5. Craig EV; Fritts HM Jr; Crass JR. Noninvasive imaging of the rotator cuff. In: Post M, Morrey BF, Hawkins RJ, eds. *Surgery of the shoulder*. Chicago : Year Book Medical Publishers, 1990:(Chap 2) 6-10. (V)

6. Ellman H. Arthroscopic subacromial decompression: a preliminary report. Paper presented at American Shoulder and Elbow Surgeons First Open Meeting. Las Vegas, NV. January 23, 1985. (Consensus/opinion)

7. Ellman H; Kay SP. Arthroscopic subacromial decompression for chronic impingement 2 to 5 year results. *J Bone Joint Surg [Br]* 1991 May; 73(3): 395-8. (V)

8. Goldman AB; Ghelman B. The double-contrast shoulder arthrogram. A review of 158 studies. *Radiology*. 1978 Jun; 127(3): 655-63. (V)

9. Hamada K; Fukuda H; Mikasa M; Kobayashi Y. Roentgenographic findings in massive rotator cuff tears. A long-term observation. *Clin Orthop*. 1990 May; (254): 92-6. (IV)

10. Harryman DT 2d; Mack LA; Wang KY; Jackins SE; Richardson ML; Matsen FA 3d. Repairs of the rotator cuff. Correlation of functional results with integrity of the cuff. *J Bone Joint Surg [Am]*. 1991 Aug; 73(7): 982-9. (IV)

11. Hawkins RJ. Impingement syndrome. *Orthop Trans*, 1979; 3:274. (V)

12. Hawkins RJ; Abrams JS. Impingement syndrome in the absence of rotator cuff tear (stages1 and 2). *Orthop Clin North Am*. 1987 Jul; 18(3): 373-82. (V)

13. Hawkins RJ; Brock RM; Abrams JS; Hobeika P. Acromioplasty for impingement with an intact rotator cuff. *J Bone Joint Surg [Br]* 1988 Nov;70(5):795-7. (V)

14. Lundberg BJ. The correlation of clinical evaluation with operative findings and prognosis in rotator cuff rupture. In: Bayley I, Kessel L, eds. *Shoulder surgery*. Berlin; New York: Springer-Verlag, 1982: (Sect II.1) 35-8. (V)

15. Mack LA; Gannon MK; Kilcoyne RF; Matsen RA 3d. Sonographic evaluation of the rotator cuff. Accuracy in patients without prior surgery. *Clin Orthop*. 1988 Sep; (234): 21-7. (IV)

16. Matsen FA III; Arntz CT. Rotator cuff tendon failure. In: Rockwood CA Jr, Matsen FA III (eds). *The shoulder*. Philadelphia: W.B. Saunders, 1990; 16:647-677. (Consensus/opinion)

17. Matsen FA III, Arntz CT. Subacromial impingement. In: Rockwood CA Jr, Matsen FA III (eds). *The shoulder*. Philadelphia: W.B. Saunders, 1990; 17:678-749. (Consensus/opinion)

18. Neer CS 2d. Anterior acromioplasty for the chronic impingement syndrome in the shoulder: a preliminary report. *J Bone Joint Surg [Am]*. 1972 Jan; 54(1): 41-50. (Consensus/opinion) & (V)

19. Neer CS 2d; Craig EV; Fukuda H. Cuff-tear arthropathy. *J Bone Joint Surg [Am]* 1983 Dec;65(9):1232-44. (V)

20. Neer CS 2d. Impingement lesions. *Clin Orthop*. 1983 Mar; (173): 70-7. (Consensus/opinion)

21. Neviaser RJ; Neviaser TJ. Observations on impingement. *Clin Orthop* 1990 May;(254):60-3. (Consensus/opinion)

22. Neviaser JS. Ruptures of the rotator cuff of the shoulder. New concepts in the diagnosis and operative treatment of chronic ruptures. *Arch Surg*. 1971 May; 102(5): 483-5. (Consensus/opinion)

23. Norwood LA; Barrack R; Jacobson KE. Clinical presentation of complete tears of the rotator cuff. *J Bone Joint Surg [Am]*. 1989 Apr; 71(4): 499-505. (IV)

24. Ogilvie-Harris DJ; Wiley AM; Sattarian J. Failed acromioplasty for impingement syndrome. *J Bone Joint Surg [Br]* 1990 Nov;72(6):1070-2. (V)

25. Post M; Silver R; Singh M. Rotator cuff tear. Diagnosis and treatment. *Clin Orthop*. 1983 Mar; (173): 78-91. (IV)

26. Rockwood CA. The role of anterior impingement syndrome to lesions of the rotator cuff. *J Bone Joint Surg [Br]* 1980 May; 62(2):274-5. (Consensus/opinion)

27. Sherman OH. MR imaging of impingement and rotator cuff disorders. A surgical perspective. *Magn Reson Imaging Clin N Am* 1997 Nov; 5(4): 721-34 (IV)

28. Wasilewski SA; Frankl U. Rotator cuff pathology. Arthroscopic assessment and treatment. *Clin Orthop*. 1991 Jun; (267): 65-70. (IV)

29. Watson M. Rotator cuff function in the impingement syndrome. *J Bone Joint Surg [Br]* 1989 May;71(3):361-6. (IV)

Frozen Shoulder

1. Bridgman JF. Periarthritis of the shoulder and diabetes mellitus. *Ann Rheum Dis*. 1972 Jan; 31(1): 69-71. (IV)

2. Grey RG. The natural history of idiopathic frozen shoulder. *J Bone Joint Surg [Am]* 1978 Jun;60(4):564. (V)

3. Harryman DT 2d; Sidles JA; Clark JM; McQuade KJ; Gibb TD; Matsen FA 3d. Translation of the humeral head on the glenoid with passive glenohumeral motion. *J Bone Joint Surg [Am]* 1990 Oct;72(9):1334-43. (II)

4. Harryman DT 2d; Sidles JA; Harris SL; Matsen FA 3d. The role of the rotator interval capsule in passive motion and stability of the shoulder. *J Bone Joint Surg [Am]* 1992 Jan;74(1):53-66. (II)

5. Murnaghan JP. Frozen Shoulder. In: Rockwood CA Jr, Matsen FA III (eds). *The shoulder*. Philadelphia: W.B. Saunders, 1990; 21:837-62. (IV)

6. Neer CS 2d ; Satterlee CC; Dalsey RM; Flatow EL. The anatomy and potential effects of contracture of the coracohumeral ligament. *Clin Orthop* 1992 Jul;(280):182-5. (III)

7. Neviaser RJ; Neviaser TJ. The frozen shoulder. Diagnosis and management. *Clin Orthop*. 1987 Oct; (223): 59-64. (III)

8. Neviaser TJ: Adhesive capsulitis. *Orthop Clin North Am* 1987;18:439-443. (IV)

9. Neviaser TJ. Arthroscopy of the shoulder. *Orthop Clin North Am*. 1987 Jul; 18(3): 361-72. (IV)

10. Neviaser TJ. Arthrography of the shoulder joint. Study of the findings in adhesive capsulitis of the shoulder. *J Bone Joint Surg [Am]*. 1962 (Oct); 44(7):1321-1330. (IV)

11. Ogilvie-Harris DJ; Wiley AM. Arthroscopic surgery of the shoulder. A general appraisal. *J Bone Joint Surg [Br]* 1986 Mar;68(2):201-7. (IV)

12. Ozaki J; Nakagawa Y; Sakurai G; Tamai S. Recalcitrant chronic adhesive capsulitis of the shoulder. Role of contracture of the coracohumeral ligament and rotator interval in pathogenesis and treatment. *J Bone Joint Surg [Am]* 1989 Dec;71(10):1511-5. (III)

13. Rowe CR; Leffert RD. Idiopathic chronic adhesive capsulitis in frozen shoulder. In: Rowe CR (ed). *The shoulder*. New York: Churchill Livingstone, 1988; 155-163. (IV)

14. Roy, S; Oldham R. Management of painful shoulder. *Lancet*. 1976 Jun 19; 1(7973): 1322-4. (IV)

Glenohumeral Instability

1. Cofield RH; Nessler JP; Weinstabl R. Diagnosis of shoulder instability by examination under anesthesia. *Clin Orthop*. 1993 Jun; (291): 45-53. (IV)

2. Gross ML; Seeger LL; Smith JB; Mandelbaum BR; Finerman GA. Magnetic resonance imaging of the glenoid labrum. *Am J Sports Med*. 1990 May; 18(3): 229-34. (IV)

3. Hawkins RJ; McCormack RG. Posterior shoulder instability. *Orthopedics*. 1988 Jan; 11(1): 101-7. (IV)

4. Jobe FW. Anterior capsulolabral reconstruction. *Techniques Orthop* 1989; 3:29-35. (V)

5. Jobe FW; Giangarra CE; Kvitne RS; Glousman RE. Anterior capsulolabral reconstruction of the shoulder in athletes in overhand sports. *Am J Sports Med*. 1991 Sep; 19(5): 428-34. (IV)

6. McGlynn FJ; Caspari RB. Arthroscopic findings in the subluxating shoulder. *Clin Orthop*. 1984 Mar; (183): 173-8. (IV)

7. Minkoff J; Stecker S; Cavaliere G. Glenohumeral instabilities and the role of MR imaging techniques. The orthopedic surgeon's perspective. *Magn Reson Imaging Clin N Am* 1997 Nov; 5(4): 767-85 (IV)

8. Mok DW; Fogg AJ; Hokan R; Bayley JI. The diagnostic value of arthroscopy in glenohumeral instability. *J Bone Joint Surg [Br]*. 1990 Jul; 72(4): 698-700. (IV)

9. Neer CS II. *Shoulder reconstruction.* Philadelphia: W.B. Saunders, 1990. (IV)

10. Neer CS II; Foster CR. Inferior capsular shift for involuntary inferior and multidirectional instability of the shoulder. A preliminary report. *J Bone Joint Surg [Am]*. 1980 Sep; 62(6): 897-908. (IV)

11. Neer CS II. Involuntary inferior and multidirectional instability of the shoulder: etiology, recognition, and treatment. *Instr Course Lect* 1985;34:232-8. (IV)

12. Nelson MC; Leather GP; Nirschl RP; Pettrone FA; Freedman MT. Evaluation of the painful shoulder. A prospective comparison of magnetic resonance imaging, computerized tomographic arthrography, ultrasonography, and operative findings. *J Bone Joint Surg [Am]*. 1991 Jun; 73(5): 707-16. (IV)

13. Neumann CH; Petersen SA; Jahnke AH. MR imaging of the labral-capsular complex: normal variations. *AJR Am J Roentgenol*. 1991 Nov; 157(5): 1015-21. (IV)

14. Rafii M; Firooznia H; Golimbu C. MR imaging of glenohumeral instability. *Magn Reson Imaging Clin N Am* 1997 Nov; 5(4): 787-809 (IV)

15. Rowe CR. Prognosis in dislocations of the shoulder. *J Bone Joint Surg [Am]* 1956; 38(5):957-77. (IV)

16. Rowe CR; Patel D; Southmayd WW. The Bankart procedure: a long-term end-result study. *J Bone Joint Surg [Am]*. 1978 Jan; 60(1): 1-16. (IV)

17. Thomas SC; Matsen FA 3d. An approach to the repair of avulsion of the glenohumeral ligaments in the management of traumatic anterior glenohumeral instability. *J Bone Joint Surg [Am]*. 1989 Apr; 71(4): 506-13. (V)

18. Tibone J.; Ting A. Capsulorrhaphy with a staple for recurrent posterior subluxation of the shoulder. *J Bone Joint Surg [Am]*. 1990 Aug; 72(7): 999-1002. (V)

19. Turkel SJ; Panio MW; Marshall JL; Girgis FG. Stabilizing mechanisms preventing anterior dislocation of the glenohumeral joint. *J Bone Joint Surg [Am]*. 1981 Oct; 63(8): 1208-17. (IV)

20. Warner JJP; Caborn DM. Overview of shoulder instability. *Crit Rev Phys and Rehab Med* 4(3,4):145-198, 1992. (IV)

21. Warner JJP; Warren RF. Arthroscopic bankart repair using a cannulated, absorbable fixation device. *Oper Tech Orth*, 1:2 (April) 1991:192-198. (V)

22. Wintzell G; Haglund-Akerlind Y; Larsson H; Zyto K; Larsson S. Joint fluid enhancement at MRI of the glenohumeral joint with intravenous injection of gadodiamide in standard and triple dose: a prospective comparative study of stable and unstable shoulders. *Skeletal Radiol* 1998 Feb; 27(2): 87-91 (III)

Arthritis of the Glenohumeral Joint

1. Barrett WP; Franklin JL; Jackins SE; Wyss CR; Matsen FA 3d. Total shoulder arthroplasty. *J Bone Joint Surg [Am]* 1987 Jul;69(6):865-72. (IV)

2. Cofield RH. Degenerative and arthritic problems of the glenohumeral joint. In: Rockwood CA Jr, Matsen FA III (eds). *The shoulder.* Philadelphia: W.B. Saunders, 1990; 17:678-749. (IV)

3. Cofield RH. Total shoulder arthroplasty with the Neer prosthesis. *J Bone Joint Surg [Am]*. 1984 Jul; 66(6): 899-906. (IV)

4. Green A; Norris TR. Imaging techniques for glenohumeral arthritis and glenohumeral arthroplasty. *Clin Orthop* 1994 Oct; (307): 7-17 (IV)

5. Neer CS 2d. Replacement arthroplasty for glenohumeral osteoarthritis. *J Bone Joint Surg [Am]*. 1974 Jan; 56(1): 1-13. (IV)

6. Neer CS 2d; Watson KC; Stanton FJ. Recent experience in total shoulder replacement. *J Bone Joint Surg [Am]* 1982 Mar; 64(3): 319-37. (IV)

7. Ranawat CS; Warren R; Inglis AE. Total shoulder replacement arthroplasty. *Orthop Clin North Am* 1980 Apr; 11(2):367-73. (IV)

8. Walch G. Primary glenohumeral osteoarthritis: Clinical and radiographic classification. *Acta Orthopedica Belgica* 1998; 64: 11 (IV)

Fibromyalgia

1. Chee EK; Walton H. Treatment of trigger points with microamperage transcutaneous electrical nerve stimulation. *J Manipulative Physiol Ther* 1986 Jun; 9(2): 131-4 (II)

2. Gam AN; Warming S; Larsen LH; Jensen B; Hoydalsmo O; Allon I; Andersen B; Gotzsche NE; Petersen M; Mathiesen B. Treatment of myofascial trigger-points with ultrasound combined with massage and exercise – a randomized controlled trial. *Pain* 1998 Jul; 77(1): 73-9 (II)

3. Gartsman GM; Brinker MR; Khan M; Karahan M. Self-assessment of general health status in patients with five common shoulder conditions. *J Shoulder Elbow Surg* 1998 May/Jun; 7(3): 228-37 (IV)

4. Mannerkorpi K; Svantesson U; Carlsson J; Ekdahl C. Tests of functional limitations in fibromyalgia syndrome: A reliability study. *Arthritis Care Res* 1999 Jun; 12(3): 193-9 (IV)

5. Norregaard J; Bulow PM; Lykkegaard JJ; Mehlsen J; Danneskiold-Samsoe B. Muscle strength, working capacity and effort in patients with fibromyalgia. *Scand J of Rehabil Med* 1997 Jun; 29(2): 97-102 (IV)

6. Simms RW; Goldenberg DL; Felson DT; Mason JH. Tenderness in 75 anatomic sites. Distinguishing fibromyalgia patients from controls. *Arthritis Rheum* 1988 Feb; 31(2): 182-7 (V)

7. Treadwell BL. Fibromyalgia or the fibrositis syndrome: a new look. *N Z Med J* 1981 Dec 23; 94(698): 457-9 (V)

Physical Therapy

1. Beckerman H; Bouter LM; van der Heijden GJ; de Bie RA; Koes BW. Efficacy of physiotherapy for musculoskeletal disorders: what can we learn from research? *Br J Gen Pract* 1993 Feb; 43(367): 73-7 (V)

2. Gam AN; Johannsen F. Ultrasound therapy in musculoskeletal disorders: a meta-analysis. *Pain* 1995 Oct; 63(1): 85-91 (II)

3. Green S; Buchbinder R; Glazier R; Forbes A. Systematic review of randomized controlled trials of interventions for painful shoulder: selection criteria, outcome assessment, and efficacy. *BMJ* 1998 Jan 31; 316(7128): 354-60 (II)

4. Levoska S; Keinanen-Kiukaanniemi S. Active or passive physiotherapy for occupational cervicobrachial disorders? A comparison of two treatment methods with a 1-year follow-up. *Arch Phys Med Rehabil* 1993 Apr; 74(4): 425-30 (III)

5. Parker RD; Seitz WH Jr. Shoulder impingement/instability overlap syndrome. *J South Orthop Assoc* 1997 Fall; 6(3): 197-203 (IV)

6. van der Heijden GJ; van der Windt DA; de Winter AF. Physiotherapy for patients with soft tissue shoulder disorders: a sustematic review of randomized clinical trials. *BMJ* 1997 Jul 5; 315(7099): 25-30 (II)

7. Winters JC; Sobel JS; Groenier KH; Arendzen HJ; Meyboom-de Jong B. Comparison of physiotherapy, manipulations, and corticosteroid injection for treating shoulder complaints in general practice: randomized, single blind study. *BMJ* 1997 May 3; 314(7090): 1320-5 (II)

Magnetic Resonance Imaging

1. Blanchard TK; Mackenzie R; Bearcroft PW; Sinnatamby R; Gray A; Lomas DJ; Constant CR; Dixon AK. Magnetic resonance imaging of the shoulder: assessment of effectiveness. *Clin Radiol* 1997 May; 52(5): 363-8 (III)

2. Boutin RD; Weissman BN. MR Imaging of arthritides affecting the shoulder. *Magn Reson Imaging Clin N Am* 1997 Nov; 5(4): 861-79 (Consensus/opinion)

3. Curtis RJ. Magnetic resonance imaging (letter; comment). *Ann Rheum Dis* 1991 Jan; 50(1): 66 (Consensus/opinion)

4. Deutsch AL; Klein MA; Mink JH; Mandelbaum BR. MR Imaging of miscellaneous disorders of the shoulder. *Magn Reson Imaging Clin N Am* 1997 Nov; 5(4): 881-95 (Consensus/opinion).

5. Ertl JP; Kovacs G; Burger RS. Magnetic resonance imaging of the shoulder in the primary care setting. *Med Sci Sports Exerc* 1998 Apr; 30(4 suppl): S7-11 (Consensus/opinion)

6. Fischbach TJ; Seeger LL. Magnetic resonance imaging of glenohumeral instability. *Top Magn Reson Imaging* 1994 Spring; 6(2): 121-32 (Consensus/opinion)

7. Gold Rh; Seeger LL; Yao L. Imaging shoulder impingement. *Skeletal Radiol* 1993 Nov; 22(8): 555-61 (Consensus/opinion)

8. Goodwin DW; Pathria MN. Magnetic resonance imaging of the shoulder. *Orthopedics* 1994 Nov; 17(1): 1021-8 (Consensus/opinion)

9. Harryman DT 2d; Mack LA; Wang KY; Jackins SE; Richardson ML; Matsen FA 3d. Repair of the rotator cuff. Correlation of functional results with integrity of the cuff. *J Bone Joint Surg [Am]* 1991 Aug; 73(7): 982-9 (IV)

10. Herzog, RJ. Magnetic Resonance Imaging of the Shoulder: Instructional Course Lectures, The American Academy of Orthopaedic Surgeons. *JBJS*. 1997 June; 79-A(6): 934 (III)

11. Ho CP. Applied MRI anatomy of the shoulder. *J Orthop Sports Phys Ther* 1993 Jul; 18(1): 351-9 (Consensus/opinion)

12. Iannotti JP; Zlatkin MB; Esterhai JL; Kressel HY; Dalinka MK; Spindler KP. Magnetic resonance imaging of the shoulder. Sensitivity, specificity, and predictive value. *J Bone Joint Surg [Am]* 1991 Jan; 73(1): 17-29 (III)

13. Iannotti JP. Evaluation of the painful shoulder. *J Hand Ther* 1994 Apr-Jun; 7(2): 77-83 (Consensus/opinion)

14. Kieft GJ; Sartoris DJ; Bloem JL; Hajek PC; Baker LL; Resnick D; Obermann WR; Rozing P; Doornbos J. Magnetic resonance imaging of glenohumeral joint diseases. *Skeletal Radiol* 1987; 16(4): 285-90 (V)

15. Meyer SJ; Dalinka MK. Magnetic resonance imaging of the shoulder. *Orthop Clin North Am* 1990 Jul; 21(3): 497-513 (Consensus/opinion)

16. Needell SD; Zlatkin MB; Sher JS; Murphy BJ; Uribe JW. Magnetic resonance imaging of the rotator cuff: peritendinous and bone abnormalities in an asymptomatic population. *Am J Roentgenol* 1996 Apr; 166(4): 863-7 (IV)

17. Neumann CH; Holt RG; Steinbach LS; Jahnke AH Jr; Petersen SA. MR Imaging of the shoulder: appearance of the supraspinatus tendon in asymptomatic volunteers. *Am J Roentgenol* 1992 Jun; 158(6): 1281-7 (Consensus/opinion)

18. Peterfy CG; Linares R; Steinbach LS. Recent advances in magnetic resonance imaging of the mussculoskeletal system. *Radiol Clin North Am* 1994 May; 32(2): 291-311 (V)

19. Resnick D. Shoulder imaging. Perspective. *Magn Reson Imaging Clin N Am* 1997 Nov; 5(4): 661-5 (Consensus/opinion)

20. Robertson PL; Schweitzer ME; Mitchell DG; Schlesinger F; Epstein RE; Frieman BG; Fenlin JM. Rotator cuff disorders: interobserver and intraovserver variation in diagnosis with MR imaging. *Radiology* 1995 March; 194(3): 831-5 (Consensus/opinion)

21. Seeger LL. Magnetic resonance imaging of the shoulder. *Clin Orthop* 1989 Jul; (244): 48-59 (Consensus/opinion)

22. Sher JS; Uribe JW; Posada A; Murphy BJ; Zlatkin MB. Abnormal findings on magnetic resonance images of asymptomatic shoulders. *J Bone Joint Surg [Am]* 1995 Jan: 77(1); 10-5 (III)

23. Tsao LY; Mirowitz SA. MR imaging of the shoulder. Imaging techniques, diagnostic pitfalls, and normal variants. *Magn Reson Imaging Clin N Am* 1997 Nov; 5(4): 683-704 (V)

24. Vellet AD; Munk PL; Marks P. Imaging techniques of the shoulder: present perspectives. *Clin Sports Med* 1991 Oct; 10(4): 721-56 (Consensus/opinion)

25. Williamson MP; Chandnani VP; Baird DE; Reeves TQ; Deberardino TM; Swenson GW; Hansen MF. Shoulder impingement syndrome: diagnostic accuracy of magnetic resonance imaging and radiographic signs. *Australas Radiol* 1994 Nov; 38(4): 265-71 (IV)

26. Wnorowski DC; Levinsohn EM; Chamberlain BC; McAndrew DL. Magnetic resonance imaging assessment of the rotator cuff: is it really accurate? *Arthroscopy* 1997 Dec; 13(6): 710-9 (IV)

Acromioclavicular Joint Disorder

1. Flatow EL; Cordasco FA; Bigliani LU. Arthroscopic resection of the outer end of the clavicle from a superior approach: a critical, quantitative, radiographic assessment of bone removal. *Arthroscopy* 1992; 8(1): 55-64 (III)

2. Fraenkel L; Shearer P; Mitchell P; LaValley M; Feldman J; Felson DT. Improving the selective use of plain radiographs in the initial evaluation of shoulder pain. *J Rheumatol* 2000 Jan; 27(1): 200-4 (II)

3. McCluskey GM 3d; Todd J. Acromioclavicular joint injuries. *J South Orthop Assoc* 1995 Fall; 4(3): 206-13 (V)

4. Yap JJ; Curl LA; Kvitne RS; McFarland EG. The value of weighted views of the acromioclavicular joint: results of a survey. *Am J Sports Med* 1999 Nov/Dec; 27(6): 806-9 (Consensus/opinion)

Outcomes

1. Bayley KB; London MR; Grunkemeier GL; Lansky DJ. Measuring the Success of Treatment in Patient Terms. *Med. Care.* 1995 Apr; 33(4-Suppl): AS226-35 (III)

2. Beaton DE; Richards RR. Measuring Function of the Shoulder. A Cross-sectional Comparison of Five Questionnaires. *J Bone Joint Surg [Am].* 1996 Jun; 78(6): 882-90 (IV)

3. Brems JJ. Rehabilitation following total shoulder arthroplasty. *Clin Orthop* 1994 Oct; (307): 70-85 (Consensus/opinion)

4. Chakravarty K; Webley M. Shoulder joint movement and its relationship to disability in the elderly. *J Rheumatol* 1993 Aug; 20(8): 1359-61 (IV)

5. Constant CR; Murley AH. A Clinical Method of Functional Assessment of the Shoulder. *Clin Orthop.* 1987 Jan. (214): 160-4 (Consensus/opinion)

6. Daum WJ; Brinker MR; Nash DB. Quality and Outcome Determination in Health Care and Orthopaedics: Evolution and Current Structure. *J Am Acad Orthop Surg.* 2000 Mar-Apr; 8(2): 133-9 (Consensus/opinion)

7. Di Fabio RP; Biossonnault W. Physical therapy and health-related outcomes for patients with common orthopaedic diagnoses. *J Orthop Sports Phys Ther* 1998 Mar; 27(3): 219-30 (V)

8. Ekberg K; Wildhagen I. Long-term sickness absence due to musculoskeletal disorders: the necessary intervention of work conditions. *Scand J Rehabil Med* 1996 Mar; 28(1): 39-47 (IV)

9. Emery DD; Schneiderman LJ. Cost-effectiveness Analysis in Health Care. *Hasting Cent Rep.* 1989 Jul-Aug; 19(4): 8-13 (Consensus/opinion)

10. Gillespie WJ; Daellenbach HG. Assessing cost effectiveness in orthopedic outcome studies. *Orthopedics* 1992 Nov; 15(11): 1275-7 (Consensus/opinion)

11. Heald SL; Riddle DR; Lamb RL. The shoulder pain and disability index: the construct validity and responsiveness of a region-specific disability measure. *Phys Ther* 1997 Oct; 77(10): 1079-89 (IV)

12. Jette DU; Jette AM. Health Status assessment in the occupational health setting. *Orthop Clin North Am* 1996 Oct; 27(4): 891-902 (V)

13. Krishnan J; Chipchase L. Orthopaedic surgery outcomes assessment model. *J Qual Clin Pract* 1997 Jun; 17(2): 109-16 (IV)

14. Kuhn JE; Blasier RB. Assessment of outcome in shoulder arthroplasty. *Orthop Clin North Am* 1998 Jul; 29(3): 549-63 (V)

15. Lirette R; Morin F; Kinnard P. The difficulties in Assessment of Results of Anterior Acromioplasty. *Clin Orthop*. 1992 May; (278): 14-6 (V)

16. Matsen FA 3rd. Early Effectiveness of Shoulder Arthroplasty for Patients Who Have Primary Glenohumeral Degenerative Joint Disease. *J Bone Joint Surg [Am]*. 1996 Feb; 78(2): 260-4 (IV)

17. Outcomes Research Resource Guide: A Survey of Current Activities, 1997-1998 Edition, (Serial). American Medical Association, published 1998 (Consensus/opinion)

18. Sledge CB. Why do outcomes research? *Orthopedics* 1993 Oct; 16(10): 1093, 1096 (Consensus/opinion)

19. Swiontkowsk, MF; Buckwalter JA; Keller RB; Haralson R. The Outcomes Movement in Orthopaedic Surgery: Where Are We and Where Should We Go. *J Bone Joint Surg [Am]* 1999 May; 81(5): 732-740 (Consensus/opinion)

20. Swiontkowski MF; Chapman JR. Cost and Effectiveness Issues in Care of Injured Patients. *Clin Orthop*. 1995 Sep; (318): 17-24 (Consensus/opinion)

21. Williams JW Jr; Holleman DR Jr; Simel DL. Measuring shoulder function with the Shoulder Pain and Disability Index. *J Rheumatol* 1995 Apr; 22(4): 727-32 (IV)

Section 8

Arthroscopy

Section Editors:
James C. Esch, MD
Armodios M. Hatzidakis, MD

Chapter 44

Arthroscopic Rotator Cuff Repair

Jeffrey S. Abrams, MD

Introduction

Open repair of full-thickness rotator cuff tears is a validated traditional treatment with well established long-term outcomes. Although not as time tested as the open repair, arthroscopic techniques are rapidly evolving in the management of rotator cuff tears. Rotator cuff tendinosis secondary to impingement syndrome can be treated effectively by arthroscopic subacromial decompression. Partial-thickness tears, especially articular-side tears (which are more common), can be evaluated, débrided, and repaired arthroscopically. Biomechanical principles outlined in the literature have enhanced the technique and security of arthroscopic rotator cuff repair. Some of these principles include the "dead-man" angle of entry of suture anchors into bone, side-to-side repairs (margin convergence), and favorable results using multiple simple sutures and anchors, compared to transosseous sutures. Small- and medium-size full-thickness tears can be repaired to the greater tuberosity with suture anchors, using all-arthroscopic techniques. Large and massive tears that involve more than one tendon can also be reconstructed with tendon-to-tendon reconstruction followed by tendon-to-bone reattachment with anchors. Irreparable tears can be evaluated and débrided, and partial repairs may reduce the size of the defect without damaging the deltoid or coracoacromial ligament. Midterm results have been encouraging.

The deltoid is an important muscle that ordinarily is split, released, mobilized, and retracted to allow visualization and fixation of the rotator cuff during surgical repair. The effective use of arthroscopic techniques can avoid trauma to the deltoid, which potentially reduces the morbidity, postoperative pain, and potential for adhesions. A unique advantage of the arthroscope includes joint visualization, which does not reliably occur when using open techniques to repair small tears, unless arthroscopy is performed followed by an open repair. Intra-articular lesions, including biceps tendon tears, articular cartilage damage, labral tears, and articular side

partial-thickness rotator cuff tears, can be seen. These associated lesions may have a significant impact on the postoperative course and eventual outcome.

There are many technical factors that must be mastered to reproduce the structural repair that is routinely obtained with open techniques. This chapter will briefly discuss the indications for rotator cuff repair, followed by a description of surgical technique and a brief review of results.

Indications

The indications for arthroscopic cuff repair are the same as for open cuff repair. The most common symptom is pain, which often interrupts sleep and limits patients' functional activities. Patients report a loss of ability to perform work-related activities, recreational activities, and activities of daily living. As the tear enlarges, a loss of active motion may occur. It is important to distinguish loss of passive motion that is caused by joint contracture from loss of active motion caused by weakness. Loss of passive motion should be corrected prior to rotator cuff repair. In the stiff shoulder, postoperative attempts at restoring range of motion will most likely undo the surgical repair.

General health assessment via standard outcomes measures is diminished in patients with a symptomatic rotator cuff tear. Nonetheless, patients begin with non-surgical treatment. The effectiveness of this treatment is unclear, as the natural history of rotator cuff tears is not well undertood. The likelihood of small tears progressing to large tears is unknown. It is logical to assume that active individuals are at risk. Repetitive tension on the edges of a torn cuff can hypothetically extend the tear. Because surgical repair is more predictable in smaller tears, it seems appropriate to repair symptomatic tears prior to tear progression.

Radiographic evaluation should include a three-view trauma series with an anteroposterior view of the shoulder including the acromioclavicular joint, a transcapular

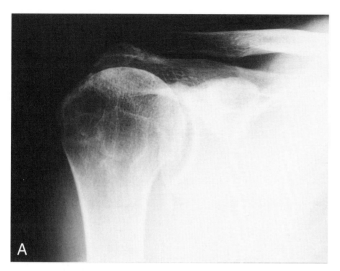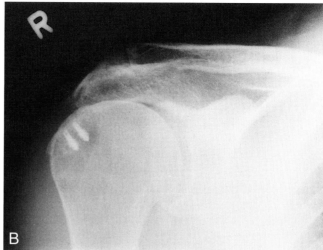

Figure 1 A, Radiograph of medium to large rotator cuff tear with mild superior head migration. **B,** Reduction of humeral head with postoperative view of rotator cuff repair.

or Y view, and an axillary view. Loss of glenohumeral articular cartilage and significant arthritis make the results of cuff repair unpredictable. Morphology of the acromion and acromioclavicular joint can be evaluated, and subacromial decompression and/or distal clavicle resection added to the preoperative plan based on the radiographs and physical examination. Preoperative evaluation of a massive chronic rotator cuff tear may demonstrate humeral head contact on an atrophic acromion. Although the arthroscope can evaluate this situation further, followed by débridement, a cuff repair is usually not possible. Partial repairs may be considered if the cuff is viable and can be mobilized. Mild superior migration can be seen preoperatively and is often reduced after repair (Fig. 1). Additional imaging studies such as MRI, arthrography, or CT can demonstrate cuff deficiency, muscular atrophy, and fatty infiltration. Higher degrees of atrophy and fatty infiltration of the rotator cuff muscles most likely lead to less functional improvement after repair, regardless of the repair technique.

Initial Arthroscopic Evaluation

The patient is placed under interscalene block and/or general anesthesia. Range of motion is assessed with the patient anesthetized. Ideally, the patient should exhibit full passive elevation and rotation preoperatively. Patients are placed in the lateral decubitus or beach chair position. Both positions can be converted to mini-open or open surgical approaches without altering the torso or upper extremity traction.

The portals include the posterior viewing portal and an anterior portal in front of the acromioclavicular joint. A lateral bursal portal is developed approximately 3 cm lateral to the acromion for access to the tear. The arthroscopic procedure is initiated with an articular

examination with the arthroscope in the posterior viewing portal. The articular surface, biceps, labrum, and the undersurface of the rotator cuff insertion should be carefully inspected. A shaver and electrocautery can be placed through an anterior portal for débridement. If adhesions or joint contracture is noted, arthroscopic release is performed.

Presence of the subscapularis tendon and its attachment to the lesser tuberosity should be confirmed visually, which is facilitated by internal rotation of the shoulder. With the viewing scope in the posterior portal, articular-sided partial tears should be débrided to a smoothed, stable edge. The surface area of the tear can be measured using the cannula, and the depth of the tear can be estimated with a probe. A spinal needle can be introduced into the tear through the deltoid approximately 2 cm lateral to the acromion and this needle can be left in place for identification of the tear when viewing from the subacromial space.

The arthroscope is then placed into the subacromial space. The lateral portal can be developed and a bursectomy is carried out. Significant adhesions should be débrided with an arthroscopic shaver and/or electrocautery device to allow full motion at the humeroacromial interface. Following needle localization of the tear, the bursal surface of the cuff should be palpated with an arthroscopic instrument such as a hook probe or switching stick. If the cuff tear is estimated to be less than 50% of the thickness of the tendon, débridement and observation is an acceptable treatment. Tears involving over half of the tendon thickness should be completed and repaired. For significant delamination lesions, passing a suture anchor percutaneously through the tendon tear and repairing the articular tear via an all-articular approach is a consideration. In high-demand patients, the superficial leaf can be divided and the cuff repaired.

Initial bleeding at the time of arthroscopy is expected, but will generally subside with irrigation. For best visualization, a saline pump should be used to distend the subacromial space. Epinephrine should be added to the saline irrigant at the beginning of the procedure. The patient's systolic pressure should be maintained at 110 mm Hg or less to minimize bleeding. A motorized shaver with limited outflow can be used to clear bursal tissue beneath the acromion so that the lateral edge of the tuberosity can be visualized. Electrocautery can be used to coagulate bleeders.

From the lateral portal, motorized instruments and a suction punch are used to improve tendon visualization. Complete bursectomy is not needed and may reduce potential vascularization and nutrition for cuff healing. A grasper can be introduced to test cuff mobilization. Many small- and medium-size tears are not significantly retracted and are adjacent to the anticipated repair site. Larger tears usually extend medially, allowing for the humeral head to migrate superiorly and further dilate the hole. These tears generally have medial extension into the substance of the infraspinatus or along the rotator interval. Clearing bursa to identify the tendon edges is essential. Cuff mobilization is not from medial to lateral, but from posterior to anterior. Anterior releases to the base of the coracoid can be carried out along the rotator interval. Generally, the posterior leaf of the cuff tear can be better mobilized than the anterior leaf, although the posterior arthroscope cannula can sometimes tether the posterior edge of the tear, diminishing its mobilization. The subacromial bursa around the posterior cannula should be débrided to minimize this effect. Tear geometry, tissue quality, and tissue mobility will determine if the cuff defect can be closed with minimal medial to lateral tension.

The treatment of rotator cuff tears associated with subacromial impingement syndrome has been acromioplasty followed by cuff repair. Subacromial decompression improves the performance of the procedure by facilitating instrument passage and knot tying. Decompression also potentially improves healing by limiting contact forces on the repair. A standard acromioplasty can be carried out to create a type I flat acromion. When the cuff cannot be repaired, débridement and smoothing of the acromion and the greater tuberosity can be done, but the coracoacromial ligament should be preserved. The undersurface of the clavicle sometimes projects inferiorly, contacting the cuff after acromioplasty is completed. This can be treated by observation, coplaning the prominence, or resection of the distal clavicle. The clinical examination combined with visualization of the distal clavicle articular surface can give the surgeon a reasonable idea if distal clavicle excision should be performed.

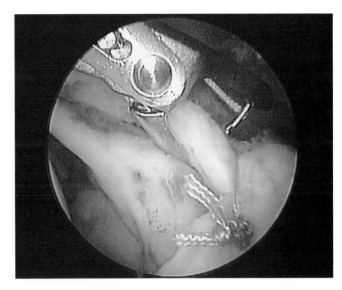

Figure 2 ArthroSew device (US Surgical, Norwalk, CT) can pass No. 2 braided suture side to side, reducing the size of the tear.

Additional information on decision-making regarding the acromioclavicular joint is available in chapters 49 and 50.

Soft tissue is carefully débrided from the greater tuberosity down to bone. Devitalized tissue can be elevated with a resector or burr up to the articular surface-tuberosity junction. Aggressive decortication should be avoided because this bone must remain strong for suture anchor purchase.

Technique of Rotator Cuff Repair

Tears of the supraspinatus and infraspinatus can often be repaired arthroscopically, even when combined with a subscapularis repair. At this time, a retracted subscapularis tear from the lesser tuberosity is better approached by the open approach through the deltopectoral interval. Tears that involve only the superior border of the tendon can be visualized and treated arthroscopically. More significant detachments are challenging to visualize and repair using arthroscopic techniques.

Initially, the medial extension found in larger tears needs to be corrected. The repair is first carried out medially at the apex of the tear. The surgeon can choose to maintain the arthroscope in the lateral or posterior portal. If the scope is maintained in the lateral portal, suture hooks can be passed via the posterior and anterior portals. Side-to-side sutures can be placed and tied. Suture choices include No. 0 or No. 1 PDS or No. 2 braided sutures. Special instruments are required to pass these sutures through the rotator cuff arthroscopically. An example is the ArthroSew device (US Surgical, Norwalk, CT), which can be moved into the subacromial space via a large cannula placed in the lateral portal (Fig. 2). Tying sutures as they are placed closes the

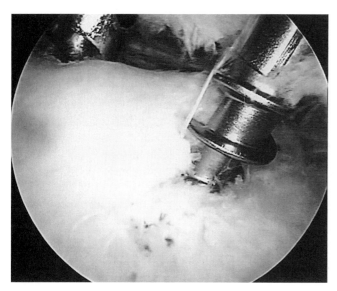

Figure 3 Suture anchor screw is placed along the edge of the tear to minimize tension.

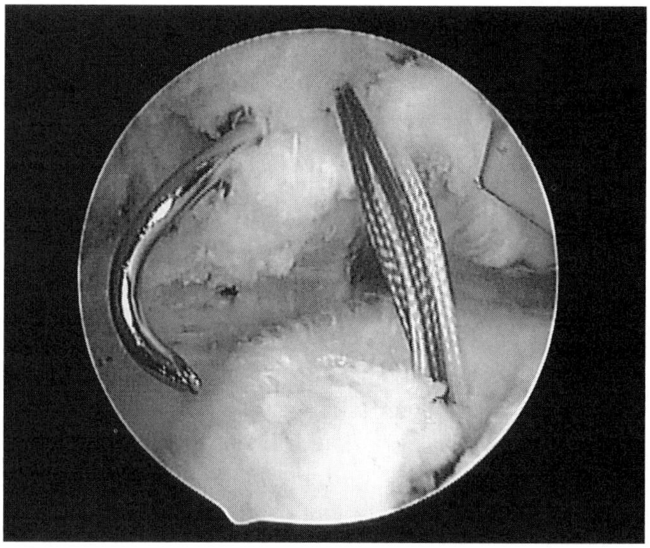

Figure 4 A spectrum suture hook can be placed through the anterior portal to retrieve sutures from anchors.

defect, depresses the head, and pulls the posterior leaf of the tear anteriorly.

A series of anchors are placed to repair the tear to the greater tuberosity. Generally, small and medium tears require two anchors. Large tears may require three or four anchors, depending on the geometry of the tear. Suture anchors should have large eyelets to allow the placement of sliding knots and multiple sutures. Anchors are placed through an accessory portal near the lateral edge of the acromion (Fig. 3). A spinal needle can be used to identify the correct entry angle. The goal is not to lateralize the cuff, but to approximate the insertion to the medial footprint of the tuberosity. After securing the anchor, the pullout strength and suture sliding should be gently tested. A multicolored suture pack allows for easier identification of suture arms. Efficient suture management is critical to avoid frustrating entanglements or unloading suture from the anchor.

With the anchor in place, one arm of the suture needs to be drawn through the rotator cuff free edge. A curved suture hook can be introduced through the anterior portal (Fig. 4). After tendon penetration, a suture shuttle (Linvatec, Largo, FL) or a PDS suture can be introduced and retrieved out the available cannula. One of the braided suture arms closest to the path of this shuttle suture can be retrieved from the same cannula. After fixing the two together, the braided stitch from the anchor can be drawn through the tendon to the bursal surface and retrieved from the anterior portal. The corresponding suture arm is retrieved from the anterior portal without passing through the cuff, and a hemostat can be used to keep them together while additional sutures are placed.

Another technique uses the lateral portal to intro-

duce a Caspari suture punch (Linvatec, Largo, FL). The shuttle is passed up through the cuff and withdrawn through the anterior portal (Fig. 5). The braided suture can be retrieved through the lateral cannula, linked to the shuttle and drawn through the cuff to the anterior portal. The second arm to suture is then retrieved. The free edge of the tendon repair is held in close proximity to the abraded bone with simple sutures that are tied with sliding knots (Fig. 6).

Arthroscopic cuff repair is only effective if secure knots can be tied arthroscopically. A series of half-hitches allows loosening of the loop, compromising the fixation. Sliding knots allow for a tight knot to be created outside of the cannula that can be easily advanced into the subacromial space to effectively secure the underlying tendon (Fig. 7). The knot can be locked by past pointing, and a series of half-hitches can be placed on the nonpost limb to prevent knot loosening. Anchor sutures are tied in sequence at the end of the case. One set of suture at a time should be retrieved through a cannula and tied seperately, so that entanglements and soft-tissue entrapment are avoided.

Patients are immobilized for 4 to 6 weeks in a sling or immobilizer. The sling is removed for daily exercises such as shoulder external rotation stretches and elbow range of motion. No active lifting should be attempted during the initial 4 weeks; after this time, assisted forward flexion is added to the protocol. Behind-the-back movements are restricted for 6 weeks. Resistive training does not begin before 8 weeks. Depending on the security of the repair, resistive exercises may be delayed 12 weeks or more after surgery. Return to functional activities is usually based on size of tear, quality of tissue, and integrity of the repair. Acceptable performance of

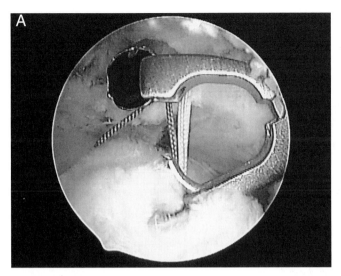
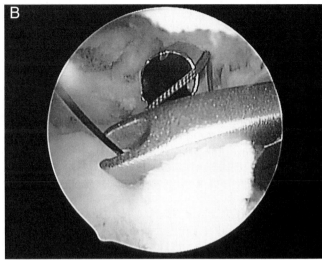

Figure 5 Caspari suture punch (Linvatec, Largo, FL). **A,** A punch can be placed through the lateral cannula. **B,** Full-thickness pass of the suture shuttle can assist suture passage.

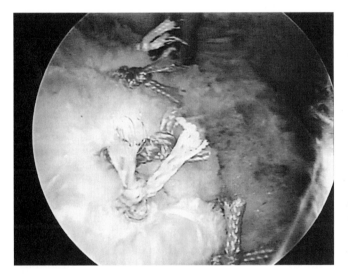

Figure 6 Completed cuff repair to the tuberosity.

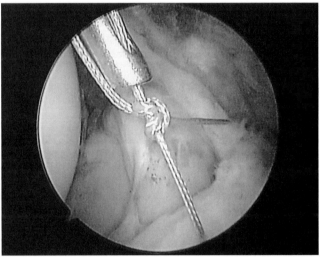

Figure 7 Simple slider knot. Underhanded and overhanded throws are passed loosely down the postsuture arm. Past pointing flips the second throw, securing the knot. Half hitches can follow to prevent late loosening.

certain activities may take from 6 months to 1 year after surgery. Many activities below the level of the shoulder and chest can be started at 4 months.

Outcomes

Midterm measures of patient satisfaction, pain relief, and functional gains have been comparable to results following open repairs, although no randomized studies have been presented. One study with 2-year follow-up demonstrated a success rate of 87% using the University of California, Los Angeles (UCLA) rating system. In another study, significantly improved outcomes were reported as measured not only by the conventional outcome scales but also by the Short Form-36 (SF-36) General Health

Survey, which measures patients' perceptions of their general health. Favorable results using arthroscopic techniques to address larger tears have also been reported. Greater mobilization of the posterior cuff allows for medial closure with multiple sutures, reducing the tension on tuberosity fixation of the cuff. This medial extension of these tears is very difficult to manage using mini-open deltoid splitting techniques. Open repair remains the gold standard for many surgeons in the management of full-thickness rotator cuff tears. Arthroscopic repair is likely to lead to long-term results that equal, and possibly exceed, open repair.

Summary

Many techniques are evolving in the arthroscopic management of rotator cuff tears. Improved visualization of larger complex tears that extend posteriorly, addressing articular pathology that may affect the outcome, and reduction of morbidity associated with deltoid incision and mobilization make arthroscopy an attractive alternative. The challenges include understanding the geometry of the tear, maximizing suture fixation, and performing repairs with minimal tension. The biologic reparative process is long and at risk for disruption during recovery and rehabilitation. As advances continue, arthroscopic repair will become an important part of the management of rotator cuff tears.

Annotated Bibliography

Introduction

Burkhart SS, Athanasiou KA, Wirth MA. Margin convergence: A method of reducing strain in massive rotator cuff tears. *Arthroscopy* 1996;12:335-338.

An explanation of how strains at the margins of a repaired rotator cuff can be decreased by the placement of side-to-side margin convergence sutures is presented. The authors hypothesized that margin convergence sutures can reduce postoperative pain, secondary to decreased mechanoreceptor stimulation at the repaired margins of the cuff.

Burkhart SS, Diaz Pagan JL, Wirth MA, Athanasiou KA: Cyclic loading of anchor-based rotator cuff repairs: Confirmation of the tension overload phenomenon and comparison of suture anchor fixation with transosseous fixation. *Arthroscopy* 1997;13:720-724.

The authors designed a biomechanical experiment testing rotator cuff repair fixation, simulating the cyclic loading conditions experienced in vivo. Rotator cuff defects measuring 1 cm × 2 cm were created in 16 cadaver shoulders. Defects were repaired with three suture anchors using simple sutures of No. 2 Ethibond. The repairs were cyclically loaded by a servohydraulic materials test system actuator at physiologic loads. A progressive gap was noted in each specimen, for a 100% rate of failure of the repairs. The central suture always failed first and by the largest magnitude, confirming tension overload centrally. Fifteen of 16 specimens failed through the tendon. Specimens from patients older than age 45 years exhibited more rapid failure of the rotator cuff repairs than the specimens from younger patients ($P < .02$). Average cycles to failure were significantly greater with suture anchor fixation than with transosseous bone tunnel fixation in a previously published study using similar methods ($P = 0.0008$).

Gartsman GM: Rotator cuff repair: Why I prefer arthroscopy. *Sports Med Arthrosc Rev* 1999;7:85-92.

The author's rationale for arthroscopic rotator cuff repair is reviewed.

Initial Arthroscopic Evaluation

Weber SC: Arthroscopic debridement and acromioplasty versus mini-open repair in the treatment of significant partial-thickness rotator cuff tears. *Arthroscopy* 1999;15:126-131.

Thirty-two patients with significant partial-thickness rotator cuff tears (tear involving at least 50% of the tendon thickness) were treated with débridement and acromioplasty. Thirty-three patients were treated with mini-open repair. Follow-up was from 2 to 7 years. Although perioperative morbidity was less in the débridement only group, follow-up UCLA scores were worse. There were 14 good, 8 fair, and 9 poor results in the débridement/decompression group versus 3 excellent, 28 good, 1 fair, and 1 poor result in the mini-open repair group. Six of the patients in the débridement/decompression group required further surgery; three cuffs had progressed to full-thickness tears and three had no evidence of healing. None of the patients in the repair group had symptoms of retearing of the rotator cuff, and none required further surgery. The author recommends repair of partial-thickness rotator cuff tears involving more than 50% of the tendon thickness.

Technique of Rotator Cuff Repair

Burkhart SS: A stepwise approach to arthroscopic rotator cuff repair based on biomechanical principles. *Arthroscopy* 2000;16:82-90.

The author linked concepts into a unified stepwise approach to arthroscopic repair of a variety of rotator cuff tear configurations, with maximum strength of fixation.

Burkhart SS, Tehrany AM: Arthroscopic subscapularis tendon repair: Technique and preliminary results. *Arthroscopy* 2002;18:454-463.

Preliminary results of 25 consecutive arthroscopic subscapularis tendon repairs are presented, with an average follow-up of 10.7 months (range, 3 to 48 months). Eight patients had isolated tears of the subscapularis and 17 patients had larger tears involving other cuff tendons. UCLA scores increased from 10.7 preoperatively to 30.5 postoperatively ($P < 0.0001$). Excellent and good results were obtained in 92% of patients, with one fair and one poor result. Forward flexion increased from 96.3° preoperatively to 146.1° postoperatively ($P = 0.0016$). Eight of 10 patients with preoperative proximal migration of the humerus had durable reversal of this migration postoperatively. Overhead arm function in these eight patients improved from a preoperative "shoulder shrug" with attempted elevation to functional overhead use of the arm postoperatively.

Gartsman GM: Arthroscopic rotator cuff repair. *Clin Orthop* 2001;390:95-106.

The author's technique and advantages and disadvantages of arthroscopic rotator cuff repair are reviewed.

Nottage WM, Lieurance RK: Arthroscopic knot tying techniques, current concepts. *Arthroscopy* 1999;15: 515-521.

Suture handling and knot tying techniques are described in addition to tips on avoiding tangles in the cannula, premature locking of knots, and inadequate knot seating. Diagrams of specific knots are depicted, including the square knot, Revo knot, Duncan loop, Roeder knot, and Tennessee slider.

Outcomes

Burkhart SS: Arthroscopic treatment of massive rotator cuff tears. *Clin Orthop* 2001;390:107-118.

The factors essential to a secure arthroscopic rotator cuff repair were reviewed and when these principles are followed, the results of arthroscopic repair of massive tears closely approximate the results of treatment of small tears.

Burkhart SS, Danaceau SM, Pearce CE Jr: Arthroscopic rotator cuff repair: Analysis of results by tear size and by repair technique-margin convergence versus direct tendon-to-bone repair. *Arthroscopy* 2001;17:905-912.

Midterm follow-up (3.5 years) of functional results of arthroscopic rotator cuff repair was reported in 59 patients, and results by tear size and repair technique (margin convergence versus direct tendon-to-bone repair) were analyzed. Tears were categorized according to size (greatest diameter, number of tendons involved, and pattern of tear [crescent versus U shape]). Crescent-shaped tears were repaired in a direct tendon-to-bone fashion and U-shaped tears were repaired by a margin-convergence technique. Good and excellent results (modified UCLA score) were achieved in 95% of the cases, regardless of tear size. Repair of large and massive tears led to the same functional outcome as repair of small and medium-sized tears ($P < 0.05$). Full overhead function was achieved rapidly (average, 4 months), and was also independent of tear size. Delay from injury to surgery, even of several years, did not adversely affect surgical outcome.

Gartsman GM, Brinker MR, Khan M: Early effectiveness of arthroscopic repair for full-thickness tears of the rotator cuff: An outcome analysis. *J Bone Joint Surg Am* 1998;80:33-40.

SF-36, UCLA, American Shoulder and Elbow Surgeons, and Constant scores were analyzed in 50 consecutive patients before and an average of 13 months after arthroscopic repair of a full-thickness tear of the rotator cuff. Patient assessment both of general health and of function of the shoulder improved after surgery. The SF-36 General Health Survey revealed significant improvements with regard to physical functioning ($P = 0.0001$), role-physical ($P = 0.0001$), bodily pain ($P = 0.0001$), vitality ($P = 0.0001$), social functioning ($P = 0.0001$), role-emotional ($P = 0.006$), mental health ($P = 0.0213$), and physical component summary ($P = 0.0001$). All shoulder rating systems were significantly improved postoperatively ($P = 0.0001$).

Gartsman GM, Khan M, Hammerman SM: Arthroscopic repair of full-thickness tears of the rotator cuff. *J Bone Joint Surg Am* 1998;80:832-840.

Arthroscopic repair of full-thickness rotator cuff tears was performed in 73 patients (average age, 60.7 years). The patients were followed up an average of 30 months and were serially evaluated with the SF-36, UCLA, American Shoulder and Elbow Surgeons, and Constant scores. Eleven tears were small (less than 1 cm in length), 45 were medium (1 to 3 cm), 11 were large (more than 3 to 5 cm), and 6 were massive (more than 5 cm). The average duration of the operation was 56 minutes (range, 35 to 90 minutes). Active and passive ranges of motion improved significantly after the procedure ($P = 0.0001$). Strength of resisted elevation improved from 7.5 to 14.0 pounds ($P = 0.0001$). SF-36 and all functional shoulder scores improved significantly ($P = 0.0001$). Fifty-seven of the 73 patients (78%) rated their postoperative pain relief as good or excellent. None of the shoulders were rated as good or excellent before the operation, whereas 61 (84%) were rated good or excellent at the most recent follow-up evaluation.

Gazielly DF, Gleyze P, Montagreen C, Ollagnier E, Thomas T: Arthroscopic fixation of distal supraspinatus tears with Revo screw anchors and permanent mattress sutures: A preliminary report, in Gazielly DF, Gleyze P, Thomos T (eds): *The Cuff.* Paris, France, Elsevier, 1997, pp 282-286.

Arthroscopic rotator cuff repair can be used effectively in the elderly. Small- and medium-size tears were repaired effectively.

Murray TF Jr, Lajtai G, Mileski RM, Snyder SJ: Arthroscopic repair of medium to large full-thickness rotator cuff tears: Outcome at 2- to 6-year follow-up. *J Shoulder Elbow Surg* 2002;11:19-24.

Forty-eight consecutive arthroscopic repairs of medium to large rotator cuff tears were performed, with mean rotator cuff tear size of 2.4 cm, mean age 57.6 years, and average pfollow-up of 39 months. UCLA Scores were 17.2 preoperatively and 33.7 postoperatively (P < 0.001). American Shoulder and Elbow Surgeons scores were also significantly improved. There were 35 excellent, 11 good, 2 fair, and no poor results. One patient had clinical evidence of failed repair. Forty-four of 45 patients (47 of 48 repairs) were satisfied with their outcomes.

Wilson F, Hinov V, Adams G: Arthroscopic repair of full-thickness tears of the rotator cuff: 2- to 14-year follow-up. *Arthroscopy* 2002;18:136-144.

Full-thickness rotator cuff tears were repaired arthroscopically by one surgeon, using two different techniques, in 100 patients. Thirty-five patients had staple fixation and 65 patients had side-to-side suture and anchor repair. Follow-up ranged from 2 to 14 years. Rotator cuffs repaired with staples (group 1) were evaluated arthroscopically at staple removal. According to the UCLA scores, in the staple group 22 patients (63%) were graded as excellent, 7 (20%) were graded good, 4 (11%) were graded fair, and 2 (6%) were graded poor. In the anchor group, 47 patients (72%) were graded as excellent, 12 (19%) were graded good, 2 (3%) were graded fair, and 4 (6%) were graded as poor. Patients with well-healed rotator cuff to bone had better overall functional results.

Classic Bibliography

Burkhart SS: Fluoroscopic comparison of kinematic patterns in massive rotator cuff tears. A suspension bridge model. *Clin Orthop* 1992;284:144-152.

Burkhart SS, Esch JC, Jolson RS: The rotator crescent and rotator cable: an anatomic description of the shoulder's "suspension bridge". *Arthroscopy* 1993;9:611-616.

Burkhart SS: The deadman theory of suture anchors: Observations along a south Texas fence line. *Arthroscopy* 1995;11:119-123.

Gartsman GM: Arthroscopic treatment of rotator cuff disease. *J Shoulder Elbow Surg* 1995;4:228-241.

Loutzenheiser TD, Harryman DT II, Yung SW, et al. Optimizing arthroscopic knots. *Arthroscopy* 1995;11:199-206.

Paulos LE, Kody MH: Arthroscopically enhanced "miniapproach" to rotator cuff repair. *Am J Sports Med* 1994;2:19-25.

Thal R: A technique for arthroscopic mattress suture placement. *Arthroscopy* 1993;5:605-607.

Chapter 45

Recurrent Anterior Dislocations

Richard K.N. Ryu, MD

Introduction

Instability of the shoulder is best classified using four parameters: mechanism (traumatic, atraumatic, repetitive microtrauma), direction (anterior, posterior, inferior, multidirectional), onset (acute, recurrent), and degree (microinstability, subluxation, dislocation). The most common sequela following acute unilateral anterior dislocation of the shoulder is recurrent anterior dislocation, which, simply stated, is recurrent symptomatic translation of the humeral head on the glenoid, resulting in a loss of articular surface contact. Although several conditions involving varying degrees of recurrent instability exist, this chapter focuses specifically on the natural history, anatomy, biomechanics, evaluation, and treatment of traumatic, unidirectional, recurrent anterior dislocations of the shoulder.

Natural History

The natural history following an initial anterior shoulder dislocation is relevant because patients typically are younger and participate in high-demand activities; both factors increase the risk of recurrence. Numerous studies, including those of young military cadets from West Point, report a recurrence rate of 50% to 90% in this high-risk population. The recurrence rate is substantially lower in individuals age 40 years or older (between 10% and 20%), but this difference may simply reflect a lower activity level. Unfortunately, this lower recurrence rate in older individuals is offset by the concomitant increased risk of neurologic and rotator cuff injury.

An understanding of the anatomy and biomechanics of the shoulder, as well as an appreciation of the numerous risk factors that can impact the success of treatment, is mandatory in determining appropriate management.

Anatomy and Biomechanics

Stability of the glenohumeral articulation requires a complex balance between static and dynamic forces.

Selective cutting studies have provided important data regarding the contribution and importance of the inferior glenohumeral ligament (IGHL). Not surprisingly, the position of the shoulder determines which static stabilizers yield the greatest contribution. The superior glenohumeral ligament (SGHL) works in conjunction with the coracohumeral ligament, which runs parallel to it, preventing inferior translation in the adducted, internally rotated position. The middle glenohumeral ligament, which may be absent in up to 30% of individuals, is most effective in providing stability in lesser degrees of abduction. In the middle ranges of abduction, the compression-concavity phenomenon, which requires an intact labrum and a well-functioning rotator cuff, provides critical dynamic stabilization. The most provocative position, abduction combined with horizontal extension and external rotation, requires that the IGHL be intact to provide adequate stability. Anatomic and biomechanical studies have shown that the IGHL is stiffest and thickest at its insertion into the glenoid. The thinner posterior band of the IGHL rotates to an inferior position and, in conjunction with the axillary pouch, provides additional support to the anterior structures when the shoulder is maximally stressed (Fig. 1).

Stress-to-failure cadaveric studies have recorded failure at the glenoid insertion site in approximately 40%, midsubstance ruptures in 35%, and failure at the humeral attachment of the glenohumeral ligaments in up to 25% of specimens tested. In addition, capsular attenuation in the form of elongation occurs within the glenohumeral ligaments prior to failure, especially with recurrent episodes of anterior instability. There is incontrovertible evidence that a solitary Bankart lesion (the "essential lesion" of acute anterior dislocations) is insufficient to cause recurrent dislocations and that associated capsular elongation is a necessary component of recurrence. Retensioning of this posttraumatic capsular laxity, as well as repair of the Bankart lesion, must be fully addressed in any surgical approach.

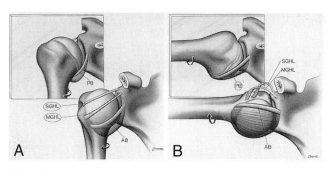

Figure 1 A, The SGHL and MGHL tighten with adduction and rotation. **B,** Tensioning of IGHL and posterior band as the shoulder is abducted and externally rotated; note relative laxity in the SGHL. SGHL = superior glenohumeral ligament, MGHL = middle glenohumeral ligament, AB = anterior band, PB = posterior band. *(Reproduced with permission from Warner JP, Boardman ND: Anatomy, biomechanics, and pathophysiology of glenohumeral instability, in Warren RF, Craig EV, Altcheck DW (eds): The Unstable Shoulder. Philadelphia, PA, Lippincott-Raven, 1999, p 65.)*

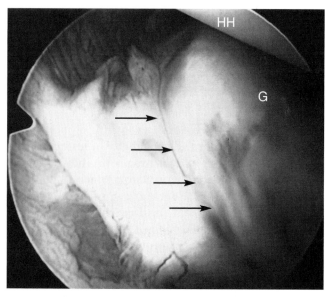

Figure 2 View from the anterosuperior portal; anterior labral-ligamentous periosteal sleeve avulsion lesion *(arrows)* is seen with medial and inferior displacement of the entire periosteal sleeve. G = glenoid, HH = humeral head.

Differing articular curvatures of the glenoid and humeral head have been discussed as a cause for recurrence. Recent imaging studies that include both subchondral bone and articular cartilage configuration, however, have shown that their radii of curvature match closely. Maximal surface-area contact of only 25% to 30% between the humeral head and glenoid at any position of rotation remains the single most significant anatomic factor contributing to instability. This limited surface-area contact has been described as a "golf ball sitting on a tee."

Evaluation

Patients with recurrent anterior dislocations have a common initiating event: a dislocation caused by significant trauma with the arm overhead or away from the side. At the time of injury, the arm is in abduction, horizontal extension, and external rotation. An indirect rotational force applied in this provocative position results in ligament failure and, ultimately, dislocation. Reduction under sedation in the emergency department is required for most patients. Subsequent episodes of instability may occur with much less force, sometimes while the patient is simply sleeping with the arm overhead.

Patients who eventually develop recurrent instability usually regain full range of motion shortly after dislocation, and pain subsides within 24 to 48 hours. In patients with persistent pain, a careful evaluation for associated rotator cuff or biceps anchor injury is warranted. On physical examination a markedly positive apprehension test elicits a grave sense of instability, rather than pain. Pain as the primary response is considered nonspecific and can be present in a variety of shoulder pathologies. A positive sulcus sign may indicate some element of associated generalized ligamentous laxity, as well as possible damage to the SGHL. The load-and-shift test in the sitting or lateral decubitus position can detect instability, although patients may resist provocative testing. Stress testing may reveal an element of posterior laxity. This phenomenon does not represent a multidirectional component; rather, it reflects recurrent posterior capsular injury that can be associated with recurrent anterior dislocation.

Diagnostic Testing

AP, axillary, and scapular "Y" views are standard. The Stryker notch view can better define the presence and size of a Hill-Sachs lesion. The West Point axillary view, obtained with the patient prone and the beam directed cephalad, detects an anterior bony Bankart lesion. With an acute injury, the patient may not be able to abduct the arm sufficiently to obtain a good axillary view. In these patients, an AP view with the beam directed 45° caudally (Garth view) also can help establish the presence of a bony Bankart lesion. Although CT can be useful in assessing glenoid version and defining bony defects, the diagnostic modality of choice in the evaluation of shoulder instability is the magnetic resonance arthrogram. Contrast within the joint enhances the evaluation of soft-tissue pathology, and there is some evidence that placement of the arm in the abducted-externally rotated position facilitates detection of capsulolabral and Hill-Sachs pathology.

Arthroscopic Evaluation

In patients with recurrent anterior dislocations, several common pathologic findings are noted at the time of arthroscopic evaluation. One prospective study evaluated intra-articular pathology in 212 patients with at

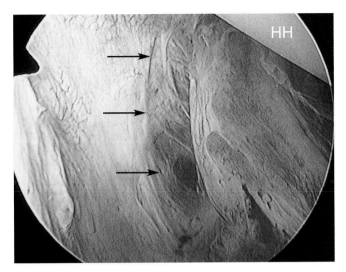

Figure 3 Outline of midsubstance capsular tear (*large arrows*) with intact labrum (*small arrows*). HH = humeral head.

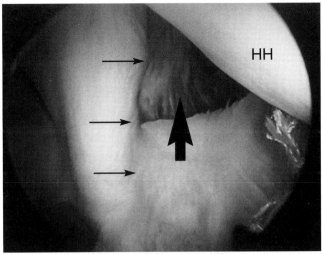

Figure 4 Outline of humeral avulsion of the glenohumeral ligament lesion (*large arrow*). Subscapularis muscle fibers are visible through the defect, while anterior band (*small arrows*) remains intact. HH = humeral head.

least one anterior dislocation, revealing Bankart lesions in 87%, Hill-Sachs lesions in 68%, glenohumeral ligament attenuation in 55%, a torn rotator cuff in 14%, and superior labral injuries in 7%.

Failure of the IGHL is the most common pathology and can take several forms. Failure usually occurs at the glenoid rim with the classic Bankart lesion. The periosteal sleeve of the IGHL attachment displaces medially and inferiorly, which then results in an anterior labral-ligamentous periosteal sleeve avulsion injury (Fig. 2). A midsubstance capsular tear, with or without a Bankart lesion, can result in recurrent instability and represents the capsular lengthening that complicates recurrent dislocations (Fig. 3). Capsular laxity and a Bankart lesion must both be addressed during surgery. A humeral avulsion of the glenohumeral ligament lesion is seen in patients in whom the glenohumeral ligaments fail at the humeral attachment (Fig. 4). Careful inspection of both sides of the glenohumeral ligament is necessary to avoid missing this lesion, which reportedly occurs in up to 8% or 9% of patients with recurrent instability.

Hill-Sachs and bony Bankart lesions often occur with anterior shoulder dislocations. A recent study has highlighted the considerable morbidity and increased surgical failure rate in patients with engaging Hill-Sachs lesions or bony Bankart lesions that result in an "inverted pear" glenoid. An engaging Hill-Sachs lesion is defined as a bony humeral lesion that engages the anterior glenoid with the shoulder in abduction and external rotation. This bony engagement is determined by the orientation of the Hill-Sachs lesion. The inverted pear glenoid is defined as a glenoid in which the normal upright pear shape of the glenoid has lost enough anterior-inferior bone to assume the shape of an inverted pear. The arthroscopic repair failure rate was noted to be 67% when either of these

lesions were present, compared to a 4% recurrence rate in patients without bony compromise. The authors recommended that in patients with an engaging Hill-Sachs lesion, an open capsular shift should be performed. In patients with an inverted pear glenoid, a Latarjet coracoid bone block glenoid reconstruction is the procedure of choice.

Superior labral anterior to posterior (SLAP) lesions may occur in up to 10% of patients with instability and may be difficult to diagnose preoperatively. Once present, SLAP lesions can further contribute to a dislocation diathesis. Type II SLAP lesions occur most frequently and should be repaired back to the superior glenoid at the time of arthroscopic instability repair. If open surgery for instability is contemplated, it is advisable to precede the open repair with an arthroscopic evaluation of the joint to rule out a SLAP lesion or other associated pathology.

Concomitant rotator cuff injury has been well documented as a potential complication of recurrent anterior dislocations, especially in middle-aged and older patients. Persistent pain and weakness following a dislocation episode mandates a meticulous evaluation of the rotator cuff, with particular attention paid to the subscapularis tendon. Injury to the subscapularis tendon occurs in at least 80% of patients age 60 years or older with an anterior dislocation of the shoulder.

Treatment

Nonsurgical Treatment

Nonsurgical treatment of recurrent anterior dislocations typically is only moderately successful and highly dependent on drastic activity modification in the younger,

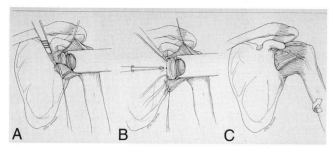

Figure 5 Open Bankart technique. **A,** Horizontal capsulotomy exposing Bankart lesion. **B,** Placement of suture anchors to facilitate labral reattachment. **C,** Capsular shifting to address attenuation. *(Reproduced from Altchek DW, Dines DM: Shoulder injuries in the throwing athlete. J Am Acad Orthop Surg 1995;3:164.)*

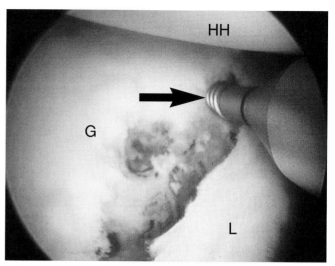

Figure 6 Drill holes and anchor are placed at the glenoid face-neck junction to recreate normal labral anatomy and capsular tensioning. The arrow indicates the most inferior anchor placement. G = glenoid, HH = humeral head, L =labrum.

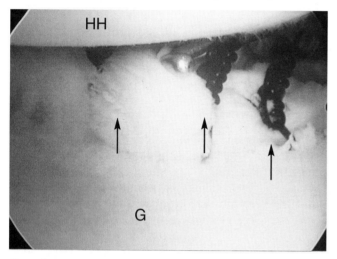

Figure 7 Reconstructed labral "bumper," enhancing concavity-compression stability (*arrows*). HH = humeral head, G = glenoid.

active population. Recent studies of these higher-risk individuals with recurrent instability who participate in a well-supervised nonsurgical treatment program have demonstrated failure rates approaching 90%. Surgical stabilization is warranted in patients who have disabling instability or are unwilling to indefinitely limit their activities.

For older, less active individuals, a short period of immobilization followed by a rehabilitation program is the appropriate treatment regimen.

Surgical Treatment

Historically, the success of open stabilization of the unstable shoulder has been judged by recurrence rates, and success rates approaching 90% to 95% have been routinely reported. The Magnuson-Stack (detachment and lateralization of the subscapularis tendon insertion) and Putti-Platt (division and shortening of the subscapularis tendon, with attachment of the lateral stump of the divided tendon to the glenoid rim/capsule) procedures are nonanatomic interventions designed to limit external rotation. The Bristow procedure was designed

to use the tip of the coracoid as a buttress for the anterior capsule while tethering the inferior half of the subscapularis tendon. Although these procedures were popular at their inception, late significant morbidity has been described, including permanent loss of external rotation, excessive constraint with premature glenohumeral arthrosis, loss of motion and velocity in the overhand athlete, and hardware loosening, migration, and breakage.

The open Bankart technique has been refined and improved. The subscapularis-splitting approach reduces subscapularis weakening and scarring. Anatomic repair of ligament to bone, facilitated by suture anchors, attempts to preserve normal anatomy (Fig. 5). Capsular tensioning is performed when appropriate to address laxity. Accelerated rehabilitation protocols, which focus on safely making gains in motion and strength, allow overhand athletes to return to a competitive level expeditiously.

Despite the low recurrence rate reported with open surgical stabilization, concerns about loss of external rotation, surgical morbidity, and difficult rehabilitation remain. Recently, arthroscopic stabilization techniques have been used to address these concerns.

Arthroscopic Treatment

Early attempts at arthroscopic stabilization initially yielded encouraging results; however, with longer follow-up, recurrence rates were alarmingly high, with some studies reporting failures in up to 50% of patients. Analysis of these failures has identified a number of risk factors, including too short a period of postoperative immobilization (eg, less than 3 weeks), use of too few anchors, anchor placement on the glenoid neck rather than the edge of the articular surface (Fig. 6), participation in contact sports, young patient age, glenohumeral ligament quality, generalized ligamentous laxity, engaging Hill-Sachs lesions, bony Bankart lesions (inverted pear glenoid), and capsular attenuation.

As with the open approach, the arthroscopic technique also has been refined, and recent studies have indicated significantly improved success rates without an increase in morbidity or loss of motion. Refinements include careful placement of at least three anchors onto the glenoid face-neck junction to recreate a labral "bumper" that deepens the glenoid concavity (Fig. 7), use of plication sutures, rotator interval closure or possible use of thermal energy to address capsular elongation, and secure repair of the Bankart lesion. These refinements have resulted in success rates that equal and, in some cases, exceed those associated with traditional open stabilization.

The current use of thermal shrinkage, radiofrequency energy that heats and shrinks elongated capsular tissue, remains controversial. Although the basic science of the tissue response has been studied and described, the long-term effects of heating capsular tissue currently are unknown. Furthermore, the appropriate postoperative rehabilitation protocol has yet to be determined. Many questions remain unanswered regarding late tensile strength, as well as potential proprioceptive deficits following thermal intervention.

The decision to use the open versus arthroscopic approach should be predicated on the surgeon's assessment of the recurrence risk factors that apply to each individual patient, the surgeon's comfort with either technique, and the patient's wishes once the combination of risk factors, surgical nuances, and potential complications have been discussed. For a successful outcome, patient selection is key, followed by meticulous surgical technique that addresses all of the pathology encountered, including Bankart lesions and capsular laxity.

Annotated Bibliography

Anatomy and Biomechanics

McMahon PJ, Dettling J, Sandusky MD, Tibone JE, Lee TQ: The anterior band of the inferior glenohumeral ligament: Assessment of its permanent deformation and the anatomy of its glenoid attachment. *J Bone Joint Surg Br* 1999;81:406-413.

Twelve fresh frozen cadaver shoulders were used to determine the mechanical and histologic properties of the IGHL in addition to testing sites of failure to tensile testing. Strength was measured by tensile testing of the glenoid–soft tissue–humerus (G-ST-H) complex. On tensile testing in abduction and external rotation, eight G-ST-H complexes failed at the site of the glenoid insertion, two at the insertion into the humerus, and two at the midsubstance.

Evaluation

Bokor DJ, Conboy VB, Olson C: Anterior instability of the glenohumeral joint with humeral avulsion of the glenohumeral ligament: A review of 41 cases. *J Bone Joint Surg Br* 1999;811:93-96.

The authors retrospectively analyzed a series of 547 consecutive shoulders treated surgically for instability. In 41 (7.5%) shoulders, the cause of instability was lateral avulsion of the inferior glenohumeral ligament from the neck of the humerus (the HAGL lesion). HAGL lesions were present in 35 of the 130 shoulders without a Bankart lesion (26.9%). Six (14.6%) of the patients with a HAGL lesion had a concomitant Bankart lesion. Patients with HAGL lesions were older on average than those with instability from other causes.

Burkhart SS, De Beer JF: Traumatic glenohumeral bone defects and their relationship to failure of arthroscopic Bankart repairs: Significance of the inverted-pear glenoid and the humeral engaging Hill-Sachs lesion. *Arthroscopy* 2000;16:677-694.

The authors analyzed 194 consecutive arthroscopic Bankart repairs, performed by two surgeons with an identical suture anchor technique. The average follow-up was 27 months (range, 14 to 79 months). Significant bone defects such as an inverted pear glenoid or engaging Hill-Sachs lesion were identified and correlated to recurrent instability. Of the 21 shoulders with recurrent instability, 14 had significant bone defects (3 engaging Hill-Sachs and 11 inverted pear Bankart lesions). For the group without significant bone defects (173 shoulders), there were only 7 recurrences (4%). For the group with significant bone defects (21 patients), there were 14 recurrences (67%). The authors suggest that failure of arthroscopic instability repair is secondary to bony lesions and not to the technique itself. They recommend that engaging Hill-Sachs lesions be treated with open capsular shift and that inverted pear glenoids be treated with the Latarjet procedure.

Cvitanic O, Tirman PF, Feller JF, Bost FW, Minter J, Carroll KW: Using abduction and external rotation of the shoulder to increase the sensitivity of MR arthrography in revealing tears of the anterior glenoid labrum. *Am J Roentgenol* 1997;169:837-844.

MR arthrography of the shoulder that included an additional oblique axial imaging sequence with the patient in the abducted-externally rotated position was performed in 256 patients. Of the 92 patients who underwent surgery, anterior glenoid labrum tears were found in 27. Conventional axial MR arthrograms revealed 13 tears (sensitivity, 48%; specificity, 91%). MR arthrograms obtained with shoulders in the abducted-externally rotated position revealed 24 tears (sensitivity, 89%; specificity, 95%). Review of the images together revealed 26 tears (sensitivity, 96%; specificity, 97%).

Sano H, Kato Y, Haga K, Iroi E, Tabata S: Magnetic resonance arthrography in the assessment of anterior instability of the shoulder: Comparison with double-contrast computed tomography arthrography. *J Shoulder Elbow Surg* 1996;5:280-285.

Forty-seven shoulders with traumatic anterior instability were studied by MR arthrography (MRA) and computed tomography arthrography (CTA). Labral damage evaluated by MRA and by CTA correlated significantly with arthroscopic findings. MRA was more sensitive in detecting torn labra (MRA, sensitivity = 87%, specificity = 75%; CTA, sensitivity = 33%, specificity = 88%). In detecting displaced labra, sensitivity and specificity were 65% and 94% for MRA and 75% and 69% for CTA. The inferior glenohumeral ligament was depicted as a lax structure in 74% by MRA but in only 21% by CTA.

Treatment

Bacilla P, Field LD, Savoie FH: Arthroscopic Bankart repair in a high demand patient population. *Arthroscopy* 1997;13:51-60.

Arthroscopic stabilization using suture anchors, nonabsorbable sutures, and a mattress configuration to allow plication was performed in 40 consecutive patients who were characterized as high risk by virtue of age and sport. All but two patients were age 23 years or younger and engaged in high-demand sports. A recurrence rate of 7% was noted, and 29 of 32 competitive athletes returned to their sport.

Bottoni CR, Wilckens JH, DeBerardino TM, et al: A prospective, randomized evaluation of arthroscopic stabilization versus nonoperative treatment in patients with acute, traumatic, first-time shoulder dislocations. *Am J Sports Med* 2002;30:576-580.

The authors performed a prospective, randomized clinical trial in which recurrent dislocation rates were compared between two groups of young athletes who had sustained an acute, traumatic shoulder dislocation—those who received nonsurgical treatment and those who had an arthroscopic Bankart repair. Fourteen patients underwent 4 weeks of immobilization followed by a supervised rehabilitation program. Ten patients underwent arthroscopic Bankart repair with a bioabsorbable tack followed by the same rehabilitation protocol as the non-surgically treated patients. Average follow-up was 36 months, and three patients were lost to follow-up. Nine of 12 nonsurgically treated patients (75%) developed recurrent instability. Six of the nine required open Bankart repair. Of the nine surgically treated patients available for follow-up, one (11.1%) developed recurrent instability.

Gill TJ, Micheli LJ, Gebhard F, Binder C: Bankart repair for anterior instability of the shoulder: Long-term outcome. *J Bone Joint Surg Am* 1997;79:850-857.

Long-term follow-up of open reconstruction of Bankart lesions, averaging 11 years, yielded excellent or good outcomes in 93% of patients. Instability recurred in 3 of 60 shoulders, each

more than 3 years postoperatively. Average loss of external rotation was 12°. A direct association between range of motion and quality of results was established in a new rating system.

Hayashi K, Massa KL, Thabit G III, et al: Histologic evaluation of the glenohumeral joint capsule after the laser-assisted capsular shift procedure for glenohumeral instability. *Am J Sports Med* 1999;27:162-167.

Capsular samples were taken from 42 patients who had undergone an arthroscopic laser capsular shrinkage procedure. Histologic analysis before and after the procedure, ranging from 0 to 38 months, demonstrated hyalinization and cell necrosis immediately postoperatively. Fibrous connective tissue with reactive cells and increased vascularity was noted at 3 to 6 months, and collagen and cell morphology returned to normal between 7 and 38 months following the procedure. Mechanical and biochemical characterization was not performed.

Hayashida K, Yoneda M, Nakagawa S, Okamura K, Fukushima S: Arthroscopic Bankart suture repair for traumatic anterior shoulder instability: Analysis of the causes of a recurrence. *Arthroscopy* 1998;14:295-301.

An arthroscopic transglenoid technique was used to treat 82 patients with traumatic anterior instability. At follow-up 2 years later, excellent results were found in 55 patients (67%), good results in 14 (17%), and poor in 13 (16%). Recurrent dislocations occurred in 13 patients, and recurrent subluxations occurred in 2 patients, for a recurrence rate of 18%. Multivariate analysis revealed that recurrence was associated with a type III Bankart lesion, return to contact sports, attenuated IGHL, and a repair using fewer than four sutures.

Hovelius L, Augustini BG, Fredin H, Johansson O, Norlin R, Thorling J: Primary anterior dislocation of the shoulder in young patients: A ten-year prospective study. *J Bone Joint Surg Am* 1996;78:1677-1684.

Two hundred forty-five patients who had 247 primary anterior dislocations of the shoulder were followed for 10 years in a multicenter study at 27 Swedish hospitals. The ages of the patients at the time of the dislocation ranged from 12 to 40 years. The patients were assigned to one of three slightly different conservative treatment groups. At the 10-year follow-up evaluation, no additional dislocation had occurred in 129 shoulders (52%). Surgical treatment was required for recurrent dislocation in 58 shoulders (23%): 34 of the 99 shoulders (34%) in patients who were 12 to 22 years old; 16 of the 57 shoulders (28%) in patients who were 23 to 29 years old; and 8 of the 91 shoulders (9%) in patients who were 30 to 40 years old. The type and duration of the initial treatment had no effect on the rate of recurrence. Radiographs of 185 shoulders were obtained at the time of initial dislocation, demonstrating a Hill-Sachs lesion in 99 shoulders (54%). This finding was associated with a significantly worse prognosis for recurrence ($P < 0.04$). Radiographs at 10-year follow-up for 208 shoulders were evaluated for postdislocation arthropathy. Twenty-three shoulders (11%) exhibited mild arthropathy and 18 (9%) moderate or severe arthropathy.

Kiss J, Mersich I, Perlaky GY, Szollas L: The results of the Putti-Platt operation with particular reference to arthritis, pain, and limitation of external rotation. *J Shoulder Elbow Surg* 1998;7:495-500.

The results of 90 Putti-Platt operations were studied with an average follow-up of 9 years. The redislocation rate was 9%. Eleven percent of the patients had pain at rest, and 35% had pain with activity. Ninety percent of the patients had restriction of external rotation both at the side of the body (average loss 24°) and in 90° abduction (average loss 23°). Osteoarthritis was moderate in 20 shoulders (29%) and severe in 1 shoulder (1%). Eighty-three percent of patients were fully satisfied, 13% were partly satisfied, and 4% were not satisfied with the result of the surgery.

Mologne TS, McBride MT, Lapoint JM: Assessment of failed arthroscopic anterior labral repairs: Findings at open surgery. *Am J Sports Med* 1997;25:813-817.

Twenty patients who had undergone open revision procedures following unsuccessful arthroscopic Bankart repairs were reviewed. At the time of the open surgery, 12 patients (60%) had healed Bankart lesions, 8 (40%) had persistent Bankart lesions, and 15 (75%) had redundant anterior capsules. The authors concluded that failure to treat either the Bankart lesion or capsular laxity at the time of an arthroscopic Bankart procedure may result in recurrent instability.

Nelson BJ, Arciero RA: Arthroscopic management of glenohumeral instability. *Am J Sports Med* 2000;28:602-614.

The authors review current technique and results of arthroscopic management of shoulder instability.

O'Neill DB: Arthroscopic Bankart repair of anterior detachments of the glenoid labrum: A prospective study. *J Bone Joint Surg Am* 1999;81:1357-1366.

Arthroscopic transglenoid stabilization was performed on 41 patients with recurrent anterior dislocations. Average follow-up was more than 4 years. Two patients (5%) experienced recurrent subluxation, and 40 of 41 (98%) returned to their preoperative sport. Twenty-two patients (54%) had full range of motion in all planes.

Pagnani MJ, Warren RF, Altchek DW, Wickiewicz TL, Anderson AF: Arthroscopic shoulder stabilization using transglenoid sutures: A four-year minimum follow up. *Am J Sports Med* 1996;24:459-467.

Thirty-seven of 41 consecutive patients with recurrent anterior instability of the shoulder were retrospectively observed for a mean of 5.6 years after an arthroscopic stabilization procedure had been performed using a transglenoid suture technique. According to the Rowe scoring system, 27 patients (74%) had good or excellent results, and 3 patients (7%) were graded as fair. Seven patients (19%) developed recurrent instability after the procedure and had failed results. Absence of a Bankart lesion at operation was associated with postoperative instability ($P = 0.03$). Four of the 13 patients who par-ticipated in contact sports or recreational skiing developed postoperative instability ($P = 0.21$). All failures occurred within 2 years of the procedure.

van der Zwaag HM, Brand R, Obermann WR, Rozing PM: Glenohumeral osteoarthrosis after Putti-Platt repair. *J Shoulder Elbow Surg* 1999; 8:252-258.

Sixty-six shoulders were treated with the Putti-Platt procedure with 22-year follow up (range, 10 to 40 years). The average age of the patients was 49.3 years (range, 33 to 74 years). The redislocation rate was low (only 3%), and 71% of the patients had no symptoms in the operated shoulder. Osteoarthrosis of the glenohumeral joint was found in 40 (61%) shoulders. Arthrosis was mild in 23 shoulders (35%), moderate in 13 shoulders (20%), and severe in 4 shoulders (6%). The number of dislocations before surgery was correlated with the severity of arthrosis but not with its incidence.

Yoneda M, Hayashida K, Wakitani S, Nakagawa S, Fukushima S: Bankart procedure augmented by coracoid transfer for contact athletes with traumatic anterior shoulder instability. *Am J Sports Med* 1999;27: 21-26.

The authors analyzed the clinical efficacy of the Bankart procedure augmented by coracoid transfer for traumatic anterior shoulder instability in athletes playing contact sports. Eighty-three athletes (85 joints) with traumatic anterior shoulder instability who underwent the combined procedure were studied. The mean patient age at surgery was 21 years, and the mean follow-up period was 5.8 years. Rowe scores were excellent in 58 shoulders (68%), good in 21 (25%), fair in 5 (6%), and poor in 1 (1%). A complete return to contact sports was achieved by 73 of the 83 patients (88%). The average loss of external rotation was 15° with the arm at the side and 7° with the arm in 90° of abduction. The complications were nonunions in two patients, screw breakage in one patient, and axillary nerve injury in one.

Classic Bibliography

Arciero RA, Wheeler JH, Ryan JB, McBride JT: Arthroscopic Bankart repair versus nonoperative treatment for acute, initial anterior shoulder dislocations. *Am J Sports Med* 1994;22:589-594.

Bankart ASB: The pathology and treatment of recurrent dislocation of the shoulder-joint. *Br J Surg* 1938; 26:23-29.

Bigliani LU, Pollock RG, Soslowsky LJ, Flatow EL, Pawluk RJ, Mow VC: Tensile properties of the inferior glenohumeral ligament. *J Orthop Res* 1992;10:187-197.

Burkhead WZ Jr, Rockwood CA Jr: Treatment of instability of the shoulder with an exercise program. *J Bone Joint Surg Am* 1992;74:890-896.

Ferlic DC, DiGiovine NM: A long-term retrospective study of the modified Bristow procedure. *Am J Sports Med* 1988;16:469-474.

Grana WA, Buckley PD, Yates CK: Arthroscopic Bankart suture repair. *Am J Sports Med* 1993;21:589-594.

Green MR, Christensen KP: Arthroscopic Bankart procedure: Two- to five-year follow up with clinical correlation to severity of glenoid labral lesion. *Am J Sports Med* 1995;23:276-281.

Hintermann B, Gachter A: Arthroscopic findings after shoulder dislocation. *Am J Sports Med* 1995;23:545-551.

Hovelius L: Anterior dislocation of the shoulder in teenagers and young adults: Five-year prognosis. *J Bone Joint Surg Am* 1987;69:393-399.

Hovelius L: Shoulder dislocation in Swedish ice hockey players. *Am J Sports Med* 1978;6:373-377.

Neviaser RJ, Neviaser TJ: Recurrent instability of the shoulder after age 40. *J Shoulder Elbow Surg* 1995;4:416-418.

O'Brien SJ, Neves MC, Arnoczky SP, et al: The anatomy and histology of the inferior glenohumeral ligament complex of the shoulder. *Am J Sports Med* 1990;18:449-456.

O'Brien SJ, Schwartz RS, Warren RF, Torzilli PA: Capsular restraints to anterior-posterior motion of the abducted shoulder: A biomechanical study. *J Shoulder Elbow Surg* 1995;4:298-308.

Rowe CR: Prognosis in dislocations of the shoulder. *J Bone Joint Surg Am* 1956;38:957-977.

Simonet WT, Cofield RH: Prognosis in anterior shoulder dislocation. *Am J Sports Med* 1984;12:19-24.

Soslowsky LJ, Flatow EL, Bigliani LU, Mow VC: Articular geometry of the glenohumeral joint. *Clin Orthop* 1992;285:181-190.

Speer KP, Deng X, Borrero S, Torzilli PA, Altchek DA, Warren RF: Biomechanical evaluation of a simulated Bankart lesion. *J Bone Joint Surg Am* 1994;76:1819-1826.

Thomas SC, Matsen FA III: An approach to the repair of avulsion of the glenohumeral ligaments in the management of traumatic anterior glenohumeral instability. *J Bone Joint Surg Am* 1989;71:506-513.

Turkel SJ, Panio MW, Marshall JL, Girgis FG: Stabilizing mechanisms preventing anterior dislocation of the glenohumeral joint. *J Bone Joint Surg Am* 1981;63:1208-1217.

Wheeler JH, Ryan JB, Arciero RA, Molinari RN: Arthroscopic versus nonoperative treatment of acute shoulder dislocations in young athletes. *Arthroscopy* 1989 5:213-217.

Walch G, Boileau P, Levigne C, Mandrino A, Neyret P, Donell S: Arthroscopic stabilization for recurrent anterior shoulder dislocation: Results of 59 cases. *Arthroscopy* 1995;11:173-179.

Wolf EM, Cheng JC, Dickson K: Humeral avulsion of glenohumeral ligaments as a cause of anterior shoulder instability. *Arthroscopy* 1995;11:600-607.

Young DC, Rockwood CA Jr: Complications of a failed Bristow procedure and their management. *J Bone Joint Surg Am* 1991;73:969-981.

Chapter 46

The Role of Arthroscopy for Acute Shoulder Dislocations

Robert E. Hunter, MD

Introduction

Over the past two decades, arthroscopy of the shoulder has progressed from a curiosity to an indispensable first-line treatment. There has been a transition from open reconstruction for all shoulder instabilities to arthroscopic management of many types of instabilities. This chapter examines the role of arthroscopy in the management of acute shoulder dislocations, reports on the outcomes of nonsurgical and surgical treatment, and discusses the advantages and disadvantages of arthroscopic intervention. The surgical technique for arthroscopic shoulder stabilization will also be discussed, in addition to follow-up care and rehabilitation.

Classification of Shoulder Instability

One way to classify shoulder instability is by the degree of instability, described as either dislocation or subluxation. Instability can be classified as either acute, meaning a single isolated situation caused the instability, or recurrent, meaning the instability is the result of repeated insults to the shoulder. Instability can also be classified based on etiology. Instability can be secondary to trauma, recurrent microtrauma, atraumatic causes, or neuromuscular etiology. Instability also should be described based on the direction of abnormal motion. The shoulder instability may be unidirectional, in which case the shoulder is unstable in either an anterior, posterior, or inferior direction, or it may be multidirectional (unstable in several directions). The surgeon must consider magnitude, direction, and etiology of instability when considering arthroscopic intervention.

Patient Factors

Age and activity levels are important factors to consider when selecting patients for arthroscopic intervention and in anticipating the incidence of recurrence of dislocation, with age being the principal variable. Recurrence rates after conservative treatment for the population younger than 25 years of age are reported to range from 60% to 95%. In a study comparing an athletic population with a nonathletic population of similar age (younger than age 30 years), the recurrence rate was 82% in the athletic population and 30% in the nonathletic population.

Imaging and Pathologic Findings

MRI is not particularly useful in evaluating acute dislocations. In a review comparing preoperative MRI assessment with findings noted at arthroscopy, MRI successfully identified labral tears in only 68% of patients and Hill-Sachs lesions in 80%. The authors concluded that MRI was only "moderately" reliable for identifying pathology in acute dislocations. Arthroscopy is a better tool for assessment of the amount and type of damage sustained at the time of dislocation.

In individuals younger than age 30 years who dislocate their shoulder anteriorly, there is almost always a traumatic avulsion of the anteroinferior labral-ligamentous complex from the anterior glenoid rim. This pathologic finding is commonly referred to as a Bankart lesion. Although a Bankart lesion is almost invariably found after acute anterior shoulder dislocations, especially in younger individuals, a number of other pathologic findings may be noted. Additional pathology that can result from dislocation of the shoulder includes capsular intrasubstance tears, articular cartilage injuries, Hill-Sachs lesions, superior labrum anterior-posterior (SLAP) lesions (Fig. 1), and rotator cuff tears. The authors of one report reviewed 24 patients ranging in age from 17 to 60 years and found a 100% incidence of hemarthrosis, labral damage, Bankart lesions, and Hill-Sachs lesions. In a study of college-aged West Point cadets who had acute dislocations, Bankart lesions were found in 97% of patients, Hill-Sachs lesions in 90%, humeral avulsions of the glenohumeral ligament complex in 2%, and hemarthroses in all patients. In patients older than 25 years of age, the incidence of capsular damage begins to increase and the incidence of labral tears, either partial or complete,

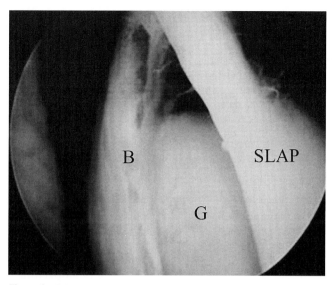

Figure 1 A SLAP lesion of a right shoulder viewed from the posterior portal. The lesion includes partial disruption of the biceps tendon. B = intact remaining biceps root; G = glenoid.

TABLE 1	Recurrence Rates of Arthroscopic and Open Techniques in Surgeries Performed by the Same Surgeon

			Recurrence (%)	
Study	Sample Size (A/O)	Mean Follow-up (A/O) (mo)	A	O
Field et al, 1999	50/50	33/30	8	0
Cole and Warner, 2000	37/22	52/55	16	9
Steinbeck and Jerosch, 1998	30/32	36/40	17	5
Guanche et al, 1996	25/12	27/25	33	8
Geiger et al, 1997	16/18	23/24	43	0

A = arthroscopic; O = open

(Reproduced with permission from Cole BJ, Warner JJP: Arthroscopic versus open bankart repair for traumatic anterior shoulder instability. Clin Sports Med 2000;19:19-48.)

decreases. A review of acute dislocations in a population of patients 30 years of age or younger found labral tears in 87% of the population and capsular tears with a normal labrum in 13%. In the group with labral tears, Hill-Sachs lesions were found in 64% of patients, rotator cuff tears in 18%, osteochondral loose bodies in 14%, and glenoid avulsion fractures in 7%.

Nonsurgical Versus Arthroscopic Treatment

Two prospective, randomized studies have examined the effectiveness of arthroscopy in acute shoulder instability compared to conservative treatment. In the first study, West Point cadets 25 years of age or younger with no prior history of shoulder pathology and who sustained traumatic dislocation requiring reduction were assessed. Thirty-six athletes (average age, 20 years) met the criteria for inclusion. One group of 15 patients was treated with immobilization for 1 month, followed by rehabilitation; full activity was allowed at 4 months. The other group of 21 patients underwent arthroscopic Bankart repair followed by the same protocol as the conservatively treated patients. Twelve of the 15 patients (80%) developed recurrent instability. Seven of the 12 patients with recurrent instability required further treatment with an open Bankart repair. Eighteen of the 21 patients (86%) treated with arthroscopic Bankart repair had no recurrent instability at last follow-up (mean, 32 months; range, 15 to 45) ($P = 0.001$). One patient eventually required an open Bankart repair to treat recurrence ($P = 0.005$). The average loss of external rotation was 3°.

In a prospective randomized study of 40 patients younger than 30 years of age followed for at least 2 years, the dislocations were traumatic in origin, caused by an abduction external rotation mechanism. All dislocations were identifiable on radiographs or required reduction. Nineteen of the 20 patients examined arthroscopically had a Bankart lesion. When an arthroscopic transglenoid suture technique was used, the authors noted a recurrence rate of 16%, compared to 47% in those treated nonsurgically. The arthroscopically treated group had statistically better scores on a quality of life index than the group treated nonsurgically. There was no significant difference between the groups for range of motion.

The timing of surgical intervention is an important issue. In a 1996 study, a comparison was made between two groups of patients whose instability was treated arthroscopically. One group included patients who were treated after the initial acute anterior dislocation and the other group included patients who were treated after recurrence of anterior dislocation. Postoperatively, the group with acute dislocations had a higher Rowe score and greater range of motion (particularly in external rotation) than the group with recurrent dislocations. This indicates that surgical intervention before recurrence of dislocations results in improved long-term outcomes. Early arthroscopic fixation is advantageous because glenoid bone that is newly injured and richly vascularized is ideal for healing; the capsular tissue is more elastic with less need for dissection; there is little or no retraction of the capsule and labrum, allowing easier reapproximation of the ligamentous tissues to the glenoid; and usually there is less intra-articular pathology, such as damage to the articular cartilage.

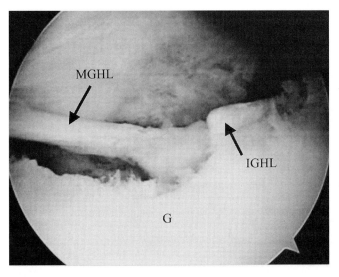

Figure 2 Right shoulder viewed from posterior portal demonstrating disruption of the inferior glenohumeral ligament (IGHL) as well as the middle glenohumeral ligament (MGHL). G = glenoid.

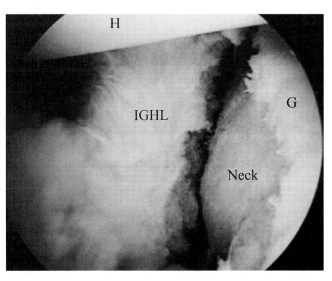

Figure 3 View of a right shoulder through an anterosuperior portal demonstrating avulsion of the IGHL from the glenoid (G) and the glenoid neck (neck). H = humeral head.

Outcomes of Nonsurgical Treatment

Although acute shoulder dislocations traditionally have been treated by reduction and nonsurgical care, this method is not particularly effective in children 16 years of age or younger. Despite the application of different nonsurgical treatment strategies, recurrence rates of 100% have been noted in this patient group. In a study of 55 West Point cadets age 25 years or younger who were treated nonsurgically in a carefully supervised program of immobilization and rehabilitation, the recurrence rate was 85%. Period of immobilization, type and intensity of rehabilitation, and time to return to function appear to offer little, if any, benefit to the young athletic population. Nonsurgical measures do not seem to impact recurrence rates or long-term outcomes. A classic study of a large population (N = 245) treated nonsurgically after acute anterior shoulder dislocation analyzed radiographs at 10-year follow-up. Mild degenerative changes were noted in 11% of patients and moderate to severe degenerative changes in 9%. It is not clear if the arthritis resulted from the trauma of the first dislocation or if it was a result of recurrent instability and continued trauma to the joint.

Open Surgical Versus Arthroscopic Treatment

Eliminating recurrence of instability is the most important measure of success, but postoperative range of motion, time and ability to return to function, and patient satisfaction must also be considered when evaluating outcomes of open or arthroscopic treatment. In one recent study of 15 patients treated with open reconstruction after primary dislocation, recurrence was reported in only 7%, leading to the conclusion that open reconstruction for young, athletic patients was the treatment method of choice. However, in more than 50% of patients, loss of external rotation was as much as 10°. Depending on the methodology and the length of follow-up of various studies, recurrence rates range from 0% to almost 50% when an arthroscopic approach is used to repair instability lesions. The wide range of reported recurrence makes outcomes difficult to predict. Recurrence rates have been higher for arthroscopic stabilization versus open techniques when surgery is performed by the same surgeon using similar postoperative protocols (Table 1). In one study, recurrence rates were found to be higher with arthroscopic repair and the loss of external rotation was not significantly greater in the population undergoing open repair. Other studies have demonstrated that loss of external rotation after arthroscopic stabilization is usually less than 5°. In a study comparing arthroscopic and open Bankart procedures, surgical time was shortened, the amount of blood loss was decreased, and the need for postoperative narcotics was dramatically reduced with arthroscopy. In addition, shorter length of hospital stay and improved return to work time were reported when the stabilization was performed arthroscopically. Also, the arthroscopic technique results in little damage to the subscapularis muscle and provides better visualization of the intra-articular structures than with the open technique. The smaller arthroscopic incisions are cosmetically more appealing than the large incisions required for open stabilization. There also is less damage to the periarticular soft tissues, resulting in a predictable return of shoulder motion, particularly external rotation. The current disadvantages associated with the arthroscopic approach are the higher recurrence rates and

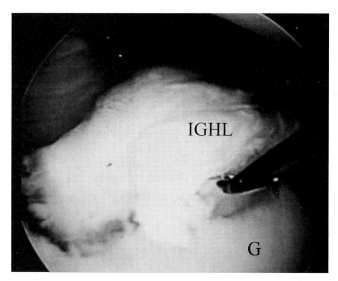

Figure 4 Right shoulder viewed from posterior portal demonstrating passage of a No. 1 PDS suture through the IGHL at the 5 o'clock position. G = glenoid.

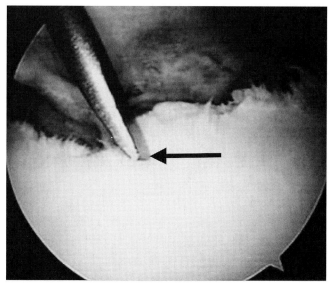

Figure 5 Positioning of the hole for anchor insertion in a right shoulder. The drill is placed 2 mm on to the glenoid surface at the 3 o'clock position (*arrow*).

the challenging technical aspects associated with arthroscopic repair. The techniques are difficult to learn initially, and require much practice and mastery before a technically expeditious and effective repair can be performed. However, once proficiency in the techniques is gained, results of the surgery can be gratifying to the surgeon and patient.

Indications for Arthroscopic Treatment

The ideal patient for arthroscopic treatment is the non-contact athlete, younger than 30 years of age, who has sustained an acute traumatic dislocation. Treatment results are better in patients with arthroscopic evidence of a Bankart lesion along with a well-developed inferior glenohumeral ligament and normal capsule, cartilage, and physiologic laxity patterns. Factors that result in increased recurrence rates include the presence of ligamentous damage in conjunction with labral damage and a very thin, ill-defined labral-ligamentous complex. The surgeon should use caution when choosing arthroscopy if the patient does not have a definite Bankart lesion, has evidence of interstitial capsular damage, has multidirectional instability, poor quality tissue, voluntary instability, and/or is noncompliant.

Arthroscopic Technique

The patient is placed in the lateral decubitus position with 10 lb each of longitudinal traction and lateral traction through the axilla. The posterior portal is used for viewing, and an anteroinferior portal becomes the working portal (Fig. 2). At times an anterosuperior portal can be of value for viewing and for suture management (Fig. 3).

Suture anchors are used for the stabilization; either two or three anchors are used depending on the size of the Bankart lesion. One anchor is placed at the 4 o'clock to 5 o'clock position, the second anchor is placed at the 3 o'clock position, and, if the lesion extends superiorly, a third anchor is used at the 1 o'clock to 2 o'clock position. No. 1 PDS or No. 2 permanent suture is placed with a single pass through the soft tissues rather than a horizontal mattress (Fig. 4). The labral-ligamentous tissues are advanced and held with a sliding knot that is reinforced with four half hitches. When positioning the drill holes on the glenoid, it is important to place the holes on the glenoid surface 1 to 2 mm in from the margin (Fig. 5). This allows for good visualization of the hole at the time of anchor insertion. It also results in a heaping of the inferior glenohumeral ligament over the glenoid at the time of stabilization recreating the bumper effect (Fig. 6). When the labral-ligamentous complex has been advanced and anchored, the surgeon should be able to see and palpate a retensioned inferior glenohumeral ligament (Fig. 7).

Follow-up Care and Rehabilitation

Postoperatively, the patient is placed in a sling and swathe with the arm held in adduction and internal rotation for 4 weeks. During that time, shoulder isometrics are performed. Elbow flexion and extension are allowed while maintaining the elbow at the side. At 4 weeks, the sling is removed and external rotation is allowed from full internal rotation to 0°. Elevation and abduction are begun with a goal of 90° in both arcs by 6 weeks after surgery. At 6 weeks, full range of motion is allowed and encouraged, and a graduated strengthening program is begun for the

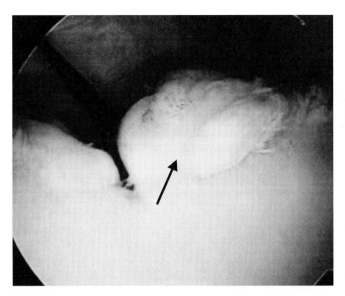

Figure 6 Reconstitution of the anterior IGHL attachment onto the glenoid with a No. 1 PDS suture. Notice the heaping of the ligamentous structures over the anterior rim of the glenoid. The arrow identifies the reconstituted bumper.

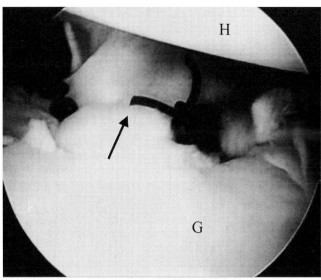

Figure 7 Restoration of tension in the superior band of the IGHL. Sutures are placed in the 3 o'clock and 5 o'clock positions. The arrow identifies the restored superior band of the IGHL. H = humeral head; G = glenoid.

shoulder girdle musculature, as well as the periscapular stabilizers. At 12 weeks after surgery, patients are allowed full unrestricted use of the shoulder for regular daily activities. Overhead throwing sports and sports that might result in a fall on an outstretched arm are restricted until approximately 6 months postoperatively, at which point full functional activities are encouraged.

Summary

It is clear that conservative treatment of acute shoulder dislocation has inferior results to those of arthroscopic stabilization in young, active patients. However, before the arthroscopic approach to acute shoulder dislocation becomes the standard accepted approach in this at-risk population, the results of arthroscopic repair must demonstrate recurrence rates that are equal to or better than those of open procedures. With standardization and mastery of arthroscopic techniques, these goals and better patient outcomes will become a reality.

Annotated Bibliography

Classification of Shoulder Instability

Baker CL: Arthroscopic evaluation of acute initial shoulder dislocations. *Instr Course Lect* 1996;45:83-89.

This is a thorough discussion of acute shoulder dislocations, including anatomy, associated injuries, arthroscopic findings, and outcomes of surgical intervention. The author calls for more research before a routine recommendation of arthro-

scopic repair of these injuries can be made.

Nonsurgical Versus Arthroscopic Treatment

Hehl G, Lang E, Hoellen I, Kiefer H, Becker LL: Arthroscopic capsule-labrum refixation in anterior shoulder dislocation: Primary or secondary management? *Unfallchirurg* 1996;99:831-835.

A comparison was made between two groups of patients whose instability was treated arthroscopically. One group included patients who were treated after the initial acute anterior dislocation and the other group included patients who were treated after recurrence of anterior dislocation. Postoperatively, the group with acute dislocations had a higher Rowe score and greater range of motion (particularly in external rotation) than the group with recurrent dislocations.

Kirkley A, Griffin S, Richards C, Miniaci A, Mohtadi N: Prospective randomized clinical trial comparing the effectiveness of immediate arthroscopic stabilization versus immobilization and rehabilitation in first traumatic anterior dislocations of the shoulder. *Arthroscopy* 1999;15:507-514.

The authors conducted a randomized, prospective study of 40 patients younger than 30 years of age who were treated with immobilization and rehabilitation or with arthroscopic stabilization. Patients treated surgically had a significantly lower rate of redislocation (15.9% versus 47%).

Outcomes of Nonsurgical Treatment

DeBerardino TM, Arciero RA, Taylor DC: Arthroscopic stabilization of acute initial anterior shoulder dislocation: The West Point experience. *J South Orthop Assoc* 1996;5:263-271.

Forty-seven of 55 patients (85%) treated nonsurgically experienced recurrence. Two of nine patients treated surgically with arthroscopic abrasion or staple repair had recurrence; 18 of 21 patients (86%) treated surgically with transglenoid sutures had no recurrence; and 35 of 39 patients (90%) treated using bioabsorbable tacks had no recurrent instability.

Hovelius L, Augustini BG, Fredin H, Johansson O, Norlin R, Thorling J: Primary anterior dislocation of the shoulder in young patients: A ten-year prospective study. *J Bone Joint Surg Am* 1996;78:1677-1684.

The authors present a prospective, 10-year follow-up of 245 patients with primary anterior shoulder dislocations treated nonsurgically. One third of patients younger than 30 years of age required surgical stabilization. Neither the type nor length of initial treatment had an effect on the recurrence rate.

Open Surgical Versus Arthroscopic Treatment

Ambacher T, Paar O: Traumatic shoulder dislocation in young athletes: Open or arthroscopic stabilization? *Sportverletz Sportschaden* 1999;13:68-73.

In this study of 15 patients treated with open reconstruction after primary dislocation, a recurrence of only 7% was found. The authors concluded that open reconstruction for young athletic patients was the method of choice. However, in greater than 50% of patients, loss of external rotation was as much as 10°.

Cole BJ, L'Insalata J, Irrgang J, Warner JJ. Comparison of arthroscopic and open anterior shoulder stabilization. A two to six-year follow-up study. *J Bone Joint Surg Am* 2000;82:1108-114.

Sixty-three consecutive patients with recurrent traumatic anterior shoulder instability were treated with an arthroscopic Bankart repair or open capsular shift. Operative decision-making was based on the findings of examination under anesthesia and arthroscopy. Thirty-nine patients with only anterior translation on examination under anesthesia and a discrete Bankart lesion underwent arthroscopic Bankart repair with use of absorbable implants. Twenty-four patients with inferior translation in addition to anterior translation on examination under anesthesia and capsular injury on arthroscopy underwent an open capsular shift. Fifty-nine of the 63 patients (94%) were examined and filled out a questionnaire at a mean of 54 months following surgery. Recurrence of dislocation or apprehension occurred after 9 of 37 arthroscopic repairs (24%) and after 4 of 22 open reconstructions (18%). There were no significant differences between the two groups with regard to the

prevalence of failure or in regard to Rowe, American Shoulder and Elbow Surgeons, or Short Form-36 scores.

Cole BJ, Warner JJ: Arthroscopic versus open Bankart repair for traumatic anterior shoulder instability. *Clin Sports Med* 2000;19:19-48.

This article extensively reviews the literature and makes comparisons between arthroscopic and open stabilization. It includes a decision-making algorithm that determines the surgical procedure to use. The authors describe specific criteria for selecting patients for arthroscopic Bankart repair.

Field LD, Savoie FH, Griffith P: A comparison of open arthroscopic Bankart repair. *J Shoulder Elbow Surg* 1999;8:195.

In this abstract, recurrence rates for shoulder instability following open or arthroscopic techniques were compared.

Geiger DF, Hurley JA, Tovey JA, Rao JP: Results of arthroscopic versus open Bankart suture repair. *Clin Orthop* 1997;337:111-117.

Sixteen patients with anterior instability were treated arthroscopically and 18 were treated with open reconstruction. The recurrence rate in the arthroscopic group was 43%. There were no recurrences in the open group. External rotation was not significantly greater in the population undergoing open repair than in the population undergoing arthroscopic repair.

Guanche CA, Quick DC, Sodergren KM, Buss DD: Arthroscopic versus open reconstruction of the shoulder in patients with isolated Bankart lesions. *Am J Sports Med* 1996;24:144-148.

Comparison of open and arthroscopic stabilization of Bankart lesions in patients with traumatic, unidirectional anterior glenohumeral dislocations. Fifteen patients had an arthroscopic Bankart repair and 12 patients were stabilized with a standard open Bankart repair. Patients were followed 17 to 42 months after surgery. In the arthroscopic group, 5 of 15 patients experienced subluxation or dislocation; 2 required reoperation. One of the 12 patients in the open repair group experienced a subluxation in the follow-up period, but no patients had dislocations or reoperations. The open group had significantly better results in regard to satisfaction, stability, apprehension, and loss of forward flexion.

Steinbeck J, Jerosch J: Arthroscopic transglenoid stabilization versus open anchor suturing in traumatic anterior instability of the shoulder. *Am J Sports Med* 1998; 26:373-378.

This article presents a prospective observational study of 62 consecutive patients with recurrent traumatic anterior instability. Thirty patients were treated with arthroscopic stabilization, and 32 were treated with open Bankart repair with a mean follow-up of 36 and 40 months, respectively (range, 24 to 60 months for both groups). Transglenoid sutures were used with the arthroscopic technique and bone anchors were used with the open technique. Recurrence occurred in five patients (17%) in the arthroscopic repair group and in two (6%) in the open repair group. According to the criteria of Rowe and associates, 24 patients (80%) who had arthroscopic repair and 29 patients (90.6%) who had open repair were rated as good to excellent. Normal or near normal functioning in sport activities was possible in 30 patients (94%) who underwent open repair and 25 patients (83%) who had arthroscopic repair.

Warme WJ, Arciero RA, Taylor DC: Anterior shoulder instability in sport: Current management recommendations. *Sports Med* 1999;28:209-220.

The authors review the evaluation and treatment of anterior shoulder dislocations. They discuss both open and arthroscopic stabilization techniques and make current management recommendations.

Arthroscopic Technique

Higgins LD, Warner JJ: Arthroscopic Bankart repair: Operative technique and surgical pitfalls. *Clin Sports Med* 2000;19:49-62.

The authors present a thorough description of arthroscopic Bankart repair techniques using both implantable fixation devices and sutures.

Classic Bibliography

Arciero RA, St Pierre P: Acute shoulder dislocation: Indications and techniques for operative management.

Clin Sports Med 1995;14:937-953.

Arciero RA, Wheeler JH, Ryan JB, McBride JT: Arthroscopic Bankart repair versus nonoperative treatment for acute, initial anterior shoulder dislocations. *Am J Sports Med* 1994;22:589-594.

Bankart ASB: Recurrent or habitual dislocation of the shoulder joint. *BMJ* 1923;2:1132-1133.

Green MR, Christensen KP: Arthroscopic versus open Bankart procedures: A comparison of early morbidity and complications. *Arthroscopy* 1993;9:371-374.

Hovelius L: Anterior dislocation of the shoulder in teenagers and young adults: Five-year prognosis. *J Bone Joint Surg Am* 1987;69:393-399.

Marans HJ, Angel KR, Schemitsch EH, Wedge JH: The fate of traumatic anterior dislocation of the shoulder in children. *J Bone Joint Surg Am* 1992;74:1242-1244.

Norlin R: Intraarticular pathology in acute, first-time anterior shoulder dislocation: An arthroscopic study. *Arthroscopy* 1993;9:546-549.

Rowe CR, Patel D, Southmayd WW: The Bankart procedure: A long-term end-result study. *J Bone Joint Surg Am* 1978;60:1-16.

Rowe CR, Zarins B, Ciullo JV: Recurrent anterior dislocation of the shoulder after surgical repair. Apparent causes of failure and treatment. *J Bone Joint Surg Am* 1984;66:159-168.

Simonet WT, Cofield RH: Prognosis in anterior shoulder dislocation. *Am J Sports Med* 1984;12:19-24.

Suder PA, Frich LH, Hougaard K, Lundorf E, Wulff Jakobsen B: Magnetic resonance imaging evaluation of capsulolabral tears after traumatic primary anterior shoulder dislocation: A prospective comparison with arthroscopy of 25 cases. *J Shoulder Elbow Surg* 1995;4:419-428.

Chapter 47

Arthroscopic Pancapsular Plication for Multidirectional Instability

Stephen J. Snyder, MD

Roger C. Dunteman, MD

Introduction

Multidirectional instability of the shoulder has become increasingly identified as a cause of shoulder disability in the young athletic population. Multidirectional instability is defined classically as involuntary excessive glenohumeral joint translation in three directions: anterior, posterior, and inferior. This instability is symptomatic and disabling. Patients exhibit global instability of three subtypes: anterior inferior dislocation with posterior subluxation, posterior inferior dislocation with anterior subluxation, and recurrent dislocation in all three directions. Multidirectional instability should be differentiated from the increased glenohumeral laxity that is found in asymptomatic individuals, especially those who participate in sports that require overhead motion. These individuals experience increased translation of the humeral head on the glenoid fossa without the disabling symptoms associated with multidirectional instability. This laxity is physiologic for these individuals and therefore surgical treatment is not indicated for them. It is unknown whether increased laxity in the asymptomatic shoulder eventually leads to multidirectional instability.

Etiology

Multidirectional instability is typically found in two different populations. The first group, patients with generalized ligamentous laxity, often present with bilateral symptoms and no history of trauma. In the other group of patients, multidirectional instability occurs secondary to a specific injury or repetitive microtrauma. This trauma injures the capsule and glenohumeral ligaments and they elongate, making the joint more unstable with time. Athletes such as swimmers, gymnasts, and those who participate in sports that require overhead motion are particularly susceptible to this type of multidirectional instability, because their shoulders are subject to excessive strains at the extremes of motion on a repetitive basis. Often a patient will present with generalized laxity that has been asymptomatic until a specific, sometimes minor event triggers the pain and dysfunction of ligamentous incompetence.

Clinical Findings

Patients with multidirectional instability may experience symptoms during normal activities of daily living when the shoulder is in the midrange of glenohumeral motion. The symptoms are exacerbated when the shoulder is in positions of extreme range of motion. These symptoms include pain, varying degrees of instability, and transient neurologic episodes. Examination will reveal involuntary subluxation or dislocation of the glenohumeral joint in three directions: anterior, posterior, and inferior. A subset of patients displays voluntary instability, in which the shoulder can be purposely dislocated. Voluntary instability can be either positional or muscular. Patients with voluntary positional instability are able to subluxate the glenohumeral joint posteriorly when the arm is placed in flexion, adduction, and internal rotation. These patients should be differentiated from those with voluntary muscular instability because the latter may be a manifestation of an emotional or psychiatric disorder. Patients with voluntary muscular instability can cause a posterior subluxation by winging the scapula with the arm at the side while contracting the internal rotators in the shoulder. This maneuver is usually not painful, and the patient can repeat it on request without apparent discomfort.

Inferior laxity is the hallmark finding for multidirectional instability and can be identified on physical examination. The sulcus test is performed by applying downward traction to the arm while it is being held at the side. If significant inferior translation occurs, a sulcus sign—a dimple in the skin just beneath the anterior lateral acromion—is observed. This implies global laxity of the glenohumeral ligaments and capsule, in addition to specific laxity of the rotator interval, which is the primary restraint to inferior translation when the arm is adducted. The redundancy of the inferior capsule can be specifically assessed when a similar downward force is applied with the arm abducted 90°. Inferior translation will be noted if there is incompetence of the inferior glenohumeral ligament (both the anterior and posterior bands). Range of motion is tested in the supine position with the arm abducted 90°. Apprehension and suppression of apprehension with a physically applied relocation force are also noted at this time. Anterior and posterior subluxation testing is performed in the lateral decubitus position. Other joints (for example, elbows, knees, finger joints) are assessed for generalized ligamentous laxity.

Plain radiographs are usually normal, but they may reveal inferior subluxation of the humeral head in relation to the glenoid. A dysplastic glenoid, a humeral head defect, or a glenoid rim fracture can also be identified. MRI is usually not indicated in the evaluation of patients with multidirectional instability because it rarely provides additional information. However, a magnetic resonance arthrogram with intra-articular gadolinium may demonstrate a redundant capsular pouch or secondary labral pathology.

Pathophysiology

The concavity-compression mechanism of keeping the humeral head centered on the glenoid is lost, and varying degrees of instability from mild subluxation to dislocation are observed. The abnormal glenohumeral mechanics associated with multidirectional instability can lead to rotator cuff and periscapular muscle overload and dysfunction.

Arthroscopy of the shoulder with multidirectional instability will always reveal an atrophic inferior glenohumeral ligament complex with a large, redundant capsule and an attenuated, rounded labrum. A capsular rent, labral tear, glenoid fracture, or humeral head defect usually is not found. However, secondary changes in the rotator interval and middle glenohumeral ligament are often present.

Nonsurgical Management

Because the rotator cuff and periscapular muscles are dysfunctional in multidirectional instability, initial treatment consists of activity modification and a structured physical therapy program. Rehabilitation focuses on strengthening and improving the neuromuscular coordination of the deltoid, rotator cuff, and scapular stabilizers. A specific, long-term physical therapy program yields a satisfactory result in 88% of patients with involuntary, atraumatic multidirectional instability. A prolonged rehabilitation program also allows time for serial examinations, leading to a bet-

ter understanding of the patient and the nature of the instability. This helps the surgeon identify voluntary dislocators and patients with secondary gain issues.

Surgical Management

Surgical intervention is indicated for compliant patients with disabling pain and involuntary multidirectional instability for whom a comprehensive therapy program has failed. Patients with voluntary muscular multidirectional instability must be identified. These patients are not good surgical candidates because their symptoms are usually secondary to an emotional or psychiatric disorder. Caution is also advised in treating patients involved in ongoing workers' compensation claims or litigation because of the high incidence of unsatisfactory results in these patients.

Open Inferior Capsular Shift

A 1980 study described the open inferior capsular shift as a surgical treatment for symptomatic patients with multidirectional instability who are unresponsive to nonsurgical treatment. Of 36 patients (40 shoulders), there was only one unsatisfactory result. Some of these patients had a concomitant Bankart repair. Since then, several studies have demonstrated the usefulness of the open inferior capsular shift, with overall patient satisfaction ranging from 80% to 95%. Again, these studies have usually included patients who required a concomitant Bankart repair.

Arthroscopic Capsular Shift Using Transglenoid Sutures

With the advancement of arthroscopic shoulder techniques, success rates are being reported with arthroscopic capsular shift for multidirectional instability. In 1993, a preliminary report of capsular shifts performed arthroscopically using a transglenoid suture technique demonstrated a satisfactory result according to Neer criteria in all 10 patients. Caspari developed this technique, in which several sutures were placed into the capsule and shuttled through a drilled hole in the glenoid neck, after which they were tied securely over the posterior scapular fascia. Four patients resumed sporting activities at their preinjury level. Another preliminary report presented a modified technique of capsular advancement for anterior and anteroinferior shoulder instability. In this technique a radial inferior capsular split in the capsule was created, allowing for more extensive advancement of the anteroinferior glenohumeral ligament complex than previously reported. Short-term follow-up in four patients revealed no recurrent subluxation or dislocation. Two-year results of the modified transglenoid, multiple suture technique described by Caspari were reported in 19 patients with

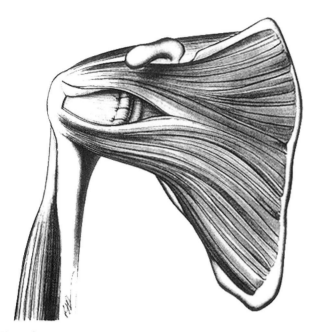

Figure 1 Neer's open extra-articular capsular plication procedure for recurrent anterior instability.

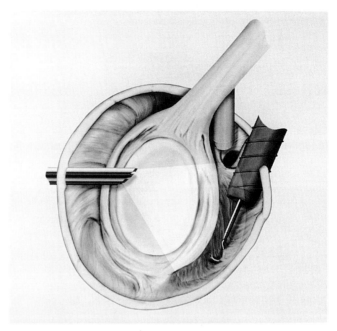

Figure 2 A full-thickness "pinch tuck" stitch of the anteroinferior capsule is created approximately 1 cm from the edge of the glenoid with a 45° suture hook.

multidirectional instability. Using the Athletic Shoulder Outcome Rating Scale, there were 13 excellent results, 5 good results, and 1 fair result. The average score was 91 out of 100. The patient rated as having a fair result reported no improvement in pain following surgery. Thirteen of 14 athletes (93%) returned to their previous level of performance. A more recent study used the same technique in 26 patients at an average follow-up of 52 months. Three patients (10%) developed recurrent instability requiring surgery. Nine of 11 high school and collegiate athletes (82%) were able to return to their previous levels of activity. Although the transglenoid technique has been shown to be effective, complications such as suprascapular nerve entrapment and pain over the suture knot posteriorly have been reported, leading to the development of alternative arthroscopic techniques.

Arthroscopic Pancapsular Plication Technique

The pancapsular plication technique was developed at the same time as the Caspari transglenoid multiple suture technique. The pancapsular plication technique enables the surgeon to accurately visualize and balance the capsular shift anteriorly, inferiorly, and posteriorly, from inside the joint. The concept of this arthroscopic pancapsular plication is similar to that of Neer's open operation for recurrent anterior subluxation, in which a deltopectoral incision is made followed by splitting the subscapularis and extra-articular plication of the capsule (Fig. 1). Several advantages are inherent to the arthroscopic technique: (1) the subscapularis tendon is

undisturbed; (2) overtightening of the capsule is avoided by maintaining the arm in abduction when the patient is in the lateral decubitus position; (3) a bumper-type effect is created by widening and deepening the glenoid labrum; (4) individual ligaments can be assessed and tightened as necessary.

Surgical Technique

A detailed examination assessing motion and stability is performed with the patient under general anesthesia. Because of the high incidence of bilateral involvement, both shoulders should be examined. The patient is supported in the lateral decubitus position and the arm is placed in 70° of abduction, 10° of forward flexion, and neutral rotation, with 10 lb of distal traction.

The joint is entered posteriorly at the midglenoid level. To allow room for later placement of the anterior midglenoid portal inferiorly, an anterosuperior portal is established in the superior aspect of the rotator interval using an outside-in technique. A 15-point glenohumeral examination is performed to document any associated intra-articular pathology. Bursoscopy is performed if preoperative MRI suggests a rotator cuff lesion or if an articular-side tear is found during arthroscopy. Using an outside-in technique, an anterior midglenoid portal is established just superior to the subscapularis tendon and lateral to the coracoid tip, approximately 2 cm distal and 2 cm lateral to the anterosuperior portal.

Anterior plication is performed with the arthroscope in the posterior portal. A manual synovial rasp is used to excoriate the synovium overlying the anterior and in-

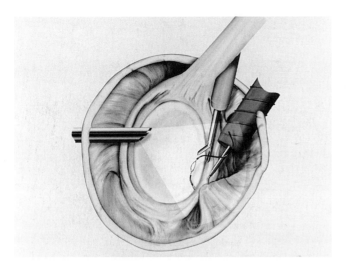

Figure 3 A suture Shuttle Relay is passed into the joint through the suture hook and retrieved through the anterior midglenoid portal.

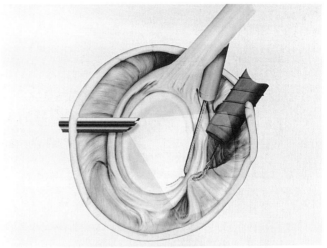

Figure 4 A No. 2 nonabsorbable suture is loaded into the eyelet of the Shuttle Relay and pulled through the labrum and the capsule and out the anterior midglenoid portal.

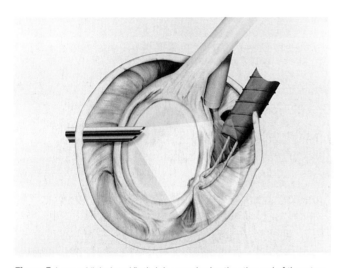

Figure 5 A second "pinch tuck" stitch is passed using the other end of the suture to create a horizontal mattress.

ferior capsule. A 45° curved suture hook is inserted through the anterior midglenoid portal and used to create a full-thickness "pinch tuck" stitch of anteroinferior capsule approximately 1 cm from the edge of the glenoid (Fig. 2). The suture hook, along with the pinch of capsule, is advanced superomedially through the anteroinferior labrum, thereby folding the tissue up to the edge of the glenoid. A suture Shuttle Relay (Linvatec, Largo, FL) or other suture transporting device/suture is passed into the joint through the suture hook and retrieved through the anterior midglenoid portal (Fig. 3). A No. 2 nonabsorbable suture is loaded into the eyelet of the Shuttle Relay and pulled through the labrum and capsule and out the anterior midglenoid portal (Fig. 4). To create a second capsular tuck, the suture hook is passed through the capsule again 1 cm away from and parallel to the pre-

vious stitch, folding the tissue up to the edge of the glenoid, and then is passed through the labrum. The Shuttle Relay is placed again and retrieved through the anterosuperior portal, where the remaining limb of suture is inserted into the Shuttle Relay eyelet. The Shuttle Relay is pulled back through the joint, carrying the suture through the labrum and capsule and out the anterior midglenoid portal, thereby creating a horizontal mattress stitch (Fig. 5). The knot is on the capsular side, and the suture bridge is on the labral side (Fig. 6). A nonsliding locked knot is tied with multiple half-hitches, placing the knot away from the articular surface. Sliding knots are not used, as they tend to cut through the labrum (Fig. 7). Additional plication stitches are placed anteriorly or inferiorly, depending on the degree of instability. Because of the proximity of the axillary nerve, care must be taken when performing the capsular tuck inferiorly.

Posterior plication stitches are performed while viewing from the anterosuperior portal. Usually, it is easier to place the posterior sutures—before the anterior plication is performed (Fig. 8). The rotator interval is imbricated if it is significantly attenuated and there is still evidence of posterior and inferior instability after completing the anterior and posterior plication. At the conclusion of the procedure, external rotation is assessed with the arm out of the lateral traction device.

Postoperative Care/Results

The arm is immobilized using an UltraSling (DonJoy Inc, Carlsbad, CA) for 4 to 6 weeks. This special sling is used because it can effectively immobilize the shoulder in a position of neutral rotation. The length of immobilization depends on patient compliance, capsular tissue quality, and direction of instability. Gentle elbow, wrist,

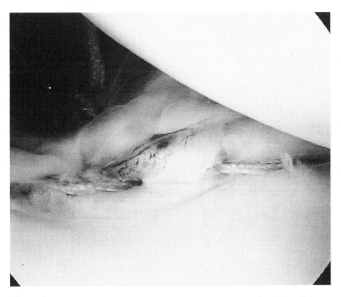

Figure 6 Arthroscopic view demonstrating the knot on the capsular side and the suture bridge on the labral side.

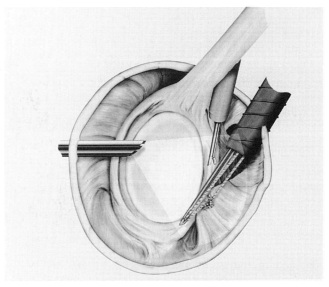

Figure 7 A nonsliding knot is tied with a loop handle knot pusher, placing the knot away from the articular surface.

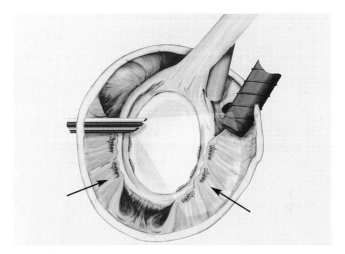

Figure 8 Additional sutures are placed anteriorly and posteriorly to create a pancapsular plication (*arrows*).

and hand exercises are started the day of surgery. At 3 weeks, pendulum and isometric exercises are begun. A formal rehabilitation program is initiated at 6 weeks and progressed until the patient has regained functional motion and strength. A throwing program is started at 3 months in throwing athletes, but contact sports are restricted for 6 months. Results at a minimum follow-up of 2 years have been reported for 24 patients who underwent pancapsular plication for involuntary multidirectional instability without a Bankart lesion. Significant functional improvement was noted as measured by the Rowe score and the American Shoulder and Elbow Surgeons 100-point Shoulder Score Index. Using the Neer criteria, 19 patients (79%) were rated satisfactory and five (21%) unsatisfactory. Of the five unsatisfactory results, three patients were involved in unresolved workers' compensation cases, and one patient was actively involved in litigation relating to a motor vehicle accident. However, only one of the five patients had any residual clinical laxity. No suprascapular or axillary nerve injuries were reported.

Summary

The results of arthroscopic pancapsular plication for the treatment of multidirectional instability, when compared with those for open techniques, appear to be comparable with respect to recurrence rates and return to athletics. The arthroscopic pancapsular plication technique selectively tightens the ligaments and widens the attenuated labrum, thereby improving the humeral head-to-glenoid surface ratio and enhancing concavity-compression without the suprascapular nerve injuries that have been noted to occur with the transglenoid

suture technique. Arthroscopy in general has the additional benefits of decreased postoperative pain, improved cosmesis, and visualization of all glenohumeral joint structures. With improved technique and attention to detail, arthroscopic methods should equal or improve on the results traditionally obtained by open surgical treatment of multidirectional shoulder instability.

Annotated Bibliography

Etiology

Mallon WJ, Speer KP: Multidirectional instability: Current concepts. *J Shoulder Elbow Surg* 1995;4:54-64.
    A review of the diagnosis, etiology, biomechanics, treatment, and results for multidirectional instability is presented.

Pathophysiology

Schenk TJ, Brems JJ: Multidirectional instability of the shoulder: Pathophysiology, diagnosis, and management. *J Am Acad Orthop Surg* 1998;6:65-72.

A review of the pathophysiology, diagnosis, and conservative versus open surgical treatment of multidirectional instability.

Surgical Management

McIntyre LF, Caspari RB, Savoie FH III: The arthroscopic treatment of anterior and multidirectional shoulder instability. *Inst Course Lect* 1996;45:47-56.

A comparison of arthroscopic versus open techniques for the treatment of multidirectional instability is presented. Seventeen of 19 patients treated with an arthroscopic repair reported good or excellent results.

McIntyre LF, Caspari RB, Savoie FH III: The arthroscopic treatment of multidirectional shoulder instability: Two-year results of a multiple suture technique. *Arthroscopy* 1997;13:418-425.

Nineteen patients with disabling multidirectional instability were treated with an arthroscopic repair. Seventeen patients reported good or excellent results. Two patients had fair results: one had recurrent instability, and one had pain during competition.

Savoie FH III, Field LD: Thermal versus suture treatment of symptomatic capsular laxity. *Clin Sports Med* 2000;19:63-75.

Twenty-six patients with multidirectional instability were treated with an arthroscopic capsular shift using a transglenoid technique. At an average follow-up of 52 months, 82% were able to return to their previous level of competition. Recurrent instability that required further surgery developed in three patients.

Treacy SH, Savoie FH III, Field LD: Arthroscopic treatment of multidirectional instability. *J Shoulder Elbow Surg* 1999;8:345-350.

Midrange follow-up (average, 5 years) in 25 patients who underwent a capsular shift with the transglenoid technique yielded a satisfactory result in 21 patients (88%) according to the Neer system. Three patients had instability after the operation.

Wichman MT, Snyder SJ: Arthroscopic capsular plication for multidirectional instability of the shoulder. *Op Tech Sports Med* 1997;5:238-243.

Twenty-four patients with multidirectional instability were treated with pancapsular plication. At an average follow-up of 2 years, 19 patients (79%) had satisfactory results using Neer criteria. Three of the unsatisfactory results were involved in ongoing workers' compensation cases.

Classic Bibliography

Altchek DW, Warren RF, Skyhar MJ, Ortiz G: T-plasty modification of the Bankart procedure for multidirectional instability of the anterior and inferior types. *J Bone Joint Surg Am* 1991;73:105-112.

Bigliani LU, Kurzweil PR, Schwartzbach CC, Wolfe IN, Flatow EL: Inferior capsular shift procedure for anterior-inferior shoulder instability in athletes. *Am J Sports Med* 1994;22:578-584.

Burkhead WZ Jr, Rockwood CA Jr: Treatment of instability of the shoulder with an exercise program. *J Bone Joint Surg Am* 1992;74:890-896.

Cooper RA, Brems JJ: The inferior capsular-shift procedure for multidirectional instability of the shoulder. *J Bone Joint Surg Am* 1992;74:1516-1521.

Duncan R, Savoie FH III: Arthroscopic inferior capsular shift for multidirectional instability of the shoulder: A preliminary report. *Arthroscopy* 1993;9:24-27.

Harryman DT II, Sidles JA, Harris SL, Matsen FA III: The role of the rotator interval capsule in passive motion and stability of the shoulder. *J Bone Joint Surg Am* 1992;74:53-66.

Lebar RD, Alexander AH: Multidirectional shoulder instability: Clinical results of inferior capsular shift in an active-duty population. *Am J Sports Med* 1992;20:193-198.

Neer CS II, Foster CR: Inferior capsular shift for involuntary inferior and multidirectional instability of the shoulder: A preliminary report. *J Bone Joint Surg Am* 1980;62:897-908.

Tauro JC, Carter FM II: Arthroscopic capsular advancement for anterior and anterior-inferior shoulder instability: A preliminary report. *Arthroscopy* 1994;10:513-517.

Warner JJ, Deng XH, Warren RF, Torzilli PA: Static capsuloligamentous restraints to superior-inferior translation of the glenohumeral joint. *Am J Sports Med* 1992;20:675-685.

Chapter 48

Thermocapsulorrhaphy

C. Thomas Vangsness, Jr, MD

Introduction

Over the last several years, there has been an increase in the clinical use of heat to help stabilize the lax shoulder. Originally, heat was applied in the form of holmium laser energy, but more recently the use of radiofrequency (RF) energy, more specifically RF thermocapsulorrhaphy, has become relatively common, with up to 50,000 operations performed annually. Many authors have expressed concern about the large number of these procedures performed without strong research to support its use. The clinical use of thermocapsulorrhaphy has been rather anecdotal. Results of some surgical studies have been published recently in peer-reviewed journals.

Pathophysiology of Collagen Shortening

Thermal changes cause the intermolecular bonds in the stable, extended, crystalline helical structure of the collagen to break, resulting in a structure that is more random, contracted, and shortened. Evaluation of various collagen tissues reveals that the density, orientation, and age of the collagen influence its ability to shorten. Contraction is increased by the amount of heat exposure.

Surgical Instrumentation

The holmium:yttrium aluminum garnet (Ho:YAG) laser is the most common laser used in orthopaedic surgery and was used in the initial studies of shoulder capsular shrinking. It has been demonstrated that lower laser fluences (J/cm^2) are preferred to decrease the risk of injury to the ligaments and adjacent structures.

RF energy has become the standard for energy transfer during thermocapsulorrhaphy. There are two types of RF probes: monopolar and bipolar. Monopolar energy travels through the body from the arthroscopy probe to a grounding pad, then exits the body. The circuit is completed as the energy travels to the RF machine and then to the wall socket. The electrons from the RF probe pass through the tissues, and the tissue resistance increases molecular movement, producing heat. Current bipolar RF devices allow the electrons to return back through the probe to the RF machine, thus preventing energy from passing through the body to the grounding pad. This action is similar to that of a bipolar electrocautery device. Both types of devices have been used to transfer heat to the tissues, but controversy remains regarding which type of probe generates more heat and thermal penetration into the tissue. Longer contact times and higher energy levels are known to increase heat production and depth of penetration. The effects of probe tip size, geometry, and manual contact pressure have not been specifically addressed.

In Vitro Studies

Several in vitro studies have established that the lower temperatures of nonablative heat applied to the capsuloligamentous surfaces inside the shoulder will shorten the tissue and tighten the joint. Thermal bath studies of ovine (sheep), bovine, and rabbit tissue, in addition to human Achilles tendon, patellar tendon, and the inferior glenohumeral ligament (IGHL) tissue, have demonstrated that shortening begins to occur at temperatures between 65°C and 75°C. The tissues shorten more at higher temperatures, and longer exposure times in the tissue baths increase the amount of contraction. Studies in which a thermistor probe is placed against bovine collagen have shown that the temperature of the tissue increases even after RF energy is no longer applied. Shortening of more than 10% to 20% causes biomechanical weakening and decreases tissue stiffness, although one study demonstrated that a 10% shortening of the human IGHL with laser energy did not appear to alter the biomechanical properties immediately after application. Decreased glenohumeral translations in a cadaver model have been demonstrated when nonablative laser heat is used.

In Vivo Studies

Few in vivo animal studies have been performed. One short-term follow-up study treating rabbit patellar tendon with laser energy showed that shortened tissue stretched over time if the knee joint was not immobilized. In a study of sheep femoropatellar joint capsules treated with laser shortening and no immobilization, stiffness decreased 14 days postoperatively. At 30 days postoperatively, normal mechanical properties returned. Another study, using a sheep knee retinacular model, demonstrated that monopolar RF energy provided an initial decrease in tissue stiffness, but normal mechanical properties returned within 6 to 8 weeks. Smaller collagen fibrils were noted at 12 weeks. Results of all of these studies suggest that after the initial shortening, shoulder motion should be protected for a period of time to prevent ligament and capsular stretching.

Indications

Currently, the surgical indications for thermocapsulorrhaphy are unclear. Thermal shortening techniques have been proposed to address laxity in symptomatic shoulder dislocations or subluxations and for addressing a lax capsule with concomitant Bankart lesions or superior labrum anterior to posterior (SLAP) lesions. RF thermocapsulorrhaphy has been used for multidirectional instability, but concerns have been raised regarding postoperative stretching of tissue over time.

Technique

Thermocapsulorrhaphy generally is performed with the patient either in the standard beach chair or lateral decubitus position. Whether traction affects the efficacy of thermal shortening has not been established. The arthroscopic fluid of choice is normal saline solution, and standard arthroscopic portals are used to access the joint. Some authors have suggested that an additional inferior posterior portal be used to access the inferior pouch. The RF probe is applied to the tissue interface with a hand-held "paintbrush" technique, sweeping over the visible interior surfaces of the glenohumeral ligaments. Between thermal applications, stripes of viable tissue should be left to allow for earlier revascularization and cellular growth into the treated areas. Heat should be applied with caution in the posteroinferior joint because the capsule thins in this area, leaving the axillary nerve vulnerable to thermal injury. The surgeon can visually observe the change in tissue color to ensure energy transfer to the tissue, but a specific appropriate end point of energy application is uncertain and unreliable. Thermal devices usually have a thermistor feedback system to measure and control temperature, but at least one of these devices has been shown to be inaccurate. This can lead to potential overheating of the tissue, unbeknownst to the surgeon, potentially increasing the risk of capsular thermal necrosis and insufficiency or axillary nerve injury.

Postoperative Care

Published studies to date have reported inconsistent methodologies for postoperative physical therapy protocols. Results of animal studies indicate that the thermally shortened tissue is weakened for 0 to 12 weeks. Range-of-motion exercises should be avoided or minimized during this time. This lengthy immobilization can result in adhesive capsulitis in some patients.

Controversies/Complications

The use of thermal energy to stabilize the shoulder is in itself a subject of considerable controversy. To date, most basic science studies have addressed only the initial reactions to thermal change. There have been very few studies on human tissue, and the effects of depth of penetration on different types of collagen in human tissues have not been examined. Inconsistent temperature monitoring makes it difficult to interpret many basic science studies.

Biologically, either the initial tissue shortening or the fibroblastic response and scar formation leads to increased shoulder stability over time. There have been many reports of difficulties in revision following failure of the procedure, secondary to insufficient ligamentous tissue for reconstruction or the complete absence of ligaments secondary to capsular thermal necrosis. Specific surgical techniques have not been adequately defined, and inconsistent delivery of energy confounds results. The anatomy of the shoulder can vary tremendously among athletes, making clinical comparisons of results difficult. Safe energy levels that prevent excessive injury or destruction of the shoulder capsuloligamentous structures have yet to be firmly established.

Nerve injury occurs at approximately 45°C, and some authors have reported that the temperatures used with RF thermocapsulorrhaphy may injure the axillary nerve as it passes beneath the inferior capsule. Sensory nerve fibers and mechanoreceptors can also be destroyed at the time of thermal application to the shoulder tissues. The proprioceptive effects of this sensory denervation are unknown.

Summary

Thermocapsulorrhaphy is an intriguing, albeit controversial shoulder procedure from both the basic science and clinical perspectives. Results of clinical trials are difficult to interpret because many variables of thermocapsulorrhaphy are difficult to control. To date, studies have failed to adequately define surgical indications and are limited by short follow-up. Thermocapsulorrhaphy has been used to treat many different types of shoulder laxity and instability, yet the reproducibility of the surgical procedure has not been established. Because the anatomy of the shoulder is variable, identification of specific structures for shortening is often difficult. For example, the deep intra-articular recesses of the shoulder are difficult to access reproducibly, and some tissues do not shrink appropriately.

Currently, the amount of energy necessary to shorten the tissues, the desired amount of contraction, and the specific methods to accomplish both have not been established. It is very difficult to determine exactly how much energy is being transferred to the tissue. Rehabilitation protocols have been inconsistent. Aggressive therapy may overstretch the weak capsule in the first 12 weeks of treatment, and some shoulders become vexingly stiff postoperatively, probably secondary to an inflammatory response to the thermal treatment.

Although not enough is known about the long-term effects of thermocapsulorrhaphy, several studies have reported clinical improvement with good measurements of clinical outcomes. Few instances of permanent nerve damage have been reported among the large volume of patients who have undergone this procedure, and strong patient satisfaction has been reported. However, well-controlled prospective human studies are lacking, and more basic science studies are needed to investigate the appropriate quality and quantity of thermal energy applied to the shoulder tissues. Good evidence-based randomized clinical trials must identify these parameters and establish results that are equal to or better than other stabilization techniques in order to justify the continued use of the procedure.

Annotated Bibliography

Introduction

Gerber A, Warner JJ: Thermal capsulorrhaphy to treat shoulder instability. *Clin Orthop* 2002;400:105-116

In this review of the literature, the authors state that although successful clinical applications have resulted in the wide use of thermocapsulorrhaphy, the indications are poorly defined. The authors conclude that additional experimental and clinical investigations are necessary to make this procedure an accepted modality in the treatment of shoulder instability.

Pathophysiology of Collagen Shortening

Hayashi K, Markel MD: Thermal capsulorrhaphy treatment of shoulder instability: Basic science. *Clin Orthop* 2001;390:59-72.

In this comprehensive review of the basic science of thermocapsulorrhaphy, the authors conclude that joint capsular tissue can be shortened significantly by thermal energy at the temperature range of 70°C to 80°C; thermal energy causes immediate loss of the mechanical properties, collagen denaturation, and cell necrosis; and thermally treated tissue is repaired actively by a residual population of fibroblasts and vascular cells, with subsequent improvement of mechanical properties. In addition, they determine that the shrunken tissue stretches with time if it is subjected to physiologic loads immediately after surgery when the tissue is weak; and leaving viable tissue between treated regions significantly improves the healing process. The authors caution that overtreatment can lead to severe immediate and permanent tissue damage. Scientific data of newly developed devices are limited, and the information from manufacturers often is unreliable and misleading. They emphasize that carefully controlled long-term clinical and scientific studies should be done to additionally clarify the advantages and disadvantages of the technique.

In Vitro Studies

Hayashi K, Thabit G III, Massa KL, et al: The effect of thermal heating on the length and histologic properties of the glenohumeral joint capsule. *Am J Sports Med* 1997;25:107-112.

The authors studied the effect of temperature variation on shrinkage and histology of glenohumeral joint capsular tissue. Seven capsule specimens were taken from different regions from each of six fresh-frozen cadaveric glenohumeral joints and were randomly assigned to one of seven temperatures (37°, 55°, 60°, 65°, 70°, 75°, and 80°C). Specimens were placed in a tissue bath set at the specific temperature for 10 minutes. Specimens treated with temperatures at or greater than 65° exhibited significantly more shrinkage compared with those treated at 37°C. The posttreatment lengths in the 70°, 75°, and 80°C groups were significantly less than the pretreatment lengths. Histologic analysis revealed significant thermal alteration (hyalinization of collagen) at 65°, 70°, 75°, and 80°C.

Lopez MJ, Hayashi K, Fanton GS, Thabit G, Markel MD: The effect of radiofrequency energy on the ultrastructure of joint capsular collagen. *Arthroscopy* 1998; 14:495-501.

The effect of RF energy with varying temperature on the histologic and ultrastructural appearance of joint capsular collagen was evaluated. Sheep patellofemoral joint capsular specimens were treated with one of three treatment temperatures (45°, 65°, or 85°C) with an RF probe, and specimens were also saved as controls. Thermal tissue damage characterized by collagen fiber fusion and fibroblastic cell death occurred at all application temperatures, with clear demarcations between treated and untreated tissue. Mean tissue thickness affected ranged from 22.5% for 45° to 50.4% for 85°C. There was a strong correlation between treatment temperature and percent area affected ($P < 0.001$). There was a general increase in cross-sectional fibril diameter and loss of fibril size variation with increasing treatment temperature. Longitudinal sections of collagen fibrils showed increased fibril diameter and the loss of cross-striations in the treated groups. Thermally induced ultrastructural collagen fibril alteration is likely the predominant mechanism of tissue shrinkage after application of RF energy.

Obrzut LS, Hecht P, Hayashi K, Fanton GS, Thabit G, Markel MD: The effect of radiofrequency energy on the length and temperature properties of the glenohumeral joint capsule. *Arthroscopy* 1998;14:395-400.

Sheep glenohumeral joint capsules were placed in a 37°C tissue bath and treated with a radiofrequency energy probe at temperature settings of 60°, 65°, 70°, 75°, and 80°C. Tissue shrinkage was found to be less than 4% for treatments at less than 65°C and increased to 14% for treatments at 80°C. Post-treatment lengths of tissues treated at 65°, 70°, 75°, and 80°C were all significantly shorter than pretreatment lengths. The maximum tissue temperatures were found directly below the probe and were 3.7° to 6.7° less than the set temperatures. As the distance from the probe was increased, the tissue temperature decreased, reaching a value of less than 45°C at 1.5 mm for all five treatment temperature settings.

Selecky MT, Vangsness CT, Liao WL, Saadat V, Hedman TP: The effect of laser-induced collagen shortening on the biomechanical properties of the inferior glenohumeral ligament complex. *Am J Sports Med* 1999;27: 168-172.

Fifty-seven bone-ligament-bone glenohumeral ligament specimens underwent uniaxial tensioning to 10% strain. Approximately one half of the specimens then underwent 10% shortening using a holmium:YAG laser. Both groups were again tensioned to 10% strain, and then loaded to failure. Ultimate strain and yield strain were significantly higher in the treated specimens. No significant difference was found for ultimate stress, yield stress, or elastic modulus between the two groups. Failure of the ligament did not appear to occur in the treated areas.

Shellock FG, Shields CL: Temperature changes associated with radiofrequency energy-induced heating of bovine capsular tissue: Evaluation of bipolar RF electrodes. *Arthroscopy* 2000;16:348-358.

Temperature changes associated with RF energy-induced heating of bovine capsular tissue using bipolar electrodes were investigated. Two different types of bipolar electrodes were used. Each electrode was activated for 3 seconds at 10 W, 16 W, and 20 W, for six separate data acquisitions. The highest mean temperatures recorded at the tissue surfaces were end

temperatures of 48.9° at 10 W, 57.0° at 16 W, and 67.3°C at 20 W. Temperature at the side of the electrode was 51.5° at 10 W, 62.1° at 16 W, and 71.2°C at 20 W. All recorded surface temperatures were within the range known to be acceptable for tissue shrinkage. None of the temperatures recorded at the different depths was excessive, suggesting that sensitive anatomic structures should not be damaged by RF energy-induced heating under the experimental conditions.

Tibone JE, McMahon PJ, Shrader TA, Sandusky MD, Lee TQ: Glenohumeral joint translation after arthroscopic, nonablative, thermal capsuloplasty with a laser. *Am J Sports Med* 1998;26:495-498.

Two anteriorly and two posteriorly directed loads were sequentially applied to the humerus of nine cadaveric glenohumeral joints, and anterior and posterior translation of the humerus on the glenoid was measured. Using the holmium:YAG laser, thermal energy was applied to the anterior capsuloligamentous structures and anterior and posterior translation measurements were then repeated. The results showed a significant reduction in anterior and posterior translation after laser anterior capsuloplasty. Anterior translation decreased from 10.9 ± 2.0 mm to 6.4 ± 1.5 mm with the 15 N load; and from 13.4 ± 2.1 mm to 8.9 ± 1.8 mm with the 20 N load. Posterior translation decreased from 7.2 ± 1.2 mm to 4.4 ± 0.6 mm with the 15 N load and from 10.4 ± 1.4 mm to 6.5 ± 0.9 mm with the 20 N load.

Vangsness CT, Mitchell W, Nimni M, Erlich M, Saadat V, Schmotzer H: Collagen shortening: An experimental approach with heat. *Clin Orthop* 1997;337:267-271.

This in vitro study examined the structural and histologic effects of heat shrinkage of human collagen. Consistent tendon shrinkage curves were found with increasing temperatures in a saline solution. A sharp increase in shrinkage to approximately 70% of resting length was noted around 70°C. Tendon shrinkage by laser-induced heat was dose related. Tensile testing of the tendons that were shortened 10% of their resting length showed a decrease in load to failure to approximately one third compared with that of control specimens. Histologic sections showed a well-demarcated site of diffuse denaturation and degeneration of collagenous elements. Normal collagen was present adjacent to thermal changes.

Wall MS, Deng XH, Torzilli PA, Doty SB, O'Brien SJ, Warren RF: Thermal modification of collagen. *J Shoulder Elbow Surg* 1999;8:339-344.

The purpose of this study was to shrink collagenous tissue thermally and then measure the mechanical property changes as a function of tissue shrinkage. Uniaxial tensile testing of normal and heat-shrunken bovine tendon was carried out. The mechanical strength decreased with increasing shrinkage. The maximal allowable shrinkage before significant material property changes occurred was between 15% and 20%. Transmission electron microscopy showed denaturation of the collagen structure.

In Vivo Studies

Hayashi K, Hecht P, Thabit G III, et al: The biologic response to laser thermal modification in an in vivo sheep model. *Clin Orthop* 2000;373:265-276.

The authors evaluated the effect of nonablative laser energy on mechanical, histologic, and biomechanical properties of joint capsular tissue in the ovine model. Femoropatellar joint capsule was treated with the holmium:YAG laser, and tissues were harvested at 0. 3, 7, 14, 30, 60, 90, and 180 days after surgery (n = 8/group). Tissue stiffness was significantly decreased from 0 to 7 days after surgery and then gradually increased after 14 days. Tissue strength was lowest 3 days after laser treatment. Histologic examination revealed immediate collagen hyalinization and cell necrosis, followed by extensive fibroblast migration and capillary sprouting. Tissue appeared to regain its mechanical properties by 30 days and was histologically normal 60 days after surgery; but collagen fibrils remained uniformly small.

Hayashi K, Nieckarz JA, Thabit G III, Bogdanske JJ, Cooley AJ, Markel MD: Effect of nonablative laser energy on the joint capsule: An in vivo rabbit study using a holmium: YAG laser. *Lasers Surg Med* 1997;20: 164-171.

The effect of nonablative holmium:YAG laser energy on the short-term histologic properties of joint capsular tissue in an in vivo rabbit model was evaluated. Specimens were processed for histology and transmission electron microscopy immediately after laser treatment (day 0), at 7 days, and at 30 days after the treatment. Immediately after surgery, histology showed diffuse hyalinization of collagen with fibroblast cell death. At 7 days after surgery, histology revealed fibroblast proliferation around and into acellular hyalinized regions of collagen. At 30 days, large reactive fibroblasts migrated and secreted matrix into the damaged areas. The authors concluded that the short-term in vivo tissue response to nonablative laser treatment is an infiltration of acellular hyalinized regions of collagen by fibroblasts, which use the treated collagen as the framework for migration and secretion of new collagen matrix for repair.

Hecht P, Hayashi K, Cooley AJ, et al: The thermal effect of monopolar radiofrequency energy on the properties of joint capsule: An in vivo histologic study using a sheep model. *Am J Sports Med* 1998;26:808-814.

The short-term tissue response of sheep joint capsule to monopolar RF energy was analyzed, and the effects of five power settings on heat distribution at 65°C was compared. The RF generator power settings were 0 W, 10 W, 15 W, 20 W, 25 W, and 30 W. Tissue was treated using a monopolar RF probe under arthroscopic control in a single uniform pass to the synovial surface. Histologic analysis at 7 days after surgery revealed thermal capsular damage at all RF power settings. The lesion's cross-sectional area, depth, vas-cularity, and inflammation increased proportionately with increases in RF power.

Hecht P, Hayashi K, Lu Y, et al: Monopolar radiofrequency energy effects on joint capsular tissue: Potential treatment for joint instability. An in vivo mechanical, morphological, and biochemical study using an ovine model. *Am J Sports Med* 1999;27:761-771.

Monopolar RF energy was applied arthroscopically to the synovial surface of the femoropatellar joint capsule of 24 sheep. The sheep were sacrificed at 0, 2, 6, and 12 weeks after surgery (six per group). Biochemical analysis revealed early collagen denaturation 0 and 2 weeks after treatment. Initially, there was a significant decrease in tissue stiffness and an increase in tissue relaxation properties, followed by gradual improvement in the tissue's mechanical properties by 6 weeks. Initial microscopic examination demonstrated collagen hyalinization and cell necrosis, which was followed by active tissue repair in the later weeks.

Pullin JG, Collier MA, Johnson LL, DeBault LE, Walls RC: Holmium: YAG laser-assisted capsular shift in a canine model: Intraarticular pressure and histologic observations. *J Shoulder Elbow Surg* 1997;6:272-285.

The initial effects of holmium:YAG laser energy on the glenohumeral joint capsules of dogs were investigated. Laser energy was applied arthroscopically to the glenohumeral joint capsule and ligaments of one shoulder in each dog. The contralateral shoulders served as controls. At 6 weeks postoperatively, marked tissue damage of the treated capsule was easily identified. Histologic evaluation revealed marked synovitis and pericapsular tissue reactivity, which was extensive and deep. The depth of the injury went beyond the joint capsule into the pericapsular tissue.

Schaefer SL, Ciarelli MJ, Arnoczky SP, Ross HE: Tissue shrinkage with the holmium:Yttrium aluminum garnet laser: A postoperative assessment of tissue length, stiffness, and structure. *Am J Sports Med* 1997;25:841-848.

The effect of laser energy treatment on the length, stiffness, and structure of rabbit patellar tendons was investigated. A holmium:YAG laser was used to deliver a calculated dose of laser energy (300 J/cm^2) to one randomly selected patellar tendon in each rabbit. The contralateral patellar tendon was used as a control. Radiopaque markers were placed in the patella and tibial tuberosity to allow for patellar tendon length measurements via standard lateral radiographs before and after laser application, and at 4 and 8 weeks. Limbs were not immobilized during the postoperative period. The tendons were harvested at 0 and 8 weeks and evaluated for stiffness, cross-sectional area, histologic changes, and electron microscopic appearance. There was significant initial tendon shrinkage (6.6% ± 1.4%) after application of the calculated laser energy dose. However, tendon length increased significantly beyond the immediate postlaser length at 4 weeks and beyond its original length by 8 weeks. At 8 weeks, the treated tendons were significantly less stiff with significantly greater cross-sectional areas than the contralateral controls. There was generalized fibroblastic response throughout the entire treated tendon characterized by a marked increase in cellularity. There was also a change from the normal bimodal pattern of large- and small-diameter collagen fibers to a unimodal pattern with predominantly small-diameter fibers in the laser treated tendons.

Controversies/Complications

Wong KL, Williams GR: Complications of thermal capsulorrhaphy of the shoulder. *J Bone Joint Surg Am* 2001; 83(suppl 2):151-155.

The rate of recurrence and the prevalence of complications related to the use of thermal energy for the treatment of glenohumeral instability were evaluated. A survey of 379 surgeons who had performed 14,277 thermocapsulorrhaphy procedures over the previous 5 years was conducted. Recurrent instability occurred after 8.0% of the procedures. Of the patients with recurrent instability, 363 required revision surgery, of which 71 (19.6%) exhibited signs of capsular attenuation at the time of the revision. Axillary neuropathy occurred postoperatively in 196 patients (1.4%). Sensory deficit only occurred in 182 patients (93%), and 14 had a combined sensory and motor deficit. Of these 196 patients, 95% recovered completely. Patients with sensory deficits recovered in an average of 2.3 months after surgery, and patients with combined deficits recovered in an average of 4 months. Ten patients (5% of the nerve injury population, 0.07% of the entire study population) had permanent nerve damage.

Clinical Studies

Levitz CL, Dugas J, Andrews JR: The use of arthroscopic thermal capsulorrhaphy to treat internal impingement in baseball players. *Arthroscopy* 2001;17: 573-577.

In this retrospective review, the authors' intent was to determine whether using arthroscopic thermal shrinkage to reduce glenohumeral translation would improve the results of arthroscopic treatment of internal impingement in baseball players. In the study, 51 patients treated with traditional arthroscopy were compared with 31 patients treated traditionally plus with monopolar thermal capsulorrhaphy. Better outcomes were found in the heat-treated group, with less loss of external rotation and no significant complications.

Levy O, Wilson M, Williams H, et al: Thermal capsular shrinkage for shoulder instability. *J Bone Joint Surg Br* 2001;83:640-645.

Short- and medium-termed clinical results of thermal shrinkage in patients were presented with multidirectional or capsular stretch-type instability. Two groups were followed for a period of 40 months and 23 months, respectively. The first group included 56 patients (61 shoulders) who were treated with laser-assisted capsular shrinkage (LACS); the second group included 34 patients (38 shoulders) treated with radiofrequency (RF) capsular shrinkage. In the LACS group, the Walch-Duplay score improved to 90 points 18 months after the operation, but declined to 80 points. In this group, 59% of the patients reported their shoulders as being "much better" or "better," but there was a failure rate of 36%. In the RF group, the Walch-Duplay and Constant scores were 80 points at the various follow-up times; 76% of the patients considered their shoulder to be "better" or "much better." RF failed in nine shoulders (24%). These results match clinical series of patients with multidirectional instability. The minimal morbidity makes this a viable alternative to open capsular shift in these patients.

Lyons TR, Griffith PL, Savoie FH III, Field LD: Laser-assisted capsulorrhaphy for multidirectional instability of the shoulder. *Arthroscopy* 2001;17: 25-30.

In this prospective study, the authors reviewed the clinical results of laser-assisted capsulorrhaphy performed on 27 shoulders in 26 patients for multidirectional shoulder instability with an average follow-up of 27 months. Holmium laser shrinkage was performed on the entire capsule. All patients were evaluated with respect to the incidence of recurrent instability, need for reoperation, and ability to return to their previous level of activity. All patients were rated as satisfactory or unsatisfactory using criteria established by Neer. At 2 years follow-up, 96% of the patients remained stable and asymptomatic, and 12 of the 14 athletes (86%) returned to their previous level of competition.

Mishra DK, Fanton GS: Two-year outcome of arthroscopic Bankart repair and electrothermal-assisted capsulorrhaphy for recurrent traumatic anterior shoulder instability. *Arthroscopy* 2001;17:844-849.

In this prospective nonrandomized study, 42 patients with recurrent traumatic anterior dislocations were evaluated. An arthroscopic capsulolabral repair along with a monopolar radiofrequency thermal shrinkage was performed on the shoulders. Of these patients, 38 returned to preinjury sports. Overall, the Rowe score improved from 38 points preoperatively to 89 points at follow-up. These results were comparable to open procedures, including in athletes involved in high-level contact and collision sports.

Chapter 49

Arthroscopic Subacromial Decompression

Armodios M. Hatzidakis, MD

R. Michael Gross, MD

Introduction

The role of arthroscopy for treatment of shoulder disorders has rapidly evolved over the last 20 years. Effective treatment of shoulder problems necessitates a good understanding of the pathophysiology and clinical diagnosis of subacromial impingement. The astute clinician must be able to distinguish the pain of pure subacromial impingement from shoulder pain related to other causes. Associated acromioclavicular (AC) joint and biceps tendon pathology must be defined for each patient. Surgeons who understand the indications and are skilled in performing the technique of arthroscopic subacromial decompression (ASD) are able to obtain results that are equivalent to those traditionally obtained with the open procedure. Techniques of ASD in the lateral and beach chair positions will be discussed, followed by results, complications, and an overview of recent ASD literature.

Anatomy/Pathophysiology

Codman proposed that rotator cuff (RC) pathology resulted from intrinsic degeneration of the tendon close to its insertion on the greater tuberosity. Neer believed in the significance of the intrinsic degenerative process, but he also believed that RC tears were caused and exacerbated by what he termed "subacromial impingement." This extrinsic process was described as the compression and abrasion of the greater tuberosity, RC, and tendon of the long head of the biceps (LHB) by the anterior acromion, coracoacromial (CA) ligament, and undersurface of the AC joint during forward flexion. Neer was the first to stress the role of the anterior acromion in shoulder pathology (as opposed to the lateral acromion), pointing out that most functional overhead shoulder activities occur not in abduction but in forward flexion.

Clinical Findings

Successful treatment of impingement begins with an accurate and thorough understanding of shoulder pathology and the three classic stages of impingement. Stage I (RC edema and hemorrhage) occurs characteristically in younger patients as a result of excessive overhead motion. Stage II (RC fibrosis and tendinitis) occurs in older patients after prolonged and repeated episodes of mechanical inflammation cause the subacromial bursa to become fibrotic and thickened. Stage III (RC or LHB rupture/bony change) is the end stage of the impingement process, usually occurring in patients older than age 40 years and increasing in frequency with every decade thereafter.

The diagnosis is made via a careful and complete history and physical examination in conjunction with appropriate radiographic evaluation. Patients in all three stages report chronic pain localized to the anterior or lateral shoulder, especially after athletic or vigorous overhead activity. This pain may awaken the patient at night and is usually localized just anterior, distal, and/or lateral to the acromion, frequently radiating distally down the lateral arm to the deltoid insertion. Active range of motion (ROM) may be reduced. Most commonly, forward flexion and abduction are limited, but sometimes internal rotation may be limited secondary to a tight posterior capsule. Characteristically, there is a painful arc between 60° and 120° of elevation, especially when letting the arm come down from the fully elevated position. There also may be reduced cross-arm adduction with pain and a feeling of tightness localized to the posterior shoulder secondary to posterior capsular contracture. In contrast, anterior shoulder pain with cross-arm adduction usually is secondary to AC arthrosis. AC joint tenderness on palpation with the patient at rest or

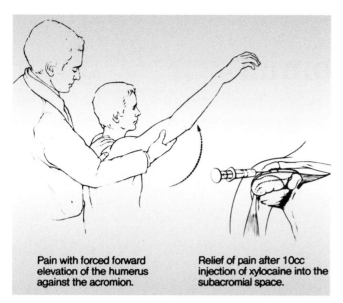

Pain with forced forward elevation of the humerus against the acromion.

Relief of pain after 10cc injection of xylocaine into the subacromial space.

Figure 1 Neer's impingement sign. Scapular rotation is prevented by one hand as the other raises the arm in forced forward elevation (somewhere between flexion and abduction), causing the greater tuberosity to impinge against the acromion. *(Reproduced with permission from Neer CS II: Impingement lesions.* Clin Orthop *1983;173:70-77.)*

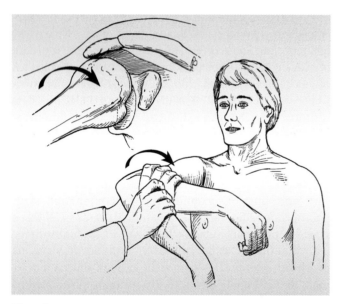

Figure 2 Hawkins' impingement sign. The arm is forward flexed to 90° and then maximally internally rotated, bringing the greater tuberosity in close contact with the acromion. Pain with this maneuver denotes a positive Hawkins' sign. *(Copyright 1997 Kevin D. Plancher, MD, New York, NY.)*

with the arm passively adducted also implicates the AC joint as a significant contributor to the patient's pain. Physical examination findings that are more specific to impingement include Neer's and Hawkins' signs. Neer's sign is best elicited by standing behind the seated patient (Fig. 1).

Anterior, lateral, or deep shoulder pain with this motion defines a positive Neer's sign. Internal rotation

of the shoulder places the greater tuberosity in a position more likely to impinge against the anterior acromion with elevation. Hawkins' sign is a variation of this concept, elicited by forward flexing the patient's arm to 90°, flexing the elbow to 90°, and then maximally internally rotating the shoulder. This motion also brings the greater tuberosity into close contact with the undersurface of the acromion, causing pain in patients with subacromial impingement (Fig. 2).

A good confirmatory diagnostic test is a subacromial injection of 10 mL of local anesthetic (Neer impingement test). Because the rotator cuff is structurally intact, pain should be relieved and strength improved in patients with stage II impingement. Persistent weakness despite pain relief after injection usually indicates that the RC is torn (stage III), although patients with full-thickness RC tears may sometimes demonstrate full strength when their pain is relieved. In patients with symptoms of AC pathology, a selective injection of the AC joint with 1 to 2 mL of local anesthetic can help differentiate the major cause of the patient's pain. Restricted shoulder ROM and AC pain typically indicate that the patient is in stage III of the impingement process.

Although subacromial impingement is primarily a clinical diagnosis, imaging techniques can be very helpful in reinforcing the clinical opinion. Shoulder radiographs should include a true AP view and an axillary lateral view to evaluate for glenohumeral and AC arthritis. A supraspinatus outlet view identifies acromial morphology, further defining the role of the acromion in the impingement process. A downward curved acromion (type II) or hooked acromion (type III) support the diagnosis of subacromial impingement. The outlet view can also be used to approximate the planned amount of anteroinferior acromial resection.

Other imaging tools that can be helpful include arthrography, ultrasound, and MRI. These tools are primarily useful when an RC tear is suspected. Glenohumeral arthrography is a relatively inexpensive and effective diagnostic test for determining a complete tear of the RC, but it does not provide much information regarding the size and location of the tear. Shoulder ultrasonography is noninvasive and cost-effective, with the added benefit of being able to accurately size and locate RC tears. A disadvantage of ultrasound, however, is that its diagnostic use depends heavily on the experience of the radiologist, technician, and surgeon. Although both of these tests are relatively inexpensive, they do not provide much additional information, such as the relationship of subacromial spurs to a torn or inflamed RC, presence of AC arthrosis with encroachment upon the RC, status of the biceps tendon, and the presence of intra-articular pathology.

MRI is the most sensitive ancillary diagnostic tool, but it is also the most expensive. MRI can identify subacromial impingement findings, including subacromial spurring, the formation of fibrotic soft tissue on the undersurface of the acromion, proliferative bursitis, AC arthrosis with medial encroachment of the AC joint on the RC, and biceps tendinitis, rupture, or dislocation. MRI also is very effective in assessing the size and location of RC tendinitis/tear and the quality of the RC musculature. In addition, MRI can be ordered to help in the diagnosis of intra-articular abnormalities. However, although MRI has many advantages, it does not supplant the clinical evaluation. Shoulder MRI findings must be coupled with findings from a thorough history and clinical examination, and treatment must be planned accordingly.

Treatment

Patients who present with stage I and II subacromial impingement should be treated initially with rest and physical therapy (RC and periscapular muscle strengthening, ice, and other modalities). With rest and physical therapy, patients with stage I impingement typically improve within 6 months of onset of symptoms. Patients with significant symptoms beyond 6 months usually are in stage II or III of the process. Adjuncts to nonsurgical therapy include anti-inflammatory medications and a subacromial steroid injection. One subacromial injection of cortisone and local anesthetic may provide temporary or more permanent relief and may be repeated up to two more times in a 1-year period. In patients who may become surgical candidates, the presence of an RC tear should be considered before subacromial injections of cortisone are given, because cortisone can have a detrimental effect on articular cartilage and tendon healing. The natural history and nonsurgical and surgical treatment of RC tears are fully covered in section 3 of this book, and the rest of this chapter will focus on the treatment of stage II subacromial impingement.

If lasting improvement does not occur after 3 to 6 months of nonsurgical therapy, subacromial decompression is indicated.

In 1972, Neer introduced the surgical treatment of subacromial impingement by decompression of the subacromial space via open anterior acromioplasty (AA). The original procedure involved a 9-cm incision from the anterior edge of the acromion to just lateral to the coracoid. Exposure of the inferior acromion was achieved by detachment of the anterior deltoid, which was repaired back to bone after completion of the acromioplasty (Fig. 3). Active forward elevation was prohibited for 10 days to allow deltoid reattachment. Satisfactory results were attained in 15 of 16 patients who had intact

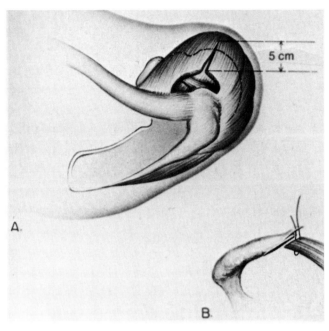

Figure 3 Deltoid detachment and repair in Neer's open anterior acromioplasty. *(Reproduced with permission from Neer CS: Anterior acromioplasty for the chronic impingement syndrome in the shoulder: A preliminary report. J Bone Joint Surg Am 1972;54:41-50.)*

rotator cuffs. Thirteen years after Neer's original work, Ellman introduced ASD as the arthroscopic method to reproduce the open operation. In one group of patients, 10 arthroscopic acromioplasties were performed, with good short-term results. These patients were able to perform active forward elevation immediately because the anterior deltoid was left intact. Further anatomic and long-term follow-up investigations have confirmed the advantages and effectiveness of ASD.

The procedure also can benefit patients in stage III of the impingement process if associated RC, LHB, and AC joint pathology are treated appropriately. Significant AC joint and LHB symptoms and signs must be completely elicited and documented preoperatively. Lack of near-complete pain relief with a subacromial injection should also prompt the surgeon to reconsider and thoroughly evaluate other possible causes of the patient's shoulder pain. Failure to identify associated pathology often will result in incomplete relief of symptoms after ASD.

Advantages and Disadvantages of ASD

It is generally accepted that after the classic open acromioplasty is performed, the patient's shoulder should be protected to allow the repair of the deltoid to heal. Most protocols describing open AA have prohibited active flexion, elevation, or abduction for 10 days to as long as 6 weeks. Conventionally, it has been accepted that ASD preserves the deltoid origin, mitigat-

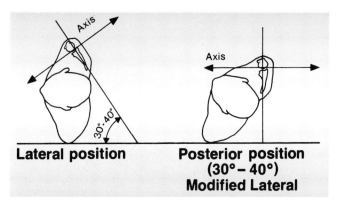

Figure 4 Lateral versus semilateral positioning. Semilateral positioning places the face of the glenoid in a position parallel to the floor. *(Reproduced with permission from Gross RM, Fitzgibbons TC: Shoulder arthroscopy: A modified approach. Arthroscopy 1985;1:156-159.)*

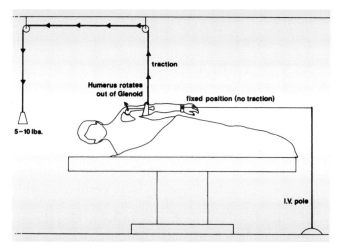

Figure 5 Perpendicular traction in the semilateral position. *(Reproduced with permission from Gross RM, Fitzgibbons TC: Shoulder arthroscopy: A modified approach. Arthroscopy 1985;1:156-159.)*

ing the requirement for postoperative protection, although a recent histologic study has suggested that a significant portion of the deltoid origin can be released, even with ASD. Computer modeling showed that a significant portion (43%) of the deltoid's direct fiber attachment to the anteroinferior acromion could be detached with just a 4-mm anterior acromioplasty. The same study also showed that most of the deltoid attachment to the acromion is direct, making subperiosteal elevation (such as described in the open procedure) impossible. The exact incidence of clinically significant deltoid dehiscence after AA or ASD is unknown. Only one case of clinical deltoid origin dehiscence after ASD has been reported in the literature, although this complication is probably underreported.

An uncontested advantage of ASD over the open procedure is that direct, comprehensive visualization of the glenohumeral joint is possible. Shoulder pain can

occur as a result of multiple etiologies, such as subtle instability, articular surface RC tears, early glenohumeral osteoarthrosis, loose bodies, labral tears, partial biceps tears/synovitis, subscapularis tears, and adhesive capsulitis. None of these processes is visualized or well addressed in the open technique. Critics of ASD have cited concerns regarding technical difficulty and lack of consistency of bony and soft-tissue resection. Visualization, orientation, and quantification of bone resection can be difficult, especially in the beginning of the surgeon's learning curve. These problems are minimized by adequate training, careful attention to technical details, and experience.

Technique/Intraoperative Decision Making

ASD can be performed with equal success whether the patient is in the lateral decubitus or beach chair position. The lateral decubitus position affords excellent exposure for visualization and instrumentation of the glenohumeral joint, and allows for arm traction with a setup of overhead pulleys and a pole for intravenous fluid. The beach chair position requires either an assistant or an articulated device to hold the extremity or apply traction. Some advantages of the beach chair position have been purported to be greater mobility of the arm, easier management of the airway, better patient tolerance of regional block anesthesia, decreased risk of traction-induced neurapraxias, orientation similar to that of the open procedure, and greater ease in conversion to an open anterior or posterior approach to the shoulder. Despite the existence of strong proponents for both forms of positioning, no controlled study has shown a clear major benefit to either. Therefore, intraoperative positioning has remained a matter of surgeon preference.

The first step in ASD is inspection of the glenohumeral joint. For the surgeon who prefers lateral positioning, a semilateral position with 30° to 40° of posterior rotation of the body positions the glenoid surface in an orientation that is parallel to the floor (Fig. 4). This position allows for easier orientation and placement of instruments, compared with the pure lateral position. Placing a light vector (5 to 10 lb) of traction perpendicular to the shaft of the humerus allows for easier inspection of the glenohumeral joint (especially the inferior one third) and obviates the need for much distal traction, virtually eliminating the risk of a traction neurapraxia (Fig. 5).

Once the patient is positioned and prepared, a posterior portal is used to visualize the glenohumeral joint. The plane of the AC joint accurately defines the plane of the glenohumeral joint. The posterior portal is made 2 to 3 cm inferior to the posterior edge of the acromion in the plane of the AC joint. The glenohumeral joint is systematically inspected. An anterior working portal is made in the plane of the AC joint, and loose bodies are removed, labral tears are débrided or repaired, undersurface partial-thickness RC tears are gently débrided or repaired, and the LHB and subscapularis are inspected carefully for inflammation/rupture. The ligamentous attachments to the glenoid rim and labrum are carefully assessed.

After glenohumeral pathology is addressed, the arthroscope is removed from the glenohumeral joint and entered into the subacromial space via the posterior portal or a lateral portal, according to the surgeon's preference. Inflow or outflow of fluid can occur through the arthroscope or a separate inflow or outflow portal. If the semilateral decubitus position has been used, the perpendicular traction rope must be cut, and the cut end must be isolated to allow proper maneuvering of the arthroscope lateral and inferior to the subacromial space.

The subacromial space can be visualized in either upside-up or upside-down fashion, depending on the surgeon's preference and the patient's positioning. With the patient in the beach chair position, the undersurface of the acromion is most easily conceptually visualized in an upside-up position. From the lateral decubitus position, the upside-down position is somewhat more natural, because the surgeon stands superior to the shoulder and visualizes the external anatomy of the shoulder in an upside-down position.

A complete ASD consists of subacromial bursectomy, release or excision of the CA ligament, and anteroinferior acromioplasty. Histologically, there is a rich supply of free nerve endings in the subacromial bursa, which can become very irritated in chronic refractory subacromial impingement. Aggressive bursectomy rids the shoulder of these pain foci while also removing a source of irritating crepitation. Conventionally, subacromial bursectomy has been completed with an arthroscopic shaver and standard ablative electrocautery. The holmium:YAG laser has been tried as a substitute, but it is unlikely that there is any significant clinical improvement linked to this device over standard electrocautery. Because the laser is more expensive to purchase and maintain, its use is not recommended at this time.

During bursectomy, the use of 1:300,000 epinephrine irrigation fluid and standard arthroscopic electrocautery controls bleeding and enhances visualization. Another effective method of improving visualization is systemic blood pressure control. A direct correlation exists between the systolic blood pressure, subacromial space pressure, and visual field. Maintaining a pressure difference of 49 mm Hg or less between the systolic blood pressure and subacromial space pressure permits good

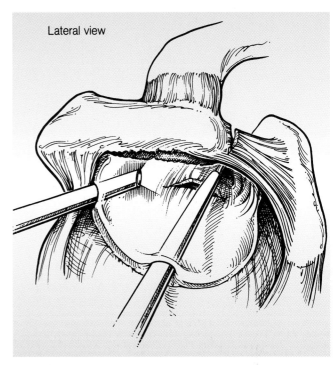

Lateral view

Figure 6 Release of the CA ligament using electrocautery. *(Reproduced with permission from Esch JC, Baker CL (eds): Arthroscopic Surgery: The Shoulder and Elbow. Philadelphia, PA, JB Lippincott, 1993, pp 151-173.)*

visualization. It is most desirable to control bleeding by hypotensive anesthesia because increasing the subacromial space pressure by turning up the arthroscopic fluid pump pressure can result in increased fluid extravasation and swelling.

The bursectomy is complete after full visualization of the anterior, posterior, and lateral subdeltoid recesses and débridement of all possible bursal tissue are achieved. Exchanging arthroscope and arthroscopic shaver portals can enhance access to these regions. When working in the subdeltoid recesses, the deltoid fascia should not be violated, because this increases extravasation of fluid into the deltoid muscle and potentiates the formation of subdeltoid adhesions. As a rule, débridement should not extend more than 5 cm distal to the deltoid origin, so that the axillary nerve is left undamaged. Leaving the deltoid fascia unviolated also minimizes this risk.

After bursectomy, attention is paid to the CA ligament. The CA ligament and underlying RC should be directly visualized and evaluated for erythema, thickening, and fraying, signs of abrasion that define the impingement process. As part of a standard ASD, the CA ligament should be directly released from its attachment to the anteroinferior acromion (Fig. 6). This step usually provokes bleeding from the acromial branch of the thoracoacromial artery, which can be stopped with arthroscopic electrocautery. This approach should be modified in the presence of an RC tear. CA ligament

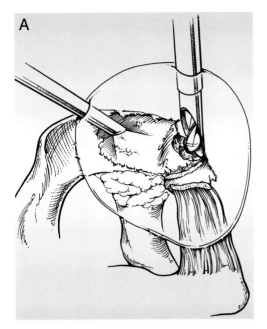

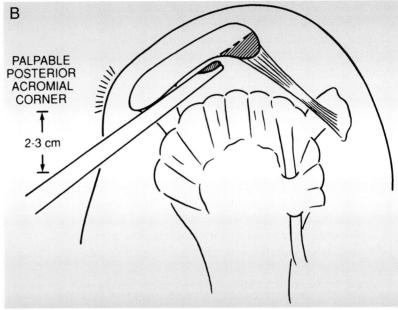

Figure 7 A, Burr lateral (anterior to posterior) technique. *(Reproduced with permission from Esch JC, Baker CL (eds): Arthroscopic Surgery: The Shoulder and Elbow. Philadelphia, PA, JB Lippincott, 1993, pp 151-173.)* **B,** Burr posterior (cutting block) technique. *(Reproduced with permission from Sampson TG, Nisbet JK, Glick JM: Precision acromioplasty in arthroscopic subacromial decompression of the shoulder. Arthroscopy 1991;7:301-307.)*

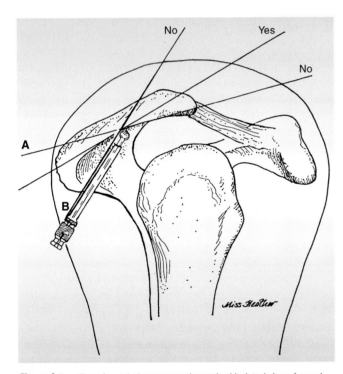

Figure 8 The effect of portal placement on the cutting-block technique. A superiorly placed portal (A) results in burr resection of too little acromion and an inferiorly placed portal (B) results in burr resection of too much acromion. *(Reproduced with permission from Caspari RB, Thal R: A technique for arthroscopic subacromial decompression. Arthroscopy 1992;8:23-30.)*

release is probably safe in patients with reparable tears and may help decompress the repair as it heals. A recent study has also shown that the CA arch has the capacity to reconstitute after arthroscopic release, via regenera-

tion and reattachment of the ligament to the anterior acromion. In the severely RC-deficient shoulder, however, the ligament should be left undisturbed because it is the most important secondary restraint to anterosuperior instability.

After subacromial bursectomy and release of the CA ligament, attention is paid to the acromioplasty. It can be performed with the burr placed in the lateral and/or posterior portal (preferably both). The burr lateral (anterior to posterior) technique involves an initial resection of bone from the anterior edge of the acromion, tapering the resection posteriorly so that the resection creates a flat, uniplanar surface (Fig. 7, *A*). The burr posterior (cutting block) technique uses the posterior acromion as a cutting block to guide appropriate bony resection from posterior to anterior (Fig. 7, *B*). When using the cutting block technique, care must be taken to use an accurate posterior portal. A portal that is too high will not allow removal of enough bone, whereas a portal that is too low may cause too much acromion to be resected (Fig. 8). Regardless of the technique used, the anteroinferior acromion should be visualized from both portals before completion of acromioplasty to ensure adequate resection of bone. A variable amount of acromial thickness is resected anteriorly, depending on the morphology of the acromion and the size of anteroinferior acromial spurs.

Acromioclavicular and Biceps Tendon Pathology

Results of a careful history, physical examination, and radiographic examination should specifically determine whether the AC joint or LHB will be addressed as part of the subacromial decompression before the patient is taken to the operating room. If the diagnosis of symptomatic AC arthrosis is made preoperatively, the distal clavicle should be completely excised. However, treatment of distal inferior clavicular spurs in patients without AC symptoms and signs is more controversial. Distal inferior clavicular spurs can cause medial encroachment of the RC, exacerbating the impingement process. Many authors address this process by flattening the undersurface of the medial acromial edge and distal clavicle with a burr, without complete distal clavicle resection. Such coplaning of the AC joint has led to favorable results in some studies. These results are in contradistinction to those of another investigation, in which 39% of patients with partial distal clavicular excision had significant postoperative AC joint pain at average intermediate term (8 to 9 month) follow-up. Patients without AC joint violation and patients who had a complete distal clavicle resection had no significant postoperative AC symptoms. The authors suggested that an "all or none" approach to the distal clavicle gives the best results; therefore, a complete distal clavicle resection should be performed or the AC joint capsule should not be violated at all.

The final structure to be addressed at arthroscopy is the LHB. Treatment of the LHB should be based on the preoperative clinical evaluation coupled with intraoperative observation of the quality of the tendon. If the structure of the tendon shows partial rupture, it is generally accepted that an LHB tenodesis or tenotomy is indicated. It is not clear, however, what should be done with the LHB that appears normal in the glenohumeral joint but is inflamed more distally.

If the biceps tendon clinically appears to be part of the impingement process, many authors believe that this pain will resolve with ASD alone. Unfortunately, this is not always the case. A new concept in LHB treatment is the subdeltoid transverse humeral ligament (THL) release. The THL is the subdeltoid covering for the LHB. Given the fixed dimensions of the bony bicipital groove, the THL may provide a source of irritation and constriction of the tendon, causing de Quervain's disease. Therefore, it has been hypothesized that subdeltoid release of the THL may remove an important component of LHB-related pain. This procedure does not destabilize the LHB because the coracohumeral and superior glenohumeral ligaments that insert at the articular entrance to the bicipital groove provide stability to the tendon (Fig. 9).

Release of the THL arthroscopically via the anterior subdeltoid recess can be performed easily with a retrograde hook from an anterolateral working portal, without damaging or destabilizing the tendon because the

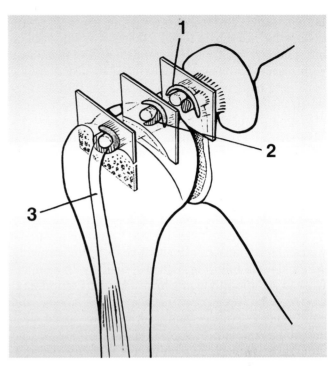

Figure 9 A schematic representation of the relations of the coracohumeral ligament and superior glenohumeral ligament to the long head of the biceps tendon. The long head of the biceps tendon is stabilized in the bicipital groove by the coracohumeral ligament (black), which forms the roof, and the superior glenohumeral ligament (hatched), which forms the floor. *(Reproduced with permission from Walch G, Nove-Josserand L, Levigne C, Renaud E: Tears of the supraspinatus tendon associated with "hidden" lesions of the rotator interval. J Shoulder Elbow Surg 1994;3:353-360.)*

coracohumeral and superior glenohumeral ligaments are left intact. In a recent uncontrolled prospective study of 49 patients, results of the subdeltoid THL release as a part of ASD were analyzed, and favorable results in patients with an inflamed but structurally intact LHB were found. Additional work is required to investigate the role of this technique in the intact inflamed LHB.

Postoperative Management

Role of Nonsteroidal Anti-inflammatory Drugs, Pain Infusion Catheters, and Physical Therapy

Postoperative management after ASD alone usually is simple. Postoperative pain control is achieved with compressive ice bandages, low-dose narcotics, and, sometimes, subacromial catheters and anti-inflammatory medications.

A prospective, randomized trial was performed to study the efficacy of a new subacromial infusion pump in controlling pain after ASD. Infusion catheters were placed directly into the subacromial space under arthroscopic visualization in 62 patients after completion of ASD and were kept in place for 48 hours postoperatively. The catheters gave a 2 mL/h constant infusion of 0.25% bupivacaine for the study group (n = 31) and normal saline for the control group (n = 31) with boluses for acute pain flares. Patients with bupivacaine infusions had significantly better pain control than those with placebo infusions, as measured by visual analog scales and narcotic pain requirements. The authors proposed that these pumps could be used postoperatively, obviating the need for and risk of interscalene blocks. There were no complications described in this study, but infections and catheter breakage have been reported anecdotally.

In another prospective, randomized, double-blinded investigation, the effect of daily ketoprofen (200 mg) was compared with that of placebo given orally to patients for 6 weeks following ASD. Forty-one patients were followed at 6 weeks and 2 years postoperatively. At the 6-week follow-up, patients treated with ketoprofen had significantly better University of California at Los Angeles (UCLA) scores, ROM, satisfaction, and pain relief, with significantly less need for narcotic analgesics. At 2-year follow-up, there was no difference in functional scores between the two groups.

One of the advantages of ASD over open decompression is that without overt deltoid detachment, patients have no significant activity precautions or restrictions. The patient is advised to gradually increase activities and wean from the sling, then progress to activities without restriction, as tolerated. Physical therapy has sometimes been used to assist in postoperative rehabilitation to optimize outcome. In an investigation from Denmark, 43 consecutive ASD patients randomized to self-training or physical therapist–guided rehabilitation were studied. Follow-up was performed by an independent observer after 3, 6, and 12 months. No significant differences in outcome as measured by the Constant Score and return to work (8 weeks) were noted between groups.

Results/Complications

Results of ASD alone are somewhat variable in the literature. This is partly a result of the multifactorial nature of subacromial impingement and the combinations of several subacromial and glenohumeral procedures that are performed on each individual patient. In addition, studies regarding ASD refer to several different shoulder scoring systems, each with its own differential focus on postoperative outcome measures. Despite this variability, it is generally accepted that for stage II impingement, ASD has a clinical success rate (good or excellent results) approximating 80% to 90%. Most studies comparing the arthroscopic to the open procedure, including two prospective randomized studies, show improved short-term results with ASD and equivalent long-term results. A 1994 study showed that patients who underwent ASD regained flexion and

strength, were discharged from the hospital, and returned to work faster than patients who underwent open decompression. The ASD patients also required less narcotic pain medicine. Open decompression patients reached the functional level of ASD patients at about 3 months postoperatively. A recent prospective randomized study done in 2002 showed that at long-term follow-up (average 25 months) subjective improvement, overall satisfaction, UCLA score, and shoulder strength were essentially equivalent in patients who underwent the open or arthroscopic procedure. Interestingly, pain and function visual analog scores improved slightly more in the open group than the arthroscopic group, but revision open surgery did not improve results in any of the failed arthroscopic cases. Unsettled compensation was a predictor of poor outcome in both open AA and ASD cases.

The most common complication of ASD is continued pain, which can be secondary to numerous factors. Inadequate resection of the anteroinferior acromion and CA ligament is an error in technique and can result in continued impingement postoperatively. Complete resection is ensured by using the arthroscope with proper orientation and hemostasis to adequately visualize the inferior acromion from both the posterior and lateral portals and by using the cutting-block technique. In questionable cases, a gloved finger may be used to palpate the undersurface through a slightly extended lateral portal hole. Another study attempted to delineate risk factors for poor results after ASD. Of 29 patients with unsatisfactory outcomes, 14 had no evidence of impingement at time of arthroscopy. Some had evidence of RC damage, but the undersurface of the acromion was smooth and undamaged, indicating lack of mechanical wear between the RC and acromial undersurface. The most significant predictor of poor outcome was a prolonged duration of symptoms before surgery. Satisfactory results were most often associated with a positive impingement test. The authors stressed proper indications for surgery and advised proceeding to ASD within 12 months of onset of symptoms. As discussed previously, missed or iatrogenic pathology can be another cause of continued pain following ASD. Other factors leading to continued pain after ASD include inappropriately treated LHB, RC, and instability lesions; these are avoided primarily by careful preoperative planning, intraoperative assessment, and decision making.

Another reason for poor results after ASD is misdiagnosis, especially in individuals younger than age 40 years. A recent investigation from Germany found a correlation between poor results after ASD and increased ultrasonically measured inferior shift of the humeral head. The authors' conclusion was that patients with hypermobile glenohumeral or unstable joints should not undergo ASD. It is also essential to distinguish the symptoms of subacromial impingement from the pain of internal impingement, which typically occurs in young athletes participating in activities requiring overhead shoulder motion. This problem typically presents with posterior shoulder pain and is exacerbated by placing the arm in the throwing or overhead position (eg, throwing athletes and tennis players). Pathophysiologically, the articular surface of the RC abrades against the posterior glenoid and labrum when the arm is abducted and fully externally rotated (Fig. 10). This form of impingement has been linked by some authors to overt glenohumeral instability, by others to occult glenohumeral pseudoinstability, and by other authors not to instability but to the repetitive nature of the activity itself. Regardless of the cause, it is important to distinguish between the different types of shoulder pain because ASD can be successful in young patients with true subacromial impingement but will fail in patients with internal impingement.

The surgeon must also be aware of secondary impingement from a tight posterior capsule. A recent investigation reported on patients with refractory impingement syndrome, all with significant restriction of internal rota-

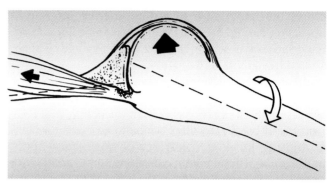

Figure 10 Internal impingement occurs when the supraspinatus contracts (narrow arrow) and the insertion impinges on the posterosuperior glenoid rim when the arm is positioned in abduction and external rotation (open arrow). This impingement is likely exacerbated by anterior shoulder instability (wide arrow). *(Reproduced with permission from Jobe FW, Screnar P, Brewster C: NATA Proceedings Book. Champaign, IL, Human Kinetics, 1998, p 202.)*

tion secondary to posterior capsular contracture. Arthroscopic posterior capsular release alone resulted in the resolution of impingement symptoms in these patients. This suggests that although posterior capsular contracture is often associated with subacromial impingement, it can sometimes actually be the primary cause of the impingement (Fig. 11). In these patients, the problem would not be addressed effectively with ASD. This under-

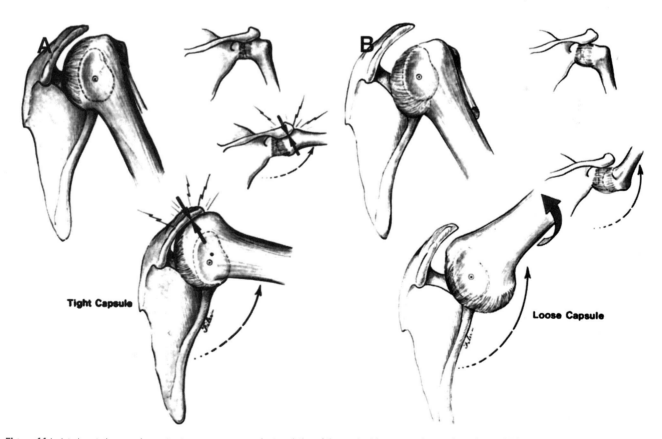

Figure 11 Isolated posterior capsular contracture can cause superior translation of the proximal humerus and secondary subacromial impingement. Releasing the capsule in selected patients can relieve the impingement. A = Tight capsule. B = Loose capsule. *(Reproduced with permission from Sampson TG, Nisbet JK, Glick JM: Precision acromioplasty in arthroscopic subacromial decompression of the shoulder. Arthroscopy 1991;7:301-307.)*

scores the importance of testing internal rotation in abduction during the initial evaluation, in addition to the importance of posterior capsular stretching after diagnosis and treatment.

Other complications of ASD occur less frequently and include infection, bleeding, neurovascular injury, captured shoulder (adhesions between the deltoid and RC), instrument breakage, reflex sympathetic dystrophy, heterotopic ossification, recurrence of subacromial spurs, and fistula. These complications do not occur with greater frequency than from the open procedure. One of the most problematic complications of ASD is acromial fracture, which is rare but very difficult to treat effectively. The best prevention of acromial fracture is to perform a tapered, uniplanar acromioplasty, without an inappropriately deepened or notched surface at any portion of the undersurface of the acromion.

Summary

ASD has become a standard of care in the treatment of patients with refractory subacromial impingement. Results are equivalent to open AA. Although nonsurgical treatment should always be tried first, prolonged lack of success with nonsurgical measures (3 to 6 months) should result in surgical treatment to optimize outcome. To ensure success of the operation, the surgeon must confirm by careful history taking and physical examination that the patient's problem is in fact subacromial impingement; ASD without clear evidence of impingement results in poor outcomes. One key to patient selection, especially in younger patients, is to distinguish the anterior pain of subacromial impingement from the posterior pain associated with internal impingement. Although posterior capsular contracture is a common coincident finding in patients with subacromial impingement syndrome, it also can be the cause of a secondary impingement process when the contracture is severe. In cases of true subacromial impingement, associated AC joint and LHB symptoms should be carefully elicited, and the preoperative plan well delineated. Strict and meticulous attention to detail must be exercised to perform complete subacromial bursectomy, CA ligament release or resection, and an adequate, uniplanar acromioplasty using proper technique. Treatment of associated LHB or AC pathology also may include an LHB tenotomy or tenodesis, subdeltoid THL release, and/or distal clavicle resection, if needed. Recent studies show promise in the use of postoperative subacromial infusion catheters and nonsteroidal anti-inflammatory drugs for improved analgesia. In the absence of an RC tear, supervised physical therapy probably is not necessary.

Annotated Bibliography

General

Altchek DW, Carson EW: Arthroscopic acromioplasty: Indications and technique. *Instr Course Lect* 1998;47: 21-28.

Clinical evaluation of subacromial impingement, ASD technique in the beach chair position, burr lateral and cutting block acromial resection, and results in throwing athletes are reviewed.

Bigliani LU, Levine WN: Subacromial impingement syndrome. *J Bone Joint Surg Am* 1997;79:1854-1868.

A comprehensive review of the literature on subacromial impingement syndrome is provided. History, etiology, acromial morphology, diagnosis, and treatment are thoroughly discussed.

Matthews LS, Blue JM: Arthroscopic subacromial decompression: Avoidance of complications and enhancement of results. *Instr Course Lect* 1998;47:29-33.

This is a review of the complications of ASD. The importance of complete preoperative workup (AC joint, acromial morphology, rotator cuff evaluation) and optimization of intraoperative factors (visualization, orientation, hemostasis, and quantification of bone resection) is stressed.

Advantages and Disadvantages of ASD

Barber FA: Coplaning of the acromioclavicular joint. *Arthroscopy* 2001;17:913-917.

In this retrospective review of 76 patients, 28 patients underwent ASD with removal of an inferior clavicular osteophyte, 27 patients had a partial resection of the distal clavicle of up to 50% of the articular surface, and 21 patients had a complete distal clavicle resection. There was no significant difference in the Constant, Rowe, American Shoulder and Elbow Surgeons, and Single Assessment Numerical Evaluation scores among the three groups of patients, and no patients required additional AC joint surgery at minimum 2-year follow-up.

Bonsell S: Detached deltoid during arthroscopic subacromial decompression. *Arthroscopy* 2000;16:745-748.

The first reported case of deltoid detachment during arthroscopic subacromial decompression is described.

Buford D Jr, Mologne T, McGrath S, Heinen G, Snyder S: Midterm results of arthroscopic co-planing of the acromioclavicular joint. *J Shoulder Elbow Surg* 2000;9:498-501.

This is a retrospective review of 37 patients with impingement syndrome, inferior AC spurs, and no significant AC tenderness who were treated with ASD and removal of 20% to 25% of the inferior clavicle. Thirty-five patients (95%) had good or excellent UCLA scores at follow-up (minimum 2 years). Only two patients (4%) had residual pain and tenderness at the AC joint at follow-up.

Fischer BW, Gross RM, McCarthy JA, Arroyo JS: Incidence of acromioclavicular joint complications after arthroscopic subacromial decompression. *Arthroscopy* 1999;15:241-248.

In this retrospective review of 183 shoulders, patients were divided into three groups: A, ASD without AC joint violation (n = 103); B, ASD with AC violation (n = 36); and C, ASD and arthroscopic distal clavicle resection (n = 44). At 8.4 months' average follow-up, substantial AC pain developed in 39% of group B patients, compared with none in group A or C (*P* = 0.0001).

Hunt JL, Moore RJ, Krishnan J: The fate of the coracoacromial ligament in arthroscopic acromioplasty: An anatomical study. *J Shoulder Elbow Surg* 2000;9: 491-494.

This article reports on a cadaveric study in which ASD was performed using the cutting-block technique. Fibers of the CA ligament and deltoid that were released as part of ASD remained attached to the acromion by a bridge of periosteum and collagenous fibers from the ligament and remaining deltoid. This remaining attachment is called the coracoacromial-deltoid-periosteal complex.

Levy O, Copeland SA: Regeneration of the coracoacromial ligament after acromioplasty and arthroscopic subacromial decompression. *J Shoulder Elbow Surg* 2001; 10:317-320.

Ten patients with RC tears treated with ASD alone required revision surgery, secondary to continued pain. In all patients, at the time of open RC repair, a ligamentous structure resembling the CA ligament was present. This structure was in the same anatomic position and possessed the same histologic features as the original CA ligament.

Morrison DS, Schaefer RK, Friedman RL: The relationship between subacromial space pressure, blood pressure, and visual clarity during arthroscopic subacromial decompression. *Arthroscopy* 1995;11:557-560.

A direct correlation between the systolic blood pressure, subacromial space pressure, and visual field was found. The authors concluded that maintaining a pressure difference of 49 mm Hg or less between the systolic blood pressure and subacromial space pressure permits good visualization.

Murphy MA, Maze NM, Boyd JL, Quick DC, Buss DD: Cost-benefit comparison: Holmium laser versus electrocautery in arthroscopic acromioplasty. *J Shoulder Elbow Surg* 1999;8:275-278.

Forty-nine stage II ASD patients were treated with standard electrocautery or the holmium:YAG laser for intraoperative débridement and hemostasis. Using the holmium:YAG laser increased hospital charges by 23% without significant difference in functional outcome or satisfaction at 1, 2, 3, 6, and 12 months postoperatively.

Ruotolo C, Nottage WM, Flatow EL, Gross RM, Fanton GS: Controversial topics in shoulder arthroscopy. *Arthroscopy* 2002;18:65-75.

The authors report on an uncontrolled, prospective study of 49 patients undergoing arthroscopic subdeltoid THL release and synovectomy of the LHB tendon, in addition to ASD. It was concluded that biceps inflammation noted at arthroscopy and correlated with clinical examination could be successfully addressed by this technique. Damage to the LHB tendon itself, whether intra-articular or in the groove, was a poor prognostic factor and is best treated by a tenotomy or tenodesis.

Torpey BM, Ikeda K, Weng M, et al: The deltoid muscle origin: Histologic characteristics and effects of subacromial decompression. *Am J Sports Med* 1998;26:379-383.

Histologic analysis of nine cadavers showed that deltoid attachments to the acromion are direct (not periosteal). Computer modeling showed 41% loss of direct fiber attachment with a 4-mm inferior acromioplasty and a 69% loss with a 6-mm acromioplasty.

Postoperative Management

Anderson NH, Sojbjerg JO, Johannsen HV, Sneppen O: Self-training versus physiotherapist-supervised rehabilitation of the shoulder in patients treated with arthroscopic subacromial decompression: A clinical randomized study. *J Shoulder Elbow Surg* 1999;8:99-101.

Results of a prospective analysis of 43 consecutive ASD patients randomized to either self-training or physical therapist–guided rehabilitation are reported. No significant differences in outcome (Constant Score and return to work) were noted between either group at 3-, 6- and 12-month follow-up.

Hoe-Hansen C, Norlin R: The clinical effect of ketoprofen after arthroscopic subacromial decompression: A randomized double-blind prospective study. *Arthroscopy* 1999; 15:249-252.

Results of an analysis of the effect of daily oral doses of 200 mg of ketoprofen (n = 21) versus placebo (n = 20) given to ASD patients for 6 weeks postoperatively are reported. Six-week UCLA scores were significantly higher and narcotic requirements lower in the ketoprofen group compared to the placebo group, but no significant difference was found at 2-year follow-up.

Savoie FH, Field LD, Jenkins RN, Mallon WJ, Phelps RA: The pain control infusion pump for postoperative pain control in shoulder surgery. *Arthroscopy* 2000;16: 339-342.

This is the report of a prospective, randomized analysis of the efficacy of subacromial infusion catheters used 48 hours after ASD. Patients with bupivacaine infusions (n = 31) had statistically significantly better pain control than those with saline infusions (n = 31) as measured by visual analog scales and narcotic pain-relief requirements (*P* < 0.05).

Results/Complications

Hawkins RJ, Plancher KD, Saddemi SR, Brezenoff LS, Moor JT: Arthroscopic subacromial decompression. *J Shoulder Elbow Surg* 2001;10:225-230.

In this study, 112 patients were treated with a standard ASD, and 28 patients (29 shoulders) were treated with a standard ASD supplemented by digital palpation through an expanded lateral portal to ensure adequate and smooth resection. Patients in the lateral portal palpation group had better results based on the Neer criteria (86% versus 48% satisfactory).

Patel VR, Singh D, Calvert PT, Bayley JI: Arthroscopic subacromial decompression: Results and factors affecting outcome. *J Shoulder Elbow Surg* 1999;8:231-237.

The authors retrospectively found unsatisfactory outcomes in 29 of 114 patients with stage II impingement treated with ASD. Poor results were linked to a questionable diagnosis (lack of evidence of subacromial impingement at arthroscopy), inadequate decompression, presence of RC calcium deposits, prolonged duration of symptoms before surgery, and presence of a partial thickness RC tear. Satisfactory results were associated with a positive impingement test (*P* < 0.05).

Schneider T, Straus JM, Fink B, Jerosch J, Menke W, Ruther W: Influence of joint stability on the results of arthroscopic subacromial decompression. *Acta Orthop Belg* 1996;62:94-99.

The authors report on ultrasonographic analysis of the shoulders of 70 ASD patients with stage I/II impingement with 3-year follow-up. Thirty-five patients with Neer score of less than 85 showed average passive humeral head inferior shift of 5.1 + 2.0 mm, compared with a 2.4 + 0.9 mm shift in patients with scores greater than 85 (*P* < 0.001).

Spangehl MJ, Hawkins RH, McCormack RG, Loomer RL: Arthroscopic versus open acromioplasty: A prospective, randomized, blinded study. *J Shoulder Elbow Surg* 2002;11:101-107.

Sixty-two patients were prospectively randomized to ASD or open acromioplasty after stratification for age (> 50 years), associated ligamentous laxity, and the presence of an ongoing compensation claim. There was no significant difference between results of the two techniques in visual analog scales for postoperative improvement (*P* = 0.30), patient satisfaction (*P* = 0.94), UCLA shoulder score (*P* = 0.69), or strength (*P* = 0.62). Open decompression patients had slightly better results than ASD patients for pain and function (*P* = 0.01). Repeat (open) acromioplasty was performed in five patients in the unsuccessful arthroscopic group without improvement. Good or excellent results were seen in 67% of patients. When unset-tled compensation claims were excluded, the good/excellent result rate was 87%.

Ticker JB, Beim GM, Warner JJ: Recognition and treatment of refractory posterior capsular contracture of the shoulder. *Arthroscopy* 2000;16:27-34.

A group of nine patients was identified in whom painful loss of internal rotation was associated with refractory impingement syndrome. The duration of symptoms averaged 18 months and a course of physical therapy specifically addressing loss of internal rotation failed in all patients. Arthroscopy revealed a thickened posterior capsule in all patients. Arthroscopic release of the posterior capsule resulted in improved motion in all patients, with substantial relief of pain.

Classic Bibliography

Codman EA: *The Shoulder: Rupture of the Supraspinatus Tendon and Other Lesions In or About the Subacromial Bursa*. Boston, MA, Thomas Todd, 1934.

Ellman H: Arthroscopic subacromial decompression: Analysis of one- to three-year results. *Arthroscopy* 1987; 3:173-181.

Ellman H, Harris E, Kay SP: Early degenerative joint disease simulating impingement syndrome: Arthroscopic findings. *Arthroscopy* 1992;8:482-487.

Gartsman GM, Blair ME, Noble PC, Bennett JB, Tullos HS: Arthroscopic subacromial decompression: An anatomical study. *Am J Sports Med* 1988;16:48-50.

Hawkins RJ, Kennedy JC: Impingement syndrome in athletes. *Am J Sports Med* 1980;8:151-158.

Lindh M, Norlin R: Arthroscopic subacromial decompression versus open acromioplasty: A two-year follow-up study. *Clin Orthop* 1993;290:174-176.

Matthews LS, Burkhead WZ, Gordon S, Racanelli J, Ruland L: Acromial fracture: A complication of arthroscopic subacromial decompression. *J Shoulder Elbow Surg* 1994;3:256-261.

Neer CS: Anterior acromioplasty for the chronic impingement syndrome in the shoulder: A preliminary report. *J Bone Joint Surg Am* 1972;54:41-50.

Neviaser TJ, Neviaser RJ, Neviaser JS, Neviaser JS: The four-in-one arthroplasty for the painful arc syndrome. *Clin Orthop* 1982;163:107-112.

Sachs RA, Stone ML, Devine S: Open vs. arthroscopic acromioplasty: A prospective, randomized study. *Arthroscopy* 1994; 10:248-254.

Sampson TG, Nisbet JK, Glick JM: Precision acromioplasty in arthroscopic subacromial decompression of the shoulder. *Arthroscopy* 1991;7:301-307.

Chapter 50

Arthroscopic Acromioclavicular Joint Resection

James P. Tasto, MD

Introduction

The acromioclavicular (AC) joint may be the isolated cause of shoulder pain or a contributing factor in impingement syndrome. A wide variety of nonsurgical and surgical approaches have been used to treat AC separations, grades I through VI, throughout the years. Conditions that affect the AC joint can be localized or systemic and may include a number of pathologies. It behooves the clinician to identify the role that the AC joint plays in shoulder pain. This chapter will discuss a number of the conditions that affect the AC joint and will specifically focus on the arthroscopic approach to AC joint disease.

Diagnosis

The history is quite important in ascertaining the possible contribution of the AC joint in a patient with shoulder pain. Any history of previous separation, a posttraumatic event, generalized osteoarthritis, and conditions isolated to sport-specific injuries, such as osteolysis in weight lifters, is needed for proper diagnosis.

The physical examination is a critical component in the assessment of AC joint pathology and must be carefully carried out prior to any attempt at surgical intervention. Differentiation between classic impingement, subcoracoid impingement, early frozen shoulder, and a variety of conditions is critical. Some of the tests and indications that have been used in that differentiation follow: (1) the cross-arm adduction test, both passive and active; (2) adduction, internal rotation, and extension to isolate posterior AC facet problems; (3) tenderness to direct palpation; (4) tenderness with attempts at AP translation; (5) localized pain at the AC joint during conventional impingement testing; and (6) a positive O'Brien test with the arm adducted, forward elevated to 90°, and in a thumb-up position.

Radiographic analysis is critical before any type of shoulder surgery to define the morphology of the acromion, AC joint involvement, and the presence or absence of an os acromiale and calcification. Radiographic views that are helpful include an AP view in internal and external rotation; a 30° tangential glenoid view; a 15° cephalic view; an outlet view; an axillary view; and, when needed, a radiograph of the opposite shoulder for comparison. Occasionally, MRI or bone scan may be indicated.

Differential injections to isolate subacromial pathology from AC joint pathology must be done in two different settings, paying careful attention to actually staying in the AC joint and not entering the subacromial space. A local anesthetic in conjunction with a steroid injection may be helpful, not only for diagnostic purposes but also as part of the treatment regimen.

Direct arthroscopic visualization often confirms the surgeon's impression that the AC joint is involved, but a relatively high percentage of AC joints will look pathologic, particularly if there are some early degenerative changes that are associated with normal aging. Therefore, this approach should not be used to determine whether or not the distal clavicle should be resected. The decision whether to resect an AC joint must be made before surgically violating the joint.

Anatomy

The AC joint is a diarthrodial joint that contains a meniscus and usually slopes medially when going from superior to inferior. There are multiple anatomic variations to this joint and preoperative radiographic evaluation is important to fully understand each anatomic variation. Preoperative evaluation may disclose conditions that result in significant hypertrophy of the distal end of the clavicle. In this case, the surgeon may choose to do a more significant bony resection on the acromion rather than take off a large amount of bone on the clavicle. Some authors have focused on creating a 5- to 10-mm space and have chosen to do most of their resection on the acromial facet rather than on the distal end of the clavicle.

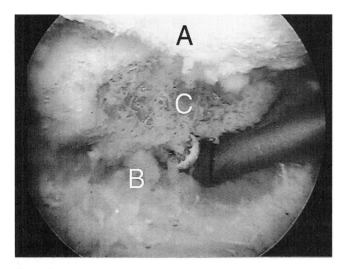

Figure 1 An RF device being used to clear soft tissue from the AC joint. A = acromion; B = rotator cuff; and C = clavicle.

Indications

There are a number of indications for arthroscopic resection of the distal clavicle, which include posttraumatic, degenerative, or rheumatoid arthritis; osteolysis; and meniscal derangement. The role of the AC joint in the impingement syndrome remains somewhat controversial. Some surgeons do a relatively large percentage of associated AC joint resections with their subacromial decompressions, whereas others remain quite selective and do only a small percentage of AC joint surgery in this syndrome. The contribution of inferior osteophytes in the production of pain remains controversial and will be discussed in the section on coplaning. Patients with old type II, III, and IV AC joint separations with obvious displacement of the distal clavicle are poorer candidates for isolated AC joint resection. A significant component of the pain syndrome in these patients often is a result of ligamentous instability, and reconstruction or reinforcement of the coracoclavicular ligaments following AC joint resection usually is necessary.

Treatment

Nonsurgical treatment of AC joint pathology usually includes nonsteroidal anti-inflammatory drugs, physical therapy, activity modification, and occasional steroid injections. The surgical treatment for recalcitrant AC joint pain has been either open or arthroscopic resection of the distal clavicle. The arthroscopic procedure has gained credibility and popularity over the years because it can be performed quite readily in conjunction with an arthroscopic subacromial decompression (ASD) or as an isolated procedure. The arthroscopic procedure carries with it a number of advantages, which include improved cosmesis, decreased pain, and more rapid rehabilitation.

Arthroscopic Techniques

The general principles used when performing arthroscopic AC joint resections are quite similar to those used with ASD. The use of a pump to control pressure and flow to better control bleeding and visualization is recommended. Before beginning the arthroscopy, the surgeon must carefully mark the anatomic landmarks so that portals can be placed accurately. The anterior portal must be well aligned with the AC joint to avoid eccentric instrument placement and difficulty with resection. It may be helpful to instill a local anesthetic with epinephrine into the area just inferior to the AC joint, the subacromial space, and the anterior coracoacromial area before working on the AC joint. Most surgeons continue to use epinephrine in the irrigant to assist them in controlling the bleeding. Occasionally, a smaller (2.7-mm) arthroscope may be necessary if the joint is extremely tight. In general, the entire surgical procedure can be done through a posterior viewing portal, without the need for the smaller arthroscope. A variety of hand instruments (curettes, rasps, and shavers with the appropriate sized burrs) are necessary.

Patient positioning can be in the lateral decubitus position with approximately 12 lb of traction, 20° to 30° of abduction, and 20° of forward flexion for all subacromial and AC work. Alternatively, the beach chair position can be used with equal success. A variety of commercial radiofrequency (RF) devices are available, which have greatly assisted the surgeon in débridement and visualization of the morphology of the acromion, as well as the AC joint (Fig. 1). These RF devices are both monopolar and bipolar and are chosen at the surgeon's discretion. These tools have largely supplanted conventional electrocautery because of ease of use, the ability for use in standard saline arthroscopic fluid (as opposed to glycine), rapid vaporization of tissue, better delineation of the bony landmarks, and a more rapid and more precise soft-tissue ablation mode.

If distal clavicle resection is performed in conjunction with ASD, the ASD should be done first so that if swelling and/or bleeding are interfering with the completion of the surgical procedure, it can easily be converted to an open distal clavicle excision if necessary. Care must be taken to thoroughly irrigate the joint after distal clavicle resection so that much of the bony debris that has been dispersed into the soft tissues and adventitia can be removed. A number of techniques are available and well described in the literature for AC joint resection. They will be listed and described as follows.

Technique I

This technique uses the conventional posterior viewing portal and an anterior portal directly aligned with the AC joint, as well as a lateral portal. The posterior viewing por-

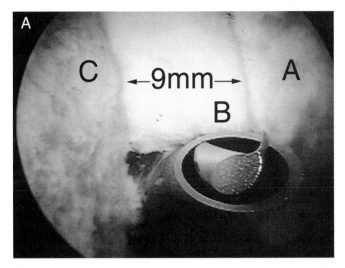

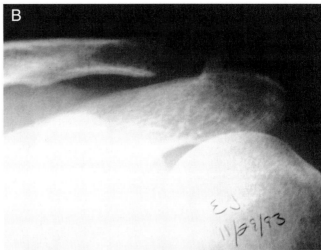

Figure 2 **A,** Arthroscopic view of the AC joint with measurement. A = acromion; B = superior AC ligament; and C = clavicle. **B,** Postoperative radiograph of an 8- to 10-mm AC joint resection.

tal can be used throughout the entire procedure, and the arthroscope generally does not have to be moved. The surgeon uses conventional burrs, shavers, and RF to delineate the AC joint, usually from the working lateral portal. A portion of the acromial facet is removed for better visualization. This is referred to as the "window to the AC joint." A small portion of the inferior distal clavicle, the size of which was determined before surgery, is resected from the lateral portal. The general recommendation for resection is between 5 and 10 mm (Fig. 2).

Once the inferior component has been removed, the outflow is changed to the lateral portal and the working portal becomes the anterior portal. At this time, the remaining component of the distal clavicle and/or a portion of the acromion is resected to a predetermined distance. Usually, the burr or shaver that is used for the resection can be used to quantitate that distance. Periscoping the arthroscope allows full visualization of the AC joint from superior to inferior and anterior to posterior (Fig. 3). Judicious use of conventional RF will help delineate the osseous margins so that no residual osteophytes or spurs are left. Most of the work on the distal clavicle is done through the anterior portal. Care must be taken to remove the entire tip of the distal clavicle to avoid residual osteophytes. Care also is taken to preserve the integrity of the superior AC joint capsule and ligamentous structures. This preservation provides for some residual stability following the surgical procedure. The entire inferior capsule and a portion of the anterior and posterior ligamentous and capsular structures have been violated during this procedure, and the maintenance of the superior component is critical to avoid long-term instability and symptoms. The completeness of resection can be further evaluated by placing the arthroscope in the anterior portal.

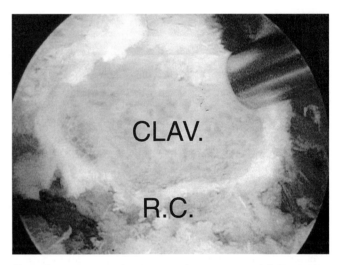

Figure 3 Full visualization of an AC resection from posterior portal. CLAV = clavicle; RC = rotator cuff.

Technique II

Technique II is similar to technique I but the clavicle is more thoroughly débrided with a central coring of the clavicle, in addition to resecting the undersurface of the clavicle. The latter reduces the amount of work that needs to be done through the anterior portal. The remaining portion of this technique is almost identical to technique I.

Technique III

The direct superior approach is somewhat more difficult because of the limited access to the AC joint, but is certainly useful in patients who do not require subacromial surgery. It is particularly helpful for those patients with osteolysis who have a wider joint space, require less resection, and can return to sports and heavy activity ear-

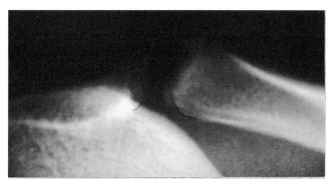

Figure 4 A widened AC joint space with osteolysis.

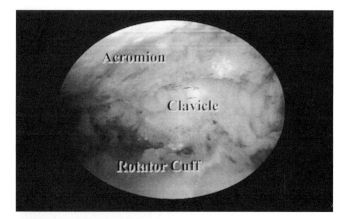

Figure 5 A symptomatic unstable AC joint 2 years after coplaning.

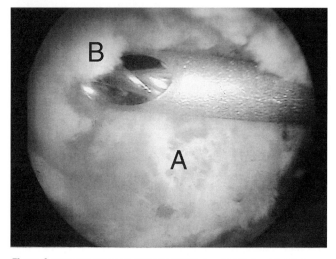

Figure 6 Residual posterior clavicular osteophyte. A = clavicle; B = osteophyte.

lier if the surgery focuses only on the AC joint with limited débridement and resection (Fig. 4). In this approach, posterosuperior and anterosuperior portals are established, usually with a conventional arthroscope, but if the space is somewhat narrow, a 2.7-mm arthroscope may be required. Often, using needles can aid in the placement of portals to localize the joint before the portal is made. This procedure may require the initial use of a small shaver to create a space for débridement of material in

the AC joint for better visualization. The arthroscope can be interchanged from anterior to posterior to gain better access to those areas of the AC joint that are directly underneath the arthroscope. An added advantage of this approach is the almost complete preservation of the circumferential stabilizing ligaments of the AC joint.

Instability and Coplaning

There has been a great deal of discussion over the past 5 years pertaining to instability in the AC joint following coplaning, as well as arthroscopic and open resection. Clinical and basic science reports have supported the fact that there is increased motion following any violation of the AC joint, be it coplaning, or arthroscopic or open resection. Clinical and laboratory cadaveric data support the principle that instability increases in the AC joint proportional to the amount of bone resected. Whether or not the increased laxity following a distal clavicle resection is of any clinical significance, however, remains untested. There currently is support for minimizing the amount resected to between 5 and 10 mm in reports of both short- and long-term follow-up.

Coplaning is defined as the resection of the inferior surface of the AC joint to include the acromial facet as well as a portion of the distal clavicle. This procedure usually is done in conjunction with a conventional ASD. A great deal of controversy exists as to the necessity of coplaning and the potential benefits and complications of adding it to ASD. Some data in the literature support avoiding coplaning of the inferior surface of the AC joint in patients with radiographic evidence of spurring. Many authors have recommended that coplaning should not be performed because it may destabilize a joint that may then become symptomatic. Coplaning should not be performed in a joint that already has early degenerative changes (Fig. 5). However, other authors believe that coplaning may add to the long-term benefits of ASD and that complications of residual AC joint symptoms do not occur in most patients who undergo coplaning. Each surgeon needs to determine whether the inferior osteophytes play a role in the creation of symptoms or are merely a reaction to the degenerative process.

Biomechanical studies have been reported that indicate significant destabilization of the AC joint following coplaning. This procedure may cause pathologic laxity in a joint that has naturally stabilized itself. The increased laxity may contribute to additional symptoms in an otherwise quiescent joint. Further studies are needed to determine the efficacy and safety of coplaning. It appears that the resection of the acromial facet during a conventional ASD violates the AC joint, but does so in a limited fashion, thereby preserving most of the capsuloligamentous structures. If the AC joint is asymptomatic during conventional workup and ASD is being performed, it may be more prudent to avoid violating this joint. If there are symptoms in the AC joint, a full distal clavicular resection should be performed.

Rehabilitation

In general, with isolated arthroscopic AC joint surgery, the rehabilitation protocol can be accelerated from the usual ASD protocol. For isolated AC joint disease, the patient can begin a passive range-of-motion (ROM) program immediately, followed in a week by active, assisted ROM and within 10 to 14 days by active ROM. Free weights may be started in 3 weeks and a return to full sports activity in about 6 weeks. If the procedure is done in conjunction with ASD, then rehabilitation needs to follow the ASD protocol.

Complications

Complications in arthroscopic AC joint resection are quite similar to those in other shoulder procedures, particularly ASD. Some complications are specifically isolated to the AC joint. Excessive bone resection generally produces symptoms and can result in destabilization of the AC joint with potential disruption of the coracoclavicular ligaments. Inadequate bone resection can result in residual AC joint symptoms (Fig. 6). Residual spurs and osteophytes, particularly in the posterosuperior and anterosuperior areas of the joint, are known to lead to poor results and continued symptoms. Excessive resection of soft tissue can result in destabilization of the AC joint and further symptoms secondary to pathologic laxity. The lack of a thorough débridement of bone fragments at the end of this procedure can result in some ectopic calcification and reactive bursitis in the subacromial space. Fractures have been reported when errant resection has been performed and a stress riser is created. Perhaps the most prevalent complication in this procedure is one of erroneous diagnosis. The shoulder is a complex joint and requires a thorough history, physical examination, and diagnostic workup prior to arthroscopic intervention to ensure that the surgeon has isolated the distinct cause of pain and disability.

Summary

Arthroscopic AC joint resection has gained popularity over the last 15 years, and its technique has been refined. Attention to detail and to the specifics of the indications and surgical technique help the surgeon avoid postoperative problems. At this time, the arthroscopic technique is a standard of care in treating AC joint disease, except in patients with instability. If the procedure is not performed correctly, the complications can certainly equal or surpass those associated with the open procedure.

Annotated Bibliography

Introduction

Shaffer BS: Painful conditions of the acromioclavicular joint. *J Am Acad Orthop Surg* 1999;7:176-188.

This is an excellent review of AC joint problems and treatment.

Diagnosis

O'Brien SJ, Pagnani MJ, Fealy S, McGlynn SR, Wilson JB: The active compression test: A new and effective test for diagnosing labral tears and acromioclavicular joint abnormality. *Am J Sports Med* 1998;26:610-613.

This is an original article describing the O'Brien active compression test. The test is performed by having the patient place his or her arm in a position of forward flexion (to 90°), adduction (10°), and internal rotation (thumb down). The examiner places his or her hand on the patient's forearm and pushes down, asking the patient to resist the force. Results are positive when there is shoulder pain that is alleviated with external rotation of the shoulder (palm up) in the same forward flexed, adducted position. Superficial or anterior pain incriminates the AC joint, but deep or posterior shoulder pain points to a possible labral tear.

Indications

Jerosch J, Schroder M, Schneider T: Arthroscopic resection of the acromioclavicular joint: Indications. Surgical technique: Outcome. *Unfallchirurg* 1998;101:691-696.

Patients who have an unstable joint should not undergo arthroscopic resection of the AC joint alone. The procedure should be combined with a stabilizing procedure.

Arthroscopic Techniques

Auge WK II, Fischer RA: Arthroscopic distal clavicle resection for isolated atraumatic osteolysis in weight lifters. *Am J Sports Med* 1998;26:189-192.

Rapid rehabilitation after limited resection for osteolysis was noted in 10 patients. Limited arthroscopic resection of the distal clavicle may suffice for osteolysis in this patient population rather than the 1 to 2 cm previously reported.

Levine WN, Barron OA, Yamaguchi K, Pollock RG, Flatow EL, Bigliani LU: Arthroscopic distal clavicle resection from a bursal approach. *Arthroscopy* 1998;14:52-56.

This is a retrospective review of 24 patients who had a distal clavicle resection through a bursal approach. Postoperative follow-up averaged 32.5 months (range, 24 to 70 months). Results were excellent in 17 patients (71%) and good in 4 (16.5%). Failure occurred in 3 patients (12.5%). The amount of bone resection did not correlate with outcome. The authors noted improved results with use of an anterosuperior portal for complete visualization.

Matthews LS, Parks BG, Pavlovich LJ Jr, Giudice MA: Arthroscopic versus open distal clavicle resection: A biomechanical analysis on a cadaveric model. *Arthroscopy* 1999;15:247-240.

The authors observed significant differences in displacement and stiffness in the intact AC joint versus the surgically resected joint.

Instability and Coplaning

Blazar PE, Iannotti JP, Williams GR: Anteroposterior instability of the distal clavicle after distal clavicle resection. *Clin Orthop* 1998;348:114-120.

Excessive AP instability of the distal clavicle can cause postoperative shoulder pain and poor surgical outcome.

Branch TP, Burdette HL, Shahriari AS, Carter FM II, Hutton WC: The role of the acromioclavicular ligaments and the effect of distal clavicle resection. *Am J Sports Med* 1996;24:293-297.

Only 5 mm of distal clavicle needs to be resected to ensure that no bone-to-bone contact occurs in rotation postoperatively. There was no difference in the end result, whether the inferior AC or the superior AC ligament was cut before removal of 5 mm of the distal clavicle.

Eskola A, Santavirta S, Viljakka HT, Wirta J, Partio TE, Hoikka V: The results of operative resection of the lateral end of the clavicle. *J Bone Joint Surg Am* 1996;78:584-587.

The authors concluded that resection of the AC joint should not exceed 10 mm.

Fischer BW, Gross RM, McCarthy JA, Arroyo JS: Incidence of acromioclavicular joint complications after arthroscopic subacromial decompression. *Arthroscopy* 1999;15:241-248.

Violation of the AC joint in the course of an arthroscopic ASD may jeopardize the outcome.

Kuster MS, Hales PF, Davis SJ: The effects of arthroscopic acromioplasty on the acromioclavicular joint. *J Shoulder Elbow Surg* 1998;7:140-143.

Preservation of the inferior capsule during arthroscopic acromioplasty is important for the integrity of the AC joint in patients who do not have severe osteoarthritic changes.

Classic Bibliography

Bigliani LU, Nicholson GP, Flatow EL: Arthroscopic resection of the distal clavicle. *Orthop Clin North Am* 1993;24:133-141.

Flatow EL, Duralde XA, Nicholson GP, Pollock RG, Bigliani LU: Arthroscopic resection of the distal clavicle with a superior approach. *J Shoulder Elbow Surg* 1995;4:41-50.

Novak PJ, Bach BR Jr, Romeo AA, Hager CA: Surgical resection of the distal clavicle. *J Shoulder Elbow Surg* 1995;4:35-40.

Patten RM: Atraumatic osteolysis of the distal clavicle: MR findings. *J Comput Assist Tomogr* 1995;19:92-95.

Snyder SJ, Banas MP, Karzel RP: The arthroscopic Mumford procedure: An analysis of results. *Arthroscopy* 1995;11:157-164.

Tolin BS, Snyder SJ: Our technique for the arthroscopic Mumford procedure. *Orthop Clin North Am* 1993;24:143-151.

Chapter 51

Arthroscopy for the Arthritic Shoulder

Theodore A. Blaine, MD

Louis U. Bigliani, MD

Introduction

Since its introduction in 1931, there has been a tremendous increase in the indications and uses of shoulder arthroscopy for diagnosis and treatment of shoulder disorders. However, the value of shoulder arthroscopy for the treatment of glenohumeral arthritis has not been clearly defined. An early study of arthroscopic débridement for glenohumeral osteoarthritis in 54 patients was successful in two thirds of patients, with only mild degeneration at 3-year follow-up. Good results were achieved in one third of patients with severe degenerative disease. Another early study described the use of the arthroscope in eight men with glenohumeral arthritis. Although all patients were believed to have benefited by the procedure, four were scheduled for additional reconstructive procedures based on the arthroscopic findings. Because of the mixed results of these early reports and partly because of the success of shoulder arthroplasty for the treatment of arthritis, there have since been few reports on the use of arthroscopy to treat glenohumeral arthritis.

The potential role of arthroscopy in shoulder arthritis has reemerged as a result of several recent developments. The widespread use of diagnostic shoulder arthroscopy has helped identify early glenohumeral arthritis in patients in whom arthroscopy was used for other indications. Improvements in medical management of rheumatoid arthritis have allowed earlier diagnosis of inflammatory arthritis of the glenohumeral joint and have made synovectomy and débridement a potential adjunct to medical management. Finally, better appreciation of the complications of shoulder arthroplasty and a recent emphasis on cartilage regeneration have made joint-preserving procedures in the shoulder a theoretical goal.

Pathophysiology

There is a potential therapeutic benefit of arthroscopic débridement for arthritis, which is better appreciated when the pathophysiology of degenerative and inflammatory joint disease is understood. Glenohumeral arthritis can be

TABLE 1 | Types and Causes of Glenohumeral Arthritis

Inflammatory	Noninflammatory
Rheumatoid arthritis	Primary osteoarthritis
Systemic lupus erythematosus	Posttraumatic osteoarthritis
Gout	Postinfectious osteoarthritis
Calcium pyrophosphate dihydrate	Postinstability osteoarthritis
Psoriatic arthritis	Postcapsulorrhaphy osteoarthritis
Ankylosing spondylitis	Charcot arthropathy

inflammatory or noninflammatory (Table 1). Although the radiographic and clinical features of inflammatory arthritis and osteoarthritis are distinctly different, both disease processes share a similar pattern of biochemical events that results in the degradation of glenohumeral articular cartilage. Alteration of these biochemical events through arthroscopic treatment may be valuable for treatment of both inflammatory and noninflammatory disease.

Inflammatory Arthritis

The most common type of inflammatory arthritis of the shoulder is rheumatoid arthritis. Other inflammatory arthritides are systemic lupus erythematosus, gout, calcium pyrophosphate dihydrate deposition, psoriatic arthritis, and ankylosing spondylitis (Table 1). Chronic inflammation is the hallmark of all of the inflammatory arthritides. The presentation of cartilage autoantigen (types II, IX, and XI collagen, aggrecan, and link protein) in conjunction with a major histocompatibility class II receptor (HLA DR-4 and HLA DR-1) by the antigen presenting cell is believed to initiate the inflammatory cascade. This is followed by a complex interplay of multiple inflammatory cells, including activated monocytes, macrophages, B and T lymphocytes, and synovial cells that together lead to

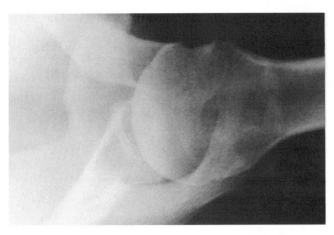

Figure 1 Axillary radiograph of the glenohumeral joint demonstrating mild loss of joint space (stage II osteoarthritis).

synovial hypertrophy and the destruction of articular cartilage. All of these cells, as well as local chondrocytes and osteoblasts, are capable of secreting proinflammatory cytokines, lymphokines, proteases, and growth factors that can initiate joint destruction. Although each cytokine plays a specific role in the process, perhaps the most important cytokines are tumor necrosis factor-alpha (TNF-α) and interleukin-1 (IL-1). Experiments using laboratory and animal models recently have demonstrated that the inhibition of these cytokines also abolishes the process of erosive arthritis that occurs with their presence. Many of the recent medical therapies for rheumatoid arthritis (eg, etanercept) are aimed at this mechanism.

The potential role of arthroscopic débridement in the treatment of inflammatory arthritis is supported by three potential mechanisms. First, the irrigation and débridement of damaged articular cartilage may decrease the amount of cartilage autoantigen available to antigen presenting cells that initiate the inflammatory cascade. Second, irrigation and washout of the cytokine-rich synovial fluid may flush out the catabolic mediators that lead to joint destruction. Finally, synovial débridement may reduce the number and capacity of inflammatory cells important in the inflammatory process. Although it is apparent that all of these potential benefits may provide only temporary relief from the inevitable series of events that occur in inflammatory arthritis, it is possible that the combination of surgical débridement with the latest medical therapies may potentiate the effects that each of these therapies would offer alone. By inhibiting the erosive process, pain may be controlled, the need for more aggressive procedures delayed, and bone stock preserved for arthroplasty.

Noninflammatory Arthritis

The pathophysiology of osteoarthritis is distinctly different

from that of the inflammatory arthritides and is perhaps less well understood. There is a cascade of cellular and biochemical events that occurs, leading to the breakdown of articular cartilage, which is followed by insufficient cartilage repair. Noninflammatory osteoarthritis of the shoulder includes both primary and secondary causes. Primary degenerative osteoarthritis of the shoulder is uncommon, occurring in less than 1% of the general population. Secondary degenerative arthritis can occur as a result of prior fracture, dislocation, instability, or infection.

The biochemical events associated with osteoarthritis include a loss of collagen matrix, resulting in an increase in water content, alterations in proteoglycan composition, and an increase in proteolytic enzymes (cathepsins B and D, metalloproteinases) and cytokines (ILs and TNF). The increase in cartilage degradation and repair processes results in an increase in cartilage breakdown products as well as an increase in the synthesis of cartilage proteoglycans. As in inflammatory arthritis, the potential benefits of arthroscopic débridement in osteoarthritis include: (1) washout of cytokines and inflammatory mediators that initiate and maintain the process of joint destruction; (2) débridement of inflamed synovium that may contribute to both cartilage degradation and pain; and (3) an improvement in joint mechanics by the removal of cartilage flaps and debris.

A biochemical analysis of the synovial fluid of 96 patients who had surgical procedures (arthroscopy or arthroplasty) for glenohumeral osteoarthritis was recently reported. In this study, cartilage breakdown products (sulfated glycosaminoglycan, keratan sulfate, and link protein) were identified and correlated with the severity (grade) of osteoarthritis. Markers of cartilage repair (3B3 epitope) were also isolated and correlated with severity of disease. These findings suggest a potential role for biochemical markers to identify early osteoarthritis and may explain the beneficial effects of arthroscopic treatment for later stages of glenohumeral osteoarthritis.

Classification

Classification of both inflammatory and noninflammatory arthritis includes staging, which is based on radiographic criteria, and grading, which is based on visual inspection of the joint cartilages through diagnostic arthroscopy. Routine radiographic evaluation of the glenohumeral joint includes AP, scapular lateral, and axillary views. CT scans can provide additional information when bone loss is present but usually are not necessary if a good axillary view is obtained (Fig. 1).

Inflammatory Arthritis

Neer classified rheumatoid involvement of the shoulder into three types: dry, wet, and resorptive. The dry form is

TABLE 2	Glenohumeral Joint Radiographic Staging Criteria

Stage	Radiographs
I	Normal
II	Mild joint space narrowing Concentric wear
III	Moderate joint space narrowing Early osteophyte formation Concentric glenoid wear
IV	Severe joint space narrowing Extensive osteophyte formation Eccentric glenoid wear

TABLE 3	Glenohumeral Joint Arthroscopic Grading Criteria

Grade	Cartilage
I	Softening or blistering
II	Fissuring or fibrillation
III	Deep ulceration
IV	Exposed subchondral bone

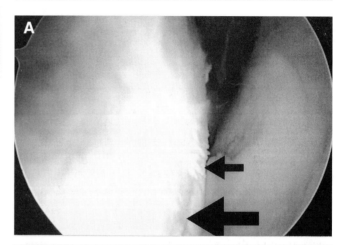

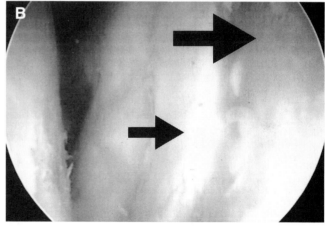

Figure 2 Arthroscopic view of the glenohumeral joint from the posterior portal. **A,** Grade II fibrillation (small arrow) and grade III ulceration (large arrow) of the humeral head. **B,** Grade I softening (small arrow) and grade IV exposed bone (large arrow) of the glenoid surface.

characterized by the absence of cyst formation and a tendency for joint stiffness. Marginal osteophytes often are present, though they are much smaller than in osteoarthritis, and minimal erosions are seen. In wet rheumatoid disease, there are severe erosions, cystic granulations, and erosion of the humeral head into the glenoid. In resorptive type disease, the bony destruction and resorption are even more severe, with compromised bone stock making reconstruction difficult.

Staging of rheumatoid disease has been defined in the elbow and could also be applied to glenohumeral disease. Stage I disease is characterized by synovitis and pain but lacks radiographic findings. In stage II disease, there is symmetric loss of joint space but good preservation of periarticular bone. Stage III disease is marked by bony erosions with mild (type A) or extensive (type B) loss of joint architecture. In stage IV disease, there is complete destruction of the joint and surrounding bone, whereas in stage V disease, there is bony joint ankylosis.

Noninflammatory Arthritis

Osteoarthritis of the glenohumeral joint is unique in its tendency to cause posterior wear of the glenoid articulation, which is best seen on the axillary radiograph. A staging system for glenohumeral arthritis that considers the importance of eccentric wear was recently described (Table 2). Stage I is characterized by the absence of radiographic findings. In stage II, there is mild joint space narrowing and concentric wear. In stage III, there is early osteophyte formation and moderate joint space narrowing, but glenoid wear is concentric. Stage IV is characterized by eccentric glenoid wear and severe joint space loss with osteophyte formation.

Shoulder arthroscopy makes grading of glenohumeral osteoarthritis possible. Grading schemes in osteoarthritis are based on Outerbridge's criteria for patellofemoral chondromalacia. This grading scheme for glenohumeral arthritis was recently modified (Table 3). Grading of both the humeral (Fig. 2, *A*) and glenoid (Fig. 2, *B*) articular cartilage should be recorded, and the most severe grade recorded should be used to determine prognosis and to guide treatment. In grade I degeneration, where there is softening or blistering of the articular cartilage (Fig. 2, *B*, small arrow), diagnosis requires direct palpation with an

TABLE 4	Indications for Arthroscopy in Glenohumeral Arthritis

Confirm diagnosis

Identify and treat additional pathology

Determine prognosis

Relieve pain

Restore motion

Improve joint mechanics

Remove loose bodies

Slow disease progression

Delay larger definitive procedure

arthroscopic probe. In grade II degeneration, there is fissuring or fibrillation (Fig. 2, *A*, small arrow), and in grade III degeneration, deep ulceration of the articular cartilage (Fig. 2, *A*, large arrow). In grade IV degeneration, there is exposed subchondral bone (Fig. 2, *B*, large arrow).

Indications and Uses

Treatment of glenohumeral arthritis is guided by both the radiographic and arthroscopic findings. Arthroscopic treatment is an accepted treatment modality in stages I and II rheumatoid disease and stages I and II osteoarthritis when there is adequate supporting periarticular bone. Management of stage III arthritis traditionally has required prosthetic replacement, but arthroscopic treatment may be considered, depending on patient factors. Stage IV arthritis, in which there is eccentric glenoid wear, has been associated with less favorable results with arthroscopic treatment and constitutes a relative contraindication to shoulder arthroscopy. In each patient, the potential benefits of arthroscopic treatment must be weighed against the potential risks of delaying prosthetic replacement, which may be significantly affected by further bone loss, soft-tissue compromise, and stiffness if the index arthroplasty is delayed. The indications and uses for arthroscopic treatment of shoulder arthritis are still being defined, and some of the accepted indications are listed in Table 4.

Arthroscopy can be a useful adjunct to other diagnostic measures in determining the extent of arthritic involvement. Visual inspection and grading using the arthroscopic system previously described can help guide treatment and determine prognosis. In a study of patients with glenohumeral arthritis confirmed by arthroscopy, preoperative radiographs rarely identified grade II osteoarthritis and correctly identified grade III in-

volvement only 50% of the time. In the future, additional diagnostic tools, such as an arthroscopic probe to evaluate cartilage structural properties and biochemical assays to evaluate cartilage metabolism, may further add to the diagnostic and prognostic utility of shoulder arthroscopy.

Arthroscopy can also identify additional pathology that is not predicted by preoperative radiographs or physical examination. A study of 54 patients who had arthroscopy and the diagnosis of osteoarthritis, showed a 9% incidence of significant biceps tendon tears and a 13% incidence of glenoid labral pathology. Similar results, specifically a 32% incidence of coexisting intra-articular pathology, including labral tears, rotator cuff tears, and lesions involving the biceps anchor were reported in another study.

Treatment of associated subacromial bursitis may also provide significant relief in patients with inflammatory and noninflammatory disease, regardless of the extent of glenohumeral involvement. In one study, a thickened subacromial bursa was a consistent finding in most patients (92%) with glenohumeral arthritis. Débridement of the subacromial inflammation and fibrosis was believed to be an important component of arthroscopic treatment. In another study of 24 patients with rheumatoid arthritis of the glenohumeral joint, open anterior acromioplasty and distal clavicle excision were performed. Nineteen of the 22 patients (86%) available for follow-up at an average of 30 months had minimal to no pain. These results suggest that subacromial bursitis may be a significant component of the pain associated with shoulder arthritis and that arthroscopic subacromial decompression even in the setting of glenohumeral arthritis may provide significant therapeutic benefit.

Pain that is not responsive to conservative treatment is a relative indication for arthroscopic débridement. For osteoarthritis, failed conservative treatment consists of a course of nonsteroidal anti-inflammatory drugs and supervised physical therapy. For rheumatoid and inflammatory arthritis, failed conservative treatment consists of an adequate course of symptom- or disease-modifying antirheumatic drugs and rheumatologic consultation indicating progression of the symptoms or disease. Progression of arthritis by radiologic criteria also may constitute an indication for arthroscopic débridement.

Arthroscopy is indicated for the release of a contracted and stiff capsule associated with arthritis. In the setting of arthritis with contracture, results have not been consistent. Neer initially reported poor results with open release, débridement, osteophyte removal, and soft-tissue balancing for osteoarthritis. Similarly, other authors indicated that best results are achieved with arthroscopic débridement when there is near-normal preoperative range of motion. In contrast, another study reported that the patients who benefited most from shoulder arthroscopy for osteoarthritis were those who had a concomitant frozen shoulder and underwent release. Another group of investigators reported decreased pain and increased range of motion in 10 patients who had open release of the subscapularis and capsule for postcapsulorrhaphy arthritis.

Shoulder arthroscopy can be used to remove loose bodies or large osteophytes that may restrict motion (Fig. 3). Although Neer found little benefit to open débridement of large osteophytes in glenohumeral osteoarthritis, a more limited débridement of smaller osteophytes as seen in stage III arthritis may be warranted. A later study reported a 38% incidence of loose bodies in patients who had arthroscopy for early degenerative joint disease and impingement. Removal of these loose bodies clearly has the potential to provide improved joint mechanics and to alleviate associated pain.

Arthroscopic treatment can be used as a second, less invasive procedure when more extensive procedures are delayed or contraindicated. Contraindications to shoulder arthroplasty include deltoid dysfunction from neurologic or neuromuscular disease, complete rotator cuff dysfunction, active infection, medical conditions that prohibit an extensive surgical procedure, or other conditions that prevent active participation in a postoperative rehabilitation program. Shoulder arthroscopy may provide a diagnostic and therapeutic benefit in these difficult situations when all other conservative treatment options have failed.

Surgical Technique

Although a detailed description of surgical technique is beyond the scope of this review, some important principles are mentioned. Following diagnostic arthroscopy of the glenohumeral joint and grading of cartilage lesions (Fig. 2), loose cartilage flaps, synovitis, and soft-tissue lesions are débrided using a combination of motorized resector and electrocautery. The goal of surgical treatment is to remove the inflammatory stimuli (cartilage breakdown products), products of inflammation (cytokines and proteases), and cells that produce inflammatory mediators (synovial and inflammatory cells). Therefore, it is important to remove all inflamed synovium in both inflammatory and noninflammatory arthritis (Fig. 4). Loose bodies should be located and removed. A recent study of washout for knee arthritis demonstrated symptomatic improvement when 3 L of hypertonic solution was used. Good results have been reported with irrigation using at least 3 L of irrigating solution.

If shoulder stiffness is present, a capsular release should be performed. This may be performed arthroscopically using hand and motorized instruments or a combination

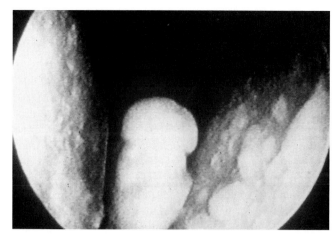

Figure 3 Arthroscopic view of the glenohumeral joint from the posterior portal showing a large loose body between the humeral head and glenoid.

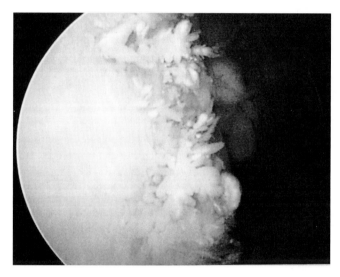

Figure 4 Arthroscopic view of the glenohumeral joint from the posterior portal demonstrating inflamed and hypertrophied synovium.

of arthroscopic dissection and closed manipulation. Circumferential release may be necessary with the dry form of rheumatoid disease in which circumferential contracture is common. Frequently, however, an anterior release alone is sufficient in the setting of osteoarthritis with anterior capsular contracture. The proximity of the axillary nerve to the inferior capsule must be remembered; occasionally, it is necessary to locate and visualize the nerve when aggressive release is required.

Associated pathology in the subacromial space and acromioclavicular joint must be addressed. Like synovial débridement in the glenohumeral joint, the goal of subacromial decompression is thorough débridement of bursal tissue, which can be a source of the cells and inflammatory mediators that mediate inflammation and produce pain. Thorough débridement of fibrous adhesions that have formed in response to inflammation also is important. Release of these adhesions can significantly improve shoulder motion in patients with stiffness.

Distal clavicle excision is necessary in patients with preoperative evidence of acromioclavicular pain. This is particularly common in patients with rheumatoid arthritis. Although it often is helpful to examine preoperative radiographs for the presence of degenerative acromioclavicular arthritis, up to 82% of patients can have radiographic evidence of degenerative disease without any symptoms. Therefore, the orthopaedist should not misinterpret radiographs to indicate a need for acromioclavicular arthroplasty. A diagnostic injection of lidocaine directly into the acromioclavicular joint as part of the preoperative workup is particularly helpful in confirming the diagnosis.

Complications

Complications of arthroscopic débridement are essentially the same as those expected with arthroscopic subacromial decompression. However, in patients with shoulder stiffness who require extensive capsular release and in patients with severe inflammatory arthritis in whom extensive synovectomy and bursectomy are performed, the complication rate may be higher. In one series of 30 patients with arthroscopic capsular release, there was only one complication, an axillary neurapraxia that recovered without further treatment.

Results

Three recent studies support the role of arthroscopic débridement in arthritis of the shoulder. In one retrospective study of 25 patients with an average 34-month follow-up, good or excellent results were reported in 80% of patients with primary or secondary glenohumeral arthritis. Improvement in both pain relief and range of motion was demonstrated, with a postoperative average forward elevation of 167°, external rotation of 53°, and internal rotation to L5. Initial pain relief lasted an average of 7 months, and only 24% of patients noted deterioration of pain relief over the follow-up period. No significant difference in improvement could be demonstrated with radiographic stage or pathologic grade of osteoarthritis.

A consistent finding in most patients (92%) in this study was the presence of a thickened subacromial bursa. Débridement of the subacromial inflammation and fibrosis was an important component of the improvement in motion and pain in these patients. These findings are consistent with a retrospective study of 36 patients with glenohumeral arthritis who had arthroscopic subacromial

decompression. Shoulder outcome scores improved from 32 to 77 points with an average 4.5-year follow-up. Results correlated with the extent of degenerative joint disease noted at the time of arthroscopy. Patients with severe (stage IV) degenerative disease noted on radiographs or grade IV changes noted on arthroscopic examination had less predictable results. The authors concluded that the presence of mild to moderate glenohumeral degenerative disease (grades I to III) did not preclude a satisfactory result from arthroscopic subacromial decompression.

The same conclusions also may apply in the setting of inflammatory arthritis. In a prospective study of 24 patients with rheumatoid arthritis, open subacromial decompression with anterior acromioplasty and distal clavicle excision was successful in 86% of patients at an average follow-up of 30 months. Average motion improved in flexion from 68° to 121° and external rotation from 23° to 52°. Although these results refer only to open decompression and include routine distal clavicle excision as a component of the procedure, similar results could be expected with arthroscopic débridement, provided that an adequate débridement is performed.

In another study of 45 patients at an average of 2 years following arthroscopic débridement for severe grade IV glenohumeral osteoarthritis, with or without capsular release, 88% of patients had satisfactory results with significant and durable (average, 28 months) improvement in pain relief. Whereas it is difficult to determine whether these results are related to the débridement performed or to concomitant capsular release, these results suggest that arthroscopic débridement may be considered even for severe stages of arthritis.

Future Directions

Although three recent studies have demonstrated the utility of arthroscopic débridement for shoulder arthritis, additional studies with long-term follow-up are necessary to prove the durability of this treatment. Basic science experiments have shown that cartilage breakdown products and inflammatory mediators are present in the arthritic shoulder joint. Additional studies should demonstrate that débridement can reduce and maintain decreased levels of these initiators and products of inflammation. In addition, the effect of anti-inflammatory and pharmacologic agents on this process should be examined. Finally, the effect of changes in the structural and material properties of the cartilage-bearing surface requires further study. The potential role of cartilage replacement, transplantation, and/or recontouring and reshaping the bearing surfaces has yet to be determined.

Annotated Bibliography

Classification

Nakagawa Y, Hyakuna K, Otani S, Hashitani M, Naka-mura T: Epidemiologic study of glenohumeral osteo-arthritis with plain radiography. *J Shoulder Elbow Surg* 1999;8:580-584.

This retrospective review of 4,035 patients who had shoulder radiographs for various indications found a 0.4% incidence of glenohumeral arthritis. In those patients with shoulder complaints, the incidence was 4.6%.

Weinstein DM, Bucchieri JS, Pollock RG, Flatow EL, Bigliani LU: Arthroscopic debridement of the shoulder for osteoarthritis. *Arthroscopy* 2000;16:471-476.

The authors report on a staging system for glenohumeral osteoarthritis and a retrospective study of 25 patients with osteoarthritis who were treated with arthroscopic débridement. The pathology and surgical technique are described. At an average 34-month follow-up, 80% of patients had good or excellent results, with improvement in both pain relief and range of motion. No significant difference could be demonstrated with radiographic stage or pathologic grade of osteoarthritis.

Indications and Uses

Naranja RJ Jr, Iannotti JP: Surgical options in the treatment of arthritis of the shoulder: Alternatives to prosthetic arthroplasty. *Semin Arthroplasty* 1995;6:204-213.

This review article outlines alternative nonprosthetic treatment options for glenohumeral arthritis. Arthroscopic débridement, synovectomy, capsular release, osteotomy, resection arthroplasty, and arthrodesis are addressed. The authors relate their own experience with arthroscopic débridement for arthritis and indicate that best results are seen in patients with concentric articulations and near-normal range of motion preoperatively.

Ratcliffe A, Flatow EL, Roth N, Saed-Nejad F, Bigliani LU: Biochemical markers in synovial fluid identify early osteoarthritis of the glenohumeral joint. *Clin Orthop* 1996;330:45-53.

The authors provide biochemical analysis of the synovial fluid of 96 patients who had surgical procedures (arthroscopy or arthroplasty) for glenohumeral osteoarthritis. The presence of cartilage breakdown products (sulfated glycosaminoglycan, keratan sulfate, and link protein) and markers of cartilage repair (3B3 epitope) correlated with severity (grade) of osteoarthritis. These findings suggest a potential role for biochemical markers to identify early osteoarthritis and may explain the beneficial effects of arthroscopic treatment for later stages of osteoarthritis.

Simpson NS, Kelly IG: Extra-glenohumeral joint shoulder surgery in rheumatoid arthritis: The role of bursectomy, acromioplasty, and distal clavicle excision. *J Shoulder Elbow Surg* 1994;3:66-69.

In this prospective study of 24 patients with rheumatoid arthritis, open subacromial decompression with anterior acromioplasty and distal clavicle excision was performed following a favorable response to subacromial injection. Nineteen of the 22 patients (86%) available for follow-up at an average of 30 months had minimal to no pain. Average motion improved in flexion from 68° to 121° and external rotation from 23° to 52°.

Complications

Harryman DT II, Matsen FA III, Sidles JA: Arthroscopic management of refractory shoulder stiffness. *Arthroscopy* 1997;13:133-147.

In this prospective study of a cohort of 30 patients (14 with diabetes) who had arthroscopic release for shoulder stiffness, 88% of patients recovered excellent function within 6 months of surgery and maintained function at an average of 33 months postoperatively. Final motion averaged 93% of the unaffected side. A single axillary neurapraxia recovered without further treatment.

Results

Bae HW, Guyette TM, Warren RF, Craig EV, Wickiewicz TL: Abstract: Results of subacromial decompression in patients with subacromial impingement and glenohumeral degenerative joint disease. *67th Annual Meeting Proceedings*. Rosemont, IL, American Academy of Orthopaedic Surgeons, 2000, p 114.

The authors report on a retrospective study of 36 patients who had glenohumeral arthritis noted at the time of arthroscopic subacromial decompression. At an average 4.5-year follow-up, results correlated with the extent of degenerative joint disease noted at the time of arthroscopy. Patients with severe (stage IV) degenerative joint disease noted on radiographs or arthroscopic examination had less predictable results.

Cameron BD, Galatz LM, Ramsey ML, Williams GR, Iannotti JP: Abstract: Non-prosthetic management of grade 4 glenohumeral osteoarthritis. *67th Annual Meeting Proceedings*. Rosemont, IL, American Academy of Orthopaedic Surgeons, 2000, p 64.

Forty-five patients were evaluated 2 years after arthroscopic débridement for glenohumeral osteoarthritis, with or without capsular release. Eighty-eight percent of patients had satisfactory results with significant and durable (average, 28 months) improvement in pain relief.

Edelson R, Burks RT, Bloebaum RD: Short-term effects of knee washout for osteoarthritis. *Am J Sports Med* 1995;23:345-349.

The authors report on a prospective study of 29 knees with symptomatic osteoarthritis that had washout with 3 L of lactated Ringer's solution. Improvement based on the HSS and Knee Society Score was seen in 86% of the knees at 1 year, with 61% improved at 2 years follow-up. No correlation between severity (grade) of osteoarthritis was demonstrated. No improvement was demonstrated in a randomized group receiving hyaluronate injection following washout.

Classic Bibliography

Burman MS: Arthroscopy or the direct visualization of joints: An experimental cadaver study. *J Bone Joint Surg* 1931;13:669-695.

Cofield RH: Arthroscopy of the shoulder. *Mayo Clin Proc* 1983;58:501-508.

Ellman H: Shoulder arthroscopy: Current indications and techniques. *Orthopedics* 1988;11:45-51.

Ellman H, Harris E, Kay SP: Early degenerative joint disease simulating impingement syndrome: Arthroscopic findings. *Arthroscopy* 1992;8:482-487.

Johnson LL: The shoulder joint: An arthroscopist's perspective of anatomy and pathology. Clin Orthop 1987; 223:113-125.

Matthews LS, LaBudde JK: Arthroscopic treatment of synovial diseases of the shoulder. *Orthop Clin North Am* 1993;24:101-109.

Neer CS II: The rheumatoid shoulder, in Cruess RL, Mitchell NS (eds): *Surgery of Rheumatoid Arthritis.* Philadelphia, PA, JB Lippincott, 1971, pp 117-125.

Ogilvie-Harris DJ, Wiley AM: Arthroscopic surgery of the shoulder: A general appraisal. *J Bone Joint Surg Br* 1986;68:201-207.

Pahle JA, Kvarnes L: Shoulder synovectomy. *Ann Chir Gynaecol* 1985;198(suppl):37-39.

Post M, Pollock RG: Operative treatment of degenerative and arthritic diseases of the glenohumeral joint, in Post M, Bigliani LU, Flatow EL, Pollock RG (eds): *The Shoulder: Operative Technique.* Baltimore, MD, Williams & Wilkins, 1998, pp 73-131.

Chapter 52

Arthroscopic Treatment of Calcific Tendinitis

Stephen C. Weber, MD

Calcific tendinitis is a common problem encountered in the shoulder. A number of issues regarding calcific tendinitis remain unclear. The exact instigating event, the predilection for patients ranging primarily from 30 to 50 years of age, and the propensity for the usual location in the supraspinatus tendon just off the greater tuberosity are all unexplained. The exact relationship to impingement remains unclear. Neer felt strongly that impingement and calcific tendinitis were unrelated disease processes, whereas Ellman's pioneering work with arthroscopic treatment initially always included an acromioplasty. Although a number of questions remain, increased understanding of the basic science of this problem is improving the orthopaedist's understanding.

Pathogenesis

Codman initially proposed a degenerative etiology, with necrosis of tendon fibers followed by dystrophic calcification. Aging or impingement would be the cause of this degeneration. This theory has come increasingly into question. Others recently have shown by electron microscopy that the intracellular calcification anticipated according to this theory does not occur. The age distribution of calcific tendinitis also is not consistent with that of rotator cuff degeneration. Calcific tendinitis peaks in the fourth and fifth decades, whereas rotator cuff disease begins in the fourth decade but becomes increasingly common with aging.

Detailed light and electron microscopic studies have suggested a reactive mechanism instead. These researchers divided the evolution of the disease into three stages: (1) precalcific, (2) calcific, and (3) postcalcific. The precalcific stage is characterized by the metaplasia of tenocytes into chondrocytes. The subsequent fibrocartilage matrix stains for proteoglycan. Although it is not proven, the predilection of chondrocytes for a low oxygen environment fits well, with multiple authors noting decreased vascularity at a so-called "critical zone" of the supraspinatus tendon

insertion into the greater tuberosity. Radiographs at this stage are normal, although the fibrocartilage can be detected by ultrasound and MRI.

The calcific phase is characterized by formation of calcium crystals in matrix vesicles. Calcium at this stage is chalk-like in consistency. The fibrocartilage matrix is gradually eroded by the deposits to form septae. Calcium deposits may remain in this state for years with few if any symptoms. Radiographs at this stage show dense, well-circumscribed deposits, which also are visible on CT scans and on ultrasound. MRI reveals a signal void on T1- and T2-weighted images, which is often missed if the scans are read without plain radiographs.

Vascular channels forming at the periphery of the deposit start the resorptive phase. Macrophages and multinucleated giant cells soon form at the periphery of the deposit and begin to remove the deposit. The calcium at this stage is the classic toothpaste-like calcification that responds to needle aspiration. On radiographs, the calcium is diffuse and can be difficult to visualize. Ultrasound continues to show the deposit. MRI is characterized by decreased signal on T1- and T2-weighted images, with increased signal on the periphery secondary to edema and increased vascularity of the surrounding tissue. Clinically, the resorptive period is the most painful, especially if the deposit ruptures into the subacromial bursa. This rupture can create the appearance of a calcific "bursogram" on plain radiographs. Given time, the phagocytes will resorb the deposit, and the tendon fibers appear to reconstitute. The occurrence of a rotator cuff tear, either spontaneously or with surgical removal of the deposit, is uncommon.

While the pathology is clear, the instigating events are not. The hypoxic environment proposed by Codman for this anatomic site may be important in the development of chondrocytes that tolerated such an environment. However, calcium also forms in the infraspinatus but rarely in the subscapularis. The trigger for resorption, often after years of quiescence, is also unknown.

Diagnosis

Plain radiographs remain the mainstay of diagnosis. Multiple views can be required to localize the calcium so that it does not project over the surrounding osseous structures. Internal and external rotation AP views are usually adequate for diagnosis, but if surgical management is contemplated, axillary and scapular lateral views will assist in localizing the deposit in the sagittal plane. Some studies have reported that ultrasound also can be used to identify these deposits, while others suggest increased accuracy of ultrasound over plain radiographs. However, in the United States, ultrasound is rarely used as a diagnostic modality. CT has been purported to be more accurate at localization when the deposits are diffuse. MRI is not routinely indicated. The unfortunate clinical practice of obtaining MRI scans without adequate radiographs creates problems, in that the signal void is often missed or the resorptive phase edema is interpreted as a tear. Surgical treatment based on these MRI readings is not likely to be successful. A combined American multicenter trial presented in 1993 and a multicenter European study reported by other authors that same year noted concomitant rotator cuff tears in fewer than 4% of patients, although another group noted a significant increase of tears in an older population. Arthrography or MRI in this setting may be of value. Preoperative radiographs before arthrography are equally important to avoid interpreting the calcium deposits as dye leakage.

The radiographic appearance of calcific tendinitis must be differentiated from that of other entities with different types of treatment. Chondrocalcinosis can show tendon calcification but is associated with joint space narrowing and spurring. Dystrophic calcification can be associated with a variety of inflammatory arthritides. This calcification usually is confluent with the greater tuberosity, an important diagnostic distinction. Extensive calcification also can be associated with hypercalcemia, which usually is associated with poorly controlled renal disease. Heterotopic ossification (HO) is not uncommon in the shoulder and behaves much like HO in other areas. Once again, appropriate history is important in differential diagnosis. Confluence of the ossification with the osseous structures is another diagnostic clue.

Treatment

Understanding the pathoanatomy and natural history of the disease provides important information to the management of calcific tendinitis. In the formative phase, pain is moderate. The calcific phase is easily diagnosed by radiographs and can, in this phase, represent an incidental finding. Aggressive treatment in the resorptive phase is usually unnecessary, because the process will take care of itself.

Nonsurgical Management

Because this process is often self-limiting, nonsurgical management is most appropriate initially. The inclusion criteria established in 1993 by the American and European studies was 6 months of both nonsurgical management prior to surgical treatment. Nonsteroidal medications can often be helpful. Range-of-motion exercises will preserve motion and prevent secondary adhesive capsulitis. Formal physical therapy rarely is indicated. Low-energy ultrasound and iontophoresis with a variety of chemicals have been suggested and continue to be widely used, but there are little data to support their use. Steroid injection continues to be of benefit to many patients. The mechanism of action seems clear in the resorptive phase but also seems to help in the calcific phase, in which inflammation is less evident.

Needle aspiration continues to be a recommended treatment. Usually, aspiration is performed under fluoroscopic control with the shoulder under local anesthesia. However, comparative studies of any type with control or any other treatment modality are unavailable. The aspiration of toothpaste-like calcification would be anticipated to be successful only in the resorptive phase; identification of this phase based on radiographs is not always possible. Needle aspiration also can be extremely painful, especially if multiple punctures fill the bursa with calcific debris that cannot be lavaged clear—a side effect not appreciated by the patient.

Applied Energy Treatments

Recently, a variety of energy applications have been suggested to break up the calcium deposits. These techniques primarily have been applied in Europe. Low-dose radiation has been suggested, but the risk of malignant transformation for this relatively benign disease process seems unwarranted. The use of ultrasound therapy has been widely reported. One prospective study showed that pulsed ultrasound several times a week over 3 weeks provided more resolution than sham ultrasound controls. Fewer than half of the patients showed complete resolution at final follow-up, however. A review by another group did not recommend the use of ultrasound. Extracorporeal shock wave treatment has also been suggested. This technique initially was used for dissolving kidney stones. The optimal dose of energy for treatment has been reviewed in a meta-analysis. In one study, this technique was used in 40 patients. Fifteen of the 40 showed no change in the size of the deposit, with 50% of patients showing incomplete resolution with one algorithm and 44% with another. Constant scores generally have improved in most series despite incomplete removal of calcium. Lower dose shock wave treatment often can be tolerated with local anesthesia; it is important to recognize that higher applications of energy require interscalene anesthesia to be tolerated by the patient. Multiple contraindications have been identified, including pregnancy, bleeding disorders, anticoagulation, and open growth plates. The most common complication was superficial hematoma, which occurred in most patients, but hypertensive crisis and hyperventilation also occurred. Comparative studies of any type contrasting energy application with surgical treatment or aspiration are not available. Extracorporeal shock wave treatment has been labeled "investigational," with more studies necessary to support its use.

Surgical Treatment

It should be emphasized that the treatment of calcific tendinitis remains primarily nonsurgical, with an anticipated success rate of approximately 80%. Open excision of calcium deposits has been commonly performed since the days of Codman. Neer continued to support this procedure 60 years later. Although he initially thought that the results might be improved by performing an acromioplasty with the excision, he later abandoned this approach. His advice to "anticipate a lengthy recovery" with open excision is of interest. Ellman first reported the arthroscopic excision of calcium anecdotally in his pioneering work on arthroscopic acromioplasty in 1987. His technique of blind needling the deposits in an attempt to identify them, followed by incision of the tendon and removal, continues to be in widespread use today. Ellman's initial technique always included a concomitant acromioplasty. Numerous other authors have substantiated his results. Surgical treatment remains the most predictable means to remove painful calcium deposits. Controversy still exists over several issues regarding treatment: (1) arthroscopic versus open excision; (2) the requirement for acromioplasty; and (3) the need to completely or at least partially remove the deposit.

Arthroscopic Versus Open Excision

In the only prospective randomized study to date, results of 16 patients treated arthroscopically were compared with 18 treated using open excision. In this limited study presented only in abstract form, both groups did well. Cosmesis was better in the arthroscopic group. The average 9-day hospital stay for both treatments makes interpreting their results difficult. Some authors continue to recommend open excision, despite findings from other studies that conclude the recovery time was shorter and functional results better with arthroscopic surgery. Although the studies do not allow rigid conclusions, the data are clear that arthroscopic removal offers no disadvantage over open treatment and will be preferred by most patients because of decreased pain and superior cosmesis.

Acromioplasty Versus Simple Excision

As noted previously, the basic science of calcific tendinitis does not readily support impingement as a cause of calcification. For this reason, most authors have recommended removing the deposit without an acromioplasty. Others, however, recommend acromioplasty if there is associated evidence of impingement. In another study, acromioplasty was thought to be of no benefit, but performed regardless in all patients with subacromial stenosis, or three fourths of the patient group. These authors recommended coracoacromial ligament resection in all patients. Concomitant acromioplasty has also been recommended if there was bony stenosis or diffusely spread deposits. The Multicentric European Study concluded that acromioplasty was of no benefit based on final scores; however, 10% of the patients without initial acromioplasty required repeat surgery. Again, firm conclusions are not possible because of the absence of well-designed studies. None of the studies have shown that acromioplasty is a detriment, and its use for patients with impingement appears to cause little harm and may, in fact, prevent reoperation.

Removal of the Deposit

The basic science would suggest that because the calcium deposit is the problem, complete removal would be ideal. Controversy over this issue persists, primarily because of the difficulty of localizing the deposits arthroscopically. The deposit is rarely visible as a whitish blister on the bursal side of the cuff; usually it is deep within the tendon. Blind needling often will locate the deposit, but every published study that neglects some form of intraoperative localization includes patients in whom the deposit could not be identified at the time of surgery.

Some authors believed that because the size of the deposit decreased in 79% of patients with acromioplasty alone, removal was not necessary. Incomplete removal was believed to be adequate in another study; although three patients required a second operation because of initial failure to remove the deposit. Most authors have noted improved outcomes with complete removal of the deposit. To make complete removal predictable, additional localization techniques will be required in some cases. Preoperative and/or intraoperative ultrasound can be used, but intraoperative fluoroscopic-assisted removal is probably the most convenient for most surgeons.

Author's Preferred Technique

The lateral decubitus position allows for convenient subsequent positioning of an image intensifier. Crowding of the equipment can be annoying, and the room setup shown in Figure 1 is useful. The image intensifier should be positioned and the calcium visualized prior to preparing the patient, both to confirm the best arm position for subsequent removal and to confirm that the deposit has

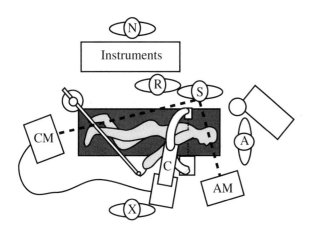

Figure 1 Standard positioning of the patient and operating room equipment for fluoroscopic-assisted arthroscopic removal of calcium. CM = C-arm monitor; N = nurse; R = assistant; S = surgeon; A = anesthesia; AM = anesthesia monitor; C = c-arm; x = x-ray technician.

not already resolved. Careful glenohumeral arthroscopy is mandatory to exclude other pathology, particularly inspection of the undersurface of the rotator cuff. Provided other findings do not alter the preoperative plan, bursoscopy is carried out next. Clearing the bursal adhesions early allows for easier localization. Once this step is complete, the fluoroscope is brought in "rainbow" fashion and the arm rotated until the deposit is best visualized, projected away from the underlying bone. Electrocautery is then used through a lateral bursal portal, and under direct visualization the deposit is incised and removed. Once complete removal is confirmed fluoroscopically, hemostasis is obtained with electrocautery.

Large defects in the rotator cuff heal slowly; complete or significantly thick partial bursal-side tears can be closed side to side arthroscopically, consistent with the recommendations for open excision. Without clear studies to guide the surgeon, acromioplasty remains the preference. Bleeding from the acromioplasty complicates removal of the deposit; therefore, the deposit should be removed first. An acromioplasty should be performed in all patients with visual or bony evidence of impingement and avoided in any patient with concomitant multidirectional instability.

Summary

Calcific tendinitis affects a significant number of patients with shoulder complaints. Recent advances in the understanding of the basic science of this disease process have helped to direct clinical management more effectively. Nonsurgical management remains the mainstay for this condition. Although newer techniques show promise, at this time surgical excision has the most predictable results for patients in whom nonsurgical management fails.

Annotated Bibliography

Pathogenesis

Uhthoff HK, Sarkar K: Calcifying tendinitis, in Rockwood CA Jr, Matsen FA III, Wirth MA, Harryman DT II (eds): *The Shoulder*, ed 2. Philadelphia, PA, WB Saunders, 1998, vol 2, pp 989-1006.

This is an excellent review of the basic science of calcific tendinitis.

Treatment

Arroyo JS, Brennan RF, Pollock RG, Flatow EL, Bigliani LU: Abstract: Calcific tendinitis of the rotator cuff: Long term follow-up of arthroscopic excision. *Arthroscopy* 1997;13:395-396.

With follow-up of 1 to 9 years, 84% of patients had good or excellent results. There were no recurrences of calcium deposits. However, 12 patients had less than 50% of the deposit removed, including three who had reoperations for retained calcium. Intraoperative fluoroscopic localization might improve these results.

Ebenbichler GR, Erdogmus CB, Resch KL, et al: Ultrasound therapy for calcific tendinitis of the shoulder. *N Engl J Med* 1999;340:1533-1538.

This is a well-designed prospective randomized study of sham versus pulsed ultrasound. In 54 patients (61 shoulders), 32 shoulders received ultrasound five or three times a week for 3 weeks. Even with multiple treatments, ultrasound completely removed calcium in only 42% of patients and decreased it in only 23% at final follow-up. At 9 months, follow-up of the control group showed that calcium deposits disappeared completely in 8% and partially in 12%, providing some support to the argument that spontaneous resolution is the rule.

Jerosch J, Strauss JM, Schmiel S: Arthroscopic treatment of calcific tendinitis of the shoulder. *J Shoulder Elbow Surg* 1998;7:30-37.

In 48 patients who were treated with removal of calcium deposits and resection of the coracoacromial ligament, 33 patients had subacromial stenosis and concomitant acromioplasty. The authors concluded that acromioplasty was of no benefit, but the study was neither prospective or randomized. A more valid conclusion might be that patients with bony impingement do as well with acromioplasty and calcium deposit removal as patients without impingement treated with ligament resection alone.

Kempf JF, Bonnomet F, Nerrison D, et al: Arthroscopic isolated excision of rotator cuff calcium deposits, in Gazielly DF, Gleyze P, Thomas T (eds): *The Cuff.* Amsterdam, The Netherlands, Elsevier Science, 1997, pp 164-167.

The authors reviewed three different surgical techniques and found no improvement by adding acromioplasty. However, an earlier study by these authors noted a 10% reoperation rate for patients in whom acromioplasty was not performed. The study confirmed that complete excision of calcium deposits offered the best results.

Loew M, Daecke W, Kusnierczak D, Rahmanzadeh M, Ewerbeck V: Shock-wave therapy is effective for chronic calcifying tendinitis of the shoulder. *J Bone Joint Surg Br* 1999;81:863-867.

In this prospective evaluation of 195 patients, 80 were randomized to either sham or three different protocols in the first part of the study. In the second part, 115 patients were randomized to a low- or high-energy treatment protocol. Results were dose dependent.

Pfister J, Gerber H: Chronic calcifying tendinitis of the shoulder: Therapy by percutaneous needle aspiration and lavage: A prospective open study of 62 shoulders. *Clin Rheumatol* 1997;16:269-274.

This recent study supports the needle aspiration treatment first proposed by McLaughlin in 1963.

Resch H, Povacz P, Seykora P: Excision of calcium deposit and acromioplasty, in Gazielly DF, Gleyze P, Thomas T (eds): *The Cuff.* Amsterdam, The Netherlands, Elsevier Science, 1997, pp 169-171.

The authors developed slightly different criteria for acromioplasty. Patients with type III acromia and diffusely spread calcium deposits benefited from acromioplasty.

Rupp S, Seil R, Kohn D: Preoperative ultrasonographic mapping of calcium deposits facilitates localization during arthroscopic surgery for calcifying tendinitis of the rotator cuff. *Arthroscopy* 1998;14:540-542.

The authors used preoperative mapping to assist in localizing the deposit. This technique minimizes theoretical radiation exposure. Many surgeons would find intraoperative localization with fluoroscopy easier.

Sistermann R, Katthagen BD: Complications, side-effects and contraindications in the use of medium and high-energy extracorporeal shock waves in orthopedics. *Z Orthop Ihre Grenzgeb* 1998;136:175-181.

In a series of 191 patients, the most common complication was superficial hematoma. Hypertension and hyperventilation also occurred. The procedure is contraindicated in patients with open growth plates, pregnancy, bleeding disorders, or in patients taking anticoagulants.

Tillander BM, Norlin RO: Change of calcifications after arthroscopic subacromial decompression. *J Shoulder Elbow Surg* 1998;7:213-217.

Providing a dissenting voice regarding the necessity of removing the calcium deposit, these authors believed that acromioplasty alone was adequate. They noted that the size of the calcium deposit was decreased at follow-up in 79% of the patients treated with acromioplasty alone, with functional results similar to those of a group of patients who received acromioplasty for impingement without calcification over the same study period. Their conclusion would have been better supported if the study included a control group in whom calcific tendinitis was treated with acromioplasty and removal.

Wittenberg RH, Rubenthaler F, Wölk T: Abstract: Chronic calcifying tendinitis of the shoulder: Prospective randomized surgical treatments. *Arthroscopy* 1998; 14:454.

The authors prospectively randomized 34 patients with calcific rotator cuff tendinitis into a open acromioplasty group (18 patients) and an arthroscopic acromioplasty group (16 patients). Outcomes were similar for both groups, with better cosmesis in the arthroscopy group.

Classic Bibliography

Ark JW, Flock TJ, Flatow EL, Bigliani LU: Arthroscopic treatment of calcific tendinitis of the shoulder. *Arthroscopy* 1992;8:183-188.

Codman EA: *The Shoulder.* Boston, MA, Thomas Todd, 1934.

Ellman H: Arthroscopic subacromial decompression: Analysis of one- to three-year results. *Arthroscopy* 1987; 3:173-181.

Ellman H, Bigliani LU, Flatow E, et al: Abstract: Arthroscopic treatment of calcifying tendinitis: The American experience, in Debeyre J, Duparc J, Patte D, et al (eds): *Fifth International Conference on Surgery of the Shoulder.* St Louis, MO, Mosby, 1993, pp 1-15.

Hsu HC, Wu JJ, Jim YF, Chang CY, Lo WH, Yang DJ: Calcific tendinitis and rotator cuff tearing: A clinical and radiographic study. *J Shoulder Elbow Surg* 1994;3: 159-164.

McLaughlin HL: Lesions of the musculotendinous cuff of the shoulder: III. Observations on the pathology, course and treatment of calcific deposits. *Ann Surg* 1946;124:354-362.

McLaughlin HL: Selection of calcium deposits for operation: The technique and results of operation. *Surg Clin North Am* 1963;43: 1501-1504.

Moke-Nancy D, Walch G, Kempf JF, et al: Abstract: Arthroscopic treatment of calcifying tendinitis: Results of the Multicentric European study, in Debeyre J, Duparc J, Patte D, et al (eds): *Fifth International Conference on Surgery of the Shoulder*. St Louis, MO, Mosby, 1993.

Neer CS II (ed): *Shoulder Reconstruction*. Philadelphia, PA, WB Saunders, 1990, pp 421-485.

Psaki CG, Carroll J: Acetic acid ionization: A study to determine the absorptive effects upon calcified tendinitis of the shoulder. *Phys Ther Rev* 1955;35:84-87.

Re LP Jr, Karzel RP: Management of rotator cuff calcifications. *Orthop Clin North Am* 1993;24:125-132.

Rompe JD, Rumler F, Hopf C, Nafe B, Heine J: Extracorporal shock wave therapy for calcifying tendinitis of the shoulder. *Clin Orthop* 1995;321:196-201.

Weber SC: Abstract: Technique and results of arthroscopic treatment of calcific tendonitis of the rotator cuff using fluoroscopic localization. *Arthroscopy* 1991;7:322.

Chapter 53

Shoulder Ganglion Cysts

Mark Pinto, MD

Ronald P. Karzel, MD

Ganglion cysts have long been recognized as a common finding around many joints. Cysts often occur because of underlying pathology; for example, meniscal cysts in the knee are associated with meniscal tears. Usually these cysts are asymptomatic. Before the widespread use of MRI, only cysts in a subcutaneous location could be readily diagnosed. Occasionally, intramuscular or intra-articular cysts were diagnosed incidentally at the time of surgery. MRI has increasingly revealed that ganglion cysts are a common finding about the shoulder. In some circumstances, these cysts cause symptoms that prompt surgical treatment.

Pathology/Etiology

The pathogenesis of ganglion cysts has not been clearly identified. Characteristically, they are found juxtaposed to joints or tendon sheaths throughout the body. Microscopic examination has shown that the outer walls of these cysts are composed of several layers of randomly organized collagen fibers. The wall is relatively acellular, with the collagen being randomly interspersed with fibroblasts and mesenchymal cells. The cyst lining lacks differentiation with no recognizable lining of epithelial cells. The cysts are filled with a clear mucinous fluid containing glucosamine, globulin, and hyaluronic acid.

According to one theory, ganglion cysts are caused by joint fluid leaking through a weak area of the capsule via a one-way valve mechanism. Studies using contrast material have shown fluid coursing from the wrist joint into a cyst but not the reverse. Theoretically, this fluid causes local irritation of the surrounding tissues. In response to the irritation, the body forms a pseudocapsule, which evolves into a ganglion cyst. Consistent with the one-way valve theory, multiple studies have demonstrated a high correlation between labral tears and ganglion cysts in the shoulder.

Another theory intimates that some ganglion cysts are the result of primary myxoid degeneration of the connective tissue near the joint. The products of this degeneration coalesce to form the cyst. This theory implies that there has been no disruption of the joint capsule, and it is used to explain why some cysts form with no visible intra-articular connection. This theory also may explain why ganglion cysts have been reported to develop in the axilla, the long head of the biceps, intraosseous locations, and the fascia of the supraspinatus and infraspinatus muscles.

Anatomy

In the shoulder, ganglion cysts often are associated with posterior glenoid labral tears. The suprascapular nerve travels around the lateral border of the scapular spine, an area called the spinoglenoid notch, where it is relatively fixed in location (Fig. 1). Cadaveric studies have shown that the motor branches of the suprascapular nerve to the infraspinatus at the spinoglenoid notch are 1.8 to 2.1 cm from the posterior glenoid rim. The relatively high incidence of posterior labral tears and the location of the associated cysts makes the suprascapular nerve particularly susceptible to compression at the spinoglenoid notch, and much less so at the suprascapular notch.

A recent cadaveric study demonstrated that the inferior transverse scapular ligament keeps the suprascapular nerve tightly constrained at the spinoglenoid notch. However, the same study also showed that even in the absence of the ligament, the nerve is tightly constrained by the right-angle turn it makes around the lateral border of the scapular spine. At this location, the nerve is susceptible to injurious compression given this tight constraint; there is insufficient space to accommodate a lesion of significant mass adjacent to the bone and nerve. Thus, even a small ganglion cyst may quickly obliterate the space through which the suprascapular nerve travels, resulting in significant nerve compression.

The anatomy of the suprascapular nerve explains the clinical findings. Cysts adjacent to the posterior labrum

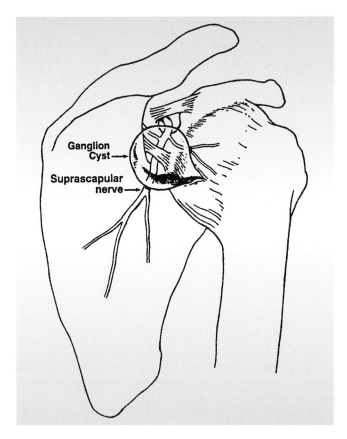

Figure 1 Illustration demonstrating the proximity of the suprascapular nerve to compression by a ganglion cyst originating from the posterior shoulder. *(Reproduced with permission from Fehrman DA, Orwin JF, Jennings RM: Suprascapular nerve entrapment by ganglion cysts: A report of six cases with arthroscopic findings and review of the literature. Arthroscopy 1995;11:727-734.)*

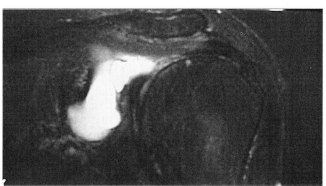

Figure 2 MRI scan demonstrating a large dumbbell-shaped ganglion cyst in the region of the spinoglenoid notch.

at the spinoglenoid notch cause isolated denervation of the infraspinatus muscle because of compression of the nerve after it has given off its branches to the supraspinatus muscle. In contrast, compression of the suprascapular nerve at the suprascapular notch occurs proximally to branches supplying both the supraspinatus and infraspinatus, causing denervation of both muscles. It is theorized that ganglion cysts grow along the path of least resistance, causing the cysts to dissect along the fibrofatty tissue overlying the suprascapular nerve and between the infraspinatus and supraspinatus muscle bellies. This dissection directs the cysts toward the spinoglenoid notch.

Diagnosis

Clinical Evaluation

Clinically, the diagnosis of suprascapular nerve compression by a ganglion cyst may be difficult. The findings are often nonspecific. Patients often report vague, dull, poorly localized shoulder pain that is aggravated by overhead activities. The most likely cause of the pain is compression of the articular branches to the acromio-

clavicular and glenohumeral joints. Patients seldom notice weakness or atrophy. However, weakness to resisted external rotation, or abduction and external rotation may be detected, depending on the magnitude and location of compression. This finding is easily confused with symptoms of a rotator cuff tear. Patients also may have painless infraspinatus atrophy because the sensory portion of the suprascapular nerve may not be affected in the distal spinoglenoid notch. In chronic cases of suprascapular nerve compression, the atrophy may be permanent, despite surgical decompression. Cross-body adduction may cause pain in the posterior shoulder in some patients. Also, direct palpation over the spinoglenoid and suprascapular notches may reproduce sharp pain in patients with suprascapular nerve compression. Finally, labral signs such as catching or locking may be elicited when a labral tear is present.

Diagnostic Imaging

Plain radiographs of the affected shoulder should be obtained, including AP, axillary, and supraspinatus outlet views, to rule out obvious bony lesions, including erosion secondary to local compression by a cyst. MRI is an excellent screening tool for evaluating soft-tissue lesions about the shoulder. Because ganglion cysts are conspicuous with foci of high signal intensity on T2-weighted images, they routinely can be identified in patients with and without suprascapular nerve compression (Fig. 2). MRI accurately shows the size and location of ganglion cysts, which is critical in planning surgical intervention. MRI also may reveal associated intra-articular pathology. However, in the absence of a large amount of native joint fluid, the labrum is not well visualized. For this reason, glenohumeral arthroscopy remains the gold standard for identifying labral tears.

Despite the fact that MRI also can detect atrophy, the diagnosis of suprascapular nerve compression is best confirmed by electromyographic and neuroconductive studies (EMG/NCS). The presence of a ganglion cyst on

MRI does not necessarily mean the nerve is compressed. Similarly, positive EMG/NCS do not confirm that the compression is the result of a ganglion cyst. Electrical studies should be ordered to specifically evaluate the suprascapular nerve in conjunction with clinical findings and the data derived from the MRI.

Treatment

Nonsurgical management of a ganglion cyst is indicated only when no evidence of extrinsic compression is present. The natural history of ganglion cysts is yet to be defined; however, it appears that they often persist or become larger. In rare instances, ganglion cysts have been shown to resolve spontaneously.

Treatment is indicated for a ganglion cyst confirmed to cause symptomatic compression of the suprascapular nerve. Image-guided aspiration has been used with mixed results. Because of occasional failure to aspirate the cyst and a high rate of recurrence even with successful aspiration, it is generally agreed that surgical excision is required. Traditionally, the surgical procedure has been performed via an open approach. A posterior approach for treatment of spinoglenoid notch ganglia and a superior approach for less common suprascapular notch ganglia have been used with good success. The advantage of these approaches is direct visualization of the cyst and nerve. This allows the entire cyst to be removed, decreasing the chance of recurrence. A drawback of the open approach is that labral pathology is not well visualized or addressed. Although MRI is an excellent modality for identifying ganglion cysts, glenohumeral labral tears are not well visualized. Because of the association of labral tears with ganglion cysts, arthroscopic evaluation has been advocated by some. Because arthroscopy has led to the identification of intra-articular pathology not seen with open surgery, arthroscopic approaches have evolved for definitive treatment of shoulder ganglion cysts. Arthroscopic excision is technically challenging but recently has been reported to have good success. Arthroscopic techniques avoid much of the morbidity associated with open approaches and facilitate comprehensive treatment of intra-articular pathology.

Technique and Results of Treatment

Several studies with small numbers of patients have demonstrated the efficacy of both open and arthroscopic treatment of shoulder ganglion cysts. Although there have been anecdotal reports of arthroscopic treatment of suprascapular nerve compression at the suprascapular notch, generally open release of the transverse scapular ligament with removal of the ganglion, if present, is used. Usually, a superior approach between the deltoid and trapezius is used. Care must be taken to avoid damaging the spinal accessory nerve during the exposure.

The treatment of ganglia at the supraglenoid notch has resulted in almost universally good results using either open or arthroscopic techniques, given proper diagnosis. Labral tears must be fully débrided and repaired to the glenoid rim when they are detached. Care must be taken to appreciate normal anatomic variants such as an anterior sublabral hole or cord-like middle glenohumeral ligament, so that unnecessary repair is avoided. The ganglion is located arthroscopically by exploring the superior, posterior, and posteroinferior capsular recesses with preoperative planning using MRI. Once the cyst wall is found, it is débrided using an arthroscopic shaver to remove as much of the synovial lining as possible. The literature has emphasized that complete removal of the cyst/lining and visualization of the nerve are not required. Recurrence rates have been minimal by "marsupializing" the cyst by making a large hole in the wall of the cyst and removing the cyst fluid—as long as labral repair is performed as required. Indications and technique of arthroscopic repair of labral tears are detailed elsewhere in this text. A combined arthroscopic and open approach to the excision of ganglia also has been reported with good results, particularly when used with large cysts.

Annotated Bibliography

Technique and Results of Treatment

Chochole MH, Senker W, Meznik C, Breitenseher MJ: Glenoid-labral cyst entrapping the suprascapular nerve: Dissolution after arthroscopic debridement of an extended SLAP lesion. *Arthroscopy* 1997;13:753-755.

This case report demonstrates complete ganglion cyst decompression with aggressive arthroscopic débridement of a large superior labral anterior-posterior (SLAP) lesion.

Fehrman DA, Orwin JF, Jennings RM: Suprascapular nerve entrapment by ganglion cysts: A report of six cases with arthroscopic findings and review of the literature. *Arthroscopy* 1995;11:727-734.

This retrospective review of six patients shows that intra-articular examination with arthroscopy is necessary when a ganglion cyst is identified. After arthroscopic evaluation and treatment of intra-articular pathology, open excision was performed with good results.

Ferrick MR, Marzo JM: Ganglion cyst of the shoulder associated with a glenoid labral tear and symptomatic glenohumeral instability: A case report. *Am J Sports Med* 1997;25:717-719.

This case report demonstrates the need for arthroscopic examination and treatment of intra-articular lesions prior to open excision of ganglion cysts. In the presence of a periarticular ganglion cyst, a labral lesion or instability should be suspected.

Hawkins RJ, Piatt BE, Fritz RC, Wolf E, Schickendantz M: Abstract: Clinical evaluation and treatment of spinoglenoid notch ganglion cyst. *J Shoulder Elbow Surg* 1999; 8:551.

This retrospective chart review of 73 patients showed that if a ganglion cyst is identified, a labral tear is almost always present as well. Furthermore, the best treatment results were achieved when the ganglion cyst and labral tear were treated surgically.

Iannotti JP, Ramsey ML: Arthroscopic decompression of a ganglion cyst causing suprascapular nerve compression. *Arthroscopy* 1996;12:739-745.

This review of three patients shows that arthroscopic excision of a ganglion cyst is well tolerated and the morbidity associated with open procedures is avoided.

Moore TP, Fritts HM, Quick DC, Buss DD: Suprascapular nerve entrapment caused by supraglenoid cyst compression. *J Shoulder Elbow Surg* 1997;6:455-462.

This retrospective review of 22 patients with suprascapular nerve compression caused by ganglion cysts demonstrates that cysts can be decompressed by either open or arthroscopic techniques with good results. Eleven of the 12 patients who underwent arthroscopy for a ganglion cyst demonstrated a SLAP lesion.

Classic Bibliography

Bigliani LU, Dalsey RM, McCann PD, April EW: An anatomical study of the suprascapular nerve. *Arthroscopy* 1990;6:301-305.

Catalano JB, Fenlin JM Jr: Ganglion cysts about the shoulder girdle in the absence of suprascapular nerve involvement. *J Shoulder Elbow Surg* 1994;3:34-46.

Fritz RC, Helms CA, Steinbach LS, Genant HK: Suprascapular nerve entrapment: Evaluation with MR imaging. *Radiology* 1992;182:437-444.

Ganzhorn RW, Hocker JT, Horowitz M, Switzer HE: Suprascapular-nerve entrapment: A case report. *J Bone Joint Surg Am* 1981;63:492-494.

Mestdagh H, Drizenko A, Ghestem P: Anatomical bases of suprascapular nerve syndrome. *Anat Clin* 1981;3: 67-71.

Murray TF, Karzel RP: Abstract: Arthroscopic treatment of suprascapular nerve palsy caused by a spinoglenoid cyst. *Arthroscopy* 1988;14:455-456.

Psaila JV, Mansel RE: The surface ultrastructure of ganglia. *J Bone Joint Surg Br* 1978;60:228-233.

Soren A: Pathogenesis and treatment of ganglion. *Clin Orthop* 1966;48:173-179.

Tirman PF, Feller JF, Janzen DL, Peterfy CG, Bergman AG: Association of glenoid labral cysts with labral tears and glenohumeral instability: Radiologic findings and clinical significance. *Radiology* 1994;190:653-658.

Warner JP, Krushell RJ, Masquelet A, Gerber C: Anatomy and relationships of the suprascapular nerve: Anatomical constraints to mobilization of the supraspinatus and infraspinatus muscles in the management of massive rotator-cuff tears. *J Bone Joint Surg Am* 1992;74:36-45.

Chapter 54

Superior Labrum Anterior and Posterior Lesions

Stephen S. Burkhart, MD

Superior labral tears were first implicated as a source of pain and dysfunction in overhead athletes in 1985. The term SLAP, referring to superior labrum anterior posterior tears, was first used in 1990. A classification system for SLAP lesions was devised according to morphology of the tear and involvement of the long head of the biceps anchor to the superior labrum. In addition, a surgical technique for repair with suture anchors was described. In contrast to a proposed mechanism of deceleration, a mechanism of acceleration during the late cocking phase of throwing was recently proposed as the mechanism that creates type II SLAP lesions, which in turn lead to the dead arm syndrome in baseball pitchers. The pathologic peel-back sign can be observed arthroscopically and is pathognomonic of posterosuperior SLAP lesions. Studies implicate a tight posterior-inferior capsule as the initiating factor in producing SLAP lesions and outlined effective surgical and rehabilitation techniques to address these lesions.

Classification

The classification system devised by Snyder and associates identifies four types of SLAP lesions (Fig. 1). A type I lesion is a degenerative superior labrum with fraying along the free margin. The surgeon should recognize that a meniscoid labrum, with a leaf of labral tissue that overlies the superior glenoid (much like a meniscus), will have more pronounced degenerative changes than a labrum that does not have a meniscoid configuration. A type II SLAP lesion occurs when the superior labrum detaches from the glenoid bone medially, leaving the superior glenoid neck uncovered for at least 5 mm from the corner of the glenoid. There is a gap between the articular cartilage and the labral attachment into bone. A type III SLAP lesion is a bucket-handle tear of the superior labrum. A type IV SLAP lesion refers to a bucket-handle superior labral tear that extends into the

biceps tendon, causing a split in the root of the biceps. This classification system was later expanded with the addition of two types. Type II SLAP lesions were subcategorized according to the part of the glenoid labrum involved (Fig. 2). A labral detachment anterosuperiorly is called an anterior type II SLAP lesion and a labral detachment posterosuperiorly is called a posterior type II SLAP lesion. Labral detachment anterosuperiorly and posterosuperiorly is called a combined anterior-posterior type II SLAP lesion.

Clinical Spectrum

Although SLAP lesions can cause significant dysfunction in the overhead athlete, they can also occur in nonathletes as a result of trauma. In the nonathlete, common mechanisms of injury appear to be: (1) an agonist force acting against an actively contracting biceps (eg, a driver with his hands on the wheel who is rear-ended in an automobile accident); (2) a sudden forced abduction-external rotation force applied to the shoulder (eg, a worker who avoids falling from a height by grabbing an overhead bar with one hand); or (3) a fall onto an outstretched hand.

In the overhead athlete, the onset of symptoms may be sudden, occurring with a single pitch, or gradual with an extended prodromal phase. In either case symptoms are similar: (1) pain with attempted overhead athletic activities and (2) inability to throw with preinjury velocity. In the throwing athlete, this combination of pain and loss of velocity is known as the dead arm syndrome.

Because pain with overhead activities is generally a feature of SLAP lesions, there is a danger of misdiagnosing a SLAP lesion as impingement syndrome. Rotator cuff tears can also occur in conjunction with SLAP lesions. The two largest series of SLAP lesions in the literature note associated rotator cuff tears (partial and complete) in 30% to 40% of patients.

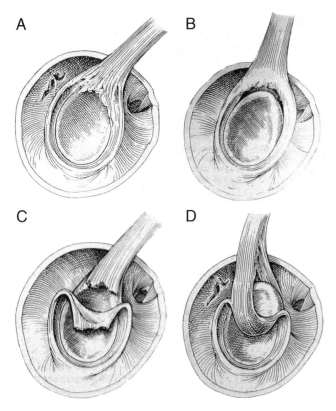

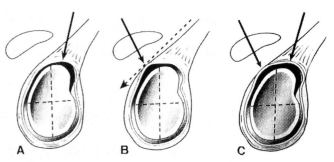

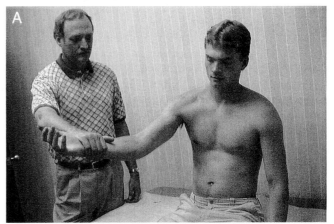

Figure 2 Burkhart and Morgan subtypes of type II SLAP based on anatomic location: Anterior **(A)**; Posterior **(B)**; and combined anterior-posterior **(C)**. *(Reproduced with permission from Burkhart SS, Morgan CD: The peel-back mechanism: Its role in producing and extending posterior Type II SLAP lesions and its effect on SLAP repair rehabilitation. Arthroscopy 1998;14:637-640.)*

Figure 1 Snyder and associates' classification of SLAP lesions. **A,** Type I lesion has degenerative fraying along its free margin, with an intact biceps root. **B,** Type II lesion is characterized by disruption of the attachments of the superior labrum and biceps to the glenoid. **C,** Type III lesion has a bucket-handle tear of the superior labrum, with an intact attachment of the root of the biceps. **D,** Type IV lesion has a bucket-handle tear of the superior labrum that extends into the biceps tendon. *(Reproduced with permission from Snyder SJ, Karzel RP, Del Pizzo W, Ferkel RD, Friedman MJ: SLAP lesions of the shoulder. Arthroscopy 1990;6:274-279.)*

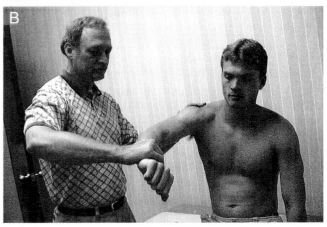

Figure 3 Tests for anterior type II SLAP lesion: **A,** Speed's test with pain in the anterior bicipital groove as the shoulder is flexed against resistance to 90° of flexion. **B,** O'Brien's cross-arm test with anterior pain elicited against resisted adduction and forward flexion across the chest with the arm at 90° of flexion.

Clinical Findings

A number of physical examination tests have been described to identify type II SLAP lesions. All of these tests in some way place either a tensile or torsional load on the biceps, stressing the loose anchor of the biceps-superior labrum complex. This stress causes pain in patients with a type II SLAP lesion. Unfortunately, correlation of physical examination findings with arthroscopic findings has been inconsistent for all of the described tests. In general, the orthopaedist should be suspicious of an anterior type II SLAP lesion if there is a positive Speed's test or a positive O'Brien cross-arm test (Fig. 3). A positive Speed's test is defined as anterior shoulder pain in the region of the bicipital groove when the examiner applies resistance to forward flexion with the patient's shoulder flexed 90° and the forearm supinated. This test can also cause anterior shoulder pain in patients with bicipital tendinitis. A positive O'Brien active compression test is defined as deep pain when the examiner applies resistance to forward flexion with the patient's shoulder adducted and flexed forward

90°, with the hand positioned thumb down. Anterior superficial pain with tenderness of the acromioclavicular joint points more to acromioclavicular pathology. Both types of pain should be relieved with external rotation of the arm (palm-up position).

For posterior type II SLAP lesions, the Jobe relocation

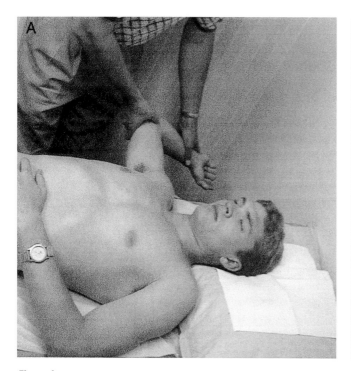
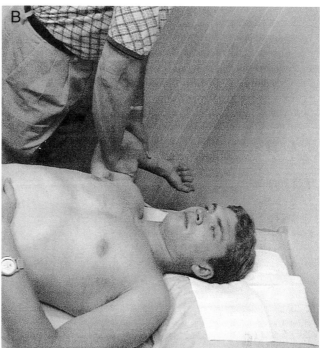

Figure 4 Jobe relocation test with posterosuperior shoulder pain in abduction and external rotation **(A)** that is relieved by posteriorly directed force on the proximal humeral head **(B)**.

test is the most reliable for diagnosis (Fig. 4). A relocation test that is positive for a SLAP tear causes posterosuperior shoulder pain (not apprehension) when the shoulder is brought into combined abduction and external rotation. This pain is relieved by a posteriorly directed force applied to the proximal humerus. This must be clearly differentiated from the response of patients with anterior shoulder instability, in whom apprehension (rather than pain) is caused by abduction and external rotation, which is also relieved by a posteriorly directed force.

For type III and type IV SLAP lesions, patients usually report mechanical symptoms such as catching and popping, but crepitus is often not reproducible on physical examination. Bucket-handle superior labral tears (types III and IV) may also have a component of disruption from bone, causing combined type II/III and type II/IV lesions. Physical examination findings in these patients may be consistent with type II lesions.

Diagnostic studies, including contrast-enhanced MRI studies, have been unreliable in diagnosing SLAP lesions.

Arthroscopic Findings

Despite the abundance of physical examination tests described for SLAP lesions, most authors agree that the definitive diagnosis can only be made arthroscopically. The bucket-handle tears of type III and type IV lesions are obvious. Type II lesions are sometimes more subtle,

and findings may vary depending on the location of the lesion (anterior, posterior, or combined anterior-posterior). Anatomic studies have shown that there is a normal superior sublabral sulcus that is up to 4 to 5 mm in depth. The critical feature of all type II SLAP lesions is medial stripping of the superior labrum, causing a sublabral sulcus of greater than 5 mm. There is a gap between the edge of the articular cartilage and the labral attachment into bone. In anterior and combined anterior-posterior type II SLAP lesions, the biceps root is disrupted and can easily be displaced by a probe. The biceps anchor does not have a firm attachment to bone. In posterior and combined anterior-posterior type II SLAP lesions, there is a positive peel-back sign. The peel-back sign is elicited by taking the arm out of traction, bringing it into 70° to 90° of abduction, and then gradually externally rotating it while viewing the superior labrum-biceps complex. With a positive peel-back sign, the entire superior labrum-biceps complex will shift medially as the arm is externally rotated. This is caused by the change in direction of the biceps pull as it twists in external rotation, displacing the superior labrum-biceps complex medially because it no longer has a firm glenoid attachment (Fig. 5).

A final arthroscopic finding in virtually all type II SLAP lesions is that of a positive drive-through sign. The arthroscope can easily be moved through the glenohumeral joint from superior to inferior. In SLAP lesions the labral ring is disrupted superiorly. Disruption of the

TABLE 1 | Arthroscopic Findings in Type II SLAP Lesions

Type of Lesion	Findings
Anterior type II	Sublabral sulcus greater than 5 mm
	Displaceable biceps root
	Positive drive-through sign
Posterior type II	Sublabral sulcus greater than 5 mm
	Positive peel-back sign
	Positive drive-through sign
Combined anterior-posterior type II	Sublabral sulcus greater than 5 mm
	Displaceable biceps root
	Positive peel-back sign
	Positive drive-through sign

posterosuperior circle of the labrum permits channeling of added laxity to the opposite side of the circle (anteroinferior). This causes an anterior pseudolaxity in the shoulder with a concomitant drive-through sign. Classic anterior shoulder instability is not present. A summary of the arthroscopic findings in type II SLAP lesions is presented in Table 1.

SLAP Lesions in Throwing Athletes

One group of investigators postulated a deceleration mechanism of injury as the biceps contracts to slow down the rapidly extending elbow in follow-through. In contrast, another group proposed an acceleration mechanism of injury in the late cocking phase of throwing. It is in this phase, with the shoulder in maximal abduction and external rotation, that the peel-back forces and shear forces are maximized, increasing the chance of a SLAP lesion. Shoulders that are particularly at risk are those with tight posteroinferior capsules. Such shoulders are prone to superior subluxation in abduction-external rotation, exposing the superior labrum to large shear forces at the point in the pitching motion where the peel-back forces are at their peak. The tight posteroinferior capsule appears to be the most critical factor in initiating the pathologic cascade that results in superior labral disruption in the throwing athlete.

Nonsurgical Treatment

Initial treatment of suspected SLAP lesions in athletes and nonathletes should be nonsurgical, consisting of anti-inflammatory medication, rest, and stretching. Throwing athletes may have a prodromal period of posterosuperior shoulder pain associated with decreased performance. Most of these throwers will have a tight posteroinferior capsule. On physical examination, they will exhibit marked scapular winging while in the prone position with their hands on their hips (Fig. 6). In addition, their total arc of rotation with the arm in 90° of abduction generally will be less than 180°. These shoulders are truly at risk and require a vigorous stretching program aimed at the posteroinferior capsule (Fig. 7).

Surgical Treatment

If nonsurgical treatment fails to eliminate symptoms after 3 months, surgery should be considered. Diagnosis of SLAP lesions requires arthroscopy with direct visualization, probing, and dynamic testing of the peel-back sign. Surgical repair of SLAP lesions is best done arthroscopically because these lesions are very difficult to approach and visualize by open surgery. The best results reported in the literature have been with repair using suture anchors. The goal of surgery is to reestablish a

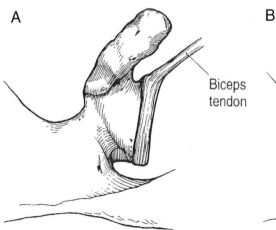

A

B

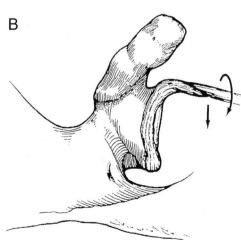

Biceps tendon

Figure 5 A, Superior view of the resting position of the biceps-superior labrum complex. **B,** Superior view of biceps-superior labrum complex in the abducted-externally rotated position, showing the peel-back mechanism as the biceps vector rotates posteriorly. *(Reproduced with permission from Burkhart SS, Morgan CD: The peel-back mechanism: Its role in producing and extending posterior Type II SLAP lesions and its effect on SLAP repair rehabilitation. Arthroscopy 1998;14:637-640.)*

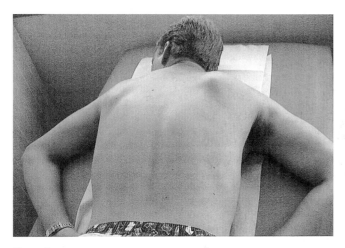

Figure 6 Scapular winging, with the hands on the hips in the prone position, is the best indicator of a tight posteroinferior capsule.

firm bone attachment of the superior labrum-biceps complex and to eliminate the peel-back and drive-through signs. At the very least, this requires placing one suture anchor beneath the biceps root with its suture looping through the posterior half of the biceps root to maximally neutralize the peel-back forces in abduction-external rotation (Fig. 8). SLAP lesions that involve the posterosuperior labrum will require a second anchor placed in the posterosuperior glenoid. Because the posterosuperior glenoid margin has a very steep angle, it cannot be effectively approached through an anterosuperior portal. Thus, a posterolateral portal must be used for anchor placement (Fig. 9). Translabral tacks have been advocated by some authors for superior labral repair, but their mechanical strength of fixation has never been compared to that of suture anchors. The surgeon should be aware that polyglycolic acid anchors lose 50% of their strength at 2 weeks in vivo.

Postoperative Treatment

After SLAP repair, the shoulder is kept in a sling for 3 weeks. During that time, the patient may externally rotate the shoulder with the arm at the side. At 3 weeks, the patient begins active and passive overhead motion. Progressive strengthening of the rotator cuff, deltoid, scapular stabilizers, and biceps begins at 6 weeks.

For throwing athletes, an interval throwing program is begun at 4 months. A focused stretching program is continued, with particular emphasis on stretching of the posteroinferior capsule. At 6 months, pitchers may begin throwing from the mound. At 7 months, they may resume full velocity throwing from the mound. Strengthening of the entire kinetic chain (legs, trunk) as well as daily stretching of the posteroinferior capsule must be continued to prevent recurrent problems.

For nonathletes, immobilization and strengthening are

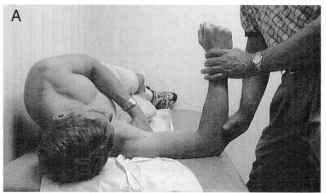

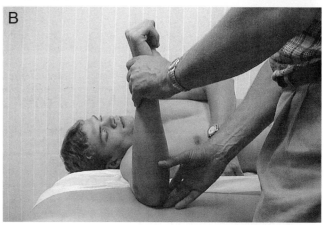

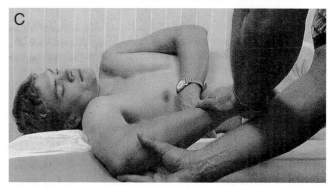

Figure 7 Starting position for posteroinferior capsular stretching. **A,** The patient lies propped up 45° on the involved side so that his body weight stabilizes the scapula. The upper arm is flexed forward at 90° to the body. **B,** In this position, the elbow is flexed 90° with the shoulder in neutral rotation. **C,** Next, the shoulder is maximally internally rotated, with the goal being to bring the forearm flat on the table, or as close as possible.

the same as for athletes. Return to full activities is usually accomplished by 4 months after surgery.

Results of Surgery

Surgical repair of SLAP lesions has yielded predictably good results, with greater than 85% good and excellent results in most series. Although subtle anterior instability has been blamed for causing the dead arm syndrome and open capsulolabral repair has been advocated to address this problem, it is likely that unrecognized

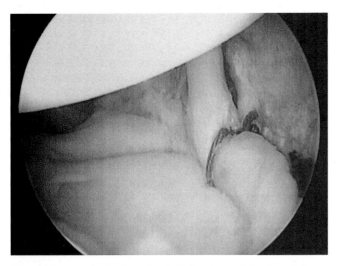

Figure 8 Suture anchor has been placed with its suture capturing the posterior half of the biceps root to neutralize peel-back forces in abduction-external rotation.

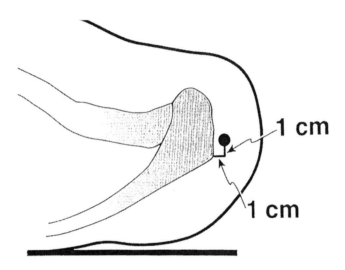

1 cm

1 cm

Figure 9 The portal used for repair of posterior type II SLAP lesions is located 1 cm lateral and 1 cm anterior to the posterolateral angle of the acromion. *(Reproduced with permission from Burkhart SS, Morgan CD: The peel-back mechanism: Its role in producing and extending posterior Type II SLAP lesions and its effect on SLAP repair rehabilitation. Arthroscopy 1998;14:637-640.)*

SLAP lesions (with their associated pseudolaxity) have often been the real culprit. Recognition of a SLAP lesion in a throwing athlete with dead arm syndrome demands SLAP repair rather than anterior instability repair. For the throwing athlete with symptoms of a dead arm in association with a type II SLAP lesion, arthroscopic repair of the SLAP lesion has produced a much higher rate of return to preinjury performance levels than open instability reconstruction procedures. In a series of 53 arthroscopic SLAP repairs for dead arm syndrome in throwing athletes, 87% were reported to be performing at their preinjury level 2 years after surgery. In the largest series (12 shoulders) of open capsulolabral instability repair for dead arm syndrome, only 50% returned to their preinjury performance level.

The Role of Internal Impingement

Internal impingement, or posterosuperior glenoid impingement, refers to the bony entrapment of the rotator cuff between the posterosuperior glenoid and the greater tuberosity of the humerus with abduction and external rotation. This internal impingement occurs in pathologic and normal shoulders. It theoretically can account for some undersurface rotator cuff damage on a mechanical basis. However, such articular surface partial cuff tears are not an indication of anterior microinstability, as has been postulated in the past. In these patients, the surgeon should not consider open or arthroscopic anterior instability surgery unless there are other significant signs of anterior instability.

Summary

Arthroscopy has added a new dimension to the surgeon's ability to more precisely diagnose and treat shoulder dysfunction, both in the high performance overhead throwing athlete and in the nonathlete. The surgeon must always consider SLAP lesions in the differential diagnosis when evaluating the painful shoulder.

Annotated Bibliography

Classification

Maffet MW, Gartsman GM, Moseley B: Superior labrum-biceps tendon complex lesions of the shoulder. *Am J Sports Med* 1995;23:93-98.

The authors add two more types to Snyder and associates' classification of SLAP lesions and note increased humeral head translation during examination under anesthesia of patients with SLAP lesions.

Snyder SJ, Banas MP, Karzel RP: An analysis of 140 injuries to the superior glenoid labrum. *J Shoulder Elbow Surg* 1995;4:243-248.

The authors report on 140 SLAP lesions, noting that 55% were type II lesions and that 40% occurred in association with rotator cuff tears. They advised suture anchor repair for type II lesions.

Clinical Findings

O'Brien SJ, Pagnani MJ, Fealy S, McGlynn SR, Wilson JB: The active compression test: A new and effective test for diagnosing labral tears and acromioclavicular joint abnormality. *Am J Sports Med* 1998;26:610-613.

The authors describe the O'Brien test as a means of diagnosing SLAP lesions and acromioclavicular pathology on physical examination.

Arthroscopic Findings

Burkhart SS, Morgan CD: The peel-back mechanism: Its role in producing and extending posterior type II SLAP lesions and its effect on SLAP repair rehabilitation. *Arthroscopy* 1998;14:637-640.

This article describes the peel-back mechanism.

Huber WP, Putz RV: The periarticular fiber system of the shoulder joint. *Arthroscopy* 1997;13:680-691.

This excellent anatomic study of the labrum demonstrates that tendon fibers from the long head of the biceps are continuous with superior labral fibers, providing a mechanism for force transmission from the biceps to the superior labrum.

Pagnani MJ, Deng XH, Warren RF, Torzilli PA, Altchek DW: Effect of lesions of the superior portion of the glenoid labrum on glenohumeral translation. *J Bone Joint Surg Am* 1995;77:1003-1010.

The authors describe the increased glenohumeral translation that occurs with disruption of the superior labrum attachments.

SLAP Lesions in Throwing Athletes

Burkhart SS, Morgan CD, Kibler WB: Shoulder injuries in overhead athletes: The "dead arm" revisited. *Clin Sports Med* 2000;19:125-158.

The authors present their perspective on the etiology and treatment of the dead arm, as well as provide a historic perspective on this problem. The pathologic cascade is proposed to begin with a tight posteroinferior capsule, leading ultimately to a posterior type II SLAP lesion. Rehabilitation is discussed in detail.

Kibler WB: Biomechanical analysis of the shoulder during tennis activities. *Clin Sports Med* 1995;14:79-86.

The author describes the biomechanics of the shoulder as a funnel for forces to the arm during overhead athletic activities. He also describes the contributions of the kinetic chain to the biomechanics of throwing.

Morgan CD, Burkhart SS, Palmeri M, Gillespie M: Type II SLAP lesions: Three subtypes and their relationships to superior instability and rotator cuff tears. *Arthroscopy* 1998;14:553-565.

The authors present their series of 102 type II SLAP lesions, both in overhead athletes and nonathletes, with repair by suture anchors. They report overall excellent results in 83% of overhead athletes returning to their preinjury level of performance.

The Role of Internal Impingement

Jobe CM: Posterior superior glenoid impingement: Expanded spectrum. *Arthroscopy* 1995;11:530-536.

The author presents his observations of impingement of the rotator cuff against the posterosuperior labrum with the arm in abduction and external rotation and proposes that this internal impingement is even worse in overhead athletes with anterior microinstability.

Classic Bibliography

Andrews JR, Carson WG Jr, McLeod WD: Glenoid labrum tears related to the long head of the biceps. *Am J Sports Med* 1985;13:337-341.

Glousman R, Jobe F, Tibone J, Moynes D, Antonelli D, Perry J: Dynamic electromyographic analysis of the throwing shoulder with glenohumeral instability. *J Bone Joint Surg Am* 1988;70:220-226.

Jobe FW, Giangarra CE, Kvitne RS, Glousman RE: Anterior capsulolabral reconstruction of the shoulder in athletes in overhand sports. *Am J Sports Med* 1991; 19:428-434.

Snyder SJ, Karzel RP, Del Pizzo W, Ferkel RD, Friedman MJ: SLAP lesions of the shoulder. *Arthroscopy* 1990;6:274-279.

Vangsness CT Jr, Jorgenson SS, Watson T, Johnson DL: The origin of the long head of the biceps from the scapula and glenoid labrum: An anatomical study of 100 shoulders. *J Bone Joint Surg Br* 1994;76:951-954.

Walch G, Boileau P, Noel E, Donell ST: Impingement of the deep surface of the supraspinatus tendon on the posterosuperior glenoid rim: An arthroscopic study. *J Shoulder Elbow Surg* 1992;1:238-245.

Chapter 55

Complications of Arthroscopic Shoulder Surgery

Wesley M. Nottage, MD

Introduction

Over the last 20 years, arthroscopy of the shoulder has changed from what initially was a diagnostic procedure into a tool for both excisional and reconstructive surgery. The first organized compilation of arthroscopic shoulder complications was completed by the Committee of Complications of the Arthroscopic Association of North America (AANA), which submitted questionnaires to the AANA membership in 1985. The Committee reported in 1986 on 395,566 arthroscopic cases, including 14,329 shoulder arthroscopies. The complication rate for all joint arthroscopic surgery was 0.56%, excluding recurrence or failure of the procedures. The highest complication rate for shoulder arthroscopy occurred with staple capsulorrhaphy (5.3%). Among 30 patients reported with complications, 19 had loose staples, 6 had impinging staples, 2 had brachial plexus stretch injuries, and 2 had bent staples. In one case, there was equipment failure. During arthroscopic surgery of the subacromial space, 4 complications (0.76%) were reported in 522 patients. Complications occurred in 3 of 73 anterior acromioplasties: 1 axillary nerve injury, 2 equipment failures, and 1 infection. Since that time, staple capsulorrhaphy has been abandoned, but subacromial decompression has become the most common arthroscopic procedure for the shoulder.

A 1987 investigation by 21 experienced arthroscopists analyzed the results of 1,184 patients undergoing shoulder arthroscopy. Complications were noted in nine patients (0.76%). Four related to staple use, two to reflex sympathetic dystrophy, one to hemarthrosis, and two were classified as nonspecific. Six of the complications were glenohumeral (0.5%) (four of the six were staple related), and three were subacromial (0.25%). Subsequent to these reports, there has been no nationwide compilation of arthroscopic shoulder complications.

Various authors have reported their individual experiences, which are often anecdotal and somewhat confusing. The highest reported complication rate was 6.4% (42 of 660 patients). Table 1 summarizes the findings. Other com-plication rates reported in the literature may be lower, because most authors would not report wound bruising, wound hematomas, or painful portals as complications.

Complications of arthroscopic subacromial decompression were analyzed in 108 patients who underwent surgery in the beach-chair position. Of these patients, seven (6.5%) had complications, including two deep infections, three frozen shoulders, one brachial plexopathy, and one acromial fracture. Reported complication rates range from 0.25% to 6.4%, but these do not accurately reflect current technical issues associated with third-generation complex arthroscopic shoulder reconstructive procedures.

In this chapter, several categories of complications

TABLE 1	Complications of Shoulder Arthroplasty in a Large Series of Patients*
Type	**Number of Patients**
Adhesive capsulitis	18
Neurologic injury	6
Minor wound bruising	6
Wound hematoma	5
Reflex sympathetic dystrophy	1
Lacerated cephalic vein	1
Pulmonary embolus	1
Heterotopic calcification	1
Corneal abrasion	1
Hardware problem	1
Painful skin portal	1

*Total number of patients = 660; total number of complications = 42 (6.4%)

are described: anesthesia-related, medical, neurologic (including positional and from direct trauma), miscellaneous complications, and those uniquely associated with a surgical technique. Fluid management and hardware failure are discussed as well.

Anesthesia-Related Complications

Anesthesia-related complications are rare. Of the 395,566 patients described in the 1986 AANA report, only 83 complications (0.02%) were reported. In two patients, complications were linked to the use of local anesthesia without epinephrine and included a superficial skin slough and a generalized seizure. Twelve complications were reported in patients who had local anesthesia with epinephrine, including five instances of blistering, four superficial infections at the injection site, two skin sloughs, and one seizure. Six complications occurred as a result of spinal anesthesia for lower extremity joint arthroscopy. These consisted of three instances of urinary retention, one cardiac arrest with mild brain damage, one temporary ascending paralysis, and one respiratory arrest. The 63 complications reported with general anesthesia included 18 patients who experienced cardiac arrhythmia while under anesthesia, 10 patients with pneumonia, 4 with aspiration pneumonitis, and 31 miscellaneous complications.

Interscalene block anesthesia has proved to be an effective alternative or adjunct to general anesthesia. Horner's syndrome (eyelid ptosis, pupil miosis, and facial anhidrosis) and hoarseness (caused by a recurrent laryngeal nerve blockade) are common side effects but are usually harmless. In addition, paralysis of the hemidiaphragm (caused by a phrenic nerve blockade) almost always occurs but usually does not result in respiratory compromise unless the patient already has a decreased pulmonary reserve. Patients rarely have a contralateral paralyzed hemidiaphragm as a preexisting condition, but in those who do, interscalene block is contraindicated. Serious complications with this type of block are rare but include hematoma, intraneural injection, pneumothorax, seizures, and cardiovascular collapse. The latter two complications are secondary to intravascular injection. The risk of major complications decreases with experienced personnel who are skilled and exhibit good judgment in performing blocks.

Medical Complications

Respiratory

Unique pulmonary complications have been reported, including spontaneous pneumothorax in four patients who did not have chest wall trauma. Their conditions were associated with preoperative cigarette smoking and asthma. Subcutaneous emphysema, pneumomediastinum, and tension pneumothorax were reported in three patients. In these patients there was not a clear understanding of the exact mechanism of injury. A single instance of complete airway obstruction caused by fluid extravasation in the retropharyngeal area was also described; this complication resolved in 24 hours with airway support.

Infection

Deep infection is relatively rare in shoulder arthroscopy. The benchmark infection rate was reported in 1982; 2% glutaraldehyde sterilization was used in 12,000 knee and shoulder arthroscopies and an infection rate of 0.04% was reported. Deep infection rates after shoulder surgery have been reported to range from 0 to 1.8%.

Neurologic Complications

Neurologic injury is the most common complication associated with shoulder arthroscopy and is of the most concern, with a complication rate reported up to 30%. Injury is caused by either positional factors or from direct trauma.

Permanent quadriparesis in conjunction with the use of general anesthesia has been reported in a patient undergoing arthroscopic decompression and mini-open cuff repair in a beach-chair position. The literature from otorhinolaryngology and neurosurgery suggests that this complication results from neck flexion in patients with variant blood supply to the spinal cord or canal stenosis, producing cord ischemia. Thus, maintaining the head, neck, and torso in a neutral position is critical during these surgical procedures.

Peripheral injuries to the axillary, median, radial, ulnar, musculocutaneous, hypoglossal, superficial radial, and posterior auricular nerves have been reported as has ipsilateral posterior and anterior interosseous nerve palsy. In the 1986 AANA report, four neurologic injuries were reported in 14,329 shoulder arthroscopies (0.02%), including three brachial plexus injuries and one axillary nerve injury. In addition, nerve injury in the contralateral lower extremity has been reported, including the lateral femoral cutaneous nerve and common peroneal nerve. These injuries often occur in patients who have been placed in the lateral decubitus position whose contralateral thigh, knee, and leg have not been well padded.

Many authors have noted a higher incidence of nerve injuries, most of which are transient. After 304 consecutive patients underwent arthroscopic surgery in the lateral decubitus position, 7% of the patients were noted to have a sensory deficit 2 weeks after surgery, and 3% had a persistent deficit 8 months postoperatively; the most common nerve involved was the axillary nerve. One study used somatosensory-evoked potentials (SSEPs) to detect nerve compression during shoulder arthroscopy of 20 patients in the lateral decubitus position. Abnormalities in the musculocutaneous nerve occurred in all 20 patients, with 10 having a varying degree of involvement in the median, ulnar, and radial nerves as well. Only 2 of the 20 had a clinical neurapraxia postoperatively, and in both patients the neurapraxia resolved within 48 hours. Results of this study show that mild nerve injury is far more common than realized, although usually it is not a significant clinical problem. Careful attention to positioning and technique can minimize this problem.

Unique position-related nerve injuries have been noted. The beach-chair position has been associated with a transient auricular nerve palsy as well as transient hypoglossal nerve palsy. The lateral decubitus position has been associated with superficial radial nerve compression caused by traction devices (6%) as well as lateral femoral cutaneous nerve injury and peroneal nerve palsy of the contralateral lower extremity.

Brachial plexopathy and brachial neurapraxia most commonly involve the musculocutaneous nerve and are associated with specific arm positions and the use of excessive traction. The brachial plexus is attached at two places along its course: the prevertebral fascia at the transverse processes and the axillary fascia in the arm. Brachial plexus strain has been measured during shoulder arthroscopy using human cadavers in the lateral decubitus position. The brachial plexus is strained the least when the arm is in 45° of flexion and 90° of abduction or in 45° of forward flexion and 0° of abduction. The highest strain occurs when the arm is in 0° of flexion and 10° of abduction. The two positions that maximize visibility and minimize brachial plexus strain are a position of 45° of forward flexion and 0° of abduction or 45° of forward flexion and 90° of abduction.

The effect of a longitudinal traction weight on brachial plexus strain during shoulder arthroscopy in the lateral decubitus position also has been studied. Longitudinal traction of 12 lb and vertical traction of 7 lb or less are not associated with alteration in SSEPs. These should be the maximum weights used, creating a balanced suspension rather than pure axial traction.

Direct Trauma

Direct nerve injury has occurred with both the creation of portals and placement of instruments during surgical procedures. Direct thermal damage to the axillary nerve has been associated with thermal capsulorrhaphy when it was used in the axillary pouch, where the nerve is immediately adjacent to the joint capsule. The exact incidence is not known but is estimated to be between 0 and 6%.

The neurapraxia usually resolves within 8 weeks, but cases of permanent nerve damage have been reported.

Portal placement may directly injure the nerves as well. Too acute an angle or too medial a superior (Caspari-Neviaser) portal through the muscle belly of the supraspinatus can directly strike the suprascapular nerve. A grossly misplaced posterior portal may traumatize the axillary nerve, and passing any portal medial to the coracoid runs the risk of direct trauma to the brachial plexus, particularly if done with an inside-out technique. Cadaveric dissections have shown that maintaining portals lateral to the coracoid provides a good margin of safety. Accessory shoulder portals have been described, including that of the anteroinferior 5 o'clock portal for shoulder arthroscopy. The average axillary-musculocutaneous nerve distance is 22 to 24 mm from this portal if it is made correctly. Subacromial portals also have been occasionally associated with nerve injury, particularly the anterolateral portal, which can damage the axillary nerve when it is brought closer to the acromion with the arm abducted.

Direct major vascular injury has not been described. One case of persistent bleeding from an anterior portal, requiring open ligation of a small subcutaneous artery, has been reported. There also has been a case report of a venous pseudoaneurysm forming after shoulder arthroscopy.

Miscellaneous Complications

Synovial cyst formation after shoulder arthroscopy has been described as well as synovial fistulas related to posterior sutures from arthroscopic suture capsulorrhaphy. These complications resolve with débridement and closure. Deep venous thrombosis of the upper extremity has been reported in a patient with hypercoagulable disease (Hodgkin's disease). Heterotopic bone has been reported and is associated with hypertrophic pulmonary osteoarthropathy, obesity, and diabetes.

Articular chondral damage is believed to be quite common, and the inability of articular cartilage to repair itself once damaged is well known. The exact incidence of significant damage, however, is unknown. Articular damage can occur with insertion of the arthroscopic trochar at the beginning of the procedure. This damage can occur particularly easily in patients with adhesive capsulitis, as the capsule can be very stiff and fibrotic, requiring more force than usual during trochar placement.

Unique Procedural Complications

Suture Capsulorrhaphy

The short-term results of transglenoid suture capsulorrhaphy have been excellent, but with longer follow-up the recurrence rate has increased. The most significant surgical complication unique to the transglenoid technique is injury to the suprascapular nerve. Its incidence is reported to range from 1.4% to 2.6%. The nerve can be damaged by the suture-passing pin traversing the glenoid from anterolaterally to posteromedially. Anatomic studies have reported that pins directed medially at the glenoid neck placed the nerve at risk, averaging a 4-mm pin-to-nerve distance, whereas anteroposterior pins aimed inferiorly had an average of 16 mm of clearance. The authors suggested that aiming at the inferior scapular tip, exiting the skin inferiorly and laterally on the scapular neck, would minimize the risk to the suprascapular nerve.

Other complications associated with this technique have been reported. In one case report advancement of the transglenoid pin by hand allowed displacement along the medial scapular neck with subsequent penetration of the chest cavity, causing a pneumothorax. In another report the suture passage pin bent and subsequently broke when advanced with a mallet, requiring open removal from the scapulothoracic joint. These problems have not been noted with power drill insertion of the pin.

Polyglyconate Tack Stabilization

Use of bioabsorbable implants has been advanced as a method of arthroscopic stabilization of the shoulder. Although using a tack does not address the issue of capsular volume reduction, it does allow attachment of soft tissues to a bony margin. The associated problems of this device include migration of the rivet, pneumothorax following posterosuperior labral repair with inadvertent pin advancement into the chest, synovitis, and marked foreign body reaction during resorption.

Suture Anchor Capsulorrhaphy

This suture technique has become more popular as anatomic repairs have gained favor. The principal complications are anchor prominence or migration with subsequent articular surface damage to the humeral head and glenoid. These complications can be minimized by adequate visualization, passage into bone, direct viewing of the anchor once seated in the bone, and testing the anchor for pull-out strength before tying the suture. The use of bioabsorbable anchors and long-term bioabsorbable suture materials may eliminate metal anchor-related complications.

Thermal Capsulorrhaphy

Recent interest in thermal capsulorrhaphy has been promulgated without significant peer-reviewed studies with measurable clinical results or complications. Significant complications reported anecdotally and by a re-

cent survey study include stiffness, recurrent instability, capsular tissue loss, transient axillary nerve injury, and occasional permanent axillary nerve injury.

Fluid Management and Complications

Shoulder arthroscopy necessitates adequate pressure from flow to distend the joint and aid in both hemostasis and visualization. Extravasation of fluid typically is associated with subacromial and glenohumeral procedures, and at times the amount of swelling can be impressive. Muscle pressures in patients undergoing shoulder arthroscopy and acromioplasty have been studied. The pressure in the deltoid muscle measured with a slit catheter measures an average of 27 to 72 mm Hg during subacromial arthroscopy, reaching a maximum of 120 mm Hg during acromioplasty. Four minutes after the procedure, however, pressure returns to the baseline of 12 mm Hg, even if there is persistent soft-tissue swelling. Electromyography at 4 to 6 weeks is normal. Although permanent damage to the deltoid or rotator cuff musculature secondary to swelling or compartment syndrome has not been reported, it is generally a good idea to keep the pump pressure as low as possible during the procedure. Maintaining the patient's blood pressure at a low level allows the surgeon to reduce the pump pressure and still maintain visualization.

The irrigating fluid chosen also may produce complications. Current recommendations include either normal saline or lactated Ringer's solution. Although it used to be a required fluid for electrocautery use in the shoulder, glycine irrigation fluid has been reported to cause transient blindness in a patient undergoing bilateral knee arthroscopy. Transient blindness with glycine irrigation also has been documented in the urology literature and is believed to be dose-related. Newer electrocautery devices no longer require glycine as the irrigant. Many arthroscopists use these newer devices, but the older devices can still be used by selectively turning on the glycine irrigation only when electrocautery is used.

Intraoperative Equipment Failure

Intraoperative equipment breakage or failure has become a less frequent cause of complications of shoulder arthroscopy. The intraoperative equipment failure rate reported by AANA in 1986 was 398 of 395,566 cases (0.1%). Subsequent redesign of instruments and improved surgical skills have decreased the intraoperative equipment failure rate significantly.

Summary

Shoulder arthroscopy has been proved to be a safe procedure with few complications. Unacceptable incidence of certain complications has led to the demise of unsafe techniques, such as staple capsulorrhaphy, and has paved the way for new techniques with better results and fewer complications. Knowledge of the frequency, magnitude, and nature of complications helps with patient education and sharpens the surgeon's attention to detail during an operation. Anesthesia-related complications are exceedingly rare. Interscalene blocks are safe but must be performed by well-trained personnel who are experienced in the technique. The risk of infection associated with shoulder arthroscopy is probably less than 0.1%. The risk of nerve injury is also less than 0.1% and is related to patient positioning, portal placement, passage of instruments, position of the arm, and the amount and type of traction used. The surgeon must also be well versed in the specific risks of particular procedures to maximize the effectiveness of treatment and minimize the incidence of complications.

Annotated Bibliography

Introduction

Berjano P, Gonzalez BG, Olmedo JF, Perez-Espana LA, Munilla MG: Complications in arthroscopic shoulder surgery. *Arthroscopy* 1998;14:785-788.

The authors conducted a retrospective study of 179 consecutive arthroscopic only (n = 141) and combined arthroscopic/open (n = 38) procedures performed by the same surgeon. Complications occurred in 10.6% of arthroscopic procedures and in 5.3% of arthroscopic/open procedures.

McFarland EG, O'Neill OR, Hsu CY: Complications of shoulder arthroscopy. *J South Orthop Assoc* 1997;6: 190-196.

The authors comprehensively reviewed the known complications and technical issues surrounding shoulder arthroscopy.

Weber SC, Abrams JS, Nottage WM: Complications associated with arthroscopic shoulder surgery. *Arthroscopy* 2002;18(suppl 1):88-95.

The authors reviewed common and unusual complications of shoulder arthroscopy.

Anesthesia-Related Complications

Borgeat A, Ekatodramis G, Kalberer F, Benz C: Acute and nonacute complications associated with interscalene block and shoulder surgery: A prospective study. *Anesthesiology* 2001;95:875-880.

The authors enrolled 521 patients undergoing elective shoulder surgery and interscalene block in a prospective study of potential complications. Patients were observed daily (for 10 days) for paresthesias, dysesthesias, pain not related to sur-

gery, and muscular weakness and were also evaluated at 1, 3, 6, and 9 months after surgery. A total of 520 patients completed the study; one was excluded after surgical axillary nerve damage. Two hundred thirty-four patients had an interscalene catheter. Acute complications consisted of one pneumothorax (0.2%) and one episode of central nervous system toxicity (incoherent speech, 0.2%). A small percentage of patients had persistent dysesthesias after surgery, but at 9 months, only one patient (0.2%) had persistence of dysesthesia. The authors estimate the incidence of short- and long-term complications to be 0.4%.

Weber SC, Jain R: Scalene regional anesthesia for shoulder surgery in a community setting: An assessment of risk. *J Bone Joint Surg Am* 2002;84:775-779.

The authors conducted a retrospective review of 218 patients who had undergone scalene block anesthesia over a 3-year period at two facilities. All blocks were performed with the patient awake and with use of preoperative nerve stimulation to localize the brachial plexus. General anesthesia also was used for 179 of the 218 patients (82%). Six complications occurred, including one generalized seizure, one episode of cardiovascular collapse, and four episodes of severe respiratory distress. Two patients had temporary neurologic injuries that persisted at least 6 weeks.

Medical Complications

Borgeat A, Bird P, Ekatodramis G, Dumont C: Tracheal compression caused by periarticular fluid accumulation: A rare complication of shoulder surgery. *J Shoulder Elbow Surg* 2000;9:443-445.

The authors described a case in which a 69-year-old woman was placed in the lateral decubitus position, and arthroscopy was performed under interscalene block only. During the first 2 hours of the procedure, both the pump pressure and flow were high, and the patient reported neck discomfort and heaviness, along with difficulty breathing. Extensive swelling was noted on the ipsilateral chest wall, neck, and face. The procedure was terminated, and the patient was brought to an upright position, at which point her breathing started to improve. The authors proposed that the patient's breathing difficulty was secondary to extravasated fluid compressing the trachea, and that the interscalene block was of great benefit in this case because the patient could warn the anesthesiologist of the impending respiratory compromise.

Dietzel DP, Ciullo JV: Spontaneous pneumothorax after shoulder arthroscopy: A report of four cases. *Arthroscopy* 1996;12:99-102.

The authors reviewed four cases of spontaneous pneumothorax that occurred after shoulder arthroscopy. All four patients had an underlying history of cigarette smoking or asthma, and the cause of pneumothorax was believed to be a rupture of an underlying bleb or bulla.

Neurologic Complications

Mohammed KD, Hayes MG, Saies AD: Unusual complications of shoulder arthroscopy. *J Shoulder Elbow Surg* 2000;9:350-353.

The authors reported on nine patients who had unusual complications after shoulder arthroscopy, including neurapraxia of the medial pectoral and anterior interosseous nerves, superficial burns, skin necrosis, and heterotopic ossification (HO) of the subacromial space. The patient with HO of the subacromial space also had prior open rotator cuff surgery complicated by infection.

Miscellaneous Complications

Scarlat MM, Harryman DT II: Management of the diabetic stiff shoulder. *Instr Course Lect* 2000;49:283-294.

The authors reported a complication caused by direct trauma when performing arthroscopic capsular release in a diabetic patient's shoulder. The arthroscopic trochar punched a hole in the humeral head, which later collapsed. Prosthetic replacement was eventually required.

Unique Procedural Complications

Burkart A, Imhoff AB, Roscher E: Foreign-body reaction to the bioabsorbable Suretac device. *Arthroscopy* 2000;16:91-95.

The authors report breakage and early loosening of the Suretac device (Acufex Microsurgical, Mansfield, MA) in four patients in whom the device was used for SLAP lesions and instability. All patients reported shoulder pain and a loss of active and passive motion. Arthroscopic examination revealed a massive synovitis without positive cultures. Loose fragments of the Suretac device were found to be dispersed in the joint cavity and had induced a foreign-body reaction histologically. The authors suggested that the fragmentation of the devices was a result of mechanical failure rather than a predisposition to an exaggerated inflammatory response.

Shaffer BS, Tibone JE: Arthroscopic shoulder instability surgery: Complications. *Clin Sports Med* 1999;18:737-767.

This is a detailed review and bibliography of the history of arthroscopic stabilization and complications associated with its use.

Silver MD, Daigneault JP: Symptomatic interarticular migration of glenoid suture anchors. *Arthroscopy* 2000; 16:102-105.

The authors summarized a case report of a patient treated with an arthroscopic Bankart repair using metal suture anchors. The patient reported painful shoulder grinding several weeks after the procedure during rehabilitation. Arthro-

scopic evaluation revealed that one of the suture anchors had migrated proud of its entry site on the glenoid rim. The proud suture anchor had worn a significant portion of the humeral articular cartilage to bone.

Wong KL, Williams GR: Complications of thermal capsulorrhaphy of the shoulder. *J Bone Joint Surg Am* 2001; 83(suppl 2):151-155.

The authors evaluated the recurrence rate and the prevalence of complications related to the use of thermal energy for the treatment of glenohumeral instability. A total of 379 surgeons who had performed 14,277 thermal capsulorrhaphy procedures over the previous 5 years were surveyed for the study. Recurrent instability occurred after 8.0% of the procedures. Of the patients with recurrent instability, 363 required revision surgery, of which 71 (19.6%) exhibited signs of capsular attenuation at the time of the revision. A total of 196 patients (1.4%) had an axillary neuropathy postoperatively, while 182 (93%) had only a sensory deficit, and 14 had combined sensory and motor deficits. Of these 196 patients, 95% recovered completely. Patients with sensory deficits alone recovered in an average 2.3 months after surgery, and patients with combined deficits recovered in an average of 4 months. Ten patients (5% of the nerve injury population, 0.07% of the entire study population) had permanent nerve damage.

Classic Bibliography

Anderson AF, Alfrey D, Lipscomb AB Jr: Acute pulmonary edema, an unusual complication following arthroscopy: A report of three cases. *Arthroscopy* 1990; 6:235-237.

Bigliani LU, Dalsey RM, McCann PD, April EW: An anatomical study of the suprascapular nerve. *Arthroscopy* 1990;6:301-305.

Burkhart SS: Deep venous thrombosis after shoulder arthroscopy. *Arthroscopy* 1990;6:61-63.

Burkhart SS, Barnett CR, Snyder SJ: Transient postoperative blindness as a possible effect of glycine toxicity. *Arthroscopy* 1990;6:112-114.

Committee on Complications of the Arthroscopy Association of North America: Complications in arthroscopy: The knee and other joints. *Arthroscopy* 1986;2:253-258.

Curtis AS, Snyder SJ, Del Pizzo W, Friedman MJ, Ferkel RD, Karzel RP: Abstract: Complications of shoulder arthroscopy. *Arthroscopy* 1992;8:395.

Goldberg BJ, Nirschl RP, McConnell JP, Pettrone FA: Arthroscopic transglenoid suture capsulolabral repairs: Preliminary results. *Am J Sports Med* 1993;21:656-665.

Johnson LL, Shneider DA, Austin MD, Goodman FG, Bullock JM, DeBruin JA: Two-percent glutaraldehyde: A disinfectant in arthroscopy and arthroscopic surgery. *J Bone Joint Surg Am* 1982;64:237-239.

Klein AH, France JC, Mutschler TA, Fu FH: Measurement of brachial plexus strain in arthroscopy of the shoulder. *Arthroscopy* 1987;3:45-52.

Lee HC, Dewan N, Crosby L: Subcutaneous emphysema, pneumomediastinum, and potentially life-threatening tension pneumothorax: Pulmonary complications from arthroscopic shoulder decompression. *Chest* 1992; 101:1265-1267.

Lee YF, Cohn L, Tooke SM: Intramuscular deltoid pressure during shoulder arthroscopy. *Arthroscopy* 1989;5: 209-212.

Moran MC, Warren RF: Development of a synovial cyst after arthroscopy of the shoulder: A brief note. *J Bone Joint Surg Am* 1989;71:127-129.

Mullins RC, Drez D Jr, Cooper J: Hypoglossal nerve palsy after arthroscopy of the shoulder and open operation with the patient in the beach-chair position: A case report. *J Bone Joint Surg Am* 1992;74:137-139.

Norwood LA, Fowler HL: Rotator cuff tears: A shoulder arthroscopy complication. *Am J Sports Med* 1989; 17:837-841.

Nottage WM: Arthroscopic portals: Anatomy at risk. *Orthop Clin North Am* 1993;24:19-26.

Pitman MI, Nainzadeh N, Ergas E, Springer S: The use of somatosensory evoked potentials for detection of neuropraxia during shoulder arthroscopy. *Arthroscopy* 1988;4:250-255.

Rodeo SA, Forster RA, Weiland AJ: Neurological complications due to arthroscopy. *J Bone Joint Surg Am* 1993;75:917-926.

Small NC: Complications in arthroscopic surgery performed by experienced arthroscopists. *Arthroscopy* 1988;4:215-221.

Wilder BL: Hypothesis: The etiology of midcervical quadriplegia after operation with the patient in the sitting position. *Neurosurgery* 1982;11:530-531.

Zuckerman JD, Matsen FA III: Complications about the glenohumeral joint related to the use of screws and staples. *J Bone Joint Surg Am* 1984;66:175-180.

Index

A

Abduction, 17, 147
Abduction and external rotation (ABER)
    position in imaging shoulder instability, 69
Accelerated postoperative shoulder rehabilitation, 403
    closed-chain axial loading for strengthening
        aquatic therapy, 406-407
        power development, 407
        rotator cuff activation, 405f, 406, 408f
        scapular control, 405-406, 406f, 407f
    principles in
        closed-chain axial loading for motion, 405, 405f
        continuous passive motion, 405
        early achievement of 90° of abduction, 405
        early postoperative motion, 404-405
        evaluation of related deficits, 403
        leg and trunk control, 403, 404f
        scapular control, 403-404
        shoulder flexibility, 404, 405f
        shoulder strength, 404
    special concerns in
        exercise machines, 407
        pain, 407
        progressions, 408
Achilles tendon allograft, 33
    in treating elbow stiffness, 329-330
Acromioclavicular joint, 3, 9-10, 37, 66
    disorders of
        arthritis in, 134, 164, 171, 224
        arthrosis in, 403
        definition of problem, 461
        expected clinical results, 461
        full-thickness tears and, 177
        inflammatory process in, 251
        osteolysis in, 118
        pathology of, 181, 182
        spurring, 182
    displacement of, 229
    motion at, 9
Acromioclavicular ligaments, 219
    injury to, 229

Acromiohumeral distance, 192, 193
Acromion, 30
    fracture of, 228-229
    full-thickness tears and, 171-172, 173f
    ossification of, 149
    surgical complications, 186
Acromioplasty, 8, 167, 186, 289, 473
    anteroinferior, 172
    complications of arthroscopic, 551
    débridement with or without, for partial-thickness rotator cuff tears, 168
    dome, 186
    full-thickness tears and, 177
    revision, 186
Acute brachial radiculitis, 439
Acute valgus instability, 313
Adhesion-cohesion, 17, 65
Adhesive capsulitis, 181, 185-186
Adson's test, 397
Age, rotator cuff tears and, 171
Alglucerase, 271
Alonso-Llames approach
    for distal humeral fracture, 359
    in total elbow arthroplasty, 362, 363f
AMBRI (Atraumatic Multidirectional Bilateral Rehabilitation Inferior)
    capsular shift, 130
    syndrome, 66, 258
American Academy of Orthopaedic Surgeons, 443
    clinical guideline on shoulder pain support document, 456-462
        definition of terms, 457
        differential diagnoses
            acromioclavicular joint disorder, 461
            fibromyalgia, 461
            frozen shoulder, 458
            glenohumeral instability, 459
            glenohumeral arthritis, 460
            rotator cuff disorders, 457-458
        future research recommendations, 462
        goals and rationale, 456
        methodology, 456-457
        scope and organization, 456
    CPT and ICD-9 Coding Committee, 412

American Shoulder and Elbow Surgeons, 412, 443
    activities of daily living functional evaluation, 178
    elbow evaluation, 428
    shoulder evaluation, 268-269, 425t, 426t, 427-428, 429
Amputation, brachial plexus injuries and, 395
Anchor placement in arthroscopy for full-thickness tears, 177
Ancillary diagnostic studies in diagnosing thoracic outlet syndrome, 399-400
Anesthesia. See also Regional anesthesia for shoulder surgery
    complications following rotator cuff surgery, 188
    examination under, 85, 106, 107
    interscalene block, 552
Aneurysms, 124-125
Angiogenesis, 251
Ankylosing spondylitis, 525
Antegrade insertion, 240-241
Anterior deltopectoral approach, 78
Anterior drawer test, 67
Anterior labroligamentous periosteal sleeve avulsion, 85-87
Anteroinferior acromioplasty, 172
Anteroinferior instability, 133
Antibiotic-impregnated cement, 287
Antimalarial agents for rheumatoid arthritis in elbow, 333
AO/ASIF/OTA Comprehensive Long Bone Classification system, 209-210
Applied energy treatments of calcific tendinitis, 534-535
Apprehension test, 68, 84, 94
Aquatic therapy in shoulder rehabilitation, 406-407
Arteriography in diagnosing thoracic outlet syndrome, 399

f indicates figure
t indicates table

Arthritis, 44-45. *See also* Osteoarthritis;
  Rheumatoid arthritis
  acromioclavicular, 134, 164, 171, 224
  in elbow, 333
  glenohumeral, 50, 98, 134-135, 164, 183,
    525
    alternative approaches, 460
    definition of problem, 460
    expected clinical results, 460
    recommendations, 460
  inflammatory, 525-527
    of the shoulder, 251-255
      clinical evaluation, 252
      incidence, 251
      nonsurgical treatment of, 252
      pathoanatomy, 251-252
      pathogenesis, 251
      pathophysiology, 251
      results of treatment, 254-255, 255*t*
      surgical treatment of, 253-254
    management of, 59
  noninflammatory, 526, 527-528, 527*ft*
  postcapsulorrhaphy, 280-281
  posttraumatic, 224
    premature, 313
  psoriatic, 525
Arthrodesis, 281
  glenohumeral, 200, 253, 279
  for osteoarthritis, 261
Arthrography
  for arthroscopic subacromial
    decompression, 508
  for inflammatory arthritis, 252
  for rotator cuff repair, 472
Arthrogryposis, 325
Arthropathy
  crystal-induced, 197
  inflammatory, 325
Arthroplasty
  for osteonecrosis and other noninflam-
    matory degenerative diseases,
    268-269
  Outerbridge-Kashiwagi, 327-328, 339
  resection, 200, 253
  semiconstrained total shoulder, 202-203,
    202*f*
  total shoulder, 59
  unconstrained total shoulder, 201
Arthroscopic acromioclavicular joint
  resection, 519-523
  anatomy, 519
  complications, 522*f*, 523
  diagnosis, 519
  indications, 520
  instability and coplaning, 522-523
  rehabilitation, 523
  techniques, 520-522, 520*f*, 521*f*, 522*f*
  treatment, 520
Arthroscopic anterior glenohumeral ligament reconstruction, 103-112
  associated pathoanatomy, 103
    capsular laxity, 104
    glenoid labrum, 103
    rotator cuff tears, 104
    rotator interval, 104

developments in arthroscopic labral
    repair, 104
  cannulated bioabsorbable implants,
    105
  metallic staples, 104
  suture anchors, 105
  transglenoid sutures, 104-105
patient selection
  diagnostic arthroscopy, 106
  examination under anesthesia, 106
  history, 105
  physical examination, 105
  radiographic evaluation, 105-106
  surgical indications, 106
postoperative rehabilitation, 112
surgical reconstruction using suture
  anchors
  anterior glenohumeral
    reconstruction, 108-109, 110*f*
  general principles, 106
  glenoid preparation and anchor
    placement, 108, 109*f*
  instrumentation, 106-107
  preparation, 107
  rotator interval, 111
  technique, 107-108, 107*f*, 108*f*
  thermal capsulorrhaphy, 111-112,
    112*f*
Arthroscopic capsular shift using transglenoid sutures, 496-497
Arthroscopic capsulorrhaphy for internal
  impingement, 121
Arthroscopic cheilectomy, 263
Arthroscopic débridement, 526
Arthroscopic drawer test, 106
Arthroscopic lavage and débridement, 200
Arthroscopic pancapsular plication, for
  multidirectional instability, 495-499
  clinical findings, 495-496
  etiology, 495
  nonsurgical management of, 496
  pathophysiology, 496
  surgical management, 496-499, 497*f*, 498*f*
    arthroscopic capsular shift using
      transglenoid sutures, 496-497
    arthroscopic pancapsular plication
      technique, 497, 497*f*
    open inferior capsular shift, 496
    postoperative care/results, 498-499
    technique, 497-498, 497*f*, 498*f*
Arthroscopic stabilization, 123-124
Arthroscopic staple capsulorrhaphy, 86, 131
Arthroscopic subacromial decompression,
  473, 507-516
  advantages and disadvantages, 510-511
    acromioclavicular and biceps tendon
      pathology, 512-513, 513*f*
    technique/intraoperative decision
      making, 510-512, 510*f*, 511*f*, 512*f*
  anatomy/pathophysiology, 507
  clinical findings, 507-509, 508*f*
  postoperative management, 513-514
  results/complications, 514-516, 515*f*
  treatment, 510, 510*f*
Arthroscopic synovectomies, 254, 261

Arthroscopy
  for acute shoulder dislocations, 487-491
    arthroscopic technique, 489*f*, 490,
      490*f*, 491*f*
    classification of instability, 487
    follow-up care and rehabilitation,
      490-491
    imaging and pathologic findings,
      487-488
    indications for arthroscopic
      treatment, 490
    nonsurgical versus arthroscopic
      treatment, 488
    open surgical versus arthroscopic
      treatment, 488*t*, 489-490
    outcomes of nonsurgical treatment,
      489
    patient factors, 487
  for anterior shoulder instability, 103
  for arthritic shoulder, 525-531
    classification, 526, 526*f*
      inflammatory arthritis, 526-527
      noninflammatory arthritis,
        527-528, 527*ft*
    complications, 530
    future directions, 530
    indications and uses, 528-529, 528*t*,
      529*f*
    pathophysiology, 525, 525*t*
      inflammatory arthritis, 525-526
      noninflammatory arthritis, 526
    results, 530
    surgical technique, 527*f*, 529-530, 529*f*
  for calcific tendinitis, 533-536
    applied energy treatments, 534-535
    diagnosis, 534
    nonsurgical management, 534
    pathophysiology, 533
    surgical treatment, 535-536
  coding for, 414-415
  complications of, 551-555, 551*t*
    anesthesia-related, 552
    fluid management and, 554
    intraoperative equipment failure, 554
    medical, 552
    miscellaneous, 553
    neurologic, 552-553
    polyglyconate tack stabilization, 554
    suture capsulorrhaphy, 553-554
    thermal capsulorrhaphy, 554
  for full-thickness tears
    indications, 176
    postoperative management, 177
    preoperative evaluation, 175-176
    results, 178
    surgical technique, 176
      glenohumeral joint, 176
      subacromial space, 176-177
  for glenohumeral joint, 182
  for internal impingement, 119-121, 121*f*
  for labrum, 104-105
    cannulated bioabsorbable implants
      in, 105
    metallic staples in, 104
    suture anchors in, 105
    transglenoid sutures in, 104-105

for multidirectional instability, 95-96
for partial-thickness rotator cuff tears, 167
for posterior instability, 99-100
for recurrent anterior dislocations, 480-483, 481*f*, 482*f*
for recurrent anterior shoulder instability, 86-87
versus open repair, 85-86
for release of elbow contracture, 327-328
for rotator cuff, 471-476
indications, 471-472, 472*f*
initial arthroscopic evaluation, 472-473
outcomes, 475-476
technique of, 473-475, 473*f*, 474*f*, 475*f*
for shoulder arthroplasty, 289
for shoulder dislocations, 487
ArthroSew device, 473
Arthrosis, 152
Arthrotomy, 253
Articular cartilage damage, 471
Articular comminution, 213
Articular conformity, 51, 57
Articular constraint, 51-52, 52*f*
Articular geometry, 13
Articular side partial-thickness rotator cuff tears, 471
Assisted passive motion exercises, full-thickness tear repair and, 174
Asymmetric posterior glenoid erosion, 56-57
Asymmetric reaming, 57
Athletes. *See also* Throwing injuries
elbow injuries from throwing in, 297-308
anterior pain, 305-306
distal biceps injuries, 306
pronator teres syndrome, 305-306
functional anatomy and biomechanics, 297
lateral collateral ligament complex, 297
medial collateral ligament complex, 297
ulnar nerve, 297
lateral pain
epicondylitis, 298-300, 299*ft*
osteochondritis dissecans, 298
radial nerve entrapment, 300
radiocapitellar overload syndrome, 300
medial pain
collateral ligament injuries and physeal injuries in children, 301
collateral ligament injuries in adults, 301-304, 302*f*, 303*f*, 304*f*
epicondylitis, 300-301
posterior pain, 306
impingement/valgus extension overload syndrome, 306-308, 306*f*, 307*f*
stress fractures, 307*f*, 308
ulnar neuropathy, 304-305
clinical presentation, 305
treatment, 305

natural history in competitive overhead, for rotator cuff disease, 152-153
reinjury in, 132
Atraumatic Multidirectional Bilateral Rehabilitation Inferior Capsular Shift/Traumatic Unidirectional Bankart Lesion Surgery classification, 91
Atraumatic sternoclavicular instability, 220
Atrophic nonunions, 223, 244-245
Avascular necrosis, 267. *See also* Osteonecrosis
Axillary nerve, injury to, 135-136, 181-182, 210, 552
risk of, 184-185
Axillary neuropathy, 181
Axioscapular muscles, 13, 18
Axon reflexes, histamine testing of, 392

B

Bag of bones fracture, 358
Bankart lesions, 103, 502
arthroscopic treatment of, 488, 502
bony, 83, 131, 481
concomitant bony, 104
evaluation under anesthesia for, 107
glenoid depth and, 15
joint stability and, 17, 19, 91-92
radiographic evaluation of, 105, 487
revision surgery and, 136
soft tissue, 83
in the throwing athlete, 123
Bankart repair
arthroscopic, 14, 74-75, 74*f*, 483, 488, 502
long-term follow-up to, 134
open, 75-76, 86, 87, 95
surgical approach to, 479
technique in, 482
T-plasty modification of, 133
Bankart tears, 71, 130
Basal coronoid fractures, 382-383
Belly press test, 87
Biceps, 43-44
long head of, 6-7, 17-18
full-thickness tears and, 173
subluxation or dislocation, 177
tears of, 177, 471
tendinopathy, 181
Bicipital groove, 6, 145
Bidirectional instability, 129
Biofeedback training, 19
Blackburn position, 42
Blood supply
to humeral head, 59
to proximal humerus, 267
Bone deficiency in recurrent anterior shoulder instability, 86, 87
Bone scan for acromioclavicular joint resection, 519
Brachial neurapraxia, 553
Brachial plexopathy, 553

Brachial plexus, 397
injuries in adults, 387-395, 552
amputation, 395
anatomy, 387-388
ancillary diagnostic studies in evaluation of closed injuries, 391-392
infraclavicular, 390
mechanisms of injury
burners, 390-391
open, 390-391
postanesthetic paralysis, 391
radiation, 391
stingers, 390-391
pain management, 394-395
peripheral reconstruction of limb, 393-394
supraclavicular
clinical examination, 388-389
common patterns of neurologic loss, 389-390
surgical treatment, neurologic reconstruction, 392-393
injuries to, 227
neuropathy, 439
Bristow procedure, 132, 280, 482
Bryan-Morrey approach to treating fractures of distal humerus, 358-359
Buntline half hitch, 109
Burners, 390-391
Burr posterior (cutting block) technique, 512
Bursa, 30-31
scapulothoracic, 10
subacromial, 7, 30, 67
subscapularis, 10
Bursectomy, 253, 511
Bursoscopy, 497

C

Calcific tendinitis, 164
arthroscopic treatment of, 533-536
Calcium pyrophosphate dihydrate depositions, 525
Cannulated bioabsorbable implants in arthroscopic labral repair, 105
Capacious inferior pouch, 92
Capitellum, fracture of, 345
Capsular acromioclavicular ligaments, 10
Capsular constraint mechanism, 15
Capsular contracture, 214
Capsular detachment in elbow stiffness, 327
Capsular insufficiency, 13
Capsular laxity, 67, 104, 106, 481
range of, 20
Capsular lesions, 20
Capsular ligament, 10
Capsular reduction by radiothermal shrinkage, 87
Capsular shift, 99
Capsular shrinkage, 95, 99, 124, 130
Capsular stretch, 19
Capsular tensioning, 482
Capsulectomy in elbow stiffness, 327
Capsulolabral augmentation, 99
Capsulolabral complex, 108

Capsulolabral repair, 19
Capsulolabral separation, 103
Capsuloligamentous laxity, 67
Capsuloligamentous restraints, 92
Capsuloligamentous structures, 15, 15*f*, 16*t*
Capsulorrhaphy, 131
    arthropathy, 87
    arthroscopic staple, 86, 131
    hardware during, 280
    posterior, 98
    suture, 104, 553-554
    thermal, 99, 131, 554
Capsulotomy in elbow stiffness, 327
Captured shoulder, 185
Carpal tunnel syndrome, 399
Carpal tunnel test, 306
Caspari suture punch, 474, 475*f*
Caspari transglenoid multiple suture
    technique, 497
Cathepsin D, 25, 27*f*
Cementing techniques, 56
Cementless tissue ingrowth, 57
Cerebral palsy, 325
Cervical radiculopathies, 171, 305, 397, 399
Cervical scoliosis, 391
Cervical spine disease, 181
Cervical spondylosis, 134
Cheilectomy, arthroscopic, 263
Chondrocalcinosis, 271, 534
Chondrocyte toxicity, 271
Chondroitin sulfate, 24
Chronic anterior dislocations, 77-79, 77*f*
Chronic elbow instability, 321
Circle concept
    of joint stability, 66
    of shoulder instability, 99
Circumflex artery, anterior, 267
    anterolateral branch of, 4
Classic impingement, 519
Clavicle, 9, 37, 388
Clavicular fractures, 219
    anatomy, 219-220, 220*f*
    classification, 220-221
    complications
        malunion, 224
        neurovascular injuries, 224
        nonunion, 223
        posttraumatic arthritis, 224
    etiology and epidemiology, 220, 220*f*
    ipsilateral, 227
    physical examination, 221
    radiologic evaluation of, 221
    treatment and results, 221-223, 222*f*, 223*f*
Clavicular shortening, 224
Clinical guidelines for shoulder pain, 443-
    462, 444*f*
    development and practice, 444-445
    development of, 443
    future, 445
Closed-chain axial loading for strengthen-
    ing, 405
    aquatic therapy, 406-407
    exercises in, 405*f*, 406
    power development, 407
    rotator cuff activation, 405*f*, 406, 408*f*
    scapular control, 405-406, 406*f*, 407*f*

Closed head trauma, 228
Closed reduction, malunions after, 275
Coding, 412
    American Academy of Orthopaedic
        Surgeons role in, 412
    for arthroscopic procedures, 414-415
    Centers for Medicare and Medicaid
        Services and, 411-412
    compliance and, 413-414
    for consultations, 413-414
    Current Procedural Terminology in, 411,
        412-413
    E/M guidelines in, 418
    handling denials, 413
    *International Classification of Diseases,
        Ninth Revision, Clinical Modification*
        and, 411
    modifiers in, 416-418
    new development in, 412
    precertification, 413
    proper billing procedures, 413
    for unlisted procedures, 415-416
Codman exercises, full-thickness tear repair
    and, 174
Codman's paradox, 37
Collagenase injection, 33
Collagen shortening, pathophysiology of,
    501
Compartment syndromes of deltoid, 185
Compass Hinge in treating posttraumatic
    arthritis of elbow, 337
Complex regional pain syndrome, 185
Compliance, coding and, 413-414
Component loosening, 59
    as complication following shoulder
        arthroplasty, 285-286
Comprehensive Classification of Fractures,
    357
Comprehensive Long Bone Classification
    systems, 210
Compression brachial plexopathy, 224
Compression neuropathy, 304
Computed tomography arthrography
    for medial collateral ligament tear, 302
    for valgus instability, 320
Computed tomography imaging
    of anterior glenohumeral ligament, 106
    of brachial plexus injuries, 392
    of calcific tendinitis, 534
    of coronoid fractures, 379
    of distal humerus fractures, 357
    of elbow, 326
    of full-thickness tears, 171
    of inflammatory arthritis, 252
    of metal implants, 132, 132*f*
    in morphometric analysis, 13
    of multidirectional shoulder instability,
        94
    of proximal humeral fractures, 211
    of radial head fractures, 344
    of repair failure, 183
    of rotator cuff repair, 472
    of soft-tissue injuries, 276
    of thoracic outlet syndrome, 399
Concavity-compression, 65, 92
Concentric reaming, 57

Conoid ligament, 10
Concomitant rotator cuff injury, 481
Congenital instability, 97
Conservative therapy for thoracic outlet
    syndrome, 400
Constant Score, 428
Constrained total shoulder arthroplasty,
    200-201
Construct validity, 426
Consultations, coding for, 413-414
Content validity, 426
Continuous passive motion, 45
    elbow stiffness and, 328-329
    full-thickness tear repair and, 174
Contralateral leg/trunk diagonal patterns,
    403, 404*f*
Convergent validity, 426
Coonrad-Morrey implant for rheumatoid
    arthritis in elbow, 335, 336*f*
Coplaning, 522-523
Coracoacromial arch, 7, 8, 23
    maintaining integrity of, 202
Coracoacromial ligaments, 7, 28, 30, 31, 227
    fibrous insertion of, 8
    hypertrophy of, 149
    role of, in pain recognition associated
        with rotator cuff disease, 30
Coracobrachialis tendons, 7
Coracoclavicular fixation, 222, 223*f*
Coracoclavicular ligaments, 7, 10, 219
    disruption of, 231
    injury to, 229
Coracohumeral ligaments, 5, 6, 7, 16*t*
    origin of, 144
Coracoid fracture, 229-230
Coracoid impingement, 98
Coracoid process, 7
    fractures of, 228
Core decompression for osteonecrosis and
    other noninflammatory degenerative
    diseases, 268
Coronal z-lengthening, 290
Coronoid fractures, 313, 317, 369, 379-383
    basal coronoid fractures, 382-383
    classification, 379
    coronoid tip fractures, 379-380
        anteromedial, 380-382, 380*f*, 381*f*,
            382*f*
    evaluation, 379, 380*f*
    postoperative management, 383
    treatment of, 372-374, 373*f*, 374*f*
Coronoid fragments, 345
Corticosteroids
    for rheumatoid arthritis in elbow, 333
    for rotator cuff disease, 158
Costoclavicular ligaments, 10, 397
Counterforce bracing for lateral epicondyli-
    tis, 299-300
Crank test, 68
Crepitus, 221, 259
Crocket hook in anterior glenohumeral
    reconstruction, 108, 110*f*
Cross-arm adduction test, 519
Crystal-induced arthropathy, 197
Cubital tunnel syndrome, 338

Cyclooxygenase-II inhibitors for rheumatoid arthritis in elbow, 333
Cytokine activity, 24-25

D

Dead-arm syndrome, 71-72, 93, 130, 399, 543
Débridement
    arthroscopic, 526
        with or without acromioplasty, 168
        for osteoarthritis, 338
        for posttraumatic arthritis of elbow, 336
        synovial, 526, 529
Decompression. *See* Arthroscopic subacromial decompression
Deep infection, 552
Degenerative failures, 30
Degenerative glenohumeral arthritis, 134-135
Deltoid muscle, 8, 471
    atrophy of, 125
    compartment syndromes of, 185
    detachment of, 186
        rotator cuff surgery and, 184
    maintaining integrity of, 202
    preservation of function in, 281
    rotator cuff disease and, 148
    as stability factor, 17
Deltoid tendon, 8
Denials, coding and, 413
Dermatan sulfate, 24
Derotational osteotomy of the humerus, 19
Diagnostic arthroscopy for anterior glenohumeral ligament, 106
Diaphyseal fractures of humerus, 237-245
    associated injuries, 237
    complex fractures, 243
    epidemiology, 237
    nonsurgical treatment for, 237-239, 238f, 239f
        contraindications to functional bracing, 237-239
        intramedullary fixation, 240-242
        plate and screw fixation, 241f, 242
        surgical exposures, 241f, 242-243
        technique of functional bracing, 239, 239f
    nonunion, 243-245, 244f
    periprosthetic fractures, 243
    surgical treatment, 239, 240f
Diaphysis, pathologic lesions of, 240f, 241-242
Digital ischemia, 124
Digital plethysmography in diagnosing thoracic outlet syndrome, 399
Digital vessel thrombosis, 124
Disabilities of the Arm, Shoulder and Hand (DASH) questionnaire, 423, 428-429
Dislocation arthropathy, 280
Dislocations
    anterior sternoclavicular, 222-223
    posterior sternoclavicular, 223, 224
Distal biceps injuries, 306
Distal clavicle, full-thickness tears and, 172-173, 174f

Distal clavicle excision, 530
Distal clavicle resection
    coplaning and, 186-187
    of shoulder arthroplasty, 289
Dome acromioplasty, 186
Doppler ultrasonography in diagnosing thoracic outlet syndrome, 399
Double crush syndrome, 399
Drawer test, 320
Drive-through sign, 85, 106
Drop sign, 42
Dumps exercises, 406, 407f
Duncan loop in anterior glenohumeral reconstruction, 109, 111f
Dynamic Joint Distractor in treating posttraumatic arthritis of elbow, 336-337
Dysplastic glenoid, 496
Dystrophic calcification, 534

E

Effort thrombosis, 399-400
Ehlers-Danlos syndrome, 91, 132-133
Elbow. *See also* Total elbow arthroplasty
    acute dislocation of, evaluation of, 315-317, 315f
    acute instability of, 313-318
    anterior pain, 305-306
        distal biceps injuries, 306
        pronator teres syndrome, 305-306
    lateral pain in
        epicondylitis, 298-300, 299ft
        osteochondritis dissecans, 298
        radial nerve entrapment, 300
        radiocapitellar overload syndrome, 300
    medial pain in
        collateral ligament injuries
            in adults, 301-304, 302f, 303f, 304f
            in children, 301
        epicondylitis, 300-301
    outcomes analysis in, 421-429
    posterior, 306
        posteromedial impingement/valgus extension overload syndrome, 306-308, 306f, 307f
        stress fractures, 307f, 308
Elbow arthritis, 333-339
    osteoarthritis, 338
        treatment, 338-339
    posttraumatic, 336
        treatment, 336-338
    rheumatoid arthritis as cause of, 333
        nonsurgical treatment, 333-334
        surgical treatment, 334-335
Elbow extension and flexion, 389
Elbow instability, 313-321
    acute, 313-318
        etiology and mechanism of elbow dislocation and fracture-dislocation, 314-315, 314f, 315t
        evaluation, 315-317, 315f, 316f
        treatment, 317-318
    chronic, 321
    constraints to, 313, 314f

recurrent, 318
    evaluation, 318-320, 319f, 320f
    treatment, 320-321, 320f
Elbow stability, assessing, 326
Elbow stiffness, 325-330
    classification, 325
        extrinsic contracture, 325
    etiology, 325
    evaluation, 325-327
    intrinsic contracture, 325
    nonsurgical treatment, 326f, 327
    surgical treatment: extrinsic contracture
        arthroscopic release, 327-328
        open capsular release, 327f, 328, 328f
        postoperative therapy, 328-329, 329f
    surgical treatment: intrinsic contracture, 329-330, 330f
Electrodiagnosis
    of brachial plexus injuries, 392
    of neurologic defects, 211
    of thoracic outlet syndrome, 400
Electromagnetic tracking technology, 39
Electromyography (EMG), 26, 39-40
    correlation of, for rotator cuff, 41-43, 42f, 43f, 44f
Epicondylitis
    lateral, 298-300, 299ft
        nonsurgical treatment of, 299-300
        surgical treatment of, 300
    medial, 300-301
Epiphyseal dysplasias, 257
ETAC (Electrothermally Assisted Capsulorrhaphy), 95
Ewald system of elbow function, 428
Examination under anesthesia
    for anterior glenohumeral ligament, 106, 107
    for recurrent anterior shoulder instability, 85
Exercise machines in shoulder rehabilitation, 407
Exercise therapy for acute anterior dislocation, 73-74, 74f
Extended Kocher approach in surgery for fracture of distal humerus, 359
Extensor carpi radialis brevis, lateral epicondylitis and, 299
External impingement, 149-150
External rotation lag sign, 42, 43f
Extracapsular scarring, 134, 134f

F

Facial anhidrosis, 552
Fasciculus obliquus, 5, 144
Fibromyalgia
    alternative approaches, 462
    definition of problem, 461-462
    expected clinical results, 462
    recommendations, 462
    rehabilitation, 462
Ficat-Arlet classification of osteonecrosis, 267-268, 270f
Finite joint volume, 65
First rib fractures, 228

Fixed-angle plate and screw devices, for proximal humeral fractures, 212-213
Floating shoulder, 227, 229, 231
    surgical indications for, 230
Fluoroscopy to evaluate implant version and loosening, 289
Four-part malunions, 277
Fracture-dislocations, malunions of, 277
Fractures
    articular segment, 213
    clavicular, 219
        anatomy, 219-220, 220*f*
        classification, 220-221
        complications, 223, 224
        etiology and epidemiology, 220, 220*f*
        ipsilateral, 227
        physical examination, 221
        radiologic evaluation of, 221
        treatment and results, 221-223, 222*f*, 223*f*
    as complication following shoulder arthroplasty, 286-287, 288*f*, 289*f*
    diaphyseal, of humerus, 237-245
        associated injuries, 237
        complex fractures, 243
        epidemiology, 237
        nonsurgical treatment for, 237-243, 238*f*, 239*f*, 241*f*
        nonunion, 243-245, 244*f*
        periprosthetic fractures, 243
        surgical treatment, 239, 240*f*
    distal humerus, 357-365
        evaluation, 357-358
        postoperative care, 363-364
        results and complications, 364-365
        surgical treatment, 358-363, 360*f*
    Monteggia, 369, 371-372, 372*f*
    radial head, 317-318, 343-352, 374
    scapular, 227-235, 229*f*, 230*f*, 231*f*, 232*f*, 233*f*, 234*f*, 235*f*
Friction neuropathy, 304-305
Frozen shoulder, 44, 183, 519
    alternative approaches, 458
    definition of problem, 458
    expected clinical results, 458
    recommendations, 458
Functional bracing, 237
    contraindications to, 237-239
    technique of, 239, 239*f*
Functional restoration, 59

G

Ganglion cysts, 121
Gaucher's disease, 267, 270-271
Generic health instruments, 422, 423*f*
Glenohumeral arthritis, 50, 98, 164, 181, 183, 230, 525
    associated with rotator cuff pathology, 197
Glenohumeral arthrodesis, 200, 253
Glenohumeral arthrography for arthroscopic subacromial decompression, 508

Glenohumeral arthroplasty
    glenoid component
        kinematics, 57-58, 58*f*
        radiolucent line and glenoid loosening, 58
        size and shape, 56-57
    goal of, 49
    humeral component, 52-54, 54*f*, 55*f*
        fixation, 55-56, 56*f*
        neck-shaft angle, 54-55, 55*f*
    results of prosthetic, 58-59
Glenohumeral index, 14
Glenohumeral instability, 5, 13-20, 65-69, 123, 181
    alternative approaches, 460
    anatomic concerns of the labrum, 130-131
    character of, 129-130
    classification of, 66
    clinical assessment of, 66
        acute dislocation, 66
        glenohumeral instability tests, 68
        glenohumeral laxity tests, 67
        recurrent instability, 66-67
    definition of problem, 459
    dynamic stability factors, 17
        deltoid muscle, 17
        long head of the biceps, 17-18
        proprioception, 18-19
        rotator cuff, 17
        scapular rotators, 18
    effect of structural lesions on
        Bankart lesions, 19
        capsular lesions, 20
        fatigue or weakness of the scapular rotators, 20
        lesions of the superior labrum, 19-20
        rotator cuff lesions, 20
        skeletal lesions, 19
    evaluation, 459-460
    expected clinical results, 460
    imaging of, 68
        magnetic resonance arthrography, 69
        magnetic resonance imaging, 68
        special views, 68
    implant complications, 132
    management of, 123
    open versus arthroscopic repair, 131
    other diagnoses, 460
    pathophysiology of, 65-66
    recurrence, 134-136
        arthritis, 134-135
        comorbidities leading to perceived failure, 134
        failure, 133-134
        infection, 136
        nerve injuries, 135-136
        reinjury, 132-133
        stiffness, 134
    rehabilitation errors, 132, 133*t*
    results of revision surgery, 136-137
    static stability factors
        adhesion-cohesion, 17
        articular conformity, 13-14, 14*f*
        capsuloligamentous structures, 15, 15*f*, 16*t*

glenoid labrum, 14-15
negative intra-articular pressure, 17
orientation of articular surfaces, 13
rotator cuff, 17
    surgical selection, 130
    technique-specific complications, 131
Glenohumeral instability tests, 68
Glenohumeral interactive factors, 65
Glenohumeral joint, 3, 13, 37, 145
    abnormalities, 176
    anatomy of, 49
    arthrodesis of, 279
    arthroscopy for, 182
        repair of full-thickness rotator cuff tears, 176
    biomechanics of, 50-51
        articular conformity, 51, 52*f*
        articular constraint, 51-52, 52*f*
        glenohumeral translations, 52, 53*f*
    capsule, 6
    glenohumeral ligaments in, 4-5
    glenoid erosion in arthritic, 50
    glenoid labrum in, 4
    long head of the biceps tendon in, 6-7
    manifestations of rheumatoid arthritis in, 251
    osseous structures in, 3-4
    rotator interval in, 5-6, 6*f*
    uniqueness of, 65
Glenohumeral kinematics, relationship between rotator cuff disease and, 156
Glenohumeral laxity, posterior, 123
Glenohumeral laxity tests, 67
Glenohumeral ligaments, 4-5, 15, 15*f*
    anterior
        arthroscopic reconstruction of, 103-112
            associated pathoanatomy, 103
            patient selection, 105-106
            with suture anchors, 106-112, 107*f*, 108*f*, 109*f*, 110*f*, 112*f*
        postoperative rehabilitation, 112
    humeral avulsion of, 20, 83, 85, 131
    static properties of, 65
Glenohumeral offset, lateral, 50, 50*f*
Glenohumeral reconstruction, anterior, 108-109, 110*f*
Glenohumeral rhythm, 38
Glenohumeral rotation, 15
Glenohumeral stability, 13, 65
Glenoid
    anteroposterior dimension of, 3
    articular surfaces of, 3
    cartilage of, 14
    dysplastic, 496
    osteoarthritic changes in, 268
    osteometry of, 19
    size and shape of, 50, 50*f*
    subchondral bone of, 50
    superoinferior parameters of, 3
Glenoid component failure, 57, 58
Glenoid concavity, 65, 67
Glenoid deficiency, anterior, 78
Glenoid depth, 51
Glenoid dysplasia, 19

Glenoid erosion in arthritic glenohumeral joints, 50
Glenoid fossa fractures, 229, 231-233, 232f, 233f, 234f, 235f
Glenoid hypoplasia, 97, 98
Glenoid labrum, 4, 14-15, 51, 103
    anatomic concerns of, 130-131
Glenoid lesion, 106
Glenoid loosening, 58, 262-263
Glenoid lucent lines, 262-263
Glenoid neck fracture, posterior, 131
Glenoid offset, 50, 50f
Glenoid opening wedge osteotomy, 19
Glenoid osteotomy, 98, 130
Glenoid resurfacing, 262
Glenoid retroversion, 19, 97
Glenoid rim fracture, 14, 496
Glenoid subchondral plate thickness, 4
Glenoplasty, 98
Global instability, soft-tissue reconstruction for, 94-95
Global shoulder laxity, 91
Glucocerebroside hydrolase, deficiency in, 270
Glycosaminoglycans, 24
Gout, 257, 525
Granuloma formation, 132
Greater tuberosity malunions, 276
Gunshot wounds, low-velocity, 393

H

HAGL (humeral avulsion of the glenohumeral ligaments) lesion, 83, 85, 131
Hawkins impingement sign, 508
    of partial-thickness rotator cuff tears, 164
Hawkins test, 67
Hematomas, postoperative, 136
Hemiarthroplasty, 58, 59, 79, 193, 201-203, 254
    for cuff tear arthropathy, 153
    humeral, 78
    for osteoarthritis, 57
    for osteonecrosis and other noninflammatory degenerative diseases, 268
    outcome following, 56-57
    postoperative rehabilitation, 279
    for progressive glenoid arthritis, 290
    for proximal humeral malunions, 278
Hemidiaphragm, paralysis of, 552
Hemochromatosis, 271
Hemopneumothorax, 227
Heterotopic ossification, 534
    examination of elbow for, 326-327
Hill-Sachs humeral head defect, 78
Hill-Sachs lesions, 19, 68, 78, 83, 94, 105, 106, 481, 487
    engaging, 83, 87
    nonengaging, 83, 85
Histamine testing of axon reflexes, 392
Hodgkin's disease, 553
Horii circle, 314, 314f
Hornblower's sign, 42-43
Horner's syndrome, 388, 438, 552

Hotchkiss fractures, management of
    type I, 345-346
    type II, 346-347, 346f, 347f
    type III, 347-348, 347f, 348f
Human experimental studies of the rotator cuff, 26-27, 28f
Humeral articular lesions, 19
Humeral avulsion of the glenohumeral ligaments, 20, 83, 85
Humeral circumflex artery
    anterior, 209
        ascending branch of, 59
    posterior, 209
        compression of, 125
        subclavian arteriography of, 125
Humeral head. *See also* Humerus
    articular surface area of, 14
    blood supply to, 59
    center, 3
    inclination, 3
    malposition of, 54
    offset, retroversion, and height, 49, 51f
    radius, 3
    replacement, 213, 213f, 263, 278-279, 278f
        total shoulder replacement versus, 262
    size and shape of, 49, 49t, 50f
    thickness, 3
    translations, 41
    vascularization of, 4
Humeral hemiarthroplasty, 78
Humeral neck-shaft angle, 49
Humeral osteotomy, 99, 130
Humeral retroversion, 19, 97
Humeral version, 55
Humeroscapular rhythm, 38
Humerothoracic motion, 39
Humerus, 37. *See also* Diaphyseal fractures of humerus; Humeral head; Proximal humerus
    derotational osteotomy of, 19
    diaphyseal fractures of, 237-245
    length of, 3
    nonunion of, 237, 243-245, 244f
Hyperabduction syndrome, 124
Hypertrophic nonunions, 243-244
Hypertrophic pulmonary osteoarthropathy, 553
Hypertrophy, isolated bursal, 253
Hypoplasia, 94

I

Iatrogenic anterior instability, 98
Idiopathic brachial plexitis, 439
Imaging. *See also* Computed tomography; Magnetic resonance arthrography; Magnetic resonance imaging; Radiographic evaluation
Immunosuppressive agents, for rheumatoid arthritis in elbow, 333
Impingement. *See also* Internal impingement
    classic, 519
    coracoid, 98

external, 149-150
internal, 119-121, 121f
internal glenoid, 51
posterior, 150
posterior internal, 119
posterosuperior glenoid, 548
rotator cuff, 287-289, 289t, 290ft
subacromial, 214
subcoracoid, 473, 519
Impingement syndrome, 30, 134, 149, 185
    subacromial, 473
Impingement tests, 94
Implant arthroplasty, 253
Implant loosening as complication following shoulder arthroplasty, 285-286
Implant wear as complication following shoulder arthroplasty, 286, 287f
Indomethacin in postoperative management of radial head fractures, 349
Infection
    after arthroscopic repairs, 188
    after glenohumeral instability, 136
    after rotator cuff surgery, 187-188
    after shoulder arthroplasty, 287
    deep, 552
    revision for, 291
Inferior capsular redundancy, 92
Inferior glenohumeral ligament, 4, 5, 103, 108-109
Inferior instability, 67
    cause of, 286
    revision surgery for, 290
Inferior laxity, 495-496
Inflammatory arthritis, 525-527
    of the shoulder, 251-255
        clinical evaluation, 252
        incidence, 251
        nonsurgical treatment of, 252
        pathoanatomy, 251-252
        pathogenesis, 251
        pathophysiology, 251
        results, 254-255, 255t
        surgical treatment of, 253-254
Inflammatory arthropathy, 325
Infraclavicular brachial plexus injuries, 171
Infraclavicular injuries, 390
    mechanisms of injury
        burners, 390-391
        open, 390-391
        postanesthetic paralysis, 391
        radiation, 391
        stingers, 390-391
Infraspinatus, 144, 147
Infraspinatus tendon, 8, 17, 26, 41
    degeneration in, 8
Infusion catheters, 513-514
Instability. *See also* Elbow instability; Glenohumeral instability; Multidirectional instability; Shoulder instability; Valgus instability
    acute valgus, 313
    anterior, 67
    atraumatic sternoclavicular, 220
    bidirectional, 129
    chronic elbow, 321

as complication following shoulder arthroplasty, 286, 286*t*, 287*f*
congenital, 97
defined, 13
global, 94-95
inferior, 67, 286, 290
joint, 258
multidirectional, 91-96
posterior, 67, 96-100, 97*t*
cause of, 286
revision surgery for, 290
posterolateral rotatory, 297, 316, 379
provocative testing for, 105
recurrent anterior shoulder, 83-87
recurrent elbow, 318
refractory, 129
revision surgery for, 290-291
superior, 286, 290
in throwing athlete, 123-124
varus-posteromedial rotatory, 313
volitional, 92
voluntary, 96, 130
Interior glenohumeral ligament complex, 16*t*
Interleukin-1, 526
Interleukin-1β, 25, 27*f*
Internal glenoid impingement, 51
Internal impingement, 31, 31*f*, 119, 150, 152
anterior, 150
in superior labrum anterior and posterior lesions, 558
in throwing athlete, 118-119, 120*f*
arthroscopic findings, 119-121, 121*f*
imaging, 119
physical examination, 119
treatment, 122, 123*f*
Internal impingement peel-back phenomenon, 120
Internal rotation lag sign, 42
Interposition arthroplasty
for elbow arthritis, 334
for osteoarthritis of elbow, 339
in treating elbow stiffness, 330
in treating posttraumatic arthritis of elbow, 336
Interscalene block anesthesia, 438, 552
Interscalene brachial plexus block, 435, 435*f*
administration, 434*t*, 435-437, 435*f*, 436*f*, 437*f*
complications and side effects, 437-438, 438t
determination of success, 439
intraoperative neurologic complications, 438-439
precautionary measures, 434*t*, 437
volume of anesthetic, 437
Intertubercular groove, 209
Intertubercular sulcus, 6
Intra-abdominal injuries, 228
Intra-articular fracture, 98
Intra-articular glenoid fracture, 229
Intra-articular lesions, 471
Intra-articular pathology, rotator cuff problems and, 182
Intra-articular pressure, 17
Intra-articular steroid injections for post-capsulorrhaphy arthritis, 280

Intramedullary fixation, 240-242, 240*f*
Intramedullary rod, placement of, 242
Intraosseous anastomosis, 59
In vitro studies of the rotator cuff, 26-27
In vivo studies
of the rotator cuff, 26, 28*f*
of shoulder motion, 37
Iontophoresis for nonsurgical management of rotator cuff disease, 159
Ipsilateral clavicle fractures, 227
Ipsilateral leg/trunk extensions, 403, 404*f*
Ipsilateral rib fracture, 227
Isolated bursal hypertrophy, 253
Isolated labral deficiency, 65

J

Jerk test, 68
Jobe position, 42
Jobe sign, 164
Joint instability, secondary osteoarthritis and, 258
Joint laxity, assessment of, 105
Joint replacement arthroplasty, for elbow arthritis, 334-335, 335*f*
Joint-specific outcomes instruments, 422, 424*f*

K

Kinematics, 57-58, 58*f*, 147
of clinical conditions, 44-45
defined, 37
glenohumeral, 156
Kinesiology
defined, 37
of sports, 45
Kinetic energy, 148
Knot typing in anterior glenohumeral reconstruction, 109
Kocher's interval, 344

L

Labral, pathology of, and rotator cuff problems, 182
Labral deficiency, isolated, 65
Labral detachment, 92
Labral tears, 181, 471
in throwing athlete, 117
Lachman test, 320
LACS (Laser Assisted Capsular Shift), 95
Langer's lines, 222
Latarjet procedure, 86, 87
Lateral collateral ligament
complex, 297
disruption of, 343, 344
injuries, 379
Lateral pivot-shift test of the elbow, 297, 319
for acute elbow dislocation, 316
Lateral scapular spine, fracture of, 228-229
Lateral ulnar collateral ligament
iatrogenic injury to, 344
as stabilizer against posterolateral rotational instability, 343-344

Laxity
capsular, 104, 106
defined, 13
global shoulder, 91
range of capsular, 20
Lesser tuberosity malunions, 276-277
Lift-off test, 87
Ligamentotaxis, 231
Light bulb sign, 76
Likert scales, 424
Limb-specific outcomes instruments, 422-423
Linked elbow prostheses for fractures of distal humerus, 357-365
Lister's tubercle, 349
Load-and-shift test, 84, 98
Localized nontraumatic neuropathy, 439
Locking intramedullary rods, 240
Long head of biceps tendon, rotator cuff surgery and, 182
Long head of biceps tenotomy, 187
Low-velocity gunshot wounds, 393
Lumbar lift-off test, 73
Luxatio erecta, 77

M

Magnetic resonance arthrography
for anterior labral pathology, 85
for glenohumeral instability, 69
for quadrilateral space syndrome, 124*f*, 125
for recurrent anterior shoulder instability, 85
Magnetic resonance imaging
for acromioclavicular joint resection, 519
for anterior glenohumeral ligament, 106
for arthroscopic subacromial decompression, 508, 509
for brachial plexus injuries, 392
for calcific tendinitis, 533, 534
for elbow, 326
for full-thickness tears, 171, 175
for glenohumeral instability, 68
for inflammatory arthritis, 252
for internal impingement, 119
for lateral epicondylitis, 299
for medial collateral ligament tear, 302
for multidirectional instability, 94, 497
for neurologic diagnosis, 181, 182
for osteochondritis dissecans, 298
for osteonecrosis, 267
for partial-thickness rotator cuff tears, 165
for proximal humeral fracture, 211
for recurrent shoulder instability, 85
for repair failure, 183
for rotator cuff disease, 155
for rotator cuff integrity, 77
for rotator cuff repair, 472
for shoulder dislocations, 487
for shoulder ganglion cysts, 539, 540-541, 540*f*
for soft-tissue injuries, 276
for thoracic outlet syndrome, 399
for valgus instability, 320

Magnuson-Stack procedure, 130, 482
Malunions, 224
    as complication of radial head fractures,
        351
    of fracture-dislocation, 277
    greater tuberosity, 276
    lesser tuberosity, 276-277
    of middle-third fractures, 224
    surgical neck, 277
    three- and four-part, 277
Marfan's syndrome, 91
Mason-Allen configuration, 173
Matrix metalloprotease-1, 25, 27*f*
Mayfield spiral fracture, 317
Mayo Elbow Performance Score, 338, 428
McLaughlin lesion, 77, 80
McLaughlin procedure, 77, 79
Medial collateral ligament, 297
    disruption of, 343, 344
    incomplete healing of, 297
    injuries in adults, 301-304, 302*f*, 303*f*,
        304*f*
        clinical presentation, 301-302, 302*f*
        evaluation of treatment, 303-304,
            305*f*
        imaging, 302, 302*f*
        postoperative management, 303
        reconstruction, 302-303, 303*f*, 304*f*
    physeal injuries in children and, 301
Medullary fixation, for proximal humeral
    fractures, 212-213
Metallic radial head arthroplasty, 352
Metallic staples, in arthroscopic labral
    repair, 104
Metaphyseal comminution, 212
Methylmethacrylate, 57
Microtraumatic injuries to the shoulder, 118
Middle glenohumeral ligament, 4-5, 16*t*
Middle-third fractures, malunion of, 224
Midglenoid transverse CT scan, 13
Milking maneuver, 320
Milwaukee shoulder syndrome/crystal-
    associated arthritis, 197, 198
Modified Bristow procedure, 130
Modifiers in coding, 416-418
Monteggia fracture-dislocations, 369-370
    treatment of, 371-372, 372*f*
Moving valgus stress test, 320, 320*f*
Multidirectional instability (MDI), 91-96,
    129, 130, 132, 133, 134, 258, 495
    arthroscopic pancapsular plication for,
        495-499
        clinical findings, 495-496
        etiology, 495
        nonsurgical management, 496
        pathophysiology, 496
        surgical management, 496-499, 497*f*,
            498*f*
    arthroscopy of shoulder with, 496
    clinical presentation
        history, 93
        physical examination, 93-94
        radiographic studies, 94
    definition and classification, 91-92
    etiology, 92-93
    failed stabilization of, 137

    nonsurgical management of, 94
    posttraumatic arthritis and, 280
    surgical management
        arthroscopic techniques, 95-96
        open techniques, 94-95
    treating, 131
Multiplane fracture, 359
Multiple neuritis, 439
Musculocutaneous nerve, injury to, 136
Myofascial balancing, preservation of, 281
Myositis ossificans, 279

N

Narrow-diameter (or flexible)
    intramedullary rods, 240
Neck-shaft angle, 3, 49
Neer classification systems, 210
Neer modification, 77
Neer position, 145, 150
Neer's impingement sign, 158, 508
    of partial-thickness rotator cuff tears,
        164
Neer's impingement test, 67, 508
Negative intra-articular pressure, 17
Nerve injuries
    antebrachial cutaneous, 303
    as complication following shoulder
        arthroplasty, 287
    glenohumeral instability and, 135-136
    peripheral, 210
    rotator cuff surgery and, 184-185
Nerve transfer techniques for treating
    brachial plexus injuries, 393
Neuralgic amyotrophy, 439
Neurapraxia as complication following
    shoulder arthroplasty, 287
Neurologic diagnosis of rotator cuff surgery
    complications, 181-182
Neuropathy, suprascapular, 181
Neurovascular injuries, clavicle fractures
    and, 224
Non-Hodgkin's lymphoma, 254
Noninflammatory arthritis, 526, 527-528,
    527*ft*
Noninflammatory osteoarthritis, 526
Nonsteroidal anti-inflammatory drugs
    for nonsurgical management of rotator
        cuff disease, 159
    for postcapsulorrhaphy arthritis, 280
    for proximal humeral malunions, 277
    for rheumatoid arthritis in elbow, 333
    for shoulder range of motion, 268
Nonsurgical management
    of calcific tendinitis, 534
    of clavicle shaft fractures, 221-222
    of cuff tear arthropathy, 200
    of diaphyseal fractures of humerus, 237-
        239, 238*f*, 239*f*
    of elbow stiffness, 326*f*, 327
    of inflammatory arthritis of the
        shoulder, 252
    of multidirectional instability, 94, 496
    of osteoarthritis, 260-261
    of osteochondritis dissecans, 298

    of postcapsulorrhaphy arthritis, 280-281
    of posterior shoulder instability, 98
    of posteromedial impingement/valgus
        extension overload syndrome,
        307-308
    of proximal humeral fractures, 211
    of proximal humeral malunions, 277
    of recurrent anterior dislocations,
        481-482
    of rotator cuff disease, 157-160
    of scapular fractures, 230-231
    of SLAP lesions in throwing athletes, 546
    of stress fractures, 308
Nonunions, 223
    atrophic, 223, 244-245
    as complication of clavicular fractures,
        223
    as complication of radial head fractures,
        351
    as complication of sternoclavicular joint
        fracture, 223
    of the humerus, 237, 243-245, 244*f*,
        364-365
    hypertrophic, 243-244
Nutritional supplements for osteoarthritis
    of shoulder, 260

O

Oblique stress fractures, 308
O'Brien cross-arm test, 105, 519, 544
Observer-based aggregate scoring systems,
    425
Ochronosis, 257
Olecranon
    fractures of, 318, 345, 369, 369*t*
    stress fractures of, 308
Olecranon osteotomy, 360-361
Open capsular release of extrinsic contrac-
    ture in elbow, 327*f*, 328, 328*f*
Open inferior capsular shift, 496
Open reduction and internal fixation, 212,
    222
    for Hotchkiss type II fractures, 346-347,
        346*f*, 347*f*
    for Hotchkiss type III fractures, 347-348,
        347*f*
    malunions after, 275
Open surgery repair. *See also* Surgical man-
    agement
    of anterior sternoclavicular dislocations,
        223
    of full-thickness rotator cuff tears
        complications and reoperations, 175,
            176*f*
        indications, 171
        postoperative support and rehabilita-
            tion, 174-175
        results and factors affecting
            outcome, 175
        surgical exposure, 171-174, 172*f*, 173*f*,
            174*f*, 175*f*
    of multidirectional instability, 94-95
    of partial-thickness rotator cuff tears,
        165

of posterior instability, 98-99, 99*t*
of recurrent anterior shoulder
  instability, 87
    versus arthroscopic repair, 85-86
of shoulder stabilization, 123-124
Open wedge osteotomy, 98
Osgood-Schlatter disease, 306
Osseous structures
  in glenohumeral joint, 3-4
  of subacromial space, 7
Ossification of acromion, 149
Osteoarthritis, 19, 56, 197, 199, 333. *See also*
  Arthritis; Rheumatoid arthritis
  biochemical events associated with, 526
  as complication of radial head fractures,
    351
  of elbow, 338
    treatment, 338-339
  hemiarthroplasty for, 57
  noninflammatory, 526
  secondary, joint instability and, 258
  of shoulder, 257-264, 258*t*
    clinical presentation, 258-259
    etiology, 257-258
    nonsurgical management of, 260
    pathophysiology, 257-258
    radiographic studies, 259-260, 259*f*,
      260*f*
    surgical management of, 260-261
      cemented versus cementless
        installation, 263
      complications, 263-264
      glenoid lucent lines and glenoid
        loosening, 262-263
      results and outcomes, 264
      soft-tissue imbalance, 263, 263*f*
      total shoulder replacement versus
        humeral head replacement, 262
Osteocapsular arthroplasty for osteoarthritis of elbow, 339
Osteochondritis dissecans, 298, 325
Osteochondromatosis, synovial, 271-272
Osteoid osteoma, 325
Osteolysis, acromioclavicular joint, 118
Osteonecrosis, 4, 59, 98, 257, 267, 275
  blood supply of proximal humerus, 267,
    268*f*
  as complication of radial head fractures,
    351
  etiology, 267, 269*f*
  four-part fractures and, 214
  management of, 268
    arthroplasty, 268-269
    core decompression for, 268
    open reduction and internal fixation,
      213
  posttraumatic, 269
  presentation and evaluation, 267
  radiographic classification of proximal
    humerus osteonecrosis, 267-268, 270*f*
  steroid-induced, 269
Osteopenia, 212, 253
Osteoporosis, 254
Osteotomy
  derotational, of the humerus, 19
  for fractures of distal humerus, 360, 360*f*

glenoid, 98
glenoid opening wedge, 19
humeral, 99
olecranon, 360-361
open wedge, 98
Outcomes analysis in shoulder and elbow,
  421-429
  application of, 423-424
    administration, 424
    assessment of pain, 424
    categorical rankings versus aggregate
      scores, 424-425, 425*t*, 426*t*
  assessing, 425
    reliability of, 426, 427*f*
    responsiveness, 426-427, 427*f*
    validity of, 426
  future developments, 429
  history, 421
  outcomes measures for, 421-422, 422*t*
    development of, 421
    disease-specific outcomes
      instruments, 423
    generic health instruments, 422, 423*f*,
      427
    joint-specific outcomes instruments,
      422, 424*f*, 425*t*, 426*t*, 427-428
    limb-specific outcomes instruments,
      422-423, 428-429
Outerbridge-Kashiwagi arthroplasty
  for elbow osteoarthritis, 339
  for elbow stiffness, 327-328
Overhead exercise test of Roos, 399
Overuse, 9, 29, 34, 34*f*, 117

P

Paget-Schroetter syndrome, 399
Paget's disease, 257
Pain
  AAOS clinical guideline on shoulder,
    456-462
  anterior elbow, 305-306
  assessment of, 424
  as indication for arthroscopic
    débridement, 528
  lateral elbow, 298-300, 299*ft*
  management of, for brachial plexus
    injuries, 394-395
  medial elbow, 300-304, 302*f*, 303*f*, 304*f*
  in rotator cuff disease, 30
  in shoulder rehabilitation, 407
  subacromial, 67
  superior shoulder, 67
Painful arc test, 67
Panner's disease, 298
Paralytic brachial neuritis, 439
Partial articular supraspinatus tendon avulsion lesion, 165*f*, 168
Passive joint positioning, range of rotational
  motion, 52
Passive range of motion, 45
  assessment of, in proximate humeral
    malunion, 275
Passive stretching, 73

Peel-back test for pathologic SLAP lesions,
  85
Periosteal elevator, 108
Peripheral nerves
  compression of, 397
  injuries to, 210
Periprosthetic fractures, 243
  treatment of, 287
Persistent instability, 129
Perthes lesion, 83
Phalen's test, 306
Phonophoresis for nonsurgical management
  of rotator cuff disease, 159
Physical examination
  for elbow, 326
  for internal impingement, 119
  for multidirectional shoulder instability,
    93-94
  for posterior shoulder instability, 97-98
  for thoracic outlet syndrome, 399
  for thrower's shoulder, 117-118
Physical therapy
  for elbow stiffness, 327
  for postcapsulorrhaphy arthritis, 280
  for proximal humeral malunions, 277
  for shoulder osteoarthritis, 260
  for shoulder range of motion, 268
Physiotherapy of inflammatory arthritis of
  the shoulder, 252
Pigmented villonodular synovitis, arthroscopic synovectomy for, 261
Pinch tuck stitch of anteroinferior capsule,
  497*f*, 498
Plate and screw fixation
  of diaphyseal fractures of the humerus,
    241*f*, 242
  of proximal humeral fixation, 211*f*, 212
Plyometrics, 73
  in shoulder rehabilitation, 407
Pneumomediastinum, 552
Pneumothorax, 131
Polyglyconate tacks, 132
  stabilization, 554
Polylactic acid implants, 132
Positional dislocator, 96-97
Postanesthetic paralysis from injury to
  brachial plexus, 391
Postcapsulorrhaphy arthritis
  etiology, 280
  evaluation, 280
  nonsurgical treatment, 280-281
  surgical treatment of, 281
  treatment, 280
Posterior capsular contracture, 66
Posterior capsular injury, 97
Posterior capsular pouch, volume of, 263
Posterior capsule, 16*t*
Posterior capsulorrhaphy, 98
Posterior drawer test, 67
Posterolateral rotation, 314
Posterolateral rotatory apprehension test, 319
Posterolateral rotatory drawer test, 319, 320
Posterolateral rotatory instability, 297, 379
  diagnosis of, 316
Posterolateral rotatory subluxation, 318-320,
  319*f*

Posteromedial impingement/valgus extension overload syndrome, 306-308, 306*f*,
307*f*
Posterosuperior glenoid impingement, 548
Postoperative fractures, treatment of, 287
Postoperative ulnar neuropathy, 326
Postreduction neurovascular check, 72
Posttraumatic arthritis, 224, 275-279
complications, 279, 279*f*
in elbow, 333, 336-338
etiology, 275
evaluation, 275-276
of fracture-dislocations, 277
nonsurgical management of, 277
surgical treatment of, 277-279, 278*f*
types of, 276-277
Posttraumatic brachial plexopathy, 389
Posttraumatic contractures, 375-376
Posttraumatic osteonecrosis, 269
Premature posttraumatic arthritis, 313
Press-fit fixation, 55-56
Press-fit glenoid prostheses, 57
Press-fit systems, 45
Primary glenohumeral osteoarthritis, 257, 258*t*
Pritchard system of elbow function, 428
Pritchard-Walker prosthesis in treating
posttraumatic arthritis of elbow, 337
Progressive glenoid arthritis, hemiarthro-
plasty for, 290
Prolotherapy for osteoarthritis of shoulder,
260
Pronator teres syndrome, 305-306
Prophylactic radiation, 376
Propionibacterium acnes as cause of infec-
tion following rotator cuff surgery, 187
Proprioception, 18-19
Proprioceptive receptors, 66
Proprioceptive training, 123
Prosthetic arthroplasty, 57
results of, 58-59
for shoulder osteoarthritis, 261
Prosthetic loosening as complication following shoulder arthroplasty, 285-286
Proteoglycans, 24
Provocative testing for instability, 105
Proximal humeral fractures, 209-214
anatomy, 209
associated injuries, 210
blood supply to the humeral head, 59
classification of, 209-210
complications, 213-214
evaluation for, 210-211
nonsurgical treatment for, 211
osteonecrosis, 59
outcomes, 214
surgical considerations, 59
surgical treatment for, 210*f*, 211*f*,
212-213, 212*f*, 213*f*
Proximal humeral malunions, 275-279
complications, 279, 279*f*
etiology, 275
evaluation, 275-276
of fracture-dislocations, 277
nonsurgical treatment of, 277
surgical treatment of, 277-279, 278*f*
types of, 276-277

Proximal humerus, 209. *See also* Humerus
anatomy of, 13
blood supply of, 267, 268*f*
geometric parameters, 3
osteometry of, 19
retroversion, 3
Proximal thrombosis with distal embolization, 124
Proximal ulna, fractures and fracture-dislocations, 345, 369
classification
coronoid fractures, 369
Monteggia fracture-dislocations,
369-370
olecranon fractures, 369, 369*t*
complications, 374-376, 375*f*
evaluation, 370
postoperative management, 374
treatment, 370-374, 372*f*, 373*f*, 374*f*
Psoriatic arthritis, 525
Pulmonary contusions, 227
Pupil miosis, 552
Push-pull test, 67
Putti-Platt procedure, 130, 135, 280, 482

Q

Quadrilateral space syndrome, 124, 124*f*,
125
Quadriparesis, 552

R

Radial collateral ligament, 344
Radial head
congenital dislocation of, 325
removal of, in treating osteoarthritis, 338
Radial head arthroplasty, 345, 348, 348*f*
Radial head fractures, 317-318, 343-352, 374
anatomy and biomechanics, 343-344,
343*f*, 344*f*
associated injuries, 345
classification, 344-345, 344*f*, 345*t*
clinical assessment, 344
complications, 350*f*, 351-352, 351*f*, 352*f*
imaging, 344
management, 345-348, 347*f*, 348*f*
postoperative, 349, 351
surgical technique, 348-349, 349*f*
Radial nerve
dysfunction, 237
entrapment, 300
Radiocapitellar overload syndrome, 300
Radiofrequency energy, 501
Radiographic evaluation
of acromioclavicular joint resection, 519
of acute anterior dislocation, 72
of anterior glenohumeral ligament,
105-106
of brachial plexus injuries, 391-392
of calcific tendinitis, 534
of clavicular fractures, 221
of coronoid fractures, 379
of elbow, 326
of glenohumeral instability, 68

of injured shoulder, 211
of internal impingement, 119
of medial collateral ligament injuries,
302
of metal implants, 132, 132*f*
of multidirectional instability, 94, 496
of osteochondritis dissecans, 298
of osteonecrosis, 267
of partial-thickness rotator cuff tears,
164-165
of posttraumatic arthritis of elbow,
336-337
of proximal ulnar fractures, 370
of radial head fractures, 344
of recurrent anterior dislocation, 480
of recurrent anterior shoulder
instability, 84-85
of rotator cuff repair, 471-472, 472*f*
of shoulder arthroplasty, 288-289
of shoulder ganglion cysts, 540
of sternoclavicular dislocations, 221
of thoracic outlet syndrome, 399
of valgus instability, 320
Radiolucent lines, 55, 58
Radiothermal shrinkage, capsular reduction
by, 87
Range of motion, 37, 44
passive, 45, 275
Reconstruction surgery of medial collateral
ligament injuries, 302-303, 304*f*
Recurrent dislocations, 129
Recurrent elbow instability, 318
Recurrent laryngeal nerve block, 438
Recurrent posterior subluxation, 96
Redundant inferior capsular pouch, 92
Reflex sympathetic dystrophy, 124, 185, 186,
439
Refractory instability, surgical treatment of,
129
Regional anesthesia for shoulder surgery,
433-440
benefits and reliability of, 433-434
choice of block, 434-435, 434*ft*, 435*t*
combined regional and general, 439
interscalene brachial plexus block, 435,
435*f*
administration, 434*t*, 435-437, 435*f*,
436*f*, 437*f*
complications and side effects,
437-438, 438*t*
determination of success, 439
intraoperative neurologic
complications, 438-439
precautionary measures, 434*t*, 437
volume of anesthetic, 437
postoperative brachial plexus blocks,
infusions and adjuvants, 439-440
Rehabilitation
exercises for nonsurgical management
of rotator cuff disease, 159-160
natural history with intervention
through, for rotator cuff disease, 153
Reliability of outcomes analysis, 426, 427*f*
Relocation test, 68, 84, 94, 120
Resection arthroplasty, 200, 253
for shoulder osteoarthritis, 261

Retrograde insertion, 241
Retroversion, 94
Reverse Bankart lesions, 97, 123
Reverse Hill-Sachs lesion, 94
Revision acromioplasty, 186
Revision surgery for shoulder arthroplasty
    preoperative planning, 288-289, 289*t*,
        290*ft*
    surgical technique, 289-291, 291*t*
Rheumatoid arthritis, 197, 199-200, 251. *See
    also* Arthritis; Osteoarthritis
    in elbow, 333
        evaluation, 333
        nonsurgical treatment of, 333-334
        surgical treatment of, 334-335, 335*f*
    in glenohumeral joint, 251
    incidence of, 251
    pathogenesis of, 251
Rheumatoid disease, 257
    staging of, 527
Rocking-horse effect, 58, 201, 254
Rotational motion, range of, during passive
    joint positioning, 52
Rotator cuff
    activation, 17, 405*f*, 406, 408*f*
    anatomy of, 23, 24*f*, 25*f*
        gross, 143-145, 143*t*, 144*t*, 145*f*, 146*f*
        histologic, 146, 147*ft*
    animal studies of, 31, 34
        intrinsic and extrinsic injury models,
            33-34, 34*f*
        overuse injury model, 34, 34*f*
        rat model, 31-32, 32*f*
        tendon healing, 32-33
    biochemical composition of, 23-25, 26*f*,
        27*f*
    biomechanical models, 25, 26-27, 28*f*
    correlation of EMG and clinical exami-
        nation of, 41-43, 42*f*, 43*f*, 44*f*
    deficiency, 58
    lesions of, 20
    microstructure of, 23
    pathology, 134
    repairing, with undue tension, 184
    routine evaluation of, 66-67
    in shoulder motion, 40-43
    as stability factor, 17
    strengthening, 73
    strength in, 404
    surgical complications
        acromioclavicular joint pathology,
            182
        acromioplasty, 186
        all-arthroscopic repair, 185
        anesthesia-related complications, 188
        deltoid detachment, 184
        distal clavicle resection and
            coplaning, 186-187
        glenohumeral arthritis and stiffness,
            182-183
        infection, 187
        labral and intra-articular pathology,
            182
        long head of biceps tendon, 182
        long head of biceps tenotomy, 187
        nerve injury, 184-185

    neurologic diagnoses, 181-182
        postoperative stiffness following
            repair, 185-186
        preoperative counseling and patient
            expectations, 183
        repair failure (reuptake), 183-184
        secondary gain, 183
    tendons of, 144
Rotator cuff cable, 145
Rotator cuff defects, full-thickness, 251
Rotator cuff disease, 8, 155
    healing patterns, 156-157, 157*f*
    incidence of, 29
    nonsurgical management, 158
        corticosteroid injection, 158
        indications for, 157-158
        iontophoresis, 159
        nonsteroidal anti-inflammatory
            drugs, 159
        phonophoresis, 159
        rehabilitation exercises, 159-160
        ultrasound, 159
    pain recognition associated with, 30
    pathogenesis of, 29, 31
    prevalence, 155-156, 156*f*
    relationship between glenohumeral
        kinematics and, 156
    use of models to study, 27-29, 29*ft*
Rotator cuff disorders, 8
    alternative approaches, 458
    biomechanical function, 146-148
        contributions from other muscles,
            148, 148*f*
        function remote to the shoulder, 148
        mechanical of (outer) scapulohumer-
            al articulation, 148
    clinical outcomes, 458
    definition of problem, 457-458
    natural history, 150-152
        in competitive overhead athlete,
            152-153
        with intervention through rehabilita-
            tion or surgery, 153
    pathogenesis, 149
        dynamic causes, 149-150, 150*t*
        static causes, 149
    recommendations, 458
    as true syndrome, 143
Rotator cuff impingement
    as complication in shoulder arthroplasty,
        287-288
    revision surgery, preoperative planning,
        288-289, 289*t*, 290*ft*
Rotator cuff injury, 29
    concomitant, 481
    extrinsic mechanisms, 30-31, 31*f*
    intrinsic mechanisms, 29-30, 30*f*
Rotator cuff tears, 7, 8-9, 9*f*, 31, 32*f*, 71, 103,
    104, 487
    arthropathy, 197-203
        arthroscopic lavage and
            débridement, 200
        clinical evaluation, 198-200, 198*f*, 199*t*
        constrained total shoulder
            arthroplasty, 200-201
        etiology, 197-198, 198*f*

    glenohumeral arthrodesis, 200
    hemiarthroplasty for, 153, 201-203
    nonsurgical management, 200
    resection arthroplasty, 200
    semiconstrained total shoulder
        arthroplasty, 202-203, 202*f*
    surgical management, 200
    unconstrained total shoulder
        arthroplasty, 201
    as complication following shoulder
        arthroplasty, 287-288
    etiology of bursal-sided, 34
    full-thickness, 253, 471
        arthroscopy, 175-177, 178
        open surgery
        complications and reoperations, 175,
            176*f*
            indications, 171
            postoperative support and
                rehabilitation, 174-175
            results and factors affecting
                outcome, 175
            surgical exposure, 171-174, 172*f*,
                173*f*, 174*f*, 175*f*
    instability and, 44
    massive, 191-194
        critical associated findings, 191, 192*t*
        disability, 192
        epidemiology, 191-192
        failed repair of, 193-194
        postoperative rehabilitation, 193
        treatment, 192-193
    partial-thickness, 471
        arthroscopy, 165*f*, 167-168
        classification, 165, 166*t*
        clinical findings, 164
        imaging, 164-165, 166*f*
        open surgical techniques, 165-167,
            167*f*
        pathophysiology, 163, 164*f*
    pathogenesis of, 8
    revision surgery, preoperative planning,
        288-289, 289*t*, 290*ft*
    in throwing athlete, 117
Rotator cuff tendinitis, 268
Rotator cuff tendinosis, 471
Rotator cuff tendons, 24
    insertions of, 209
Rotator interval, 5-6, 6*f*, 7, 104
    in anterior glenohumeral reconstruction,
        111
    defects in capsule, 92
    integrity of, 67
    laxity or incompetence of, 67
    lesions of, 92
    tissue deficiency in, 92

S

Scalenotomy, anterior, 397
Scalenus anticus syndrome, 397
Scapula, 9, 10, 37
    upward rotation of, 148
Scapular clock exercises, 405-406, 406*f*
Scapular dyskinesias, 118

Scapular dyskinesis, 403
Scapular fractures, 227-235
    anatomy, 227
    associated injuries, 227-228
    classification, 228
        acromion and lateral scapular spine,
            228-229
        coracoid process, 228
        glenoid, 229, 229f
        scapular neck, 229, 230f
    evaluation, 229-230, 231f
        complications, 230
        surgical indications, 230
    neck, 229
    nonsurgical treatment and results,
        230-231
    surgical management
        floating shoulder, 231
        glenoid fossa fractures, 231-233, 232f,
            233f, 234f, 235f
        results, 233-234
Scapular-plane elevation, 27
Scapular rotators, 18
    fatigue or weakness of, 20
Scapular strengthening, 73
Scapular winging, 98
Scapulohumeral articulation, 145
    mechanics of, 148
Scapulothoracic abduction and elevation,
    220
Scapulothoracic articulation, 10, 37, 93
Scapulothoracic bursa, 10
Scapulothoracic crepitus, 230
Scapulothoracic dysfunction, 20
Scapulothoracic rotation, 18
Scapulothoracic space, 3
Screw fixation of proximal humeral fixa-
    tion, 211f, 212
Semiconstrained total elbow arthroplasty,
    365
Semiconstrained total shoulder arthroplas-
    ty, 202-203, 202f
Serial arthrography to illustrate progression
    of partial-thickness tear to a complete
    tear, 163
Serratus anterior, 18, 40
Shoulder. *See also* Accelerated postopera-
    tive shoulder rehabilitation; Floating
    shoulder; Frozen shoulder; Regional
    anesthesia for shoulder surgery; Total
    shoulder arthroplasty
    acute anterior dislocations of, 66, 71-76
        exercise therapy for, 73-74, 74f
        imaging of, 72, 73f
        natural history, 71, 72f
        pathology, 71
        patient presentation/evaluation,
            71-72
        postimmobilization assessment of,
            73, 73f
        postreduction immobilization of,
            72-73
        reduction of, 72, 72f
        surgical intervention in, 74-75, 74f
        treatment algorithm in, 75-76, 75f,
            76f

acute dislocation of
    inferior, 77
    posterior, 66, 76-77, 77f
acute dislocations of, arthroscopy for,
    487-491
angular velocity of, 117
anterior instability of, 67, 103
    subscapularis rupture and, 286
anterior internal impingement of, 150
chronic posterior dislocations of, 79-80,
    79f, 80f
description of positions, 37, 38f, 39f, 40f
inflammatory arthritis of, 251-255
    clinical evaluation, 252
    incidence, 251
    nonsurgical treatment of, 252
    pathoanatomy, 251-252
    pathogenesis, 251
    pathophysiology, 251
    results, 254-255, 255t
    surgical treatment of, 253-254
kinematics of clinical conditions
    rotator cuff tears and instability, 44
    stiffness, 44-45
kinesiology of sports, 45
microtraumatic injuries to, 118
muscle function in, 39-40
    biceps, 43-44
    prime movers, 40, 41f
    rotator cuff, 40-43
normal motion in, 37-38
    axial rotation, 39
    elevation, 38-39
outcomes analysis in, 421-429
pathomechanics of, 119
recurrent anterior dislocations, 80,
    479-483
        anatomy and biomechanics, 479-480,
            480f
        arthroscopic evaluation of, 480-481,
            481f, 482f
        arthroscopic treatment, 482-483, 482f
        diagnostic testing, 480
        natural history, 479
        nonsurgical treatment, 481-482
        surgical treatment for, 482
    rehabilitation of, 45
    in vivo study of motion in, 37
Shoulder arthroplasty, 263, 285-291
    complications, 285, 286t
        fractures, 286-287, 288f, 289f
        implant loosening, 285-286
        implant wear, 286, 287f
        infection, 287
        instability, 286, 286t, 287f
        nerve injuries, 287
        rotator cuff tears and impingement,
            287-288
    revision surgery, preoperative planning,
        288-289, 289t, 290ft
    surgical technique, 289-291, 291t
Shoulder ganglion cysts, 539-541
    anatomy, 539-540, 540f
    clinical evaluation, 540
    diagnostic imaging, 540-541, 540f
    pathology/etiology, 539

    technique and results of treatment, 541
    treatment, 541
Shoulder immobilizer following full-thick-
    ness repair, 174
Shoulder instability
    circle concept of, 99
    classification of, 487
    posterior, 96-100, 97t
        arthroscopic techniques, 99-100
        clinical presentation, 97
        definition and classification, 96-97
        etiology, 97
        nonsurgical treatment, 98
        open techniques, 98-99, 99t
        physical examination, 97-98
    recurrent anterior, 83-87
        arthroscopic repair, 86-87
        arthroscopic versus open repair,
            85-86
        bone deficiency, 86
        classification of, 83
        complications, 87
        evaluation of, 83-84, 83f, 84-85, 84f,
            85, 85f
        open repair, 87
Shoulder Pain and Disability Index
    (SPADI), 428
Shuttle Relay, 498, 498f
Shuttle relay device in anterior gleno-
    humeral reconstruction, 109, 110f
Sickle cell disease, 257, 267, 269-270
Simple Shoulder Test (SST), 428
SLAP lesions, 4, 85, 103, 105, 106, 481, 487,
    502
    in throwing athletes, 546
        nonsurgical treatment, 546
        postoperative treatment, 547
        results of surgery, 547-548
        surgical treatment, 546-547
    type I, 543
    type II, 543, 544-545, 545, 546
    type III, 543, 545
    type IV, 543, 545
Sling immobilization, 112
    following full-thickness repair, 174
Soft-tissue abnormalities, 98
Soft-tissue reconstruction for global insta-
    bility, 94-95
Soft-tissue stretching, degree of, 263
Speed's test, 544
Sphingolipid, 270
Spinoglenoid notch, 539, 540
Spinoglenoid notchplasty, 123
Splenectomy in treating Gaucher's disease,
    270
Splinting/range-of-motion regimen for
    elbow stiffness, 327
Spondyloarthropathies, 251
Spontaneous pneumothorax, 552
Sports. *See also* Throwing injuries
    kinesiology of, 45
Spurling's maneuver, 181
Staphylococcus, as cause of infection follow-
    ing rotator cuff surgery, 175, 187
Staple capsulorrhaphy, 87
Step-ups/step-downs, 403

Stereophotogrammetry, 9, 14, 148
Sternoclavicular joint, 3, 10, 37, 66, 219
    dislocations of, 219
        anatomy, 219-220, 220*f*
        anterior, 222-223
        classification, 220-221
        complications, 223, 224
        etiology and epidemiology, 220, 220*f*
        physical examination, 221
        posterior, 223, 224
        radiologic evaluation of, 221
        treatment and results, 221-223, 222*f*,
            223*f*
Sternoclavicular ligament, 10
Steroid-induced osteonecrosis, 269
Steroid injections for proximal humeral
    malunions, 277
Stiff shoulder, treatment of, 185
Stingers, 390
Streptococcus, as cause of infection follow-
    ing rotator cuff surgery, 187
Stress fractures about the elbow, 307*f*, 308
Stryker notch view, 68, 85, 480
Subacromial bursa, 7, 30, 67
Subacromial bursitis, treatment of, 528
Subacromial crepitus, 66
Subacromial decompression. *See*
    Acromioplasty
Subacromial impingement, 214
Subacromial impingement lesions, 30
Subacromial impingement syndrome, 473
Subacromial pain, 67
Subacromial space, 3, 23
    arthroscopy for
        acromioclavicular joint, 177
        acromioplasty, 177
        anchor placement, 177
        repair site preparation, 177
        suture placement, 177
        tear classification, 176-177
    coracoacromial ligament in, 7
    decompressing, 8
    deltoid muscle in, 8
    osseous structures in, 7
    rotator cuff in, 8-9, 9*f*
    subacromial bursa in, 7
Subacromial steroid injections, 186
Subacromial/subdeltoid bursa, full-thickness
    tears and, 173
Subchondral bone of the glenoid, 50
Subclavian arteriography of posterior
    humeral circumflex artery, 125
Subclavian artery, 227, 397
Subclavian-axillary aneurysm, 399
Subclavian veins, 397
    occlusion of, 399-400
Subcoracoid impingement, 519
Subcutaneous emphysema, 552
Subscapularis, 17, 26, 147
    advancement, 290
    rupture of, 73
        anterior instability and, 286
    structure of, 143
    tears of, 171, 177
Subscapularis bursa, 10
Subscapularis splitting approach, 134

Subscapularis tendon, 146, 209
    degeneration in, 8
    failure of, 87
    integrity of, 67
    Z-plasty of, 78
Subscapularis transfer as adjunct to rotator
    cuff repair, 174
Subscapular tendon rupture, 87
Sulcus, 30
Sulcus sign, positive, 20
Sulcus test, 67, 93, 495
Superior deltoid splitting approach, 212
Superior glenohumeral ligament, 4, 5, 6, 16*t*,
    65
Superior instability
    cause of, 286
    revision surgery for, 290
Superior internal impingement, 119
Superior labrum, lesions of, 19-20
Superior labrum anterior and posterior
    lesions, 543-548
    arthroscopic findings, 545-546, 546*ft*
    classification, 543, 544*f*
    clinical findings, 544-545, 544*f*, 545*f*
    clinical spectrum, 543
    role of internal impingement, 548
    SLAP lesions in throwing athletes, 546
        nonsurgical treatment, 546
        postoperative treatment, 547
        results of surgery, 547-548
        surgical treatment, 546-547
Superior shoulder pain, 67
Superior shoulder suspensory complex, 227
Superoinferior translation, 18
Supraclavicular injuries
    clinical examination, 388-389
    common patterns of neurologic loss,
        389-390
Suprascapular artery
    branches of, 4
    circumflex scapular branch of, 4
Suprascapular nerve
    anatomy of, 539-540
    compression, 540, 540*f*
    direct compression of, 121
    injury to, 136
        incidence of iatrogenic, 175
Suprascapular neuropathy, 181
    in throwing athlete, 121-123, 123*f*
    outcomes, 122-123
Supraspinatus, 5, 17, 26, 41, 144
    compressive stiffness of, 27-28
    structure of, 143
    tears of, 42
Supraspinatus tendon, 8, 23
    degeneration in, 8
Suretac bioabsorbable device, 105, 107, 131
Surgical management. *See also* Open reduc-
    tion and internal fixation; Open surgery
    repair; Revision surgery
    for acute anterior dislocations, 74-75, 74*f*
    for anterior glenohumeral ligament, 106
    for brachial plexus injuries in adults
        neurologic reconstruction, 392-393
        peripheral reconstruction of limb,
            393-394

for calcific tendinitis, 535-536
for clavicular fractures, 222
for contaminated or infected fractures,
    362-363
for cuff tear arthropathy, 200
    arthroscopic lavage and
        débridement, 200
    constrained total shoulder
        arthroplasty, 200-201
    glenohumeral arthrodesis, 200
    hemiarthroplasty, 201-203
    resection arthroplasty, 200
    semiconstrained total shoulder
        arthroplasty, 202-203, 202*f*
    unconstrained total shoulder
        arthroplasty, 201
for diaphyseal fractures of the humerus,
    239-243, 240*f*, 241*f*
for extrinsic contracture in elbow
    arthroscopic release, 327-328
    open capsular release, 327*f*, 328, 328*f*
    postoperative therapy, 328-329
for floating shoulder, 231
for glenoid fossa fractures, 231-233, 232*f*,
    233*f*, 234*f*, 235*f*
for inflammatory arthritis of the
    shoulder, 253-254
for intrinsic contracture in elbow,
    329-330, 330*f*
lateral exposure, 358
for multidirectional instability, 94-96,
    496-499, 497*f*, 498*f*
    arthroscopic techniques, 95-96
    open techniques, 94-95
    natural history with intervention
        through, for rotator cuff disease,
        153
for osteoarthritis, 260-261
for osteochondritis dissecans, 298
for osteoporotic bone, 361
for partial-thickness rotator cuff tears
    arthroscopy, 167-168
    open techniques, 165-167, 167*f*
for postcapsulorrhaphy arthritis, 281
posterior exposures in, 358-361, 360*f*
for posterior instability, 98-100, 99*t*
for proximal humeral fractures, 59, 210*f*,
    211*f*, 212-213, 212*f*, 213*f*
for radial head fractures, 348-349, 349*f*
for recurrent anterior dislocation, 482
for rheumatoid arthritis in elbow,
    334-335, 335*f*
for scapular fractures, 233-234
for SLAP lesions in throwing athletes,
    546-547
for thoracic outlet syndrome, 401
in total elbow arthroplasty, 361-362
Surgical neck angulation and malunion, 214
Surgical neck malunions, 277
Suture anchors, 131
    in arthroscopic labral repair, 105
    surgical reconstruction using
        anterior glenohumeral reconstruc-
            tion, 108-109, 110*f*
        general principles, 106

glenoid preparation and anchor
placement, 108, 109*f*
instrumentation, 106-107
preparation, 107
rotator interval, 111
technique, 107-108, 107*f*, 108*f*
thermal capsulorrhaphy, 111-112,
112*f*
Suture capsulorrhaphy, 104, 553-554, 554
Suture hook, 111
in anterior glenohumeral reconstruction,
108, 110*f*
Suture placement in arthroscopy for full-
thickness tears, 177
Suture shuttle, 474
Swallow tail sign, 43
Symptomatic laxity, surgery on throwers
with, 123
Symptomatic subluxation, 130
Synovectomies, 253
arthroscopic, 254
for elbow arthritis, 334
Synovial chondromatosis, arthroscopic syn-
ovectomy for, 261
Synovial cyst formation, 131
Synovial débridement, 526, 529
Synovial osteochondromatosis, 271-272
Synovitis, 120, 251
in elbow, 333
Systemic lupus erythematosus, 251, 267, 525

T

T-capsulorrhaphy, 134
Tendinitis, 30
calcific, 164
rotator cuff, 268
Tendinopathy, 23, 31
Tendinosis, 30, 33*f*, 34
Tendon transfers, long-term results of, 153
Tenotomy, long head of biceps, 187
Tensile keel strain, 57-58
Tension pneumothorax, 552
Teres minor, 8, 17, 40, 41, 147
atrophy of, 125
dysfunction of, 42-43
lesions, 177
Terrible triad, 379
Thermal capsular modifications, 20
Thermal capsular shrinkage, 5
Thermal capsulorrhaphy, 20, 99, 124, 131,
554
for anterior glenohumeral ligament
reconstruction, 111-112, 112*f*
Thermal energy, 112
for multidirectional instability, 95-96
Thermal shrinkage, 483
Thermocapsulorrhaphy, 501-503
controversies/complications, 502
indications, 502
pathophysiology of collagen shortening,
501
postoperative care, 502
surgical indications for, 502
surgical instrumentation, 501

technique, 502
in vitro studies, 501
in vivo studies, 502
Thoracic kyphosis, 403
Thoracic outlet syndrome, 124, 125, 181,
182, 224, 397-401
anatomy, 397
ancillary diagnostic studies, 399-400
clinical presentation, 398-399
conservative therapy, 400
diagnosis of, 124
history, 397-398, 398*f*
indications for surgery, 400
paresthesias due to, 404
physical examination, 399
surgical procedures for, 401
complications, 401
results of, 401
Three-part malunions, 277
Thrombocytopenia, 333
Thrombosis, effort, 399-400
Throwers' paradox, 123
Throwing injuries, 117-125, 118*t*
history, 117
instability as, 123-124
internal impingement, 118-119, 120*f*
arthroscopic findings, 119-121, 121*f*
imaging, 119
physical examination, 119
treatment, 122, 123*f*
physical examination of, 117-118
rehabilitation of, 129
in shoulder, 117, 118*f*
SLAP lesions in, 546
suprascapular neuropathy, 121-123, 123*f*
outcomes, 122-123
vascular lesions, 124-125
quadrilateral space syndrome, 124*f*,
125
vessel aneurysms, 124-125
Tinel's sign, 326
Tobacco use, osteonecrosis in, 267
Total elbow arthroplasty, 361-362
semiconstrained, 365
for treatment of fracture of distal
humerus, 357
Total shoulder arthroplasty, 56, 58, 59, 79,
254, 263, 411
component loosening after, 3-4
humeral head replacement versus, 262
for osteonecrosis and other noninflammatory degenerative diseases, 268
for proximal humeral malunions, 279
semiconstrained, 202-203, 202*f*
for shoulder osteoarthritis, 261
unconstrained, 201
T-plasty modification of the Bankart technique, 133
Trabecular bone, 4
volume fraction of, 4
Traction paresthesias, 93
Transglenoid labral repair, 86, 87
Transglenoid sutures in arthroscopic labral
repair, 104-105
Transolecranon fracture-dislocations, 369
Transverse olecranon stress fractures, 308

Triceps reflecting anconeus pedicle
approach in surgery for fracture of distal
humerus, 359
Trispiral tomography, 326
Trochlear notch
comminution of, 382
realignment of, 370-371
Trunk extension strength, 403
T-shaped capsulotomy, 131
Tuberosity reconstruction, postoperative
rehabilitation after, 279
TUBS (Traumatic Unidirectional Bankart
Surgery) lesion, 66, 130, 258
Tumor necrosis factor-alpha, 526
Turnbuckle splint, 351
for elbow stiffness, 327

U

Ulna. *See also* Proximal ulna
realignment of, 370
Ulnar nerve, 297
dysfunction of, 364
injury to, as complication in medial
collateral ligament injuries, 303
Ulnar neuropathy, 304-305, 338-339, 399
clinical presentation, 305
treatment, 305
Ulnar tunnel, fracture of, as complication in
medial collateral ligament injuries, 303
Ulnohumeral arthroplasty, for osteoarthritis
of the elbow, 338
Ulnohumeral instability, 375, 375*f*
Ulnohumeral joint
anterior dislocation of, 371
incongruity of, 313
Ultrasound
for arthroscopic subacromial
decompression, 508
for rotator cuff disease, 155, 159
Unconstrained total shoulder arthroplasty,
201
Unidirectional (anterior) instability, 92
University of California, Los Angeles End-
Result Score, 428
University of Pennsylvania Shoulder Score,
428

V

Valgus impacted fractures, 210
four-part, 212*f*, 213
Valgus instability, 320, 320*f*
as complication of radial head fractures,
351-352
medial collateral ligament tear and, 304
treating, 321
Valgus stem alignment, 54-55
Valgus stress test to assess medial collateral
ligament stability, 301-302, 302*f*
Valgus testing for acute elbow dislocation,
316
Validity of outcomes analysis, 426
Varus malposition, 56
Varus malunion, 212

Varus-posteromedial rotation injuries, 314-315, 317
Varus-posteromedial rotatory instability, 313
Varus stem alignment, 54, 55f
Varus testing for acute elbow dislocation, 316
Vascular injuries, 210
Vascular lesions in throwing athlete, 124-125
    quadrilateral space syndrome, 124f, 125
Vessel aneurysms, 124-125
Vessel compression, 124
Viscoelastic stiffening, 20

Visual analog scales, 424
Volitional instability, 92
Voluntary dislocation, 96
Voluntary instability, 96, 130

W

Wave plate osteosynthesis, 245
Wedge sign, 317
Western Ontario Shoulder Instability Index, 129, 423
West Point (axillary) view, 84, 94, 260, 480
    for glenohumeral instability, 68
    for recurrent anterior shoulder instability, 84-85

Whole-limb questionnaires, 423
Windmill softball pitch, 45
Wright's test, 397, 399
Wrist extension, examination of, 389

Y

Yersinia enterocolitica, risk for infections with, 271

Z

Z-plasty of the subscapularis tendon, 78